Neurology

FOR THE

Non-Neurologist

Holle Janeski
313 - 900 - 8002
282-4121

Neurology
FOR THE
Non-Neurologist

• • •

Third Edition
Edited by
William J. Weiner, M.D.

Professor of Neurology
Director of the Movement Disorders Center
Department of Neurology
University of Miami
School of Medicine
Miami, Florida

and

Christopher G. Goetz, M.D.

Professor of Neurology
Department of Neurological Sciences
Rush Medical College
Rush Presbyterian-St. Luke's Medical Center
Chicago, Illinois

With 33 additional contributors

• • •

J. B. Lippincott Company
Philadelphia

Acquisitions Editor: Mary K. Smith
Assistant Editor: Anne Geyer
Indexer: Lillian R. Rodberg
Cover Designer: Lou Fuiano
Production Manager: Janet Greenwood
Production Editor: Mary Kinsella
Production: Editorial Services of New England
Compositor: Circle Graphics
Printer/Binder: R. R. Donnelley & Sons, Inc.

Third Edition

Library of Congress Cataloging-in-Publication Data

Neurology for the non-neurologist / edited by William J. Weiner and
   Christopher G. Goetz ; with 33 contributors.—3rd ed.
        p.   cm.
     Includes bibliographical references and index.
     ISBN 0-397-51288-0
     1. Neurology.   2. Nervous system—Diseases.   I. Weiner, William
J.   II. Goetz, Christopher G.
     [DNLM: 1. Nervous System Diseases.   WL 100 N49515 1994]
   RC346.N453   1994
   616.8–dc20
   DNLM/DLC
   for Library of Congress   93-36306
                                                                 CIP

The authors and publisher have exerted every effort to ensure that drug
selection and dosage set forth in this text are in accord with current
recommendations and practice at the time of publication. However, in view
of ongoing research, changes in government regulations, and the constant
flow of information relating to drug therapy and drug reactions, the
reader is urged to check the package insert for each drug for any change
in indications and dosage and for added warnings and precautions. This is
particularly important when the recommended agent is a new or
infrequently employed drug.

To our families

Contributors

David A. Bennett, M.D.
Assistant Professor
Department of Neurological Sciences
Clinical Director, Rush Alzheimer's Disease Center
Rush Medical College
Rush Presbyterian-St. Luke's Medical Center
Chicago, Illinois

Donna C. Bergen, M.D.
Associate Professor
Director, EEG Laboratory
Department of Neurological Sciences
Rush Medical College
Rush Presbyterian-St. Luke's Medical Center
Chicago, Illinois

Joseph R. Berger, M.D.
Professor of Neurology
Department of Neurology
University of Miami School of Medicine
Miami, Florida

Thomas P. Bleck, M.D.
Associate Professor of Neurology and Neurological Surgery
Director, Nerancy Neuroscience Intensive Care Unit
University of Virginia Health Science Center
Charlottesville, Virginia

Cynthia L. Comella, M.D.
Assistant Professor
Senior Attending
Department of Neurological Surgery
Rush Medical College
Rush Presbyterian-St. Luke's Medical Center
Chicago, Illinois

Charles M. D'Angelo, M.D.
Associate Professor
Senior Attending
Department of Neurological Surgery
Rush Medical College
Rush Presbyterian-St. Luke's Medical Center
Chicago, Illinois

Larry E. Davis, M.D.
Professor and Vice Chairman
Department of Neurology
Albuquerque VA Medical Center
Albuquerque, New Mexico

John A. Difini, M.D.
Neurological Center
Gastonia, North Carolina

Stewart A. Factor, D.O.
Associate Professor of Neurology
Department of Neurology
Albany Medical College
Albany, New York

Morris A. Fisher, M.D.
Professor of Neurology
Department of Neurology
Loyola University Medical Center
Maywood, Illinois

Jacob H. Fox, M.D.
Jean Schweppe Armour Professor and Chairman
Co-Director, Rush Alzheimer's Disease Center
Department of Neurological Sciences
Rush Medical College
Rush Presbyterian-St. Luke's Medical Center
Chicago, Illinois

Russell H. Glantz, M.D.
Associate Professor
Director, Electromyographic Laboratory
Department of Neurological Sciences
Rush Medical College
Rush Presbyterian-St. Luke's Medical Center
Chicago, Illinois

Christopher G. Goetz, M.D.
Professor and Associate Chairman
Director, Section of Movement Disorders
Department of Neurological Sciences
Rush Medical College
Rush Presbyterian-St. Luke's Medical Center
Chicago, Illinois

James A. Goodwin, M.D.
Associate Professor of Ophthalmology and Neurology
Director, Neuro-Ophthalmology Service
Department of Ophthalmology and Visual Sciences
The University of Illinois at Chicago
Chicago, Illinois

Lawrence Honig, M.D.
Assistant Professor of Neurology
Department of Neurology
Stanford University Medical School
Stanford, California

Judd M. Jensen, M.D.
Assistant Professor of Neurology
Department of Neurological Sciences
Rush Medical College
Rush Presbyterian-St. Luke's Medical Center
Chicago, Illinois

Roger E. Kelley, M.D.
Professor of Neurology
Department of Neurology
University of Miami School of Medicine
Miami, Florida

William C. Koller, M.D., Ph.D.
Professor and Chairman
Department of Neurology
University of Kansas Medical Center
Kansas City, Kansas

Ružica Kovačević-Ristanović, M.D.
Assistant Professor
Department of Neurological Sciences
Medical Director of Sleep Disorder Service
*   and Research Center*
Rush Medical School
Rush Presbyterian-St. Luke's Medical Center
Chicago, Illinois

Steven L. Lewis
Assistant Professor
Department of Neurological Sciences
Rush Medical College
Rush Presbyterian-St. Luke's Medical Center
Chicago, Illinois

Bernard B. Megaffin, M.D.
Chief Resident
Department of Neurology
University of Kansas Medical Center
Kansas City, Kansas

Hans E. Neville, M.D.
Professor of Neurology
Neuromuscular Division
Department of Neurology
University of Colorado Health Sciences Center
Denver, Colorado

Lois M. Nora, M.D., J.D.
Assistant Professor, Neurological Sciences
Department of Neurological Sciences
Assistant Dean, Clinical Curriculum
Rush Medical College
Rush Presbyterian-St. Luke's Medical Center
Chicago, Illinois

Peter Portegies, M.D.
Clinical AIDS Department
Department of Neurology
University of Amsterdam
Amsterdam, The Netherlands

Ruth G. Ramsey, M.D.
Professor of Radiology
Head, Section of Neuroradiology
Department of Radiology
The University of Chicago Hospital
Chicago, Illinois

Steven P. Ringel, M.D.
Professor of Neurology
Neuromuscular Division
Department of Neurology
University of Colorado Health Sciences Center
Denver, Colorado

Joel R. Saper, M.D., F.R.C.P.
Founder and Director
Michigan Head-Pain and Neurological Institute
Ann Arbor, Michigan

Kathleen Shannon, M.D.
Assistant Professor
Department of Neurological Sciences
Rush Medical College
Rush Presbyterian-St. Luke's Medical Center
Chicago, Illinois

William A. Sheremata, M.D., F.R.C.P.
Associate Professor of Neurology
Department of Neurology
University of Miami School of Medicine
Miami, Florida

Lisa M. Shulman, M.D.
Clinical Fellow in Movement Disorders
Department of Neurology
University of Miami School of Medicine
Miami, Florida

Carlos Singer, M.D.
Assistant Professor of Neurology
Department of Neurology
University of Miami School of Medicine
Miami, Florida

Susan Miguel Snodgrass, M.D.
Assistant Professor of Neurology
Department of Neurology
University of Miami School of Medicine
Miami, Florida

Jordan L. Topel, M.D.
Assistant Professor of Neurology
Department of Neurological Sciences
Rush Medical College
Rush Presbyterian-St. Luke's Medical Center
Chicago, Illinois

William J. Weiner, M.D.
Professor of Neurology
Director of the Movement Disorders Center
Department of Neurology
University of Miami School of Medicine
Miami, Florida

Robert S. Wilson, Ph.D.
Professor
Department of Neurological Sciences
and Department of Psychology
Rush Medical College
Rush Presbyterian-St. Luke's Medical Center
Chicago, Illinois

Preface

The third edition of *Neurology for the Non-Neurologist* maintains its focus on educating those who deal with nervous system disease but who have not committed their careers to neuroscience. This includes internists, family practitioners, psychiatrists, geriatricians, rehabilitation specialists, and advanced nurses. As neurology has broadened its scope and depth over the past years, we have not only updated the second edition of this book, but also expanded it to encompass new areas of interest and clinical concern. We have prepared this book not as a comprehensive text but rather as a series of focused and concise essays on major topics in neurology. As such the book might be read in its entirety to give an overview of contemporary clinical neurology, or alternatively, it may be used as a selective reference source on individual topics.

The initial chapters of this edition deal with topics of general pertinence and cover the basic neurologic examination and the ordering of neurologic tests. The repertoire of diagnostic tests has increased recently, as has their expense, and an overview of the usefulness and expected yield of various examinations will help to guide the treating physician in a logical evaluation sequence. A common and difficult decision is "When should a neurologist be called?" Although there is no simple textbook answer, these early chapters are written to help front-line physicians maximally utilize the neurologic examination and testing opportunities in a clinical context to arrive at diagnostic, treatment, and referral decisions.

Subsequent chapters guide the reader through the frequently encountered neurologic problems of medically ill patients. Some of these chapters are based on contributions from the second edition but have been largely written to incorporate colleagues' comments and feedback that we received in using this book in various educational contexts. As in the second edition, the authorship represents faculty of national reputation from our two institutions, with added experts from several other university and practice centers.

Some chapters are completely new and reflect our decision to include areas of growing interest in neurologic diagnosis and treatment. The chapter on central nervous system infections has been completely rewritten to address the ever-changing use of medications, resistant forms of infectious agents, and newly evolving illnesses. We have added a chapter on AIDS because this disease is a major source of neurologic disability, and neurologic abnormalities may be the initial symptoms of patients who present to their primary care physician. The chapter on the neurologic complications of pregnancy has been added because as the population expands and women have children in early puberty as well as late middle age, neurologic complications are seen with alarming frequency and need to be identified and diagnosed accurately. Furthermore, patient populations that formerly did not become pregnant because of infertility problems or social and medical constraints are now bearing children, and neurologic complications of their underlying conditions superimposed on pregnancy can lead to a wide variety of problems. The chapter on medicolegal issues in neurology has been included because of the increasing interest and importance of this subject to both treating physicians and their patients. The questions of brain death and the seizure patient who wishes to drive are just two of these important topics.

We think that this edition is our best and most comprehensive effort, that it capitalizes on our strong university faculties, and that it reflects our experience in the field of continuing medical education that extends over many years. It is with shared pride that we offer this edition of *Neurology for the Non-Neurologist* as a symbol of our mutual commitment to neurology and to continuing medical education.

William J. Weiner, M.D.
Christopher G. Goetz, M.D.

Preface
to the First Edition

Neurology for the Non-Neurologist is an outgrowth of over 20 years of continued participation in the education and training of undergraduate neuroscience students, postgraduate residents, and practicing physicians. Our experience has been that despite the diverse backgrounds and interests of these groups, there is a common point at which they begin to acquire their working knowledge of neurology. Based on this assumption, this text has been designed to be valuable to both pre- and postgraduate physicians, as well as to students, and concisely covers the implications of neurologic disease for clinical medicine and neuroscience.

Most neurology texts are organized by anatomy (diseases of the hemispheres, brain stem, peripheral nerves, and muscles) or etiology (genetic, infectious, autoimmune neurologic diseases). Some entities are more easily and clearly discussed from the former vantage and others are better understood when approached from the latter. This text integrates both approaches, emphasizing the anatomic method of organization in some chapters (peripheral neuropathy, muscle disorder, neuroophthalmology, and so forth) and the etiologic organization in others (epilepsy, infections, and tumors). Other chapters are descriptive and aim to guide the physician in a reasonable and satisfying therapeutic approach to common neurologic dilemmas: trauma, behavioral neurology, minimal brain dysfunction, sleep disorders, and so forth.

We have not attempted to write a comprehensive neurologic textbook, but instead to collect a series of concise essays concerning areas of current clinical relevance to neurology. Each chapter includes a description of a clinical disorder with emphasis on signs, symptomatology, pathophysiology, clinical therapeutics, and an overall view of research trends in that particular field. At the conclusion of each chapter there are several self-study questions with appropriate discussion provided for the reader. The book may be read in its entirety to give an overview of clinical neurology to medical students and beginning neurology residents, psychiatrists, students in related fields or neurosciences, and practicing physicians in internal medicine or family practice. *Neurology for the Non-Neurologist* may also be used as a selective reference work, since each chapter can stand entirely by itself.

William J. Weiner, M.D.
Christopher G. Goetz, M.D.

Acknowledgments

We wish to thank Maynard M. Cohen, M.D., Ph.D., for his enthusiasm, dedication, and interest in this book when the first edition was being prepared. His guidance was instrumental in the publication of this series. We also thank Raiza Perez, Rebeca Barquero, and Marilynn Payton, who provided invaluable help in the preparation of this manuscript.

Contents

Neurology
FOR THE
Non-Neurologist

The Neurologic Examination

Carlos Singer
William J. Weiner

Despite the widespread use of very sophisticated diagnostic procedures, neurology remains a clinical specialty. The history and neurologic examination remain at the core of a neurologic consultation. They should guide the physician to the localization of the neural dysfunction and the appropriate diagnosis. The history and examination should dictate whether or not further diagnostic procedures are required and, if so, which ones should be utilized. The inappropriate use of diagnostic aids such as magnetic resonance imaging (MR) scanning, computed tomography (CT) scanning, electroencephalogram (EEG), and electromyogram (EMG) as screening procedures to look for disease should be avoided.

The history should be elicited with care. The nature of the symptoms, their duration, whether or not the symptoms are progressive in severity, and the anatomic region affected must all be elicited. The time course of the initial onset of the symptoms should also be noted. The description of the onset of a hemiparesis will yield valuable information (*e.g.*, sudden onset suggests a vascular event such as a cerebrovascular accident [CVA], whereas a slow onset suggests a space-occupying lesion such as a tumor). In eliciting the history one should try to inquire about associated symptoms that may help make the diagnosis. For example, if a patient complains of loss of consciousness (LOC), whether or not there were associated tonic–clonic movements,

tongue laceration, or incontinence would be very valuable information in diagnosing a generalized seizure as the etiology for the patient's LOC. Finally, the history should be very instrumental in guiding the neurologic exam to a particular area of investigation. If a patient complains of burning dysesthesias in both feet from the ankles down, the examination should focus more on the peripheral nervous system than on aspects of higher cortical function.

The neurologic examination consists of an evaluation of mental status, cranial nerves, motor system, sensory system, cerebellar system, reflexes, and gait. Each of these aspects of the evaluation will require more or less detailed examination depending on the information obtained from the clinical history.

While eliciting the history, the clinician generates a hypothesis regarding the site in the nervous system that has been affected and the nature of the lesion. The neurologic examination is particularly useful in the localization process, whereas the history is frequently pivotal during consideration of the nature of the illness (etiology).

In some instances the history has to be obtained from others. The patient who has had a generalized seizure or an episode of impairment of consciousness will not be able to provide a complete history of the event. The patient with cognitive deficits or speech difficulties will also be unable to provide adequate historical information. It is important to

1

question the spouse, a relative, or witnesses to a specific event in order to obtain a more complete and often more accurate history.

Certain neurologic conditions are commonly associated with a normal neurologic examination (*e.g.*, primary generalized epilepsies, transient ischemic attacks [TIAs], migraine, and other headaches). In these and other disorders initial diagnostic considerations depend on a good history. If the neurologic examination detects abnormalities, additional diagnostic alternatives may be raised. For example, a positive Babinski sign days after a grand mal seizure suggests that the seizure may have been of focal onset and that a search for a structural brain lesion has to be considered. The finding of mild hand clumsiness after an acute event points to a stroke rather than a TIA. Therapeutic choices may be different for a patient with a TIA rather than a completed CVA.

Since the neurologic examination is often crucial in establishing the correct diagnosis, it is important for all physicians to be able to perform a complete, albeit often brief, evaluation of the nervous system. The often-written chart note for the neurologic examination found on non-neurology services (Neuro-WNL) should be avoided; most often, WNL is interpreted as "we never looked." The neurologic examination should be conducted following a consistent routine so that portions of the evaluation are not forgotten. Obviously, the history will guide the examining physician as to where the emphasis in the conduct of the neurologic examination should be. A good neurologic examination does not require the performance of every clinical test of a given system.

The neurologic examination can be further complemented with aspects of the general physical examination. The examination of the heart and carotid arteries is particularly relevant in patients with TIA or stroke, and auscultation of the head (a bruit suggests an arteriovenous malformation) and palpation of the frontal, paranasal, and maxillary sinuses are of importance in the headache patient. The infant with developmental delay needs to be examined for organomegaly.

This chapter presents a method of performing a concise, focused, and complete neurologic evaluation. We have emphasized certain diseases that are associated with particular pathologic signs. These examples have been chosen because of their common occurrence and do not exclude the possibility that the same sign may be caused by other etiologies.

MENTAL STATUS

The mental status examination begins the moment the physician first greets the patient. It should be recognized that a patient who fully participates in the history taking and provides a coherent accurate history interspersed with accurate references to current social or political events and who follows instructions during the examination may not require a formal evaluation of mental status, memory, and language functions. The physician should carefully observe to what extent the patient participates during the interview. A withdrawn, nonparticipating patient may have cognitive dysfunction (with or without dementia) or may be depressed. A patient with significant cognitive deficits in the area of memory or language will not be able to provide adequate information even while trying hard to communicate. The physician should also note other aspects of behavior. Avoidance of eye contact and depressed facies suggest depression. Irritability, distractibility, aimless picking on clothing or surrounding objects, and indifference to serious symptoms being discussed suggest cognitive impairment. One of the clearest indications that a formal mental evaluation should be conducted is the often-seen clinical situation in which the spouse or caregiver asks to give the history and then proceeds to do so. In these instances the patient often sits quietly, not speaking spontaneously, while an entire discussion ensues of how his personality and behavior have changed.

As the history unfolds, the clinician makes the judgment as to whether to proceed with a formal mental status examination. This aspect of the examination is particularly relevant in patients with a history suggestive of forgetfulness, word-finding difficulty, or changes in behavior. When the history suggests memory dysfunction or changes in behavior, historical information from relatives, friends, coworkers, and employers may be required. Often patients with early, mild dementing processes may still be "smarter" than their evaluators and often use various tricks of social grace and convention to evade specific questions. Patients may become belligerent if deficits are revealed, and this should be done cautiously. For example, specific mental status testing may be performed by telling patients in a nonthreatening manner that silly questions have to be asked and will they please cooperate. On the other hand, in the instance of a patient who gives a perfectly coherent and detailed account of noncognitive symptoms, other parts of the neurologic exam are likely to be more pertinent to the patient's problem.

A final caution before beginning the mental status evaluation is to take into consideration the educational and language background of the patient. Although patients with dementing processes often explain their inability to answer specific questions by stating that they have no interest in that subject, it may be that a specific patient's background precludes accurate answers to commonly employed questions.

The formal examination of mental status starts with questions related to orientation to time, place, and person. Orientation to time should progress from year through season, month, and date to day of the week. Orientation to space starts with the current actual location (e.g., Dr. Smith's office) and city, then goes to county, state, and country. The patient should be asked to state his full name and to identify any person accompanying him. Memory evaluation should be divided into tests of immediate and recent call. Immediate recall is tested by asking the patient to immediately repeat a random sequence of numbers (digit span). Digits can be presented in groups of increasing numbers (from three to six). Normal adults can readily repeat without errors sequences of five to six numbers. Most adults are able to reverse the number sequence successfully, and great difficulty in reversing the sequence may be a subtle sign of cognitive impairment. Many patients with early to moderate dementing illnesses can successfully perform digit spans. Recent recall is tested by presenting the patient with three to four unrelated words, asking the patient to remember them, and then proceeding with other elements of the mental status evaluation. After 3 to 5 minutes the patient should be asked to repeat the previously given words. Unimpaired patients will be able to recall at least two to three of the words. Impairment of recent recall is often affected early in dementing processes and may reflect the frequent historical complaint that the patient has to be repeatedly told things and does not seem to remember recent events.

Concentration and calculating ability are evaluated by the use of serial 7s. The patient is asked to subtract 7 in a sequential manner from 100 (100, 93, 86, 79, 72, 65, and so on). Finger gnosis, right–left orientation, and ability to perform three-step commands can be assessed by asking the patient to take his right index finger and touch his right ear and then close his eyes.

Language can be quickly assessed by evaluating spontaneous speech, repetition, comprehension of spoken and written material, and the ability to write. Speech may be fluent or nonfluent, and this observation may be very useful in localizing a potential cortical lesion. Nonfluent speech (Broca's aphasia) is localized to the dominant posterior inferior frontal region and is often associated with a hemiparesis, whereas fluent aphasic speech (Wernicke's aphasia), which sounds "normal" in delivery but makes little or no sense, is localized to the posterior superior temporal area and is not associated with a marked paresis. The presence of aphasia may prevent adequate memory and other cognitive testing.

Apraxia (difficulty in performance of motor acts independent of motor or primary sensory impairment) can be evaluated by asking the patient to demonstrate how he would comb his hair, salute, or use a screwdriver. The apractic patient may use his hand as a tool instead of pretending to hold the object or may simply be unable to demonstrate the essential movement involved in the act. Apraxia can also be suspected if the patient displays difficulties in the execution of motor tasks such as finger tapping or hand pronation or supination that appear to be out of proportion to mere slowness, clumsiness, or weakness. Language disturbances (aphasia), calculation difficulties (dyscalculia), and the apraxias may each represent involvement of the dominant hemisphere or be a sign of more widespread cognitive impairment (dementia).

The ability to draw a clock and to copy a three-dimensional representation of a cube can be interpreted as a function of visual spatial orientation. This ability may be impaired due to focal disease (nondominant hemisphere) or a dementing illness. Clock drawing may also detect a visual field deficit when the patient repeatedly draws only half or a quarter of the clock.

The use of a quantifiable standardized tool for screening in the office for dementing processes is useful. The Folstein Mini-Mental Status evaluation is widely used and provides not only scores that can be compared with normals but also a record by which to judge the patient's future performance.

CRANIAL NERVES

The olfactory nerve (cranial nerve I) may be tested by presenting the patient with a selection of two or more distinct and nonirritating aromas (e.g., coffee, tobacco, mint). Each nostril should be alternately occluded while testing the other. Isolated hyposmia (decrease in olfactory function) or anosmia results more frequently from local nose and sinus disease and from post-traumatic olfactory damage than from central nervous system dysfunction. The clinician finding an olfactory nerve deficit in a patient whose history or behavior suggests frontal lobe dysfunction should suspect a subfrontal neoplasia (*e.g.*, olfactory groove meningioma). Patients with Parkinson's disease often exhibit degrees of anosmia. Testing of this cranial nerve is most useful in patients with a subjective decrease in sense of taste or smell and in those patients in whom subfrontal pathology may be present (*e.g.*, dementia). Loss of sense of smell significantly affects the sense of taste, although the ability to distinguish primary tastes is preserved. Testing of olfaction is not routinely performed.

The optic nerve (cranial nerve II) examination encompasses the testing of visual function subserved by the optic chiasm, optic radiations, and occipital lobes. Office testing of central vision starts by determining the patient's ability to read normal-sized printed material with each eye separately. Use of corrective lenses is allowed. If unable to distinguish letters, then the ability to count fingers, detect hand motion, or detect light will allow for assessment of the degree of impairment of central vision.

Visual fields can be tested by confrontation. The examiner faces the patient and has the patient look at his nose. The examiner then moves his own fingers into each of the four visual quadrants. The patient is asked to report when the fingers are first seen. The examiner will also be able to evaluate the response because he will see the finger moving as well. If an abnormality is detected (hemianopia, quadrantanopia), the screening procedure should be repeated, testing each eye separately (cover the other eye). Visual field deficits restricted to one eye suggest ophthalmologic or optic nerve pathology. Visual field deficit in both eyes may represent involvement of posterior visual pathways (between the optic chiasm and the occipital lobe). Involvement of the temporal half of each visual field (bitemporal hemianopia) suggests chiasmatic pathology. A deficit of the temporal half of the visual field of one eye and nasal of the other (homonymous hemianopia) suggests involvement of optic radiations or occipital lobe (see Chap. 22).

The fundoscopic exam visualizes the optic nerve head, the vessels arising through its center, and the retina. An optic disk with blurred margins raises the possibility of optic neuritis or papilledema. Optic neuritis is frequently unilateral and always associated with a decrease in visual acuity that cannot be corrected with glasses. It is also associated with an afferent pupillary defect (Marcus–Gunn pupil), in which the pupil of the affected eye fails to constrict to a light stimulus as the stimulus is moved from the uninvolved eye to the involved eye. This results in the seeming paradox of the affected pupil dilating in response to a light stimulus. Papilledema is bilateral and associated with preservation of visual acuity except for extremely advanced cases. The presence of papilledema suggests increased intracranial pressure and can be seen with brain tumors, occlusions of the cerebral venous drainage, and benign intracranial hypertension. The absence of venous pulsations and presence of vessel engorgement and disk hyperemia allow the clinician to distinguish papilledema from pseudopapilledema (a benign familial condition). Optic disk pallor implies optic atrophy and represents a sequela of optic nerve disease.

The examination of cranial nerves III (oculomotor), IV (trochlear), and VI (abducens) covers ocular motility and pupillary function. The position of the eyes on straight-ahead gaze is noted first. The patient is asked to follow the observer's finger in all four quadrants. The observer notes if any limitation seen is conjugate (symmetrical) or dysconjugate. Nystagmus may also be noted during this part of the exam. Pupillary size and equality are observed. A difference of up to 1 mm between pupils (anisocoria) is accepted as normal. The pupillary direct and consensual reaction to light and to near and far objects is tested. The latter can be tested by asking the patient to look alternately at the observer's finger placed at the level of the patient's nose (near object) and at the observer's nose (far object). Constriction and dilatation, respectively, should be the normal responses.

Pupillary abnormalities may be unilateral or bilateral. Bilateral small pupils unreactive to light but reactive to accommodation (light–near dissociation) can be seen in neurosyphilis (Argyll–Robertson pupils), diabetes, and other autonomic neuropathies. Miosis with ptosis suggests involvement of central or peripheral sympathetic pathways (Horner's syndrome). Unilateral mydriasis without associated ptosis or abnormalities of eye movement is due to local eye disease (*e.g.*, after trauma).

Involvement of cranial nerves III, IV, and VI or of the muscles they serve is almost invariably accompanied by diplopia except in long-standing squints and progressive external ophthalmoplegia (a rare muscular disorder). Involvement of cranial nerve III distal to its nucleus may present with unilateral ptosis and deficits of adduction, depression, or elevation of the eye with or without associated mydriasis. Bilateral asymmetrical extraocular movement deficits without pupillary involvement may represent disease of the ocular muscles (Graves' disease) or the neuromuscular junction (myasthenia gravis). A lesion of cranial nerve VI will result in a deficit of abduction of the eye and will be accompanied by medial deviation of the eye on straight-ahead gaze. A lesion of cranial nerve IV will result in a deficit of intorsion (internal rotation) of the eye (superior oblique weakness) when the affected eye is attempting to look down and in. (See chap. 22 for further details of ocular examination.)

Impairment of conjugate eye movements implies pathology of the cerebral centers controlling eye movements. This may be seen in cerebral hemisphere strokes or basal ganglia degenerative diseases (*e.g.*, progressive supranuclear palsy). These disorders are not accompanied by diplopia.

Examination of cranial nerve V (trigeminal nerve) includes testing facial sensation for light touch and pin, assessing the presence and symmetry of the corneal reflex (gentle stroke of the cornea with a wisp of a cotton while the patient is looking away from the observer), and the strength of the masticator muscles. The latter is checked by examining jaw-opening strength, palpating jaw muscles while the teeth are being clenched, and evaluating side-to-side jaw movements. Unilateral weakness will cause the jaw to deviate to that side upon jaw opening. The jaw jerk is a jaw closure movement elicited by tapping the partially opened jaw at its midline. This reflex may become hyperactive in conditions affecting connections between cortex and the cranial nerves subserving mastication, speech, and deglutition (*e.g.*, bilateral hemispheral CVAs).

Cranial nerve VII (facial) is evaluated by examining the symmetry of facial movements with attention paid to the excursion of the nasolabial folds on spontaneous or forced smiling, ability to whistle or blow the cheeks, the forcefulness of eye closure, and the ability to wrinkle the forehead. The ability to wrinkle the forehead is often used to distinguish between upper and lower motor neuron involvement of the facial nerve. If the forehead is spared when the lower face is paralyzed it is suggestive of upper motor neuron involvement such as is seen in cortical lesions (CVA). If the forehead is involved in the paralytic process then the lesion is likely to be lower motor neuron (the nucleus or the nerve itself) as in Bell's palsy.

The eighth cranial nerve is composed of an auditory and a vestibular component. The auditory component can be assessed by separately whispering a word in either ear or comparing the maximum distance from either ear at which the ticktack sound of a watch may still be heard. A tuning fork placed on the midfrontal region should be equally perceived in both ears (Weber test). If it is better perceived in one ear than the other, either the former ear has defective air conduction or the opposite ear has a neurologic deficit. The sound of the tuning fork conducted by air should be perceived long after it has stopped being transmitted through the mastoid bone (Rinne test). An air conduction defect is otherwise suggested. Involvement of the vestibular component is suggested by symptoms of vertigo and the findings of nystagmus. Vertical nystagmus on up or down gaze suggests brain-stem dysfunction.

Symmetry of soft palate elevation while performing the gag reflex assesses the glossopharyngeal and vagus nerves (cranial nerves IX and X) while the same movement on command reflects vagal nerve function exclusively. Voice nasality and swallowing difficulties with liquids also suggest bilateral vagal involvement or neuromuscular disease of the palatal and deglutition muscles (*e.g.*, myasthenia gravis). The gag reflex need not be performed in every patient. There exists a wide range of response to this test, and many normal people are hypersensitive to it. Some patients will start to gag as soon as they see the tongue blade. The gag reflex may also be almost absent in a normal patient. A history of swallowing difficulties and speech changes and assorted neurologic abnormalities need to be present before the gag reflex assumes meaning. Isolated reports that the gag reflex is hypersensitive or absent are usually meaningless.

Cranial nerve XI (spinal accessory nerve) subserves rotation of the head toward the opposite side (sternocleidomastoid muscle function) and ipsilateral shoulder shrugging (trapezius). A lower motor neuron lesion of cranial nerve XII (hypoglossal nerve) will result in the protruded tongue deviating to the same side of the lesion and atrophy of that same half of the tongue. Lesions involving connections between the cortex and the nucleus of XII, particularly if bilateral, will give rise to slow in-and-out or side-to-side tongue movements. Lingual consonant sounds will be affected.

MOTOR EXAMINATION

The motor examination assesses strength, tone, efficiency and rapidity of movement, muscle bulk, reflexes, and the presence of abnormal involuntary movements. The motor examination should be approached in a logical manner. Assessment of muscle strength should proceed in a manner which allows asymmetries to become apparent. Muscle groups should be isolated in a side-to-side manner, allowing hemiparesis to become apparent. Muscle groups should also be assessed for proximal and distal discrepancies. For example, proximal symmetrical weakness often reflects a myopathic process, whereas distal symmetrical weakness reflects a neuropathic process. Associated signs accompanying weakness which may help to establish a diagnosis include whether the deep tendon reflexes are increased or decreased, whether tone is spastic or hypotonic, whether muscle bulk appears normal or exhibits atrophy and fasciculations, and whether the Babinski sign is present or absent.

Although the patient may remain dressed while the motor examination is conducted, it is better to have him disrobe in order to fully evaluate by inspection whether any focal atrophy is present. In addition, it will be much easier to observe large muscle areas for the presence of fasciculations (spontaneous contractions of multiple muscle fibers which are often not noticed by the patient and do not produce muscle movement). Arm drift is evaluated with the patient seated before the examiner. The patient holds his arms outstretched, palms up, and with eyes closed is asked to maintain this position. If one arm asymmetrically drifts down, this is a subtle indication of paresis. In fact, in very mild weaknesses of the upper extremity a drift may be detected before individual focal muscle group weakness is apparent. The physician then proceeds to focal muscle group testing in the upper extremities, comparing groups side to side and proximal to distal. In addition to looking for patterns of distribution of weakness as already discussed, there are patterns of weakness which reflect particular involvement of cervical and thoracic nerve roots. Without being overly detailed in regard to the particular root that supplies each muscle, the following provides a convenient summary: C5 innervates the deltoid and biceps, C6 wrist extensors, C7 wrist flexion, C8 finger flexion and hand group, and T1 finger adduction and abduction.

The lower extremities should be evaluated in a similar manner. Attention should be directed to laterality of paresis and to proximal–distal distribution. L1, L2, and L3 innervate the iliopsoas (tested by opposing elevation of the extended leg in a supine position); L2, L3, and L4 innervate the quadriceps (tested by opposing knee extension); L5 subserves dorsiflexion, eversion, and inversion of the foot (tested by opposing these actions); and S1 subserves plantar flexion (tested by opposing this action).

Gradations of muscle weakness may be recorded as mild, moderate, or severe. Strength can also be assessed using a clinical scale of 0 to 5 (0 = absence of movement; 1 = flicker of movement; 2 = movement only if gravity is removed [e.g., knee flexion and extension in the horizontal plane]; 3 = segment examined can move against gravity but not against active resistance [e.g., knee flexion and extension in the vertical plane]; 4 = able to move against active resistance but eventually overcome by it; 5 = active resistance cannot overcome the movement).

Tone is operationally defined as the resistance offered by the limb or other body segment when it is passively mobilized. Tone is assessed as the examiner passively moves the limb through a full range of flexion and extension movements at the elbow, wrist, knee, ankle, and neck. Tone may be normal, decreased (in lower motor neuron or cerebellar lesions), or increased (in upper motor neuron and extrapyramidal disorders). The increase in tone may be perceived as a ratchety feeling of intermittent tone releases like the cogs of a wheel (cogwheel rigidity), or as an increase in tone that suddenly gives way reminiscent of a razor blade (spastic), or a more diffuse feeling of resistance to movement without any "give" feeling to it (lead pipe rigidity as seen occasionally in dystonias and akinetic rigid syndromes or the "gegenhalten" of the demented patient).

The rhythm and flow of movement should be tested by asking the patient to perform finger tapping, hand opening and closing, hand pronation and supination (rapid alternating movements), foot stomping, and foot tapping. One observes the speed, amplitude, and regularity of these movements. Abnormalities include slowness, decreased amplitude, interruptions in the flow of movement, movement breakdown, and incompleteness of movement. This aspect of the motor exam may be impaired in cerebellar or basal ganglia diseases with preservation of strength.

With the patient sitting quietly, the examiner should review his earlier observations regarding the presence or absence of abnormal involuntary movements (AIMs). A tremor may appear when the patient's hand is outstretched, or various abnormal movements, including chorea, dystonia, myoclonus, and tics, may become apparent while the patient sits (see chap. 10).

Evaluation of pathologic reflexes and the deep tendon reflexes is described in a separate section of this chapter.

SENSORY SYSTEM

The sensory examination can be performed with the patient seated and facing the examiner. The patient does not have to be completely undressed, but removal of the shoes and socks, exposure of the legs at least to the knees, and exposure of the arms to the elbows facilitate the examination. If a spinal cord sensory level is suspected because of the history or motor findings on examination, the trunk must also be exposed for testing. The sensory examination is very dependent on the subjective responses of the patient to various stimuli. If the patient is confused, aphasic, or demented, or has an altered level of consciousness, then the response to testing will be unreliable and this portion of the neurologic examination should be omitted. On the other hand, if the patient is anxious, seems to have limited tolerance to testing or a limited but not totally impaired attention span, and the history suggests that the sensory examination will be important in reaching a diagnosis, the examination should begin with sensory testing.

The sensory examination should be divided into the evaluation of the so-called primary sensations and the cortical sensations. The primary sensations that are evaluated include pain, temperature, and light touch, which are transmitted via the sensory nerve endings, spinothalamic tracts, ventroposteriolateral (VPL) nucleus of the thalamus, and postcentral sensory cortex. Vibration and position sense are also evaluated, and these sensations are transmitted via the sensory nerve endings, posterior columns of the spinal cord, the medial lemniscus, thalamus, and sensory cortex. Cortical sensations that can be evaluated include double simultaneous stimulation, two-point discrimination, stereognosis, and graphesthesia. These cortical sensations can only be evaluated in the presence of normal primary sensation. For example, if a patient has a sensory neuropathy and has impaired sensation to pinprick over the hands, it would not be possible to test two-point discrimination. On the other hand, in a patient with intact primary sensory modalities impaired two-point discrimination may be a valuable clue to parietal lobe dysfunction.

The same organization and logic that were used to conduct the motor examination should be employed in carrying out sensory testing. In particular, side-to-side and proximal-to-distal comparisons should be made. Decreased sensation to pin (hypesthesia) on one-half of the body (hemihypesthesia) is due to a lesion in contralateral sensory pathways in the brain stem or cerebral hemisphere. Involvement of the distal limbs, particularly if bilateral, has been described as "stocking" or "glove" distribution of a sensory deficit and suggests involvement of the sensory fibers in the peripheral nervous system (peripheral neuropathy). In fact, peripheral neuropathies most commonly begin with distal sensory loss. A very useful examination technique is to quickly compare the patient's appreciation of pinprick from proximal to distal and from side to side. If a particular area of decreased sensation to pin is identified in a part of a limb, careful attention to its boundaries will suggest either root (dermatomal), plexus, or peripheral nerve involvement. Although considerable confusion can arise in interpreting the sensory exam to pin because of the difference between cutaneous nerve sensory patterns and radicular involvement, the examiner should attempt to accurately define the borders of the involved area. It is sometimes useful to ask patients to quantify the sensation that is reported as decreased or increased. For example, the patient can be told that the good area (side to side, or focal) is worth one dollar and then asked what the bad area is worth. In anxious patients small and insignificant changes in perception of the pinprick may then be disregarded as probably insignificant. The examination should be conducted with disposable pins. Pins should not be used from patient to patient.

Considerable individual variation occurs in the radicular or segmental innervation pattern. However, a useful guideline to remember is that in the upper extremity sensation is supplied by roots C5–T1 and that lower extremity sensation is supplied by roots L1–S2 (see Chap. 12 for further description and figures). Sensation to temperature will parallel although not exactly overlap the findings on sensation to pin. It can be tested by the use of the back of the tuning fork or some other cold metallic stimulus. It has confirmatory value when the findings of sensation to pin are questionable.

Vibratory sense is tested with a tuning fork. Comparisons are made in a similar fashion as with sensation to pin, with similar conclusions derived as to site involved. It may be a particularly sensitive test in peripheral neuropathies preferentially affecting large myelinated fibers where distal decreases in sensation to vibration may be the only sensory abnormalities noted. The patient's perception of the sensation perceived is judged by determining if there are any differences in terms of the length of time the vibration is perceived while the tuning fork is held against a particular surface. The tuning fork can be positioned so that the examiner can also feel the vibration. The examiner's own perception of the vibration may also be used as a control to judge the patient's response. If there is no vibratory deficit distally then there is no need to test more proximal sites. Allowance is made for decreased sensation to vibration in toes of elderly individuals, which is a normal finding. If lateralized deficits are noted on examination it is wise to test the validity of the finding by testing vibratory sensations over the forehead and sternum. Since these sites are in reality single structures, laterality to the right or left side of the forehead and/or sternum indicates that the patient's response is unreliable.

Proprioception is partially evaluated by testing position sense. This is performed by gently grasping a toe or finger on its lateral surfaces and performing up and down movements. The patient's eyes should be closed during this maneuver. Initially small excursions are increased if a deficit is detected to determine the degree to which this modality is affected. Testing more proximal sites becomes necessary only if toes or fingers are affected. A subtle clue to a sensory deficit in this modality is the patient's slight movement of the toe or finger in an attempt to perceive additional sensory clues.

As discussed previously, evaluation of higher cortical sensory functions can be performed accurately only when primary sensations are intact. Unilateral loss of cortical sensation indicates dysfunction of the contralateral parietal lobe. Double simultaneous stimulation consists of simultaneously touching a part of a limb or the face on each side of the body with the patient's eyes closed. If the patient consistently fails to identify one side (*e.g.*, right face, right arm) when the primary modalities of sensation on that side are normal (pin, touch, vibration, and position), a lesion affecting the contralateral parietal hemisphere or its connections should be suspected. The failure to perceive one of the double stimuli may quickly extinguish. It should be recognized that the patient may accurately identify the same stimulus to the arm or face when it is delivered independently. Graphesthesia can be evaluated by checking the ability of the patient to identify a number or letter "written" on the hand of the affected side without looking at it. Finally, stereognosis can be tested by examining the ability of a patient to accurately identify objects placed in the hand without visual cues. Keys or coins are often used for this purpose. If the hand is paretic, stereognosis can still be evaluated by moving the object around in the patient's palm.

CEREBELLAR FUNCTION EXAM

Although the cerebellum is not primarily a motor organ, its dysfunction results in disorders of muscular coordination, speech, equilibrium, and gait. The clinical manifestations of these disorders can be evaluated by listening to the patient's speech; using examination techniques to demonstrate incoordination, kinetic tremor, and decomposition of movement; and observing the gait. The presence of weakness in the limbs, involuntary movements, or any other concomitant neurologic deficit will affect the cerebellar examination. In evaluating specific motor functions the patient's ability to judge the speed, power, and distance to carry out the act should be noted. If these are faulty, dysmetria is present. If the patient has difficulty carrying out repetitive successive acts or difficulty stopping one motor maneuver and immediately starting an opposite motor act, dysdiadochokinesia is present.

Appendicular ataxia is tested by having the patient perform finger-to-nose-to-finger and heel-to-knee maneuvers. Finger-to-nose-to-finger testing is carried out with the patient sitting and facing the examiner. The patient's eyes should be open as he touches the examiner's finger and then his own nose, back and forth as quickly and smoothly as possible. The examiner should place the target finger at arm's length from the patient, since this will exacerbate any terminal kinetic tremor. The examiner should observe the patient's hand for the appearance of a tremor, pastpointing, or missing the target. The heel-to-knee maneuver is carried out with the patient supine. The heel is raised into the air and then placed on the opposite knee. The patient is then asked to move the heel up and down the shin. The examiner should observe for tremor and/or ataxia.

Rapid alternating movements in the upper and lower extremities should be evaluated. Each limb is tested separately. Tasks for the upper extremities include rapidly supinating and pronating the hand, tapping a tabletop with the palm of the hand, or repeatedly touching the index finger and thumb. Tapping of the toes will evaluate this function in the lower extremities.

Abnormalities discussed so far on the cerebellar examination are reflections of cerebellar hemisphere dysfunction. Midline cerebellar dysfunction which produces truncal ataxia will not be detected by these maneuvers. Truncal ataxia is observable when the patient sits upright or walks. Typical abnormalities present on gait testing with cerebellar dysfunction include a wide-based, slightly unsteady walk. "Cerebellar speech" is described as scanning in multiple sclerosis and staccato in Friedreich's ataxia. The speech is slow, slurred, jerky, and occasionally explosive.

REFLEXES

Of the numerous deep tendon reflexes (DTRs) described, the biceps, brachioradialis, triceps, knee, and ankle reflexes have been incorporated into the routine neurologic exam. A variety of reflex hammers are available. The choice of any of them is less important than the proficiency that comes with experience. The patient is examined in the seated or supine position and is made to relax the body segment being tested. The examiner should use the hammer to deliver a light but firm tap on the tendon of the muscle being tested, and observation of the elicited movement should be recorded. There is a wide range of responses to tendon taps that must be learned.

Asymmetrical decrease or loss of a particular reflex or reflexes is seen with radiculopathies, plexopathies, or mononeuropathies. Examples include ipsilateral loss of biceps and brachioradialis reflexes in pathology of the sixth cervical root, or the loss of the knee reflex in a femoral neuropathy. Decrease or loss of reflexes in the upper extremities with hyperreflexia in the lower extremities suggests spinal cord pathology at the cervical level or amyotrophic lateral sclerosis. Bilateral decrease or absence of distal DTRs suggests peripheral neuropathy.

Hyperreflexia is seen in diseases affecting the upper motor neuron (motor cortex or corticospinal tract) and is associated with increase in tone (spasticity) and a positive Babinski reflex. It is seen with degenerative, neoplastic, inflammatory, vascular, and post-traumatic disease affecting the brain, brain stem, or spinal cord.

The Babinski response is normal only in children up to the age of 2 and otherwise represents disease of the upper motor neuron. Slow and deliberate stroking of the sole of the foot in its lateral half should normally elicit a flexor response of all toes. A sustained extensor response of the big toe, at times accompanied by fanning out of the other four toes, represents the classic Babinski sign. At times the finding is less clear-cut, and the clinician may have to qualify its presence with the words *possible* or *questionable*. Dystonic involvement of the lower extremities may bring about the presence of a spontaneous upgoing toe, which should not be confused with a positive Babinski reflex.

GAIT EXAMINATION

Just as with the mental status examination, the gait examination starts the moment the physician greets the patient. The gait exam is best interpreted after the symptoms and signs have been gathered and diagnostic hypotheses have been framed.

The patient is asked to arise from a chair with his arms crossed. The patient may display mild difficulties by performing this task slowly, flexing the knees while bringing the upper body forward, or sliding the buttocks forward over the seating surface before trying to stand up. A measure of more difficulty in rising is the need for repeated attempts before accomplishing the task or the need to use the hands to push the body up. More severe degrees of impairment are indicated by the need for assistance. Difficulties in this area can be due to proximal muscle weakness, basal ganglia disease, or pain in the low back or proximal lower extremities.

The patient's posture is observed. Parkinson's disease patients exhibit a stooping posture (simian posture) which may be associated with thoracic kyphosis and additional lateral bending. Patients with progressive supranuclear palsy—another extrapyramidal disorder causing bradykinesia and rigidity—frequently display an erect or hypererect posture. An exaggerated lumbar lordosis may be seen in patients with proximal lower extremity weakness, as seen in muscular dystrophies and other myopathies.

The patient's ambulation is analyzed as to speed, stride length, turning, and associated movements. Diseases affecting the pyramidal tract or the extrapyramidal system may shorten the stride length, slow ambulation, decrease the vertical displacement of the advancing foot, and be associated with a decrease or absence of the associated arm movement on the same side. It is sometimes impossible to distinguish, on gait exam alone, the patient who has only partially recovered from a stroke from a patient with early Parkinson's disease. Patients with cerebellar disease, progressive supranuclear palsy, or labyrinthine disease may exhibit a cautious, wide-based stance with consequent slowing of ambulation. The festinating gait of the parkinsonian patient is characterized by rapid, increasingly accelerating short steps where the patient may have difficulty coming to an immediate halt at will.

Weakness of the tibialis anterior muscle results in inability to adequately dorsiflex the foot as the foot is being advanced and a resultant compensatory marked elevation of the leg in what is called a *steppage gait* (seen in common peroneal neuropathy or L5 radiculopathy). Weakness of the same muscle may be manifested by an inability to heel walk (also seen in pyramidal tract disease). Toe walking difficulty is indicative of gastrocnemius weakness (seen in posterior tibial neuropathy or S1–S2 radiculopathies).

Efficient turning is accomplished by an act of sequential pivoting of both legs. The leg opposite to the desired direction of turn is the one making the final advance prior to the turning moment, and the posteriorly placed leg is the first to pivot. Difficulties in this area are manifested by the substitution of multiple steps or the appearance of sudden interruptions of the movement (freezing). It is at this juncture that falls are more likely to occur, and the examiner should be reasonably close to the patient to prevent this. Adequate turning or pivoting may be affected in disorders of basal ganglia, cerebellar disease, or labyrinthine disease. Freezing is viewed exclusively as an extrapyramidal (basal ganglionic) dysfunction.

The patient is then asked to stand with one foot next to the other. Patients with cerebellar disease, advanced basal ganglia disease, or acute labyrinthine disease may be unable to successfully accomplish this task and may find it necessary to separate the distance between the feet. Only after a standing stance has been successfully accomplished can the clinician proceed to perform the Romberg test. The patient is asked to close his eyes while trying to stand still. Oscillations in the lateral or anteroposterior direction may normally appear, but the feet will not move. Wider oscillations culminating in a loss of equilibrium suggest proprioceptive

difficulties in the lower extremities, implying dysfunction in the posterior columns, although it can also be seen with severe sensory neuropathies.

Postural stability can be checked in the anteroposterior direction by having the clinician place himself behind the standing patient and firmly push the patient on the midsternal area or the anterior aspect of both shoulders. A normal response results in quick return of the displaced upper body to its preperturbation position. At times, a normal subject may have to take one or two steps back to avoid a fall. Abnormal responses are variable, ranging from the need for multiple steps, to the failure of multiple steps to avoid the fall, to the loss of generation of these multiple steps with a tendency to fall *en bloc* sometimes without the compensatory forward elevation of the upper extremities. The most severely affected patients are those who need to be held while standing or walking. Basal ganglia and cerebellar disease are the most frequent causes of problems in this area.

Postural stability is checked in the lateral direction by asking the patient to walk in tandem. Difficulties in this area include cerebellar disease, labyrinthine disease, proprioceptive difficulties in the lower extremities, and basal ganglia disease.

QUESTIONS AND DISCUSSION

1. A 62-year-old man has had a feeling of generalized weakness for the preceding 3 weeks associated with difficulty in chewing and swallowing and a change in the quality of speech. Further questioning reveals that he has been suffering from intermittent diplopia and droopiness of one eyelid for the preceding year. The examination reveals ptosis of the left eye associated with deficit of abduction. There is weakness of jaw opening and nasality of speech. Gag reflexes are present. The soft palate shows decreased symmetrical excursion to both reflex and command. Weakness is generalized, affecting both proximal and distal muscles. There are no cognitive findings (including no emotional lability) and no sensory findings. Reflexes are symmetrical and normoreactive, there are no Babinski responses, and the tone is normal. The likely site of the lesion is:

    A. Both cerebral hemispheres
    B. The neuromuscular junction

C. The brain stem affecting cranial nerves III, V, VI, IX, and X

D. The peripheral nerves in a diffuse fashion as seen in Guillain–Barré syndrome

The correct answer is not (A). Bilateral hemisphere dysfunction capable of causing difficulty in chewing, swallowing, and speaking is known as a *pseudobulbar state*. It implies bilateral involvement of corticobulbar fibers, that is, a dysfunction of those connections between the cerebral hemispheres and the brain-stem nuclei. This may be seen in the setting of individuals who have suffered multiple strokes. This patient had diplopia, a symptom that cannot be explained by lesions proximal to the brain-stem nuclei. He also lacked cranial hyperreflexia (hyperactive jaw jerk and gag reflexes), limb hyperreflexia, Babinski responses, limb spasticity, or cognitive changes (slowness of mental function, emotional lability).

(B) is the correct answer. Myasthenia gravis is the most commonly seen disease of the neuromuscular junction. It can affect eye movements in an asymmetrical fashion, with diplopia being a frequent early complaint. This patient had difficulty in chewing due to jaw muscle weakness but no evidence of direct cranial nerve V involvement (no sensory findings over the face). The patient's difficulty in swallowing and nasality of voice were expressive of involvement of the soft palate musculature. The fact that gag reflexes and jaw jerk were not hyperactive spoke against the involvement of corticobulbar fibers. The fact that the generalized weakness was not accompanied by reflex, tone, or sensory abnormalities spoke against involvement of central (corticospinal tracts at brain, brain-stem, or spinal cord level) or peripheral motor fibers.

(C) is not the correct answer. A brain-stem event may in fact be associated with diplopia by affecting cranial nerve nuclei or fibers connecting them (medial longitudinal fasciculus). Ptosis of the one eye in such a context could be due to Horner's syndrome, but the ipsilateral pupil was not miotic. It could also be due to involvement of cranial nerve III or its fibers before they emerge from the brain stem, but cranial nerve III–dependent functions were not affected (no deficit of eye adduction, elevation, or depression, no pupillary dilatation). A brain-stem event could also be associated with dysphagia. Dysarthria (deficit in articulation) or anarthria (absence of articulation) rather than nasality of voice is a more likely speech difficulty. An acute brain-stem event (*e.g.*, CVA) may be associated with quadriparesis but would also be associated with flaccidity

of tone and hyporeflexia. As the patient recovers, spasticity and hyperreflexia will appear. Neither feature was present in this case.

(D) is not the correct answer. An acute inflammatory polyradiculoneuropathy (Guillain–Barré syndrome) can be associated with rapid onset of generalized weakness including bulbar dysfunction (dysphagia, difficulty with mastication, voice nasality) but is not likely to be preceded by diplopia for months, as was the case of this patient. Areflexia is a very important feature of this condition. Sensory findings may also be present, such as distal loss or decrease of sensation to light touch, pin, temperature, vibration, or position.

2. A 55-year-old woman has noticed gradual loss of dexterity of her left hand and increasing difficulty with ambulation. Examination discloses a wasted left hand and bilateral lower extremity spasticity. The left lower extremity is weaker than the right, while pin is better perceived on that same side. The decrease in sensation to pin on the right side extends to the midtrunk. There are no cranial nerve findings, and cognitive functions are intact. The likely site of the lesion is:

A. An asymmetrical polyneuropathy affecting the left median nerve and both sciatic nerves

B. A cervical cord–compressive syndrome

C. A diffuse motor neuron disorder (amyotrophic lateral sclerosis)

Polyneuropathy does not cause lower extremity spasticity, which is a sign of upper motor neuron dysfunction. (A) is not the correct answer.

(B) is the correct answer. An asymmetrical spasticity with the weaker lower extremity on the left and the decreased sensation to pin on the opposite side places the site of pathology in the spinal cord, predominantly on the left side. The reason pinprick is diminished on the right is that the sensory fibers cross to the opposite side shortly after entering the spinal cord. Thus, a lesion that affects the pathways for pain sensation (spinothalamic tracts) on one side of the cord will be experienced as decreased sensation to pin on the opposite side. The precise location of the lesion is given by the wasting of the left hand, a lower motor neuron lesion that suggests involvement of the lower motor neurons at the C8 segment. The sensory level in this case falsely localizes the process to the midthoracic area.

(C) is not the correct answer. Motor neuron disease can present with a combination of upper and motor neuron signs such as in this case. But there is no sensory involvement.

3. A 35-year-old female presents with complaints of painful burning feet and difficulty with ambulation. The examination discloses severe loss of position and vibration sense in the lower extremities—distal more than proximal—associated with spasticity, hyperreflexia, and Babinski responses. The upper extremities disclose a similar sensory deficit but of a milder degree. There are no cranial nerve or cognitive deficits. The likely site of the lesion is:

   A. The posterior columns and corticospinal tracts at the level of the spinal cord
   B. The peripheral nerves, particularly the large myelinated fibers which conduct proprioceptive information
   C. The brain stem, affecting the proprioceptive fibers (medial lemnisci) and corticospinal tracts

(A) is the correct answer. The loss of proprioceptive information can be due to a peripheral neuropathy affecting large myelinated fibers or to disease affecting the posterior columns in the spinal cord. The concurrent presence of upper motor neuron signs (spasticity, hyperreflexia, and Babinski responses) points to the spinal cord as the site of pathology.

(B) is not the correct answer. A peripheral neuropathy could be associated with selective or preferential involvement of those fibers conducting proprioceptive information, but it would not be the cause of the associated upper motor neuron syndrome.

(C) is not the correct answer. The patient does not have evidence of involvement of other brain-stem structures such as cranial nerves, gaze centers, or other sensory modalities.

4. A 25-year-old myopic woman presents with the complaint of blurred vision of the left eye associated with eye pain for the preceding 7 days. Past history reveals that she has been experiencing amenorrhea for the preceding 6 months. There is a very strongly positive history of glaucoma in the family. The extraocular movements are intact, and there is no ptosis. The eye examination discloses no overt abnormalities of the cornea, iris, or lens. Visual acuity of the left eye is 20/80, uncorrected by glasses, while it is 20/25 on the right eye with glasses. The left pupil dilates as a light is directed from the right to the left eye. Fundoscopic exam reveals blurred margins of the left disk. There are no other findings on neurologic exam. The likely site of the lesion is:

   A. The optic chiasm as a result of compression by a pituitary gland tumor
   B. The right occipital lobe or right optic radiations
   C. This represents an acute attack of glaucoma
   D. The left optic nerve

(A) is not the correct answer. Although the patient's amenorrhea warrants investigation, it is unlikely to explain her symptoms and signs because a lesion at the level of the optic chiasm would cause loss of both temporal fields of vision and not a uniocular decrease in visual acuity.

(B) is not the correct answer. A lesion of the right occipital lobe or the optic radiations would cause a loss of vision in the nasal field of the right eye and the temporal field of the left eye (left homonymous hemianopia).

(C) is not the correct answer. Sudden loss of vision due to an acute attack of glaucoma can be associated with eye pain and even with an unreactive pupil. It is not associated with swelling of the optic disk. The patient's positive family history for glaucoma proves to be a "red herring" rather than a clue in this particular case.

(D) is the correct answer. The patient's picture is very characteristic of an acute optic neuritis with a decrease of central vision in one eye, associated with an afferent pupillary defect and swelling of the optic disk. Sometimes the swelling of the optic nerve may occur more posteriorly and the disk may appear normal (retrobulbar neuritis). Approximately 30% of patients who suffer optic neuritis will go on to develop multiple sclerosis.

SUGGESTED READING

Bradley WG, Daroff RB, Fenichel GM et al (eds): Neurology in Clinical Practice. Boston, Butterworth–Heinemann, 1991

Haerer AF: DeJong's—The Neurologic Examination, 5th ed. Philadelphia, JB Lippincott, 1992

Medical Research Council: Aids to the Examination of the Peripheral Nervous System. London, HMSO, 1976

Clinical Use of Neurologic Diagnostic Tests

Thomas P. Bleck

The diagnostic tests used in neurologic practice are most effectively employed as adjuncts to the history and physical examination. Prior to the advent of computerized imaging studies, the noninvasive electrodiagnostic tests were often ordered as a battery to determine whether invasive radiologic studies or diagnostic cranial exploration was indicated. As computed tomography (CT) and magnetic resonance imaging (MR) have advanced, the electrophysiologic studies are less important anatomically; however, as pathophysiologic studies they remain unchallenged. Similarly, cerebrospinal fluid (CSF) examination is less often indicated in the work-up of mass lesions but is prominent in the study of neuroimmunologic disorders. Hence, diagnostic studies can now be more appropriately tailored, with a considerable decrease in risk, time, and expense. However, if these tests are used indiscriminately, rather than to include or exclude specific clinical hypotheses, they can increase costs and delay diagnosis and treatment.

Cerebrospinal fluid examination and electrodiagnostic procedures are considered in this chapter. Neuroradiologic studies are discussed in Chapter 3 and are mentioned only as an alternative means of acquiring data.

CEREBROSPINAL FLUID EXAMINATION

Since Quincke introduced the diagnostic lumbar puncture (LP) at the end of the 19th century, CSF evaluation has been applied to most neurologic disorders. As other diagnostic tests have become more sophisticated, CSF examination is no longer a standard part of the analysis of all central nervous system (CNS) disorders. This procedure is most commonly indicated for the diagnosis of CNS infection, neoplastic invasion of the subarachnoid space, multiple sclerosis (MS), acute inflammatory demyelinating polyneuropathy (Guillain–Barré syndrome), other neuroimmunologic disorders, and pseudotumor cerebri.

TECHNIQUE

An LP is usually performed with the patient lying on his side, with the knees flexed as close to the chest as possible. The patient should be informed about each stage of the procedure and he should be positioned with the back as close to the edge of the bed as possible. The location of the intended puncture should be determined before cleansing the skin. A line connecting the posterior iliac crests crosses the L3–L4 interspace, which is usually the most rostral space employed. The caudal end of the spinal cord is at L2 in most adults. After palpating the spinous processes, the examiner can mark the L4–L5 and L5–S1 interspaces with thumbnail pressure prior to gloving. The skin is cleansed with iodine followed by alcohol, and sterile drapes are positioned around the area to be punctured. The skin is anesthetized with 1% lidocaine, using a 25-gauge needle, which is then exchanged for a 22-gauge needle. This longer, stiffer needle is used to anesthetize the

William J. Weiner and Christopher G. Goetz, eds. *Neurology for the Non-Neurologist*, Third Edition. Copyright © 1994, 1989 by J. B. Lippincott Company. Copyright © 1981 by Harper and Row Publishers, Inc.

deeper tissue down to the epidural space. As the needle is advanced, the syringe is aspirated to avoid intravascular or subarachnoid injection. The epidural space is recognized by the sudden loss of resistance to injection.

A 20- or 22-gauge spinal needle is adequate for most LPs; smaller caliber needles make pressure measurements difficult. The needle should always be advanced with the stylet in place (to avoid subarachnoid introduction of epidermal tissue). Although some experts replace the stylet when withdrawing the needle to avoid entrapping a spinal nerve root, there is a no apparent difference in the rare incidence of this complication with either technique. The needle should be advanced with the bevel up, to separate the fibers of the ligamentum flavum. The needle is angled 15 degrees cephalad to avoid the spinous processes. Dural puncture produces a "pop"; the stylet is then withdrawn. If free CSF flow does not occur, rotating the bevel toward the head is often useful (with all movements of the needle, the stylet should be replaced). Should it be necessary to redirect the needle, it must be withdrawn almost to the skin. Newer spinal needles, which have a conical tip and a side port rather than a beveled tip, may produce less of a dural tear and therefore fewer, less severe postprocedural headaches.

When free flow has been established, the CSF pressure is measured with a manometer attached to the needle by means of a stopcock. The patient's legs should be extended to prevent a falsely increased reading. The respiration and pulse should both fluctuate.

For accurate pressure readings, if possible, patients on ventilators (especially those receiving positive end-expiratory pressure) should be transiently disconnected to lower the transmitted intrathoracic pressure. The Queckenstedt jugular compression test is unreliable and dangerous. Following pressure measurement, four tubes of CSF are withdrawn and processed for cell counts (at the start and end), biochemical and immunologic studies, and microbiologic analysis. The usefulness of closing pressure measurement is uncertain.

Following the withdrawal of the needle, pressure should be applied to the site of entry and the patient should be placed in the prone position. Although the evidence is inconclusive, many experts feel that 1 to 3 hours prone is the most effective method of preventing a post-LP headache, which is the major complication of the procedure.

If the physician is unable to enter the subarachnoid space with this technique, the patient should be placed in a sitting position. With the patient leaning forward on a support, the spinous processes will be palpable in the midline. When the needle is in the subarachnoid space, the patient should be returned to the recumbent position for a pressure measurement.

When lumbar spine disease or the question of an intraspinal mass prevents the lumbar approach, a lateral cervical approach can be performed by a physician trained in this technique. Fluoroscopic guidance can be employed with either approach.

CONTRAINDICATIONS

Prior to LP, the physician must be certain that the patient does not have an intracranial or intraspinous mass. A CSF examination is rarely useful in this situation, and the withdrawal of CSF may alter the CNS pressure dynamics sufficiently to cause herniation.

The absence of papilledema does not exclude an intracranial mass, although its presence mandates a CT scan prior to LP (as does an asymmetry on neurologic examination). It is *not* necessary that all patients be scanned before an LP is performed, especially if acute bacterial meningitis is suspected. If LP is delayed for CT scanning when bacterial meningitis is suspected, one should consider a single dose of empirically chosen antibiotics prior to the CT scan (after blood cultures have been obtained).

Coagulopathy is a relative contraindication to LP, because epidural hematomas can arise at the puncture site. Infusions of fresh frozen plasma or platelets, as appropriate, should be given prior to the procedure if possible. If the coagulopathy is discovered after the LP, therapy should still be given because bleeding may occur for many hours. The patient should be examined frequently for signs of cauda equina dysfunction, which may necessitate surgical extirpation of the extravasated blood.

Cutaneous infection at the intended puncture site requires that a different approach (*e.g.*, lateral cervical) be used.

INTERPRETATION OF RESULTS

Normal lumbar CSF is under a pressure of no more than 180 mm (of CSF) with the patient in a recumbent position. An elevated pressure suggests the presence of infection, a mass lesion, increased CSF production, or its diminished resorption. Normal pressure does not exclude an infection or a mass.

The glucose concentration in CSF is normally at least two-thirds of the serum glucose; as glucose takes time to equilibrate in the subarachnoid space, the CSF value tends to lag behind the serum by about 30 minutes. Low CSF glucose concentrations are seen with meningeal inflammatory processes (*e.g.*, infection or meningeal spread of neoplasms). The protein concentration primarily reflects albumin derived from the serum; in the lumbar space, it is usually 15 to 45 mg/dl. Elevation usually reflects an increased transudation of albumin, generally as a consequence of inflammation. The protein concentration may be low or low-normal in pseudotumor cerebri.

High-resolution electrophoretic studies of CSF proteins reveal the presence of *oligoclonal antibodies* in over 90% of multiple sclerosis patients. This finding is also seen in other settings in which immunoglobulins are produced in the subarachnoid space (*e.g.*, infections), and rarely in the presence of primary brain tumors. They are also frequently present in the Guillain–Barré syndrome.

A cytologic examination of normal CSF should reveal no more than 5 lymphocytes per fl, and no polymorphonuclear leukocytes (PMNs). The presence of PMNs indicates an acute inflammatory process; lymphocytes predominate generally in aseptic, chronic, or resolving conditions.

Cultures and stains for microbial agents should be obtained if any possibility of infection arises. These include Gram stains, India ink preparations, stains for acid-fast bacilli (AFB), routine bacterial cultures, fungal cultures, and AFB cultures. Various newer studies are available for the analysis of bacterial infective agents; these studies include counterimmunoelectrophoresis (CIE) for specific bacterial antigens and the limulus test for endotoxin. Routine viral cultures of CSF seldom reveal the etiology of aseptic meningitis or encephalitis except for HIV-1, but antibody titers in the CSF and serum may be helpful. Serologic testing for syphilis is an increasingly important test.

Although subarachnoid hemorrhage is usually diagnosed by CT, an LP may be necessary to confirm the diagnosis. The scan may not detect small amounts of subarachnoid blood in patients without atrophy; in this case, LP is required. The procedure may also be used to reduce CSF pressure, and thus symptoms, if there is no intraparenchymal extension of bleeding.

Tables 2-1 and 2-2 summarize the expected CSF findings associated with the more common indications for LP.

ELECTROENCEPHALOGRAPHY

Indications for electroencephalography (EEG) have varied during the 60-year history of this technique. Imaging studies have supplanted it as a method for localizing anatomic pathology. This has freed EEG to develop as a pathophysiologic tool, detecting abnormal cerebral *function* that cannot be visualized radiographically or magnetically. Thus, the use of EEG is greatest in the evaluation of transient states (*e.g.*, seizures), evolving conditions (*e.g.*, herpes simplex encephalitis), global disorders (*e.g.*, dementia), and neonates. As with the other procedures considered in this chapter, the usefulness of EEG data depends on the clinical hypothesis being tested. Only a few EEG patterns are diagnostic of particular diseases, but the test is helpful in deciding among diagnostic alternatives.

TECHNIQUE

The quality of EEG recording and interpretation varies dramatically among laboratories. In evaluating the standards of practice used, the physician should expect the following:

1. The technologists are trained specifically in EEG and are either eligible for, or have obtained, certification by the American Board of Registration in Electrodiagnostic Technology.
2. The technologists participate in regular continuing education activities, both locally and nationally.
3. The electroencephalographers are neurologists certified by both the American Board of Psychiatry and Neurology and the American Board of Clinical Neurophysiology.
4. The laboratory meets the accreditation standards of the American Electroencephalographic Society.
5. The patient's head is always measured prior to the application of electrodes, according to the International 10–20 System.
6. The equipment employed has at least 16 channels and is calibrated prior to each use.
7. Each record performed includes both wakefulness and sleep (and states this clearly).
8. Hyperventilation and photic stimulation are used routinely as activation procedures unless contraindicated.
9. Extra electrodes (*e.g.*, sphenoidal) are employed when indicated.

TABLE 2-1. Cerebrospinal Fluid Abnormalities in Common Meningitides

	ACUTE BACTERIAL MENINGITIS	ASEPTIC MENINGITIS	TUBERCULOUS MENINGITIS	CRYPTOCOCCAL MENINGITIS	PARTIALLY TREATED BACTERIAL MENINGITIS	NEOPLASTIC MENINGITIS	ACUTE HIV-1 INFECTION
Pressure (mm CSF)	Up to 1000	Up to 350	300–500	300–500	Up to 500	Up to 500	Up to 350
Glucose (mg/dl)	0–40 (<35% of serum)	10–40	1–40	5–40	May be low	5–40	Usually normal
Protein (mg/dl)	Up to 1000	Up to 200	Up to 1000	Up to 500	May be elevated	Up to 500	Up to 200
WBCs (per fl)	500–50,000	15–200	100–500	100–500	Often elevated	20–500	Up to 500
Polys (%)	>90	May predominate early	5–15	5–15	Up to 30%	Occasional	Rare
Lymphs (%)	10	Predominant later	85–95	85–95	Predominant	Predominant	Predominant
Microbiologic studies	Gram stain culture	Culture (rarely)	AFB smear culture	India ink culture	Gram stain culture		Culture
Immunologic studies	CIE; limulus test	Antibodies; VDRL		Cryptococcal antigen	CIE; limulus test	β-2 microglobulin	Antigen, antibody studies
Other						Cytology	

AFB = acid-fast bacilli; CSF = cerebrospinal fluid; CIE = counterimmunoelectrophoresis; VDRL = Venereal Disease Research Laboratory test; WBC = white blood cell count.

TABLE 2-2. Cerebrospinal Fluid Abnormalities in Other Disorders

	HERPES SIMPLEX ENCEPHALITIS	SUBACUTE SCLEROSING PANENCEPHALITIS	ACUTE INFLAMMATORY DEMYELINATING POLYNEUROPATHY	CYSTICERCOSIS	ACUTE TOXO-PLASMOSIS	MULTIPLE SCLEROSIS	SUBARACHNOID HEMORRHAGE
Pressure (mm CSF)	Up to 450	Normal	Normal	Up to 250	Normal	Normal	Up to 500 (may be normal)
Glucose (mg/dl)	30–70	Normal	Normal	Normal	Normal	Normal	Usually normal
Protein (mg/dl)	Up to 200	Up to 100	Up to 100 (rarely, to 1000)	Up to 50	Up to 100	Up to 60	Often elevated
WBCs (per fl)	Up to 1000	6–500	0–5	Up to 300	10–50	Up to 20	Acutely, proportional to blood entry; later, elevated
Polys (%)	Up to 30	Rare	Rare	Rare	Rare	Rare	Acutely
Lymphs (%)	Predominant	Predominant	Up to 100	Predominant	Predominant	Predominant	Predominate later
Immunologic studies	Viral antibodies (late)	Measles and oligoclonal antibodies	Oligoclonal antibodies	Antibody titers	Antibody titers	Oligoclonal antibodies	
Other					Occasional eosinophils		Gross blood within 1–2 hours; xanthochromia

CSF = cerebrospinal fluid; WBC = white blood cell count.

10. The EEG report includes both a technical description and a clinical interpretation. This interpretation attempts to correlate the EEG with the patient's history. Although it may contain suggestions for further evaluation (*e.g.*, a sleep-deprived EEG), management recommendations beyond the scope of an EEG (*e.g.*, the suggestion of specific medications) are inappropriate.

TOPOGRAPHIC MAPPING

Many manufacturers have adapted computer interpolation techniques to produce colorful "brain maps" of EEG (and evoked potential) data. Although these maps have a great deal of emotional appeal and may eventually be found to aid in EEG interpretation, they currently require expert technologists and electroencephalographers to be certain that the data entered are free of artifacts. The statistical analysis of these maps is in its initial stage. At present, they cannot substitute for a standard EEG.

INTERPRETATION

EEG interpretation attempts to answer clinical questions about the cerebrum in light of the electrophysiologic data; thus, the interpretation is most useful when the questions are well defined and are appropriate for the examination. An EEG is one of the most useful studies in the evaluation of suspected seizures, for example, but is seldom valuable in the analysis of headaches or dizziness. The most commonly encountered EEG abnormalities are epileptiform events, slowing of normal rhythms, and disorders of age-specific patterns.

EPILEPTIFORM EVENTS

The term *epileptiform* is used because spikes and other sharp activity on the EEG rarely represent actual seizures. The usual EEG signature of a seizure disorder is the *interictal spike*. Such irritative events do occur (albeit rarely) in individuals without seizures, and their presence does not diagnose a seizure disorder (unless the actual seizure is recorded). Similarly, the absence of epileptiform abnormalities never excludes the diagnosis of a seizure disorder; this is a clinical decision.

Epileptiform activity may be divided broadly into *focal*, *multifocal*, and *generalized* events. In complex partial seizures of temporal lobe origin, for example, the abnormality is often localized over one anterior temporal region. In absence epilepsy, the 3-Hz discharges are typically widespread and bilaterally synchronous. This distinction is most crucial in the patient with a generalized convulsion, for whom the work-up, treatment, and prognosis depend on an accurate distinction between *primary generalized epilepsy* and *partial epilepsy with secondary generalization*. Other syndromes with specific EEG patterns, such as benign Rolandic epilepsy of childhood, have predictable courses and seldom require imaging studies or further work-up.

Several special EEG techniques are helpful in the diagnosis of epilepsy. Partial sleep deprivation may bring out otherwise undetected epileptiform abnormalities and should be performed whenever the routine EEG is unrevealing. Various extra electrodes have been developed and are most useful when a focal EEG abnormality is detected but is not definitely epileptiform. The most commonly employed are nasopharyngeal electrodes; however, studies have shown that extra true temporal (T1 and T2) electrodes are just as valuable and are less noxious. Sphenoidal electrodes or double-density electrode arrays may be suggested by the electroencephalographer in particular clinical situations, but they are not indicated routinely. Ambulatory 24-hour EEG technology is improving and can contribute to the differential diagnosis of intermittent behavioral episodes. Prolonged inpatient recordings, sometimes employing intracranial electrodes, are occasionally necessary for a definitive diagnosis.

The normal EEG contains several benign variants that may be confused with truly epileptiform activity. Small sharp spikes, positive occipital sharp transients of sleep, 14 and 6 Hz–positive spikes, "phantom" spikes, and "psychomotor variant" are imbedded in the older literature but are of dubious significance. EEG reports that stress their association with epilepsy or "neurovegetative disorders" should prompt the clinician to find another electroencephalographer.

SLOW WAVE ABNORMALITIES

As with epileptiform activity, the crucial distinction is among focal, multifocal, and diffuse abnormalities. A focal abnormality may result from gray or white matter dysfunction in that area; this distinction is based on other EEG characteristics. Recall here that the EEG is a physiologic test; postictal slowing from a recent seizure and the constant slowing emitted by cerebral tissue adjacent to a brain tumor may be indistinguishable on a single EEG. Imaging and electrophysiology are thus complementary, and unexplained focal slowing should prompt a radiologic or magnetic investigation.

Diffuse abnormalities are commonly a consequence of a toxic (*e.g.*, drug), metabolic (*e.g.*, hepatic), degenerative (*e.g.*, Alzheimer's disease), infectious (*e.g.*, encephalitis), or postictal condition. Pure diffuse slowing has few characteristics that distinguish among these possibilities; EEGs are most useful when acquired serially to monitor change in the patient's condition. Specific patterns, such as triphasic waves that exhibit temporospatial lags in hepatic encephalopathy, may suggest an etiology but are rarely diagnostic of a particular metabolic cause. Some forms of dementia (*e.g.*, subacute spongiform encephalopathy) have specific EEG signatures that are usually diagnostic of that particular disorder. A paucity of EEG abnormality in an apparently demented patient raises the possibility of depressive pseudodementia.

The combination of focal and diffuse disturbances is often a useful finding. In herpes simplex encephalitis, the EEG is the earliest diagnostically useful test to become abnormal and is often used to determine the site of brain biopsy before radiologic studies are abnormal. Multifocal abnormalities, especially if intermixed with epileptiform discharges, may suggest the embolic origin of a stroke.

Electrocerebral silence ("flat EEG") is the most extreme diffuse abnormality. If hypothermia and hypnosedative drug intoxication are excluded, this finding may be used to diagnose cerebral cortical inactivity. As the EEG does not reflect brain-stem activity, the EEG is not a substitute for a physical examination in the diagnosis of "brain death." The American Electroencephalographic Society has strict published criteria for these recordings. Such a study is only supportive, however, and is subject to false-negative interpretation due to artifacts. Studies that image intracranial blood flow are more useful in this setting.

AGE-SPECIFIC PATTERNS

Neonatal EEG recordings provide the clinician with the opportunity to assess cerebral development, as well as to detect the abnormalities previously described. The more subtle manifestations of seizures in newborns may only be detected by EEG.

A modest degree of focal slowing in the temporal regions commonly accompanies normal aging and may be overread by inexperienced interpreters.

EVOKED POTENTIALS

The role of evoked potential studies (EPs) has been in flux during the past decade. Prior to the wide availability of MR and CSF oligoclonal antibody studies, EPs were often essential in the diagnosis of MS because of their ability to detect subclinical lesions. Although they still play an ancillary role here, they are being applied increasingly to other areas.

Several sensory modalities can be investigated by evoked potentials; the most commonly studied are the visual, auditory, and somatosensory systems. "Cognitive" potentials and the cerebral events associated with motor output are areas of current research interest that may find a clinical application in the next several years.

TECHNIQUE

EPs rely on computer averaging to eliminate signals that are not related temporally to the stimulus used. Many reliable commercial systems for acquiring and displaying EP data are now available; problems arise due to variability in stimulus parameters, data manipulation, and interpretation. Standardization of techniques and interpretation is currently poor. At a minimum, the clinician should expect that the laboratory performing EPs has validated its technique and normative data by testing at least 20 normal subjects. Since the definitions of abnormality in EPs are based on numerical differences of latency and amplitude from a control population, the criteria of abnormality employed must be clearly stated. The number of falsely positive and negative studies depends on how these criteria are defined, rather than on a qualitatively abnormal measurement. In order to reduce false-positive results, most laboratories now use three standard deviations from the control mean as the definition of abnormality.

VISUAL EVOKED RESPONSES

Visual evoked responses (VERs) can be elicited with various stimuli; the most commonly employed are reversing checkerboard patterns, sinusoidal gratings, and repetitive flashes. The size of checks (or the spatial frequency of the grating), the luminance of the pattern, the ambient light, and the repetition rate of the stimuli are all important variables. Thus, norms derived in one laboratory may not apply to another.

The response is recorded over the occipital region. Each eye is tested separately to examine for prechiasmal lesions; stimulation of individual fields may also be performed if postchiasmal dysfunction is suspected.

Visual acuity is an important determinant of the response; if the patient wears glasses, they should be used during pattern testing.

For pattern reversal and sinusoidal gratings, the major potential of interest is a surface positive wave occurring about 100 msec after the stimulus (termed P100). Flash responses elicit a surface negative wave approximately 80 msec after the stimulus (N3).

BRAIN-STEM AUDITORY EVOKED RESPONSES

Although the auditory evoked response can be followed up to the cortex, the major use of this test on brain-stem auditory evoked responses (BAERs) is the evaluation of brain-stem structures. The stimuli are clicks, delivered monaurally through headphones. The frequency spectra of the clicks, their intensity, their duration, and their repetition rate influence the latency and amplitude of the responses.

Five waves are routinely recorded. Wave I originates from the VIII nerve, wave II from the cochlear nucleus, wave III from the superior olivary complex, wave IV from the lateral lemniscus, and wave V from the inferior colliculus. All of these responses normally occur within 6 msec of the stimulus.

SOMATOSENSORY EVOKED RESPONSES

Upper extremity somatosensory evoked responses (SSERs) are recorded following stimulation of the median nerve, and lower extremity SSERs from the posterior tibial nerve. The stimulus intensity is adjusted according to the motor response. These stimuli travel in the posterior column/medial lemniscal system, so that digit movement, rather than discomfort, is used to determine the stimulation level. Repetition rate and stimulus intensity affect the latency and amplitude of the responses.

From the upper extremity, responses are recorded over the brachial plexus, at the dorsal root entry zone, and over the contralateral primary sensory cortex. Lower extremity responses are measured at the popliteal fossa, the dorsal root entry zone, and the midline scalp over the somatosensory cortex (the foot area being located in the interhemispheric fissure).

INTERPRETATION

The major use of EPs is in the detection of subclinical lesions. Within the visual system, asymptomatic optic neuritis is easily detected; its presence may aid in the diagnosis of MS. Abnormalities of the optic nerves are poorly visualized by MRI, making VERs an important adjunct when the diagnosis of demyelinating disease is in doubt. Similarly, BAERs and SSERs can detect physiologic lesions below the limit of resolution of imaging techniques. This is especially true for MS plaques in the spinal cord, another area where MRI has been disappointing.

In infants, VERs have been used to assess the integrity of the visual system when blindness is suspected. Paradigms to determine refractive error are under investigation.

In addition to detecting asymptomatic brain-stem lesions in MS, auditory evoked responses are an excellent screening procedure when tumors of the eighth nerve are suspected. The sensitivity of BAERs in the setting is over 90%. BAERs are often employed in the operating room to help protect the eighth nerve during resection of posterior fossa lesions. The test is also useful when neuromuscular junction blockade or large doses of hypnosedative drugs have abolished the clinically testable brain-stem reflexes. The presence of BAERs (beyond wave I) confirms the activity of the brain stem and can also help to localize brain-stem lesions producing coma.

Analysis of BAER wave latencies as a function of intensity serves as a useful marker of auditory acuity in infants. This technique allows the early selection of hearing-impaired children for hearing aids and helps prevent their misdiagnosis as autistic or mentally retarded.

SSERs are also useful in suspected MS, because they allow the documentation of unsuspected or poorly defined sensory dysfunction. As the technique evolves, dermatomal SSERs may allow better definition of nerve root compression (e.g., by a herniated disc). SSERs also have a place in the operating room, guiding the degree of tension on distracting rods during scoliosis surgery.

ELECTROMYOGRAPHY AND NERVE CONDUCTION STUDIES

These procedures are valuable primarily in the analysis of peripheral nerve and muscular disorders. They serve as adjuncts to the patient's history and physical examination and must be tailored to a specific clinical question.

TECHNIQUE

Electromyography (EMG) demands a high degree of clinical and technical skill from the physician performing the study. The laboratory should be directed by a member of the American Association of Electromyography and Electrodiagnosis. Many variables influence the interpretation of results, including anatomic variations and the cooperation of the patient.

The usual EMG study involves recording spontaneous, voluntary, and electrically stimulated muscle activity by way of small intramuscular needle electrodes. Since the voluntary contraction of muscles is crucial for some parts of the study, the procedures should be clearly explained to the patient. Some discomfort is unavoidable during the test. Patients can be premedicated with codeine or anxiolytic agents without altering the data obtained; this often results in better cooperation and tolerance.

Some conditions indicate special studies. Myasthenia gravis and the myasthenic (Eaton–Lambert) syndrome exhibit characteristic responses to repetitive stimulation; the requesting physician must communicate such suspicions to the electromyographer.

Nerve conduction velocity (NCV) studies can be performed by trained technologists under the electromyographer's supervision. These tests involve electrical stimulation of a peripheral nerve, measuring the rate of transmission and the amplitude of the response along the nerve. These results are compared to statistically derived normal ranges. Careful attention to variables such as limb temperature and length is required for a valid interpretation.

INTERPRETATION

Abnormalities of the EMG can be produced by disease anywhere in the motor unit, from the lower motor neuron cell body to the muscle fiber. Characteristic patterns have emerged which allow the electromyographer to suspect diagnoses, but the test results are only meaningful with reference to a particular clinical problem. The analysis of the EMG and NCV data best illuminates questions of primary motor neuron or muscle disease, demyelinative *vs* axonal neuropathy, nerve root *vs* plexus disorders, and the localization of a mononeuropathy.

Motor neuron disease (*e.g.*, amyotrophic lateral sclerosis) results in abnormal spontaneous activity of motor units and individual muscle fibers. This activity is seen throughout the body. Muscle disorders (*e.g.*, myotonic dystrophy) produce characteristically different patterns of spontaneous activity.

Polyneuropathies cause EMG and NCV abnormalities according to their pathophysiology. Demyelinative neuropathies produce slowed conduction with preserved amplitude, whereas axonal neuropathies reduce amplitude with little effect on NCV. Chronic axonal neuropathy produces diffuse denervation responses in muscle (similar in nature to those seen focally in mononeuropathies). These tests can thus narrow the diagnostic spectrum in polyneuropathy and should be performed early to help plan the subsequent work-up. In acute demyelinative neuropathies (*e.g.*, the Guillain–Barré syndrome), special studies of conduction through the nerve roots (F responses and H reflexes) are often confirmatory when the routine NCV studies are normal.

The correct localization of a lesion along the course of a peripheral nerve (root, plexus, or at distal sites) is usually required for diagnosis and therapy. Root lesions produce denervation in paraspinal muscles in addition to distal changes; thus, a herniated disk can be separated from other pathologic lesions. Denervation changes require from 1 to 6 weeks to appear following an injury; thus, these studies are rarely indicated acutely. Such a study is important when multiple sites of pathology are detected along the course of a nerve. Some surgeons require EMG confirmation of focal lesions prior to removing a disk or transposing a peripheral nerve.

Entrapment syndromes are often diagnosed best by EMG and nerve conduction studies. The most common disorder is the carpal tunnel syndrome; this is also a situation in which clinical judgment in interpretation is crucial. Asymptomatic median nerve compression in the carpal tunnel is common; if the electrical studies are limited only to the wrist, pathology in the neck may be overlooked and the wrong therapy may be undertaken.

The routine use of EMG and NCV studies in the evaluation of neck, shoulder, or low back pain in the absence of neurologic deficits is costly, time-consuming, and seldom benefits the patient. The test is best used to confirm and define abnormalities seen on examination. Only if the clinical suspicion of a discrete lesion is high, or confirmation of equivocal imaging studies is required, should these tests be performed in such a situation.

SUMMARY

Neurodiagnostic studies can provide critical data for the evaluation of diagnostic alternatives. The preceding discussion has hopefully served to place these tests in their proper clinical perspective. One must use the information obtained as an extension of the history and physical examination, or incorrect diagnosis and improper therapy are likely.

The future of electrophysiologic studies is bright; improvements in automated data analysis and artificial intelligence will elicit more data from the available tests. As the power of these techniques increases, however, so does their potential for error. As the clinician becomes more dependent on other people's interpretation of data, it becomes increasingly important to be certain that the clinical laboratories used are appropriately certified.

QUESTIONS AND DISCUSSION

1. A patient presents with paraparesis and a history of optic neuritis in the left eye. An MR study reveals no cerebral lesions and no evidence of spinal cord pathology. Which of the following tests is most likely to help confirm or refute the diagnosis of multiple sclerosis?

    A. NCV studies
    B. CSF evaluation for oligoclonal antibodies
    C. Contrast myelography
    D. BAERs
    E. EEG

The answer is (B). Oligoclonal antibodies are present in over 90% of MS patients. Nerve conduction velocity is not affected in multiple sclerosis. Contrast myelography is unnecessary if the MR is normal. BAERs might be abnormal but would be superfluous if oligoclonal antibodies are present. The EEG is not helpful in diagnosing MS.

2. A patient with suspected complex partial seizures has a normal routine EEG. Which of these procedures would be most useful diagnostically?

    A. VERs
    B. LP
    C. Repeat EEG with sleep deprivation and extra electrodes
    D. 24-hour EEG monitoring
    E. EMG studies

The answer is (C). Sleep deprivation and extra electrodes often demonstrate epileptiform activity when the routine EEG is unrevealing. Evoked response studies are not specifically abnormal in epilepsy. 24-hour EEG monitoring is helpful in special circumstances but is seldom necessary in routine practice. An EMG would not shed light on possible epilepsy.

3. Which of the following is *not* a contraindication to LP?

    A. Papilledema, stiff neck, and fever
    B. Cutaneous infection of the lower back
    C. Suspected intraspinal mass
    D. Posterior fossa tumor
    E. Coagulopathy

The answer is (A). Papilledema is seen in states of increased intracranial pressure but does not necessarily imply a risk of herniation. In the setting of fever and stiff neck, papilledema is suggestive of meningitis so that a lumbar puncture is necessary. Patients with pseudotumor cerebri usually benefit symptomatically from an LP, and the test is necessary for the diagnosis. A CT scan, however, should precede an LP in the presence of papilledema. The other situations are all contraindications to an LP.

4. Which of the following tests is the most useful screening procedure for cerebellopontine angle tumors?

    A. Skull films
    B. EEG
    C. VERs
    D. BAERs
    E. SSERs

The answer is (D). Although MR is probably the most sensitive diagnostic test for cerebellopontine angle tumors, its expense is prohibitive for screening. BAERs are sensitive and are relatively inexpensive. Skull films and EEGs may be abnormal if the tumor is large, but not early in the course. VERs and SSERs are not characteristically affected by these lesions.

5. Nerve conduction studies in axonal neuropathies are characterized by:

   A. Slow conduction and normal amplitude
   B. No changes in either conduction velocity or amplitude
   C. Loss of amplitude, with relative sparing of velocity
   D. Increased conduction velocity
   E. High amplitude responses

The answer is (C). The amplitude reflects the number of nerve impulses that arrive at the neuromuscular junction; axonal neuropathies primarily reduce this number. Those impulses that are transmitted have a relatively normal conduction velocity. Demyelinative neuropathy slows conduction but does not reduce the number of fibers carrying impulses.

SUGGESTED READING

American Electroencephalographic Society: Guidelines in EEG and evoked potentials. J Clin Neurophysiol (Suppl 1) 3, 1986

Aminoff MJ (ed): Electrodiagnosis in Clinical Neurology, 2nd ed. New York, Churchill Livingstone, 1986

Chiappa K (ed): Evoked Potentials in Clinical Medicine, 2nd ed. New York, Raven Press, 1990

Cracco RQ, Bodis–Wollner I (eds): Evoked Potentials. New York, Alan R. Liss, 1986

Daly DD, Pedley TA: Current Practice of Clinical EEG. New York, Raven Press, 1990

Fishman RA: Cerebrospinal Fluid in Diseases of the Nervous System. Philadelphia, WB Saunders, 1980

Liveson JA: Peripheral Neurology, 2nd ed. Philadelphia, FA Davis, 1991

Niedermeyer E, Lopes da Silva F (eds): Electroencephalography, 2nd ed. Baltimore, Urban and Schwarzenberg, 1990

Schaumburg HH, Spencer PS, Thomas PK: Disorders of Peripheral Nerves. Philadelphia, FA Davis, 1983

Scheld WM, Whittley RJ, Durach DT (eds): Infections of the Central Nervous System. New York, Raven Press, 1991

Neuroradiology—Which Tests to Order?

Ruth G. Ramsey

Magnetic resonance imaging (MR), introduced in 1983, is the latest in several technological advances that have occurred in recent years. MR has already had a definite impact on the evaluation and diagnosis of neurologic disease. The technique is now a permanent part of our diagnostic armamentarium and, although used for body imaging, it is most useful for the evaluation of the central nervous system (CNS). The earliest impact was on brain imaging; however, it now appears that a significant contribution of MR will be in the evaluation of the spine. MR uses a magnetic field and radio frequency waves (not radiation); it is totally noninvasive and is based on the principle of imaging of the hydrogen proton. Short spin-echo (SE) sequences (T1-weighted images) best illustrate the anatomy, whereas long SE sequences (T2-weighted images) best demonstrate pathologic areas that become bright or increased in signal intensity. Other imaging sequences are also available; however, in-depth discussion is beyond the scope of this chapter.

Computed tomography (CT), introduced in 1973, revolutionized the approach to diagnosis and rapidly became an integral and necessary part of the diagnostic armamentarium. Positron emission tomography (PET), a technique that uses various compounds tagged with radioactive (positron-emitting) radionuclides, and nuclear medicine scanning techniques are also available. PET remains primarily a research tool. Single photon emission computed tomography (SPECT) is becoming more widely available. Newer nonionic contrast materials have been introduced for both myelography and intravascular use. Metrizamide (Amipaque) was introduced in 1978 and rapidly became the standard myelographic contrast agent. Iohexol (Omnipaque) and iopamidol (Isovue) were introduced in 1986; both are nonionic contrast agents for intrathecal and intravascular use. All of the nonionic contrast agents are less painful than standard ionic contrast agents when injected intravascularly, and they have less cardiovascular effect. The common clinical procedure is to use nonionic contrast agents in pediatric patients and those patients with cardiovascular compromise and also in those who have exhibited an anaphylactoid reaction to standard contrast agents. Ioxaglate (Hexabrix) is a new, low-osmolality, ionic contrast material for intravascular use. Ioxaglate is less nephrotoxic and less cardiotoxic than standard contrast agents and less painful; it is not used intrathecally.

Despite the tremendous technological advances that have occurred in neuroradiology, the plain roentgenogram continues to be a useful part of the diagnostic work-up. Skull roentgenograms are better than other techniques for the evaluation of (1) skull fractures; (2) metastatic disease; (3) general alterations in the appearance of the skull, such as changes seen with primary hyperparathyroidism or Paget's disease; (4) the size and configuration of the sella turcica; and may also be diagnostic for (5) hemangioma (well-defined, *nonsclerotic* margin, spoke-wheel pattern), epidermoid (well-defined, *sclerotic* margin), and eosinophilic granuloma (ill-defined, irregular margin, often with a beveled edge because either the inner or the outer table is affected more than the other).

NEUROIMAGING AND SPECIFIC DIAGNOSES

STROKE

Ischemic and hemorrhagic stroke is one of the most common clinical problems evaluated by neuroimaging techniques. CT is the preferred initial examination procedure, although it is not uncommon that a CT which is performed shortly after ischemic infarct is normal. Approximately 70% of ischemic infarcts will be visible as areas of low density 7 days post ictus. Although ischemic infarction itself is not usually an indication for emergency CT scanning, if anticoagulants are under consideration, CT can provide valuable evidence concerning the presence of hemorrhage. CT is sensitive to the presence of blood, and hemorrhagic infarcts are immediately apparent; MR is less accurate for the diagnosis of acute hemorrhage and may miss the presence of blood in the subarachnoid space. Other processes may mimic the clinical presentation of stroke. These processes include subdural hematoma, primary or secondary brain tumor, intracerebral hematoma secondary to hypertensive basal ganglia hemorrhage, arteriovenous malformation (AVM), or even subarachnoid hemorrhage.

Most infarcts identified by CT scanning are typically confined to a single vessel distribution and are most common in the middle cerebral artery distribution. Lacunar infarcts occur in the basal ganglia, and so-called watershed infarcts occur typically at the junction between the anterior and middle cerebral artery distribution. When visualized, acute infarcts appear as varying shades of gray and are usually non–space occupying. Maximum edema occurs at 2 to 4 days, and a large infarct may exhibit a significant mass effect with compression of the ipsilateral ventrical, subfalcian herniation, and transtentorial herniation (Fig. 3-1). Transtentorial herniation results in compression of the brain stem and may cause slit-like (duret) hemorrhages in the brain stem, resulting in the patient's death.

Old or ancient infarcts may be associated with focal dilatation of the lateral ventricle that becomes

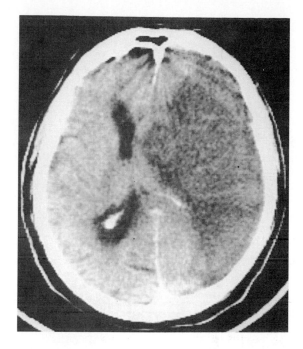

FIG. 3-1. Acute infarct. There is lucency involving the entire left hemisphere, with marked mass effect and shift to the contralateral side. An infarct with this amount of mass effect is approximately 2 to 4 days old and may occasionally mimic the appearance of a chronic subdural hematoma.

apparent after 1 month. Many older infarcts, because of necrosis and brain loss as well as a progression to postinfarct porencephaly, appear lucent and will be similar to cerebrospinal fluid (CSF) in density (Fig. 3-2).

MR scanning reveals that areas of infarction are readily identified as areas of increased signal intensity on the T2-weighted images. However, MR is *much* more sensitive than CT, and infarcts will be demonstrated earlier by MR; additionally, many small infarcts not seen on CT will be identified by MR. This is particularly true of the small vessel, end-artery infarcts seen in a deep white matter distribution. The patient who is in an advanced stage of this disease has a "bat-wing," periventricular distribution of increased signal intensity on the T2-weighted images (Fig. 3-3). It appears that there is a bell-shaped curve of these changes in the aging population, even in the nor-

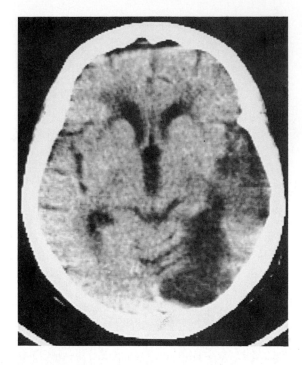

FIG. 3-2. Chronic and superimposed acute infarct. The left occipital infarct has progressed to an area of porencephaly containing material of CSF density. There is a new infarct in the left middle cerebral artery distribution that is lucent, but not the density of CSF.

motensive patient, who has a variable number of periventricular infarcts secondary to arteriosclerotic cerebrovascular disease.

Although occasional infarcts are identified in the midbrain and pons with CT scanning, MR is more sensitive in this region. The lack of artifact and degradation by bone artifact make MR the ideal modality for the evaluation of the midbrain, pons, and medulla. Approximately 1 to 6 weeks post ictus, an infarct may demonstrate enhancement following the infusion of iodinated contrast material. This enhancement may exhibit various appearances and is secondary to the breakdown of the blood–brain barrier. As there is no additional information to be gained, and because patients with enhancing infarcts do less well clinically, an infusion scan is not recommended in patients with infarct. Hemor-

rhagic infarcts may also occur, but they are far less common than ischemic infarcts.

The work-up of transient ischemic attacks and occasionally a stroke includes CT and MR scanning as well as standard angiography or intra-arterial digital subtraction angiography (IADSA) for an evaluation of both extra- and intracranial carotid stenosis. Intravenous digital subtraction angiography has been largely replaced by magnetic resonance angiography (MRA).

MAGNETIC RESONANCE ANGIOGRAPHY

MRA is a recent addition to the diagnostic armentarium of some MR equipment. MRA relies on the intrinsic properties of moving substances such as intravascular blood flow. The technique is totally noninvasive and does not require the injection of contrast material. A variety of imaging sequences are available, and their use depends upon the pathology and the anatomic area that is to be examined. MRA is ideal for evaluation of the carotid arteries in the neck (Fig. 3-4) but may also be used for the intracranial vessels, not just for evaluation of atherosclerotic disease but also for processes such as AVMs, aneurysms, and venous abnormalities such as superior sagittal sinus thrombosis.

Various sequences are used in these evaluations; they include two-dimensional time of flight, three-dimensional time of flight, and phase contrast techniques. Each has a specific indication so that an accurate prestudy diagnosis is helpful for directing the examination of each patient. In occasional cases re-examination will need to be performed for complete evaluation. MRA is an ideal noninvasive method of evaluating the patient with transient ischemic attack or stroke. At the University of Chicago, each patient who presents with signs or symptoms of cerebral ischemia is studied with a routine MR examination of the brain as well as MRA of the neck and circle of Willis (Fig. 3-5).

BRAIN TUMORS

Brain tumors are readily diagnosed by CT or MR scanning. If an enhancing lesion is suspected, contrast enhanced MR (CEMR) is the initial preferred procedure. Both MR and CT provide accurate localization of the tumor, although CEMR is proving to be the more sensitive method of evaluation. When the posterior fossa is to be examined, CEMR is the preferred technique since there is no bone

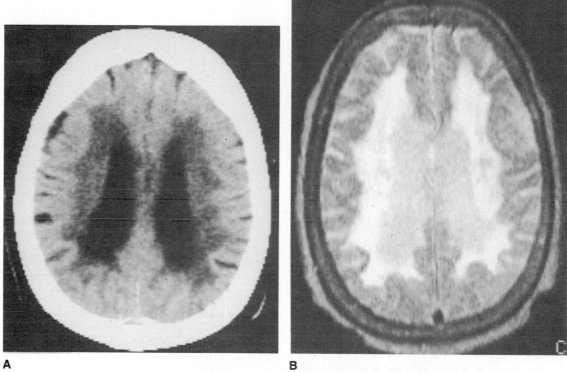

FIG. 3-3. Multiple deep white matter infarcts. (*A*) Computed tomography scan reveals the typical "bat-wing" distribution of lucency around the lateral ventricles. (*B*) T2WI demonstrates increased signal intensity in the areas of small, end artery infarction.

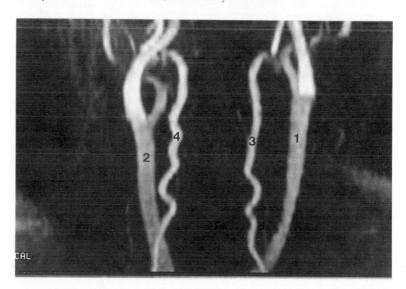

FIG. 3-4. Normal MRA of the neck. The vessels are readily seen and identified: 1 = left carotid artery; 2 = right carotid artery; 3 = left vertebral artery; 1 = right vertebral artery.

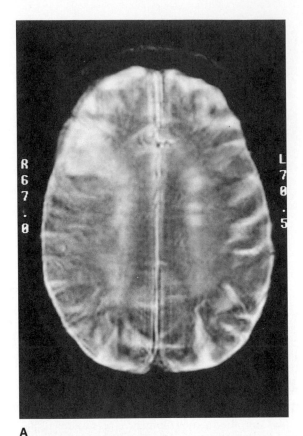

FIG. 3-5. Infarct with occluded right common carotid artery. (*A*) T2WI reveals a wedge-shaped area
of increased signal intensity in the right frontal region, consistent with an area of infarction. There are
also other scattered areas of increased signal intensity consistent with scattered areas of infarction.

A

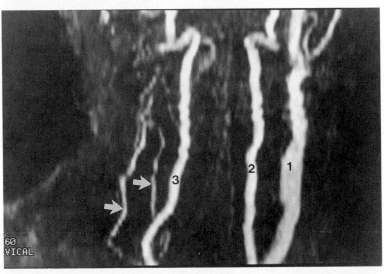

FIG. 3-5. (*continued*) (*B*) MRA
reveals complete occlusion of
the right common, internal,
and external carotid artery.
Only the left carotid (*1*), left
vertebral (*2*), and right vertebral artery (*3*) are demonstrated. The left carotid artery
is diffusely irregular secondary
to atherosclerotic plaques.
Small vessels identified on the
right side are attempts at collateral vessels (*arrows*).

B

artifact and the anatomy is easily evaluated. The multiplanar imaging capability of MR is particularly helpful in the evaluation of the posterior fossa. CEMR readily identifies the presence of multiple enhancing lesions; therefore, it easily detects metastatic disease and is more sensitive than CECT.

GLIOBLASTOMA MULTIFORME

Glioblastoma is a tumor seen most frequently in the third through fifth decades. These tumors are often large at the time of presentation (Fig. 3-6). Patients not uncommonly present with headache only, although at other times there may be a neurologic symptom such as seizure, hemiparesis, or paralysis. Plain skull films are usually normal, although amorphous calcification may rarely be seen. CT

and MR scans typically reveal a large low-density mass involving primarily the white matter. There is typically a dense enhancement of an irregular rim of tissue on the postinfusion portion of the examination. There may be an extension to the contralateral hemisphere via the corpus callosum; this has been called the "butterfly" appearance of glioblastoma. A large amount of irregular edema usually surrounds the mass and will be noted to follow the white matter pathways. The low-density center of a glioblastoma was originally thought to reflect tumor necrosis secondary to growth of the tumor that exceeded its blood supply. Surgery, however, often reveals viable tumor in the center, and a delayed CT or MR scan performed after 30 to 45 minutes may demonstrate homogeneous enhancement of the entire tumor mass. Occasionally, CT

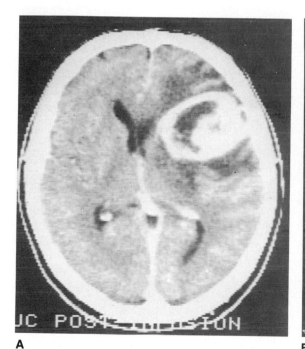
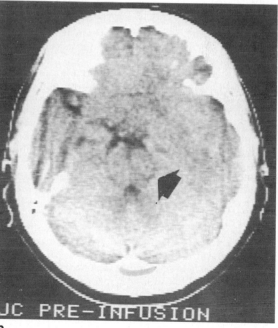

A

B

FIG. 3-6. Glioblastoma multiforme. (*A*) Computed tomography scan obtained postinfusion reveals a dense ring of enhancement with a nodule of enhancement, a low-density center, and surrounding edema. There is a marked shift to the contralateral side with transtentorial herniation of the medial portion of the temporal lobe and compression of the midbrain (*arrow in B*). Although the appearance is typical of glioblastoma multiforme, metastatic disease or abscess may have a similar appearance.

may reveal areas of amorphous calcification within the tumor not visible on plain skull radiography; calcification is difficult to identify on MR evaluation. Rarely, there may be a sizable tumor that does not demonstrate enhancement in any portion of the tumor. Since a large infarct may occupy space and would also not enhance, differentiation between the two may be difficult. In this instance, the clinical history should be helpful to separate these two possibilities; in some cases follow-up scans may be necessary for complete evaluation. Histologic grading of a tumor cannot be determined based upon enhancement characteristics.

MENINGIOMAS

Meningiomas arise from arachnoid cells embedded in the dura. They are most common in the frontal convexity region and become progressively less common in the lower convexity and at the skull base. These tumors are often higher than normal brain density on the preinfusion CT scan because they contain psammomatous calcification. Meningiomas do not have a blood–brain barrier and thus they usually demonstrate dense, homogeneous enhancement on the postinfusion portion of the examination. Plain skull roentgenograms may reveal an enlargement of the middle meningeal artery groove, since this vessel usually supplies a meningioma; both skull films and CT may demonstrate reactive bone formation. In some cases there is no mass effect (apparently because of slow growth and pressure atrophy) whereas in others there is marked surrounding edema and midline shift.

Bone and calcification contain a low number of mobile protons and are therefore poorly visualized by MR. Because meningiomas contain areas of calcification, they often appear decreased or isointense on T1WI and remain low signal intensity on T2WI. A densely calcified skull base meningioma without surrounding edema may be missed by MR. CEMR reveals dense homogeneous enhancement of the meningioma and may also demonstrate a central area of flow void secondary to the enlarged meningeal artery vessel supplying the meningioma. Angiography with selective internal and particularly external carotid studies are recommended to outline the specific vascular supply.

METASTASES

Although metastatic disease may present as a solitary ring or homogeneously enhancing mass, multi-plicity of lesions is characteristic of metastatic disease. Breast and lung cancer are the most common primary sources. Melanoma commonly metastasizes to the brain and is both vascular and hemorrhagic and therefore has a high density on the preinfusion scan with homogeneous enhancement postinfusion (Fig. 3-7). MR reveals the metastatic lesions as areas of increased signal intensity on the T2-weighted images. CEMR is presently the procedure of choice for evaluation of cerebral metastases. Metastatic lesions frequently have marked surrounding edema. Metastases may masquerade clinically as transient ischemic attacks, and in those cases the postinfusion CT or MR scan often reveals a myriad of tiny metastatic foci. It should be noted that contrast enhancement is necessary as the T1WI and T2WI without contrast may appear normal.

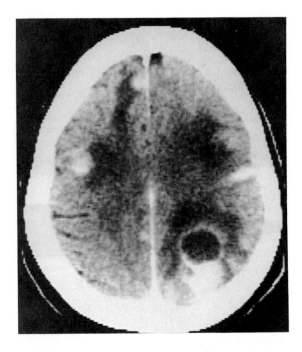

FIG. 3-7. Multiple metastases. Postinfusion computed tomography scan reveals multiple rounded areas of enhancement, with one cystic area of enhancement in the left posterior parietal region, probably reflecting a necrotic center. There is marked surrounding edema. The appearance is typical of metastatic disease.

ACQUIRED IMMUNODEFICIENCY SYNDROME

Acquired immunodeficiency syndrome (AIDS), initially identified in 1983, is an increasingly common problem. AIDS is caused by the HIV lymphotrophic virus and is most commonly seen in homosexual males and intravenous drug abusers. CT brain scanning not uncommonly demonstrates an appearance of diffuse atrophy for the patient's age in the absence of any other abnormality. Because of the depressed immune mechanisms in these patients, they also develop unusual infections of the CNS with opportunistic organisms such as toxoplasmosis or cytomegalovirus, and there is an increased incidence of brain tumors such as CNS lymphoma. The multiple enhancing lesions of disease processes such as toxoplasmosis may mimic metastatic disease. AIDS encephalomalacia is seen in association with AIDS dementia complex (ADC). It affects the white matter, does not enhance, and is best evaluated by CEMR. Contrast enhanced CT is frequently the initial imaging procedure; however, CEMR should be performed if CT is negative since MR better demonstrates the white matter abnormalities (Fig. 3-8).

TRAUMA

CT scanning has greatly aided our ability to evaluate the intracranial abnormalities in patients who have craniocerebral trauma. CT provides a more accurate evaluation than any previously available method. Skull roentgenograms are more accurate for an evaluation of the presence of a skull fracture of the cranial vault, whereas CT is preferable for skull-base fractures. The time factor is essential in

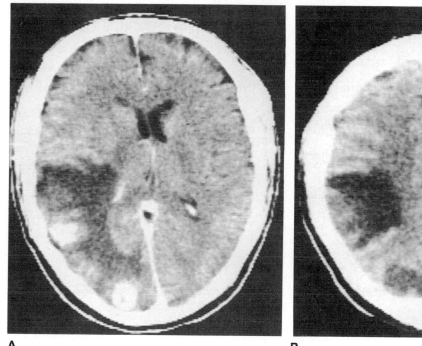
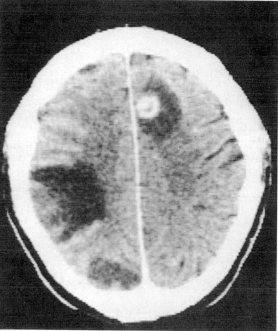

A   B

FIG. 3-8. Toxoplasmosis in a patient with AIDS. (*A* and *B*) Postinfusion computed tomography scans reveal multiple ring enhancing lesions with marked surrounding edema. In the correct clinical setting, the findings are typical of toxoplasmosis, although multiple metastases have a similar appearance.

an evaluation of the patient who has acute craniocerebral trauma, because processes such as acute subdural or epidural hematoma are life threatening and may lead rapidly to the patient's death.

Subdural hematomas are more common in the extremes of life (the young and the elderly), whereas epidural hematomas are more common in middle-aged groups. Subdural hematomas result from tearing of the bridging veins in the subdural space and are usually crescentic in configuration. Acute subdural hematomas are increased density on CT and are usually readily identified as extracerebral collections. Usually unilateral, subdural hematomas vary in size from skim collections that mimic a thickened calvarium to large collections with a marked shift of the midline structures and either subfalcine or transtentorial herniation or both. There is no midline shift when bilateral, symmetrical subdural hematomas are present. Subacute subdural hematomas may settle in a "hematocrit" appearance or may have a mottled density (Fig. 3-9). Chronic subdural hematomas, probably greater than 2 weeks in age, have a low density on CT; however, because of their increased protein content, they are higher than CSF density. Elderly patients with bilateral isodense subdural collections may have an appearance of a "hypernormal CT scan for age" because there is obliteration of the cortical sulci and bilateral symmetrical compression of the lateral ventricles. Rarely, this appearance may also occur in the younger age-groups, and the index of suspicion must be high. Although a postinfusion CT scan is not generally recommended for most patients who have cerebral trauma, the

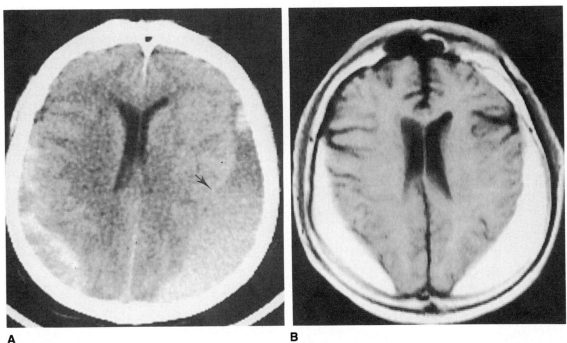

A **B**

FIG. 3-9. Bilateral subdural hematomas. (*A*) Computed tomography scan reveals mottled density extracerebral collections bilaterally. There is a "hematocrit" level on the left side (*arrow*), secondary to settling of the heavy hemoglobin molecule. The lateral ventricles are compressed toward the midline and elongated, reflecting the bilateral nature of the problem. (*B*) MR better demonstrates the increased signal intensity extracerebral collections on this T1-weighted image. The increased signal is secondary to the formation of methemoglobin and is present only after the first 48 hours.

chronic or isodense subdural hematoma may be identified only by the enhancing membrane and displaced cortical veins on a postinfusion scan, or by MR scanning.

Epidural hematomas are usually secondary to arterial bleeding and are frequently associated with a fracture of the calvarium that crosses the groove of the middle meningeal artery. The dura forms the periosteum of the inner table of the skull and, therefore, is closely applied to the calvarium. The dura is thus peeled away from the bone by an epidural hematoma and this, therefore, results in the typical lentiform configuration. These epidural hematomas are life threatening, and prompt diagnosis and treatment are essential.

Other lesions that may occur are cerebral contusions, subarachnoid hemorrhage (which often ac-

companies other traumatic lesions), edema, and shearing injuries with tearing of the nerve fibers at the gray—white junction.

MR is excellent for an evaluation of patients with craniocerebral trauma after the initial 48 hours, and in the subacute and chronic injury cases. The acutely injured patient is probably not a candidate for MR because there is often multiorgan involvement, and most life support systems cannot be brought into the MR scanning room. While many CT scan slices are sub–5-second scans, the relatively long scanning times necessary with MR (5 to 10 min) also dictate that the patient be cooperative. Furthermore, an acute hemorrhage less than 48 hours old appears decreased in signal on the T1-weighted images (0.5T magnet) and is therefore similar in appearance to edema or tumor; it could not be

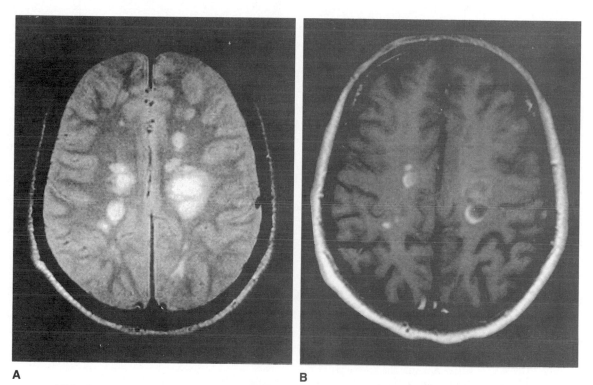

A   B

FIG. 3-10. Multiple sclerosis. (*A*) T2WI reveals multiple deep white matter and periventricular areas of increased signal intensity secondary to plaques of multiple sclerosis. (*B*) T1WI postcontrast reveals multiple solid and ring-shaped enhancing plaques, reflecting acute demyelination. Note that the areas of enhancement do not involve all of the plaques demonstrated on the T2WI.

properly identified. Therefore, acute hemorrhage is better demonstrated by CT than by MR. By MR evaluation blood appears increased in signal intensity after 48 hours and is readily identified. It is not uncommon that small subdural collections are identified by MR even though they are not visible on CT.

The changes of chronic injury such as might be seen with a shearing injury, or diffuse axonal injury, reveal areas of increased signal intensity on T2WI as well as areas of decreased signal intensity on all scanning sequences secondary to hemosiderin deposition.

DEGENERATIVE TOXIC AND METABOLIC DISEASES

Multiple sclerosis (MS) is a common neurologic disease; it is an acquired myelinoclastic disease that results in demyelination of the nerves of the CNS but never affects the peripheral nerves. The results of CT scanning are often normal, but when they are abnormal, the scan reveals diffuse atrophy and may demonstrate periventricular areas of decreased density representing the areas of demyelination. The postinfusion CT scan may occasionally demonstrate enhancement in the areas of acute demyelination. MR is sensitive to these areas of demyelination and, although not specific, the typical periventricular distribution of increased signal intensity plaques on T2-weighted SE images is often diagnostic (Fig. 3-10). The MR scan will frequently be grossly abnormal when the CT scan is normal or shows minimal abnormality. In the patient with clinical and laboratory-proved MS and a normal MR scan, the demyelinating plaques are presumably in the brain stem and spinal cord, and these are seen only occasionally with MR (Fig. 3-11). Involvement of the corpus callosum is frequently seen in MS and results in varying degrees of atrophy of the corpus callosum.

Carbon monoxide poisoning results in necrosis of the globus pallidus bilaterally. This then appears as areas of decreased density on CT.

Adrenoleukodystrophy, a hereditary disease, is one of several diseases of the myelin sheath in which there is both dysmyelinogenesis and poor myelin maintenance. Adrenal insufficiency may be the presenting symptom in some patients, and occipital lobe involvement typically leads to blindness. MR is the preferred procedure and reveals increased signal intensity on T2-weighted images in the areas of involvement.

Many other demyelinating and dysmyelinating processes are also readily evaluated by MR.

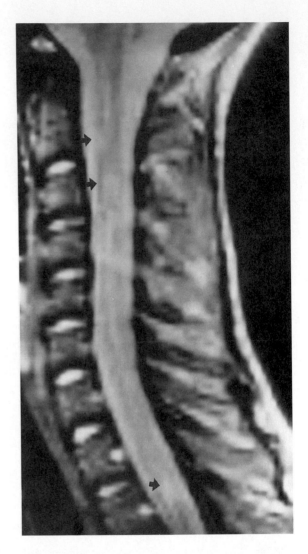

FIG. 3-11. Spine multiple sclerosis. T2WI of the cervical spine reveals multiple oval areas of increased signal intensity secondary to plaques of multiple sclerosis (*arrows*).

VASCULAR LESIONS

AVMs are the most common vascular malformations seen. Other types include occult (so named because, although they may hemorrhage, they cannot be demonstrated angiographically) vascular

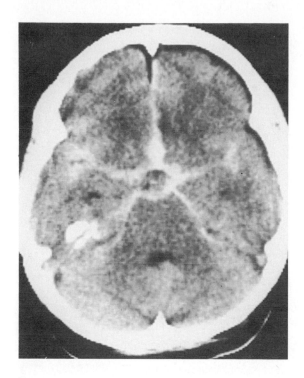

FIG. 3-12. Subarachnoid hemorrhage. A computed tomography scan reveals a large accumulation of high-density blood in the basilar cisterns and outlines the sylvian fissures bilaterally. The optic chiasm appears as a negative filling defect.

malformations; venous angiomas, and vein of Galen aneurysms. Vein of Galen aneurysm is a misnomer because this is really a deep AVM draining to the vein of Galen or rarely a direct arteriovenous fistula between the posterior cerebral artery and the vein of Galen. MR is the preferred initial diagnostic procedure and is frequently pathognomonic for many of these abnormalities.

Venous angiomas are deep malformations that form from a coalescence of enlarged medullary veins into a large trunk-like vein that drains superficially. Rarely, they may calcify. CT reveals a linear enhancing structure extending from the deep white matter to the cortex, while MR reveals a similar defect, now appearing as a linear area of negative flow defect. Angiography is pathognomonic, with the lesion appearing only on the venous phase.

Subarachnoid hemorrhage (SAH) may result from bleeding of an AVM; however, the most frequent source is a berry aneurysm, and CT is diagnostic in greater than 95% of patients with acute SAH (Fig. 3-12). However, CT is almost never able to demonstrate the aneurysm itself, and angiography is necessary for a complete evaluation (Fig. 3-13). Because 20% of patients have multiple aneurysms, an evaluation of both carotid and vertebral circulations is usually necessary. More recently, MRA has shown promise for identification of aneurysms 4 mm or larger.

Both MR and CT scanning (Fig. 3-14) are useful in the diagnosis of AVM. MRA may also be used for evaluation of AVMs or for such processes as superior sagittal sinus thrombosis.

SPINE

While the initial emphasis of MR was on brain evaluation, its ultimate significant clinical impact may be with spine scanning. Multiple abnormalities can be evaluated; these included disc disease (Fig. 3-15),

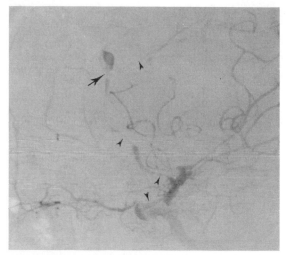

FIG. 3-13. Aneurysm with hemorrhage. Carotid angiogram reveals a typical appearance of a berry aneurysm at the bifurcation of the pericallosal and callosal marginal arteries (*arrow*), although the location is rare. There has been a rupture of the aneurysm, with blood in the subarachnoid space and a marked spasm of multiple blood vessels (*arrowheads*). Blood is irritative and creates vascular spasm.

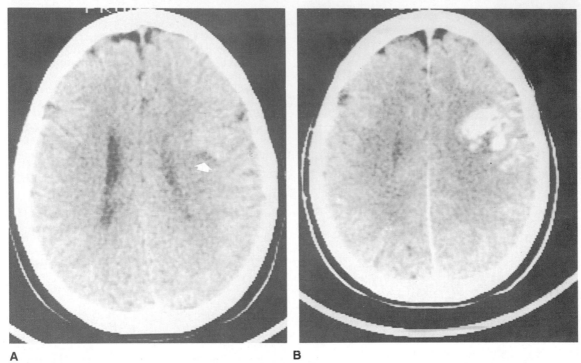

A   **B**

FIG. 3-14. Arteriovenous malformation. The patient is a 26-year-old woman with a clinical history of one grand mal seizure. (*A*) A preinfusion computed tomography scan reveals a poorly defined area of higher-than-normal brain density with a small area of lucency posterior to this (*arrow*). There is a slight mass effect with compression of the body of the lateral ventricle. (*B*) Postinfusion there is dense serpiginous enhancement of this area. Adjacent curvilinear areas of enhancement are enlarged arteries and draining veins.

spinal stenosis, spine metastases, congenital abnormalities such as the Chiari malformation (Fig. 3-16), syringohydromyelia, discitis, tuberculosis, AVMs of the cord, tethered cord, meningiomyelocele, lipoma, and spinal cord tumors (Fig. 3-17). MR has largely replaced other diagnostic methods for the evaluation of spinal abnormalities and is the initial procedure of choice for evaluation of all spinal abnormalities.

Lumbar disks and hypertrophic changes are readily evaluated by CT scanning. With a herniated disc there is a tear in the annulus fibrous and the nucleus pulposus protrudes through this tear into the vertebral canal, resulting in compression of the thecal sac or nerve roots. CT scanning of the spine can be performed before or after the instillation of

water-soluble contrast material. Myelography is approximately 85% accurate in the diagnosis of a herniated lumbar disc. Myelography is performed using nonionic, water-soluble contrast materials such as iohexol or iopamidol. An initial evaluation should always begin with plain spine roentgenograms to determine the number of lumbar vertebrae, bony destructive changes, spondylolysis, or spondylolisthesis and loss of vertebral or disc space heights. MR easily demonstrates herniated discs in most cases and has largely replaced other diagnostic methods.

Spinal cord tumors may be categorized into three major classes, each with a typical myelographic appearance (Table 3-1). *Intramedullary lesions* cause a diffuse expansion of the cord. *Intradural lesions* dis-

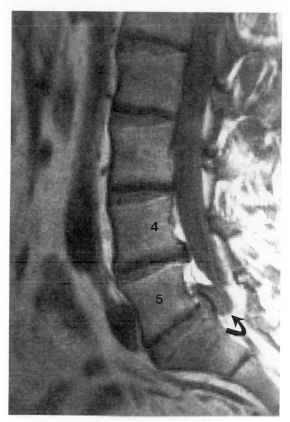

FIG. 3-15. Herniated disc. (*A*) Sagittal T1WI reveals a herniated disc at the L5–S1 level (*arrow*) and a bulging disc at the L4–L5 level.

A

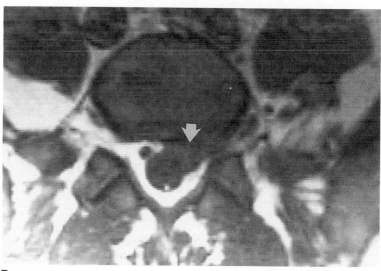

FIG. 3-15. (*continued*) (*B*) Axial T1WI reveals the disc on the left side (*arrow*). There is interruption of the bright epidural fat and encroachment on the left intervertebral foramen.

B

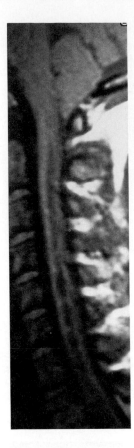

FIG. 3-16. Chiari malformation with syrinx. Sagittal T1WI reveals that the pointed cerebellar tonsils extend below the level of the foramen magnum. There is a multiloculated syrinx cavity in the cervical spinal cord.

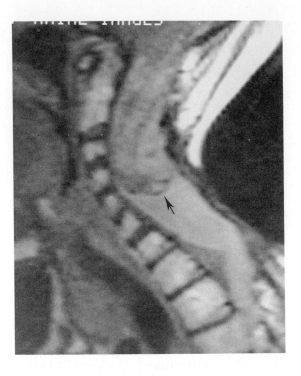

FIG. 3-17. Intramedullary tumor. Midsagittal, T1-weighted magnetic resonance image reveals marked expansion of the cervical spinal cord by a mottled signal intensity tumor. The lower margin of the tumor appears to end in a curvilinear fashion (*arrow*), although the cord is expanded and kinked below this level. Because of the long-standing nature of this tumor there is pressure erosion of the posterior margin of the vertebral bodies in the cervical region.

place the cord to the contralateral side and compress the cord; there is "capping" of the lesion by the contrast material in a typical meniscal appearance. *Extradural lesions* cause compression of the subarachnoid space and compression of the cord in one plane with an appearance of widening of the cord in the orthogonal plane.

Myelography can also be used to evaluate the presence of spinal cord tumors; however, MR has replaced myelography for evaluation of these ab-

TABLE 3-1. Types of Spinal Cord Tumors

INTRADURAL	INTRAMEDULLARY	EXTRADURAL
Neurofibroma	Ependymoma	Metastases
Schwannoma	Astocytoma	Herniated disc
Meningioma	Syringohydromyelia	Extradural
Drop		hematoma
metastases		

normalities. The anatomic location and morphology of these tumors are readily identified, while the CSF behaves similar to contrast material used for myelography. MR is superior, however, because it is totally noninvasive. Essentially all spinal cord tumors enhance after contrast infusion in MR imaging.

MR is the preferred procedure for the evaluation of metastatic diseases to the vertebral column. An initial screening can be performed with the body coil, followed by surface coil images of any areas of interest. After radiation therapy, there is a relative increase in the amount of adipose tissue in the bone marrow included in the treatment port (Fig. 3-18). MR can also be used to follow the response to treatment. CEMR is used for evaluation of meningeal carcinomatosis where the tumor appears as nodules or sheet-like areas of enhancement (Fig. 3-19).

ORBIT

CT is ideal for an evaluation of the bony orbit and its contents. Multiple entities can be evaluated with CT, including facial bone fractures, hyperthyroid exophthalmopathy (unilateral or bilateral), hemangioma of the orbit, lacrimal gland tumors, optic glioma or meningioma, and orbital pseudotumor. Accurate evaluation of sinusitis and orbital or periorbital cellulitis can also be made. The bony destructive changes of tumor can also be readily evaluated as well as the invasion of adjacent structures, particularly the invasion of the brain.

SUMMARY

The work-up of patients with neurologic disease often includes several neurodiagnostic imaging tests. Over the preceding 10 years, there has been a gradual evolution of the order of testing. However, as a general statement it is best to begin with noninvasive studies, such as plain skull films or spine roentgenograms, and then proceed to more invasive studies. CT has become an essential diagnostic tool, and MR has rapidly established itself in the evaluation of both the brain and the spine. MR has replaced other diagnostic tests for several problems, particularly in the area of degenerative and demyelinating diseases of the brain. MR complements other tests for the evaluation of some spine problems and has become the sole diagnostic test in the majority of abnormalities involving the spine. There has been a definite decrease in the need for

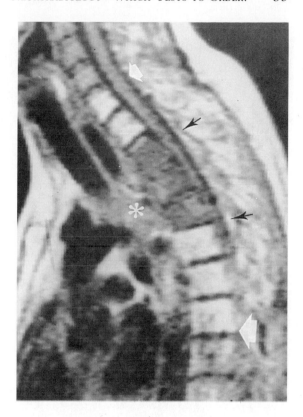

FIG. 3-18. Metastatic disease with radiation therapy effect. Midsagittal T1-weighted image of the spine reveals a decreased signal intensity tumor replacing three vertebral bodies (*black arrows*) and increased signal intensity involving the two vertebrae above and three vertebrae below (*white arrows*) because of a relative increase in the adipose tissue following radiation treatment. A prevertebral mass secondary to tumor (*asterisk*) is also noted.

angiography for the diagnosis of tumors, and more recently MRA has become available for the evaluation of cerebrovascular atherosclerosis, superior sagittal sinus thrombosis, cerebral aneurysms, and AVMs.

QUESTIONS AND DISCUSSION

1. Magnetic resonance angiography is a new technique that (choose 1 item or more):

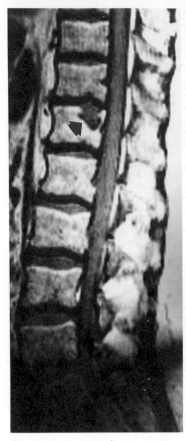

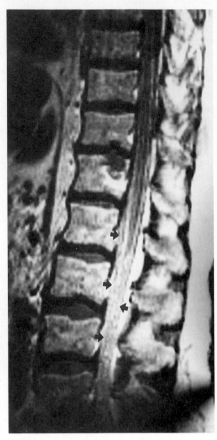

A   B

FIG. 3-19. Spinal meningeal carcinomatosis. (*A*) Sagittal T1WI without contrast reveals a small, low signal intensity metastatic deposit in the superior aspect of L1 (*arrow*). The subarachnoid space appears homogeneous in signal intensity. (*B*) T1WI postcontrast reveals diffuse enhancement of the meninges of the spine and nerve roots of the cauda equina secondary to meningeal carcinomatosis (*arrowheads*).

A. Requires the infusion of contrast material
B. Is useful for extracranial carotid stenosis
C. Is useful for arterial abnormalities, but is not useful for lesions involving the venous system.
D. Cannot yet be used for diagnosis of aneurysms
E. Is frequently used independent of routine MR scanning

The answer is (B) only. MRA does not require the use of contrast material and is based upon the properties of normal blood flow. MRA can be used for diagnosis of both arterial as well as venous abnormalities; MRA is useful in the diagnosis of aneurysm and is a good screening tool for aneurysms.

MRA is always used in conjunction with routine MR scanning.

2. For the evaluation of acute cerebral ischemic disease (stroke) which of the following is/are true?

A. MR is more sensitive than CT for the diagnosis of acute subarachnoid hemorrhage.
B. CT is the initial exam of choice.
C. A postinfusion study should be performed immediately.
D. MR is more sensitive than CT; it often reveals ischemic infarcts earlier than CT and demonstrates additional infarcts.

E. CT is more sensitive than MR for evaluation of the midbrain and brain stem.

The answers are (B) and (D). CT is more accurate than MR for the evaluation of acute subarachnoid hemorrhage as well as hemorrhage in other locations. MR is useful after hemorrhage has been ruled out as it is more accurate in evaluating the presence of acute infarcts and is more sensitive in identifying additional areas of infarction. Generally a postinfusion study is not recommended acutely, enhancing infarcts are apparent after 1 week, and the enhancement persists for approximately 6 weeks.

3. For the diagnosis of primary and secondary brain tumors:

   A. A postinfusion study is not necessary with MR as the metastases are apparent on the T2WI as areas of increased signal intensity.
   B. CT is the procedure of choice for diagnosis.
   C. MR is much more sensitive than CT for the diagnosis of areas of calcification.
   D. MR reveals a different pattern of enhancement than CT scanning and may result in inaccurate tumor localization.
   E. CT is more accurate than MR for the diagnosis of bone metastases

The answer is (E). In general, CT is more accurate than MR for the diagnosis of bony metastases as bone is poorly demonstrated on MR scans. (A) is false. Although metastases are frequently demonstrated on the T2WI, this is not always the case, and a postinfusion scan must be performed for complete evaluation. (B) Although a very good technique of diagnosis, CEMR is a more sensitive technique and should be used if available. (D) The pattern of enhancement is essentially the same for CT and MR scanning, although MR is more sensitive and may reveal more dense enhancement than CT and in the case of metastases may reveal additional lesions not seen by CT. (C) Calcification is much more accurately diagnosed by CT than by MR.

4. MR of the spine has become the diagnostic procedure of choice for all lesions of the spine. Of the following statements regarding MR of the spine, which are true?

   A. Approximately 50% of spinal cord tumors exhibit enhancement.
   B. Plaques of multiple sclerosis are not visible by MR as they are usually too small to be demonstrated.
   C. Herniated discs are visible on the sagittal MR images; however, the lateralization of these discs is more accurately evaluated by CT scanning.
   D. MR is the procedure of choice for diagnosis of bony metastatic disease.
   E. MR, even with contrast enhancement, cannot diagnose spinal meningeal carcinomatosis.

The answers are (D) and (E). MR is the procedure of choice for bony metastases, readily demonstrating the level of involvement, the amount of soft tissue abnormality, and the amount of cord compression. CEMR is the most accurate method of demonstrating spinal meningeal carcinomatosis. (A) It appears that essentially all spinal tumors enhance on the CEMR. (B) MS plaques are not common in the spinal cord but may be identified by MR as areas of increased signal intensity. (C) Herniated discs are accurately demonstrated on MR scans on both the sagittal and axial images. Surgery is frequently based on the MR findings alone.

5. Regarding the use of MR in the diagnosis of various abnormalities of the brain and spine:

   A. MR uses a slightly greater amount of ionizing radiation than CT and less than standard radiographic techniques
   B. Contrast material in the subarachnoid space enhances on the T2WI.
   C. MR and MRA will result in a decrease in the number of angiograms needed for diagnosis of many vascular abnormalities.
   D. MR is useful for diagnosis of superior sagittal sinus thrombosis.

The correct answers are (C) and (D). MR and MRA will definitely result in a decrease in the number of standard angiograms. A normal MRA evaluation of the extracranial carotid arteries will probably preclude the need for standard angiography, MRA provides very good evaluation of the circle of Willis in the evaluation of possible aneurysms, and MR and MRA are very accurate for the evaluation of sagittal sinus thrombosis. (B) This is false, and at this point no contrast material is available for instillation in the subarachnoid space. (A) MR does not use ionizing radiation.

SUGGESTED READING

Barkovich AJ. Pediatric Neuroimaging. New York, Raven Press, 1990

Becker DH, Townsend JJ, Kramer RA, Newton TH: Occult cerebrovascular malformations: A series of 18 histologically verified cases with negative angiography. Brain 102:249, 1979

Bryan RN, Levy LM, Whitlow WD, Killian JM et al: Diagnosis of acute cerebral infarction: Comparison of CT and MR imaging. AJNR press, 12:611, 1991

Edelman RR, Shoukimas GM, Stark ED et al: High resolution surface coil imaging in lumbar disk disease. AJR 144:1123, 1985

Fayad PB, Brass LM: Single photon emission computed tomography [SPECT] in cerebrovascular disease. Stroke 22:950, 1991

George AE, deLeon MJ: Computed tomography, magnetic resonance imaging and positron emission tomography in aging and dementia. In Latchaw RE (ed): MR and CT Imaging of the Head, Neck and Spine, 2nd ed, 413. St. Louis, CV Mosby, 1991

Keller PJ, Drayer BP, Fram EK et al: MR angiography with two-dimensional acquisition and three-dimensional display. Radiology 173:527, 1989

Kelly AB, Zimmerman RD, Snow RB et al: Head trauma: Comparison of MR and CT—experience in 100 patients. AJNR 9:699, 1988

Litt AW, Eidelman EM, Pinto RS et al: Diagnosis of carotid artery stenosis: Comparison of 2D time-of-flight MR angiography with contrast angiography in 50 patients. AJNR 11:449, 1991

Marchal G, Bosmans H, Van Fraeyenhoven L et al: Intracranial vascular lesions: Optimization and clinical evaluation of three-dimensional time-of-flight MR angiography. Radiology 175:443, 1990

Pech P, Haughton VM: Lumbar intervertebral disk: Correlative MR and anatomic study. Radiology 156:699, 1985

Ramsey RG, Geremia GK: CNS complications of AIDS: CT and MR findings. AJR 151:449–454, 1988

Ross JS, Delamarter R, Hueftle MG et al: Gadolinium-DTPA enhanced MR imaging of the postoperative lumbar spine: Time course and mechanism of enhancement. AJNR 10:37, 1989

Sze G, Abramson A, Krol G et al: Gadolinium-DTPA in the evaluation of intradural extramedullary spinal disease. AJNR 9:153, 1988

Sze G, Krol G, Zimmerman RD, Deck MDF: Intramedullary disease of the spine: Diagnosis using gadolinium-DTPA-enhanced MR imaging. AJNR 9:847, 1988

Sze G, Krol G, Zimmerman RD, Deck MDF: Malignant extra dural spinal tumors: MR imaging with Gd-DTPA. Radiology 167:217, 1988

Taphoorn MJB, Heimans JJ, Kaiser MCRLE et al: Imaging of brain metastases: Comparison of computerized tomography (CT) and magnetic resonance imaging (MRI). Neuroradiology 31:391, 1989

Yousem DM, Patron PM, Grossman RI: Leptomeningeal metastases: MR evaluation. J Comput Assist Tomogr 14:255, 1990

Examination of the Comatose Patient

Jordan L. Topel

Steven L. Lewis

DEFINITIONS AND CLINICAL SYNDROMES

The discussion of the evaluation and treatment of the comatose patient necessitates the definition of certain terms regarding different states and levels of consciousness and unconsciousness. Although the examination and diagnostic studies must be carried out in a rather organized and systematic procedure, the definitions of different levels of consciousness are, by themselves, confusing and often contradictory. When one physician's definition of terms such as lethargy, stupor, or obtundation differ from those of his colleagues, he may think that the patient's condition has deteriorated when only the terminology has changed between observers. It is better to describe specifically a patient's reactions to external stimuli, and the presence of spontaneous movements and the respiratory patterns, for example, rather than to categorize the patient as being stuporous, lethargic, or semicomatose.

Consciousness is the awareness of one's self and the environment. This is a poor definition, because one can argue that a sleeping person is unconscious, that is, unaware of himself and his environment. Clinically, however, no one regards a sleeping person as unconscious; he can be aroused to appropriate physical and mental activity with appropriate, non-noxious stimuli.

Consciousness comprises a continuum from full alertness to deep coma, or total unresponsiveness. Drowsiness or lethargy is characterized by easy arousability with light stimuli. There may be a verbal response or appropriate limb movements to pain. Stupor reflects arousability by persistent or vigorous stimuli only, and the arousal is incomplete. There is little verbal response, but limb movements may still be appropriate to the stimulus. Mental and physical activity are reduced to a minimum. Coma reflects the state in which the patient cannot be aroused to make purposeful responses. This is subgrouped into light coma, in which there may be reflex, primitive, or disorganized responses to noxious stimuli (*e.g*, decorticate and decerebrate responses), and deep coma, in which there is no response to painful stimuli.

Hysterical coma is feigned or assumed depression of consciousness. The patient appears unresponsive but is physiologically awake. The heart and respiratory rates are usually normal. The patient lies with the eyes closed, and the eyelids are frequently difficult to separate. Muscle tone is normal. Although there may be little resistance to passive movement, holding the hand over the face usually results in its falling to the side instead of directly downward. Pupils are equal and reactive unless certain eyedrops have been used. Ice water caloric testing produces nystagmus, a sign seen only in awake

43

patients. The electroencephalogram reveals a waking record.

The "locked-in" syndrome, also termed "pseudo coma," is an important condition to recognize. The patient appears to be in coma but has essentially all higher mental activity intact. The syndrome is most frequently related to basilar pontine destruction or infarction. There is an interruption of the descending corticobulbar and corticospinal tracts, resulting in quadriplegia and paralysis of lower cranial nerves. The patient is unable to talk, breathe, or move his extremities. Since the ascending reticular activating system is spared, however, arousability and wakefulness are present. There is also sparing of fibers controlling eye blinking and vertical eye movements. Thus, the patient's only means for communication may be using eye blinks (Morse code). The ramifications of not recognizing this disturbing clinical condition are obvious. Every patient, no matter how deep in coma he appears to be, should be asked to open and close the eyes, or to move the eyes up and down.

The vegetative state appears clinically to be the opposite of the "locked-in" syndrome. The patient is actually in coma and unable to attain higher mental functions (wakeful unresponsiveness). Although the patient may visually track the examiner, there is essentially no other appropriate response. Sleep–wake cycles may have returned, but there is no return of higher mental activity. The syndrome occurs in the setting of severe cortical dysfunction with relative brain-stem sparing (*e.g.*, from anoxia).

It is not uncommon to see patients with the acute onset of global aphasia to be initially diagnosed as being in coma. The patient is indeed unable to comprehend, communicate, or carry out simple verbal commands. The diagnosis may be established by noting that the patient frequently appears to be awake and alert, with roving eye movements or deviation of the eyes to the left, and he most often has a right hemiplegia.

COMA

ANATOMY

In the evaluation of the comatose patient, it is necessary to consider the physiologic and anatomic abnormalities that result in a decreased level of consciousness. Simply stated, coma results from bilateral, diffuse cerebral hemisphere dysfunction or involvement of the brain-stem (midbrain and pons) ascending reticular activating system, or a combination of the two.

Coma is unusual with unilateral cerebral hemisphere disease unless there is a dysfunction of the other hemisphere or secondary pressure or destruction of brain-stem structures. Most large cerebral hemisphere infarctions will result in a slightly decreased level of consciousness, but the patient can still be aroused to elicit some purposeful movements or higher mental activity. Exceptions may be patients with large, acute lesions affecting the dominant cerebral hemisphere. In contrast, profound coma may result from very small infarctions in the brain stem affecting the ascending reticular activating system.

A unilateral hemispheral mass lesion, such as a tumor, abscess, or expanding hemorrhage, will frequently present with unilateral focal neurologic symptoms and signs. Upon continued enlargement of the mass, there may be a compression of the contralateral cerebral hemisphere or a downward herniation of the ipsilateral temporal lobe, creating distortion and compression of the brain-stem ascending reticular activating system. At this point, coma will ensue. There is also evidence that horizontal displacement of the brain at the level of the pineal body may correlate more closely with levels of consciousness than downward displacement with brain-stem compression.

Metabolic processes usually affect both brain-stem and cerebral hemispheres to produce coma. This likely reflects a direct interference of the metabolic activity of the neurons. Initially, the patient is drowsy, but coma ensues as the metabolic process worsens.

ETIOLOGY

Coma is not an independent disease entity but a reflection of some underlying disease process. The causes of coma can be divided into two main categories: (1) those of primary central nervous system (CNS) disease and (2) those of metabolic or systemic depression (see Table 4-1). The latter group is the most common cause of a depressed level of consciousness.

Metabolic or systemic disorders generally cause depressed consciousness without focal neurologic findings. Primary CNS disorders may or may not produce focal abnormalities on examination. A previous neurologic injury, however, may render cer-

TABLE 4-1. Causes of Coma

COMA SECONDARY TO PRIMARY BRAIN INJURY OR DISEASE

Infection

Meningitis	Nuchal rigidity; CSF shows pleocytosis, increased protein; glucose may be decreased
Encephalitis	May have focal findings; CSF shows mild increased protein, increased lymphocytes, normal glucose (unless mumps or herpes simplex).
Abscess	Focal findings; positive CT scan; history of ear or sinus infection; CSF shows mild increased protein, increased cells, negative cultures.

Tumor

Primary or metastatic	Focal findings; progressive course; papilledema
Infarction	Usually no coma unless bilateral or acute, large, dominant hemisphere, or involving brain-stem reticular activating system

Hemorrhage

Subarachnoid	Sudden onset; headache; nuchal rigidity; vomiting; positive CT scan; bloody CSF
Intracerebral	Sudden onset; headache; nuchal rigidity; vomiting; focal findings; abnormal CT scan; history of hypertension

Trauma

Concussion, contusion	Positive history, evidence of injury on examination; uncomplicated concussion leaves no residual
Subdural hematoma	Depressed level of consciousness can occur before focal findings; may have trivial or no trauma history
Epidural hematoma	Lucid interval; skull fracture over middle meningeal artery

Seizures

	Convulsive or nonconvulsive status epilepticus; postictal progressive improvement in level of consciousness unless other factors are involved

COMA SECONDARY TO METABOLIC AND SYSTEMIC DISEASES

Exogenous Toxic Substances

Sedatives, hypnotics, antidepressants	Positive blood or urine screens; may cause pupillary abnormalities
Alcohol	Breath odor may not be apparent; seizures, delirium tremens on withdrawal
Acid poisons—methyl alcohol, paraldehyde	Metabolic acidosis; visual symptoms with methyl alcohol
Enzyme inhibitors—heavy metals, cyanide, arsenic, lead, salicylates	Lead encephalopathy common in children, not in adults, salicylate blood level

Endogenous Toxic Substances

Hepatic coma	Fetor hepaticus, jaundice, ascites, asterixis; triphasic waves on electroencephalogram
Uremic coma	Uriniferous breath; seizures; asterixis; increased BUN
CO_2 narcosis	Increased P_{CO_2}; positive physical chest findings, electrolytes
Endocrine—pituitary, thyroid, pancreas (diabetes), adrenals	Urine and serum osmolalities; thyroid studies

(continued)

TABLE 4-1. Causes of Coma (cont.)

Hypoxia	
Pulmonary disease, carbon monoxide intoxication, anemia	Abnormal blood gases; carboxyhemoglobin
Ischemia	
Decreased cardiac output	Congestive heart failure, myocardial infarction, arrhythmia, cardiopulmonary arrest
Hypertensive encephalopathy	Papilledema; proteinuria; headaches; seizures
Hypoglycemia	Reversed with D_{50} unless prolonged
Thiamine Deficiency	Wernicke's encephalopathy potentially reversible
Electrolyte Imbalance	Water, sodium, acidosis, alkalosis, calcium
Temperature Regulation	
Hypothermia	Exposure; myxedema; barbiturates; circulatory failure
Hyperthermia	Heat stroke; phenothiazines (neuroleptic malignant syndrome)

BUN = blood urea nitrogen; CSF = cerebrospinal fluid; CT = computed tomography.

tain neurons more susceptible to a metabolic insult. A metabolic encephalopathy could thus produce focal neurologic findings. These signs may disappear after the metabolic disturbance has been corrected.

EVALUATION AND TREATMENT

Initial emergency treatment for a comatose patient is essentially the same as with all other medical emergencies. An adequate airway should be established. Endotracheal intubation and artificial ventilation may be necessary. The cardiovascular status must be promptly evaluated, and shock and blood pressure should be controlled. The temperature should be noted, since hypo- or hyperthermia may play a prominent role in the identification of the underlying problem.

A history should be taken, but unfortunately this is often incomplete, nonexistent, or misleading. A search for "less likely" causes for the coma is necessary when the treatment procedures for the "obvious" cause from the history obtained do not change the patient's clinical status. Nevertheless, aggressive management of the unconscious patient includes an aggressive pursuit of the history. Friends or family of the patient often do not realize the value of the information that they can offer.

There should be a search for evidence of trauma. Battle's sign (purple and blue discoloration of the mastoid skin area), blood in the external auditory canal, or blood noted behind the tympanic membranes may signify a temporal bone or basal skull fracture. Raccoon eyes (purple discoloration of the eyelid and orbital regions) may signify orbital or basal skull fractures.

One should check carefully for nuchal rigidity, but several factors must be considered in doing so. If there is any suspicion of a cervical neck fracture, there should be no manipulation of the neck. In deep coma, nuchal rigidity may be lacking despite its presence in a lighter level of consciousness. Finally, some patients with a CNS infection or subarachnoid hemorrhage may not manifest nuchal rigidity initially in the course of their illness.

The odor of the patient's breath may indicate the cause for the coma. Alcohol gives its characteristic smell; hepatic coma is often associated with a musty odor, and a fruity or acetone smell is characteristic of ketoacidosis.

After a screening general physical examination, an orderly, systemic neurologic examination is undertaken. The goal of the neurologic examination is essentially to determine the presence, location, and nature of the underlying process creating the decreased level of consciousness and also to give some prognosis of the patient's condition.

Respiratory patterns yield information regarding the activity of different cerebral areas. When one develops bilateral cerebral hemisphere dysfunction (essentially functioning at the diencephalic level), Cheyne–Stokes respiration may occur. This respiratory pattern is associated with periods of hyperpnea alternating with periods of apnea. There is a regularity to the respirations: first a gradual build-up of respirations to the level of hyperpnea and then a gradual tapering off of respirations to apnea.

The periods of apnea may last up to 30 seconds or more. It is believed that Cheyne–Stokes respiration relates to an abnormal response of carbon dioxide–sensitive respiratory brain centers. There is an increased ventilatory response to carbon dioxide stimulation, creating hyperpnea. After the concentration of carbon dioxide drops below the level at which the centers are stimulated, the apnea phase appears and continues until the carbon dioxide reaccumulates and the cycle repeats itself. Because sleep induces further cerebral depressing mechanisms, Cheyne–Stokes respiration may be seen in some patients during sleep, whereas they exhibit normal breathing patterns while awake.

Cheyne–Stokes respiration is, by itself, not a serious prognostic sign. Although it can be seen in focal primary CNS problems, it can also be seen early in many metabolic and systemic problems.

Central neurogenic hyperventilation appears when lower brain centers are involved; it is noted with dysfunction at the midbrain or the upper pons. There are continuous, regular, and rapid respirations up to 40 or 50 times/minute. Arterial blood gases reveal a respiratory alkalosis with decreased Pco_2 and increased pH. The PO_2 must be greater than 70 or 80 millimeters of mercury (mm Hg). If the PO_2 is not above that level, it raises the possibility of an extracerebral cause (hypoxemia) for the respiratory problem. Cardiac, pulmonary, and metabolic (e.g., diabetes, uremia, hepatic, salicylates) problems must be ruled out as possible causes of the hyperventilation.

Apneustic respiration is noted in lower pontine lesions and consists of a prolonged inspiratory phase with a pause at full inspiration. Cluster breathing, also signifying lower pontine damage, is characterized by a disorderly sequence of closely grouped respirations followed by apnea.

Ataxic respirations signify a lower pontine or medullary respiratory center problem. The breathing pattern is chaotic and haphazard with irregular pauses. It may, and usually does, lead to gasping and eventual cessation of breathing. Ataxic breathing is a forewarner for respiratory arrest, and prompt endotracheal intubation is necessary at the time of its discovery.

The examination of the pupillary responses, eye movements, and fundus must be undertaken. In a patient with a decreased level of consciousness, but who is not yet in coma, visual threat (forceful movements of the hand toward either side of the eyes) may be helpful. Blinking in response to a threat from one side, but not from the other side, suggests a hemianopsia. The abnormality would thus be in the cerebral hemisphere opposite to the side that did not blink. A funduscopic examination may reveal papilledema or retinal hemorrhages.

The pupillary response is recorded. The light reflex is mediated, in succession, through the optic nerve, the optic chiasm, the optic tract, the posterior diencephalon, and the Edinger–Westphal nuclei of the midbrain, and then to the sphincter pupillae by way of the parasympathetic nerve fibers in the oculomotor nerve (cranial nerve III). Thus, it is not surprising that the most significant abnormalities of the pupils are seen with dysfunction at the level of the midbrain or oculomotor nerve.

Diencephalic pupils, the result of bilateral hemispheral dysfunction, are small and reactive. The small size likely reflects sympathetic nerve dysfunction at the level of the takeoff of the sympathetic fibers from the hypothalamus.

Midposition, unreactive (4 mm to 7 mm) pupils result from direct midbrain (tectal region) damage. The pupillary size likely reflects an involvement of both the descending sympathetic fibers and the parasympathetic fibers of the oculomotor complex.

A widely dilated, fixed pupil is usually seen as a result of direct oculomotor nerve involvement, with unopposed dilator sympathetic tone. In addition to the pupillary abnormalities, ptosis and extraocular muscle paralysis (especially adduction of the eye) are frequently present. Since the oculomotor nerve is strategically situated at the temporal incisura, temporal lobe herniation will result in a widely dilated, fixed pupil, and possibly total cranial nerve III paralysis.

Pinpoint pupils are seen with pontine damage but may be a transient finding for only the first 24 or 48 hours. The pupils are small and can be seen occasionally to react slightly to light if viewed through a magnifying glass. It is thought to relate to damage of the descending sympathetic tracts. Frequently, however, midposition and fixed pupils are noted with pontine dysfunction.

Of great importance is the fact that metabolic processes do not alter pupillary response until late in their course, if at all. For example, a deeply comatose patient with no spontaneous or reflex movements and no respirations, but with reactive pupils, must be considered to be in metabolic coma until proved otherwise.

In addition, certain drugs can alter pupillary size and response. Opiates characteristically produce pinpoint pupils (reversed with naloxone). Glutethimide produces midposition or widely dilated and frequently fixed pupils. Atropine may result in widely dilated and fixed pupils. Various eyedrops may also alter pupillary size and reaction.

The position and movements of the eyes are observed, and certain procedures are undertaken to evaluate cerebral hemisphere and brain-stem integrity. The neural pathways for the control of horizontal conjugate eye movements are outlined in Figure 4-1. Cortical control originates in the frontal gaze centers (Brodmann's area 8). Descending fibers controlling horizontal conjugate gaze cross the midline in the lower midbrain region and descend to the paramedian pontine reticular formation (PPRF) in the pons. The PPRF is thus the major area of confluence of pathways controlling horizontal eye movements. Neurons from the PPRF project to the nearby abducens nerve (cranial nerve VI) nucleus and thereby stimulate movement in the lateral rectus muscle of the eye ipsilateral to the

PPRF and contralateral to the frontal gaze center. In addition, impulses from the abducens nerve nucleus cross the midline and ascend the median longitudinal fasciculus to the medial rectus nucleus of the oculomotor nerve (cranial nerve III) in the midbrain. This stimulates adduction of the eye ipsilateral to the frontal gaze center. Horizontal conjugate gaze is thus completed.

By following these pathways, it can be seen that stimulation of fibers from the frontal gaze center of one cerebral hemisphere results in horizontal, conjugate eye movements to the contralateral side. If one frontal gaze center or its descending fibers are damaged, the eyes will tend to "look" toward the involved cerebral hemisphere due to unopposed action of the remaining frontal gaze center. For example, a destructive lesion in the right cerebral hemisphere, involving descending motor fibers and frontal gaze fibers, will cause a left hemiplegia

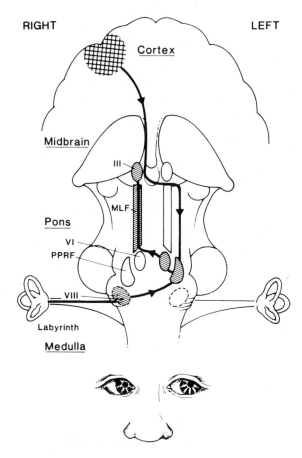

FIG. 4-1. Diagram of the conjugate vision pathways; nuclei and paths are shaded to include those important to left conjugate gaze: fibers from the right frontal cortex descend cross the midline, and synapse in the left paramedian pontine reticular formation (PPRF). Fibers then travel to the nearby left cranial nerve VI nucleus (to move the left eye laterally) and then cross the midline to rise in the right medial longitudinal fasciculus (MLF) to the right cranial nerve III nucleus (to move the right eye medially). In addition to the cortical influence on the left PPRF, there is vestibular influence. With vestibular activation from the right, the left PPRF is stimulated, and the eyes conjugatively move to the left. Instillation of ice water into the right ear canal will test the integrity of this vestibular-PPRF-cranial nerve-VI-cranial nerve-III-circuit, and if the eyes move to vestibular stimulation, the brain stem from medulla to midbrain must be functioning.

with head and eyes deviated to the right. In other words, the eyes "look" at a destructive hemispheral lesion and "look" away from the resulting hemiplegia.

By contrast, a destructive left pontine lesion, for example, will damage the left PPRF. The eyes, therefore, cannot go to the left and will tend to deviate to the right. Since descending pyramidal tract fibers cross the midline in the medulla, damage to the pyramidal tract fibers in the pons on the left results in a right hemiplegia. Thus, the eyes "look" away from a destructive pontine lesion but "look" toward the hemiplegia.

If the abducens nerve or nucleus is destroyed, there will be a loss of abduction of the ipsilateral eye (cranial nerve VI palsy). With destruction of the tract of the medial longitudinal fasciculus, disconjugate gaze results, with loss of adduction of the ipsilateral eye (same side as the tract of the medial longitudinal fasciculus). Abduction of the contralateral eye is preserved, but there is nystagmus. This type of disconjugate gaze abnormality is also termed *internuclear ophthalmoplegia* (see Chap. 22). The pathways for vertical eye movements are less well understood. Lower centers likely exist in the midbrain (pretectal and tectal) regions.

If a patient cannot follow verbal commands, two useful tests are employed to determine brain-stem integrity. An oculocephalic (doll's head) maneuver is performed by turning the patient's head rapidly in the horizontal or vertical planes and by noting the movement or position of the eyes relative to the orbits. This maneuver should obviously not be performed if a cervical neck fracture is suspected. If the pontine (horizontal) or midbrain (vertical) gaze centers are intact, the eyes should move in the orbits in the direction opposite to the rotating head. An abnormal response (no eye movement with doll's head maneuver) implies pontine or midbrain dysfunction and is characterized by no movement of the eyes relative to the orbits, or an asymmetry of movement.

Horizontal oculocephalic maneuvers are a relatively weak stimulus for horizontal eye movements. If a doll's head maneuver is present, it is not necessary to continue with oculovestibular testing. If, however, a doll's head response is lacking, ice water calorics should be performed, since it is a stronger stimulus than oculocephalic maneuvers.

Oculovestibular responses (ice water calorics) are reflex eye movements in response to irrigation of the external ear canals with cold water. The head is raised to 30° relative to the horizontal plane, and the external canals are inspected for the presence of cerumen or a perforated tympanic membrane. Fifty to 100 ml cold water is instilled into the canal (waiting 5 min between each ear), and the resulting eye movements are noted. Ice water produces a downward current in the horizontal semicircular canal and decreases tonic vestibular input to the contralateral PPRF. Simplistically, one can think of this as an indirect means of stimulating the ipsilateral PPRF. Hence, after cold water instillation, there is a slow, tonic, conjugate deviation of the eyes toward the irrigated ear. In a waking patient, there is a correction of the eyes to the opposite side, resulting in a fast nystagmus away from the stimulated ear. In an unconscious patient, there is a loss of the fast-phase nystagmus, and only tonic deviation of the eyes is seen if appropriate pontine–midbrain areas are intact. Thus, if nystagmus is noted in a seemingly unconscious patient, the patient is either in a very light coma or a hysterical coma.

A lack of oculovestibular responses thus suggests pontine–midbrain dysfunction. Ice water calorics can help to differentiate between the conjugate gaze weakness or paralysis caused by either cortical (cerebral hemisphere) or brain-stem (pontine) damage. Oculovestibular responses should not be altered in patients with only hemispheral pathology.

Movement of the ipsilateral eye toward the irrigated ear, but no movement of the contralateral eye, suggests an abnormality of the contralateral medial longitudinal fasciculus (see Chap. 22).

Severe metabolic coma (*e.g.*, barbiturate overdose) may result in a lack of oculocephalic and oculovestibular responses. Reactive pupils may signify that the coma is of metabolic origin.

Ocular bobbing is characterized by a rapid downward eye movement with a slow return to the horizontal plane. This is seen most often in pontine destruction and is thought to relate to the loss of horizontal eye movements with preservation of midbrain-mediated vertical eye movement pathways.

Roving eye movements signify intact brain-stem mechanisms for horizontal gaze. The movements should be distinguished from those seen in patients with seizures. In the latter, the eye movements are of a jerking quality and frequently tend to lateralize to one side. In reference to Figure 4-1, it can be seen that an irritative cortical focus in the area of the frontal gaze center will deviate the eyes away from the side of the lesion (and possibly toward a hemiplegia). Oculovestibular responses will usually be able to overcome the eye deviations because of the strong direct input into the pons, "bypassing" the cortical effects on eye movements.

Motor movements may be spontaneous, induced, reflex, or totally absent. It is important to note not only the type of response but also the symmetry of response. An asymmetrical induced motor movement may be the only indication of an underlying focal problem.

It may be necessary to observe the patient for several minutes to note the presence or lack of spontaneous or reflex motor movements. The position of the extremities (e.g., a persistent externally rotated leg secondary to weakness of that extremity) may indicate focal pathology.

The most favorable prognostic sign related to the motor system is symmetrical, spontaneous movements of all four extremities. Appropriate motor response to noxious stimuli (e.g., pain) signifies that sensory pathways are functional and there is at least partial integrity of corticospinal tracts. It is not necessary to use unusually noxious stimuli, but rather mild supraorbital pressure, pinching of the skin of the neck, or mild sternal pressure.

Reflex motor movements can frequently be elicited by light, painful stimuli; flexion of the neck; or during routine care of the patient, such as tracheal suctioning. Decorticate posturing consists of flexion of the arms, wrists, and fingers, and adduction of the upper extremities. In the legs, there is extension, internal rotation, and plantar flexion. Decerebrate (extensor) posturing consists of extension of the arms as well as adduction and hyperpronation of the arms. There may be opisthotonic posturing of the neck. The movement of the lower extremities is similar to that seen in decorticate posturing. Although not completely anatomically specific, bilateral decerebrate posturing is often seen in lesions of the midbrain and pons, while decorticate posturing often implies a higher corticospinal tract lesion. Decerebrate posturing, often seen secondary to structural processes involving or compressing the high brain stem, is generally a poorer prognostic sign than decorticate posturing. However, decerebrate posturing can also occasionally be seen in the setting of severe, although potentially reversible, metabolic encephalopathies.

A common mistake regarding the interpretation of motor responses is that of relating a withdrawal response in the legs as representing an appropriate cortical response. When the bottom of the foot is stroked, or a noxious stimuli is applied to the leg, there may be hip flexion, knee flexion, and dorsiflexion of the foot (triple flexor response). This signifies spinal cord reflex integrity and does not signify an intact cerebral response.

Asymmetrical extensor toe signs (i.e., flexion on one side, extensor response on the other) are of moderate value in localizing a focal cerebral lesion. Bilateral extensor toe signs can be seen in any form or at any level of coma, and are, of themselves, neither prognostic nor localizing. For example, transient extensor toe signs are common in hypertensive encephalopathy.

LABORATORY EVALUATION AND TREATMENT

Following the establishment of an airway, assisting of respirations, and maintenance of circulation, certain laboratory tests and therapeutic measures are undertaken, often occurring simultaneous to obtaining a history and performing a neurologic examination.

Blood is drawn for a complete blood count (CBC), electrolyte, glucose, calcium, and blood urea nitrogen (BUN) determinations, liver function tests, arterial blood gas determinations, and a drug–toxin screen. Urinalysis and urine drug screening are performed. An electrocardiogram and chest roentgenograms are obtained. If hypoglycemia is suspected, or if the cause of the coma is uncertain, 25 ml to 50 ml of 50% dextrose in water is given intravenously (IV). Hypoglycemia is an extremely important potentially reversible cause of coma which if not treated promptly will lead to irreversible cerebral damage. For suspected opiate overdose, naloxone 0.4 mg IV is given and is repeated every 5 to 15 minutes as needed. Repeated infusions should be instituted if the response to glucose or naloxone is incomplete. Other medications can be given for specific drug overdoses when appropriate, such as intravenous physostigmine for severe anticholinergic toxicity or intravenous flumazenil for benzodiazephine overdose. If chronic or acute ingestion of alcohol is suspected, thiamine should be given IV to treat or prevent the Wernicke–Korsakoff syndrome. Correction of any other underlying metabolic process (e.g., hyponatremia) must be undertaken. If there is significant evidence for increased intracranial pressure, intubation with hyperventilation, and the use of mannitol must be considered. Corticosteroids may be beneficial to reduce vasogenic edema related to neoplasms, but their effect is not immediate.

Seizure activity may be generalized or focal and necessitates prompt treatment and a search for a cause. Myoclonic jerks (symmetric or asymmetric rapid, brief movements of the extremities) are frequently seen in metabolic encephalopathies and are common following anoxia (*e.g.*, after cardiac arrest). Unfortunately, myoclonic jerks in the setting of severe anoxic coma are often difficult to treat, and their appearance following anoxia is a poor prognostic sign.

It may be necessary to proceed with further neurologic studies if the cause of the coma remains unclear. Computed tomography (CT scan) will demonstrate intracerebral or extracerebral blood, mass lesions, infarctions, and abscesses, as well as skull fractures. Magnetic resonance imaging (MR scan) is less useful in the evaluation of the comatose patient. Patients will need to be left unattended for a longer scanning time. Unconscious patients are often on ventilators, which usually cannot be placed near the MR scanner. If a CNS infection or subarachnoid hemorrhage is suspected, a lumbar puncture is indicated, though a CT or MR scan will identify most subarachnoid hemorrhages sufficient to cause coma. A CT scan should usually be obtained prior to the lumbar puncture in order to rule out a focal mass lesion or increased intracranial pressure.

The electroencephalogram may be helpful in the diagnosis of an overdose from sedatives (excessive fast activity), hepatic or uremic encephalopathy (triphasic waves), hysteria (normal EEG), or in differentiating focal from diffuse disease. It can be used to rule out subclinical seizure activity as a cause for prolonged, unexplained coma. An electroencephalogram with no evidence of cerebral activity can be reversibly noted secondary to barbiturate intoxication (and occasionally other drugs) and also with hypothermia.

PROGNOSIS

Several studies that have dealt with postanoxic coma have revealed that the prognosis is generally better for the patient with spontaneous motor movements or appropriate movements in response to noxious stimuli, and present pupillary reactions and oculocephalic or oculovestibular responses. Patients studied after cardiopulmonary arrest reveal that depth and duration of postarrest coma correlated significantly with poor neurologic outcome. Motor unresponsiveness, lack of pupillary responses, and lack of oculocephalic and oculovestibular responses were associated with a poor

prognosis for neurologic functional recovery. In addition, the prediction of survival and outcome could be based on a loss of consciousness alone within 3 days after cardiopulmonary arrest. Those patients not awakening within 72 hours had the worst prognosis.

Prognosis for patients with metabolic encephalopathies or drug overdose cannot be based upon the level of consciousness. For example, patients with barbiturate overdose in deep coma may have no spontaneous respiration, absent oculovestibular responses, and absent cerebral activity on the electroencephalogram, yet have a complete neurologic recovery.

QUESTIONS AND DISCUSSION

1. A 24-year-old man is brought to the emergency room with a decreased level of consciousness. Upon arrival, he suffers a respiratory arrest and is intubated. An examination reveals small, reactive pupils (2 mm), a lack of oculocephalic and oculovestibular responses, and no response to painful stimuli. Which is the best answer?

   A. The most likely diagnosis is a pontine hemorrhage.
   B. A CT scan should be obtained immediately.
   C. The pupils should be pharmacologically dilated to obtain a good funduscopic examination.
   D. Neurosurgical consultation should be sought immediately to evacuate a subdural hematoma.
   E. Drug screen and other blood tests should be obtained immediately, and glucose and naloxone should be given IV.

The correct answer is (E). Metabolic encephalopathies can result in a lack of oculocephalic and oculovestibular responses, with preserved pupillary responses.

2. Cheyne–Stokes respiration:

   A. Is associated with irreversible brain disease
   B. Is pathognomonic of midbrain dysfunction
   C. Is characterized by sustained inspirations
   D. May occur in noncomatose patients while they are asleep
   E. Is associated with decerebrate posturing

The correct answer is (D). Cheyne–Stokes respirations are related to bilateral hemispheral dysfunction. During sleep, increased inhibitory influences may create this pattern of respiration.

3. A right hemispheral destructive lesion may produce:

   A. Lack of caloric responses, eyes conjugately deviated to the left, and left hemiplegia
   B. Right eye deviated to the right, left eye midline, and left hemiplegia
   C. Eyes conjugately deviated to the right, left hemiplegia, and present caloric responses
   D. Ocular bobbing and left hemiplegia
   E. Present caloric responses, eyes conjugately deviated to the left, and left hemiplegia

The correct answer is (C). Eyes "look toward" a destructive hemispheral lesion. Caloric responses are preserved because the pathway for the oculovestibular responses does not involve hemispheral connections.

4. Lack of caloric (oculovestibular) responses bilaterally:

   A. Signifies marked suppression of both cerebral hemispheres
   B. Is pathognomonic of pontine hemorrhage
   C. Is frequently associated with Cheyne–Stokes respiration
   D. Can be seen in metabolic encephalopathy
   E. Is always reversible

The correct answer is (D). Oculovestibular responses are mediated by brain-stem (*i.e.,* pontine) pathways. The responses are reversible if a metabolic encephalopathy is corrected in appropriate time.

5. Decerebrate posturing:

   A. May be associated with central neurogenic hyperventilation

   B. Is seen in patients with bilateral frontal lobe dysfunction
   C. Consists of flexion of the arms and wrists
   D. Signifies integrity of spinal cord and occipital lobe synapses
   E. Is a good prognostic sign

The correct answer is (A). Decerebrate posturing, which partially consists of extension and hyperpronation of the upper extremities, is often associated with midbrain dysfunction (as is central neurogenic hyperventilation).

SUGGESTED READING

Bates D: Predicting recovery from medical coma. Br J Hosp Med 33:276, 1985

Buettner UW, Zee DS: Vestibular testing in comatose patients. Arch Neurol 46:561, 1989

Fisher CM: The neurological examination of the comatose patient. Acta Neurol Scand 45(Suppl 36):1, 1969

Jennett B, Teasdale G, Braakman R et al: Prognosis of patients with severe head injury. Neurosurgery 4:283, 1979

Krumholz A, Stern BJ, Weiss HD: Outcome from coma after cardiopulmonary resuscitation: Relation to seizures and myoclonus. Neurology 38:401, 1988

Leigh RJ, Hanley DF, Muschauer FE et al: Eye movements induced by head rotation in unresponsive patients. Ann Neurol 15:465, 1984

Levy DE, Caronna JJ, Singer BH et al: Predicting outcome from hypoxic-ischemic coma. JAMA 253:1420, 1985

Lewis SL, Topel JL: Coma. In Weiner WJ (ed): Emergent and Urgent Neurology. Philadelphia, JB Lippincott, 1992

Plum F, Posner JB: The Diagnosis of Stupor and Coma, 3rd ed. Philadelphia, FA Davis, 1980

Ropper AH: Lateral displacement of the brain and level of consciousness in patients with an acute hemispheral mass. N Engl J Med 314:953, 1986

Cerebrovascular Disease

Roger E. Kelley

Cerebrovascular disease can be classified into several categories depending upon whether there is a primary ischemic or primary hemorrhagic insult. The former category includes arterial thrombosis, venous thrombosis, and arterial embolism. The latter includes primary intracerebral hemorrhage (ICH) and subarachnoid hemorrhage (SAH). Arterial thrombosis consists of large-artery thrombosis, which is often called *lacunar infarct*, a term that has become somewhat controversial. The "classic" teaching implied that lacunae were small infarcts secondary to occlusion of subcortical penetrating arteries and that the pathogenesis, in the vast majority of cases, was related to lipohyalinosis from long standing hypertension. This appears to be an oversimplification. Clearly, hypertension is a major factor in the pathogenesis of stroke, but not all small strokes are "lacunar" in nature. Figure 5-1 is a schema that outlines the most common stroke types with the frequencies found in a prospective consecutive series of stroke patients seen at Temple University Hospital in Philadelphia.

The term *transient ischemic attack* (TIA) implies a neurologic deficit, on an ischemic basis, which resolves within 24 hours. This is a clinically useful concept, but it may be somewhat artificial. A number of patients have mild residual deficits which might persist for days or weeks. In such instances, the term *minor stroke* or *reversible ischemic neurologic deficit* (RIND) is often used. From a practical standpoint, TIA and minor stroke are often lumped together as a clinical presentation which identifies a population at relatively high risk for a major stroke. It is estimated that between 5% and 10% of subjects per year, with TIA or minor stroke, will go on to have a major stroke. There are a number of caveats to this statement. The risk of recurrent stroke is related to the stroke mechanism. For example, a subject with atrial fibrillation and rheumatic heart disease will have a very high risk of stroke. On the other hand, this risk can be substantially reduced with the judicious use of anticoagulant therapy.

EPIDEMIOLOGY

Stroke affects approximately 500,000 people per year in the United States. The prevalence of stroke is on the order of 1.7 million, and stroke remains the leading cause of chronic disability in the adult population. The frequency of stroke in a particular population will be directly related to demographic characteristics. There is a strong relationship between increasing age and stroke risk, for example. The incidence of stroke more than doubles for each successive decade beyond age 55. Thus, a retirement community will be expected to have a clustering of stroke-prone individuals.

The major and minor risk factors for stroke are summarized in Table 5-1. Men have a 30% higher

William J. Weiner and Christopher G. Goetz, eds. *Neurology for the Non-Neurologist*, Third Edition. Copyright © 1994, 1989 by J. B. Lippincott Company. Copyright © 1981 by Harper and Row Publishers, Inc.

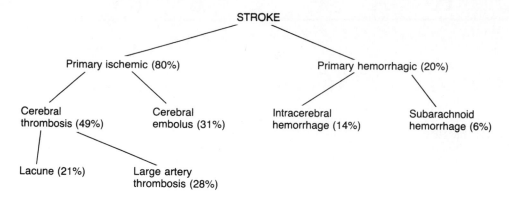

FIG. 5-1. Schematic representation of stroke type with frequencies found in a hospital-based consecutive series of stroke patients.

rate of stroke than women, and blacks have a higher incidence than whites. In a study comparing stroke frequency in blacks and whites, the rate was 109/100,000 for whites and 208/100,000 in blacks. Blacks also have a higher incidence of ICH and SAH. Hypertension, especially if poorly controlled, is an important risk factor for both thromboembolic stroke and ICH. There is a two- to four-fold increased risk of stroke with isolated hypertension and an approximately two-fold increased risk with diabetes mellitus.

Elevation of the hematocrit is associated with increased blood viscosity and a reduction in cerebral blood flow (CBF). Stroke is a not uncommon complication of polycythemia vera. There is increasing evidence that cigarette consumption is associated with cerebral atherosclerosis and propensity to cerebral infarction. The secondary polycythemia that can be seen in heavy smokers might also play a role in this enhanced stroke risk. Asymptomatic bruit is a marker for stroke risk, but this risk is not necessarily in the vascular distribution where the bruit is heard. Similarly, there is an increased risk of stroke in subjects with peripheral vascular disease; this is reflective of the often diffuse nature of the atherosclerotic process.

Prior stroke appears to be the greatest risk factor for recurrent stroke. In one study, the cumulative 5-year recurrence rate for stroke was 42% for men and 24% for women. The risk of major stroke for patients with TIA is roughly one in three over 5 years. The actual risk is very dependent upon attention to ongoing risk factors and the efficacy of interventional therapy. It is also important to note that patients with TIA are more likely to die of cardiac disease than of stroke.

Cardiac disease, independent of other risk factors for stroke, is associated with a two-fold increased risk. Some of the more important potential cardiogenic sources of embolism are outlined in Table 5-2 along with an estimate of the risk of recurrent stroke. The risk of recurrent stroke tends to be greatest around the time of the initial insult. In nonvalvular atrial fibrillation, for example, the risk of recurrent stroke is reported to be as high as 20% within 11 days of the first stroke. The Framingham study found, however, that beyond the acute period the risk of recurrence diminished progressively to the point that it is not significantly greater than in those without atrial fibrillation by

TABLE 5-1. Risk Factors for Stroke

Major Risk Factors

Age	Hypertension
Gender	Polycythemia
Race	Sickle cell diseases
Genetic predisposition	Transient ischemic attack
Diabetes mellitus	Prior stroke
Cigarette smoking	Cardiac disease
Asymptomatic bruit	Hypercoagulable state

Minor Risk Factors

Hypercholesterolemia	Alcohol consumption
Oral contraceptive use	Physical inactivity
Obesity	Mitral valve prolapse

TABLE 5-2. Relationship of Type of Cardiac Disease to
Risk of Stroke and Risk of Recurrent Stroke

CARDIAC DISEASE	RISK OF STROKE	RISK OF RECURRENT STROKE
Nonvalvular atrial fibrillation	5% per year	20% at 11 days
Atrial fibrillation plus rheumatic heart disease	17 ×	At least 50%
Acute myocardial infarct	1.7–2.4%	Unknown
Left ventricular thrombus	5–7%	Unknown
Prosthetic mechanical valve*	21.1% at 12 yrs	Unknown
Prosthetic porcine valve	26.4% at 12 yrs	Unknown

*With anticoagulant therapy.

6 months. Myocardial infarct, which is associated with a 1.7% to 2.4% risk of cerebral embolism, displays a similar pattern in that the risk of embolization, directly related to the myocardial infarct, becomes negligible at approximately 6 months.

A dilated cardiomyopathy associated with a markedly impaired ejection fraction is an important cause of cerebral embolus. The demonstration of a mural wall thrombus with or without significant left ventricular hypokinesis is also a major risk. This risk is compounded by coexistent factors such as atrial fibrillation. Lone atrial fibrillation in subjects under 60 years of age is not a significant risk factor. Beyond age 60, especially if there are associated factors such as hypertension or recent congestive heart failure, the risk is 5% per year or greater.

The importance of paradoxical cerebral embolism has recently been emphasized. This usually implies thromboembolism from a peripheral source with transmittance, through the heart, via a patent foramen ovale. This is now recognized as a not uncommon presumptive mechanism especially in younger individuals who do not have readily identifiable risk factors for stroke.

Mitral valve prolapse continues to pose somewhat of a dilemma in terms of its importance in the pathogenesis of ischemic stroke. This entity is found in up to 6% to 10% of the normal population, and its confirmation depends largely on the interpretation of the echocardiogram. Cardiac auscultatory findings can certainly be indicative of the presence of prolapse, but the exact degree, possible redundancy of the valve, and other important factors necessitate cardiac imaging. One study found that 40% of stroke patients under age 45 had mitral valve prolapse, and a population-based study concluded that there was a four-fold increased risk of stroke with mitral valve prolapse. Despite this, large hospital-based stroke series, including those composed of young stroke victims, have found a prevalence for mitral valve prolapse of between 0% and 5%. It appears, therefore, that to attribute an ischemic stroke to mitral valve prolapse then etiologies must be excluded.

There is a 4- to 13-fold increased risk of cerebral infarction in women on oral contraceptives. This risk is compounded by cigarette smoking. Ethanol has been implicated as a risk factor for stroke. It can be a direct factor, especially in cases of excessive binge drinking with alteration of fluid status. It can also have a secondary effect by promoting noncompliance of antihypertensive medication or through the development of Laennac's cirrhosis.

More esoteric causes of stroke include meningovascular syphilis, systemic lupus erythematosus, and polyarteritis nodosa. Stroke-like episodes have been reported in acquired immunodeficiency syndrome, but the pathogenesis requires clarification. A hypercoagulable state can be seen in association with antithrombin III deficiency, protein C deficiency, and protein S deficiency. In addition, a prothrombotic state can be seen in association with antiphospholipid antibodies. These are immunoglobulins which are usually of the IgG or IgM class; they include anticardiolipin antibodies and lupus anticoagulants. These antibodies can be seen in association with systemic lupus erythematosus, malignancy, acquired immunodeficiency or with certain drugs, or they can occur spontaneously. Despite their increased prevalence in thrombotic states, their exact role in the pathogenesis of ischemic stroke requires further research.

Bleeding diathesis can result in ICH. Thrombocytopenia, from various causes, can promote intracranial bleeding when severe. Anticoagulant administration can be complicated by intracranial bleeding. Hemophilia remains the most common congenital bleeding disturbance associated with ICH.

DIAGNOSTIC EVALUATION

The diagnostic evaluation of any stroke or TIA patient should include a complete blood count (CBC), prothrombin time, partial thromboplastin time, platelet count, syphilis serology, electrocardiogram, chest x-ray, and computed tomography (CT) brain scan. The latter study is mandatory to distinguish ischemic from hemorrhagic stroke and to exclude other possible diagnoses. The evolution of a subcortical ischemic infarct is demonstrated in Figure 5-2. Tumor, brain abscess, cerebritis, subdural hematoma, epidural hematoma, and focal seizure activity can mimic spontaneous stroke or TIA.

A CBC allows for an evaluation of possible polycythemia that can be associated with increased blood viscosity, decreased CBF, and a predisposition to ischemic stroke. An elevated white blood cell count should alert the clinician to pay particular attention to the temperature curve and to the heart because bacterial endocarditis remains a not uncommon cause of stroke. On the other hand, a low white blood cell count may alert the clinician to immunodeficiency. An elevated erythrocyte sedimentation rate can also be helpful in screening for atrial myxoma, metastatic disease, or a connective tissue disorder. Coagulation parameters are helpful for detection of a bleeding diathesis in hemorrhagic stroke or a hypercoagulable state in ischemic stroke. Furthermore, baseline coagulation parameters are important if a cerebral arteriogram, lumbar puncture, or anticoagulant therapy is being contemplated. The possibility of sickle cell disease necessitates a sickle cell preparation and possibly a hemoglobin electrophoresis. An inverse relationship has been reported between hyperglycemia and outcome in stroke.

The routine performance of an electrocardiogram in stroke patients emphasizes the importance of the heart in patients with cerebral ischemia. The heart is not only the most likely source of cerebral embolus, but also patients with TIA are more likely to die of cardiac disease than of stroke disease. If there is any evidence of cardiac disease by history, physical examination, electrocardiogram, or if the person is 45 years of age or younger, further cardiac evaluation is probably necessary. This evaluation should include two-dimensional echocardiography and, in selected cases, cardiac monitoring. It is becoming increasingly clear that a transesophageal echocardiogram is superior to transthoracic echocardiography in the detection of a possible cardiogenic source of cerebral embolism. Approximately one-third of patients with ischemic stroke and TIA have significant coronary disease. This finding has led some stroke specialists to recommend stress electrocardiography as part of the evaluation in patients with TIA or minor ischemic stroke.

The need for cerebral angiography depends on the patient's neurologic status and the type of treatment considered. The arteriogram can provide an-

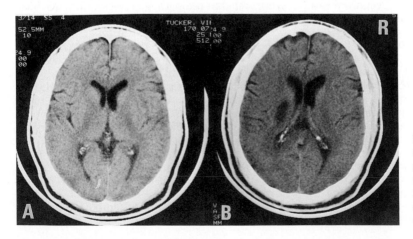

FIG. 5-2. (*A*) Initially normal CT brain scan in a patient presenting with right hemiparesis. (*B*) Follow-up CT brain scan, 3 days later, which demonstrates a discrete left subcortical ischemic infarct.

swers to questions about possible extracranial or intracranial vascular occlusive disease. Figure 5-3 demonstrates a high-grade internal carotid artery stenosis in a patient experiencing TIAs. The nature of the symptoms, the degree of stenosis, and the medical stability led to the performance of a carotid endarterectomy. Several studies have indicated that there is a definite relationship between the degree of internal carotid artery stenosis and the likelihood of stroke disease. A symptomatic internal carotid artery stenosis of 70% or greater is most likely to be associated with the development of ischemic stroke.

Cerebral arteriography can also demonstrate intracerebral occlusive vascular disease including arteritis. It can also be used to document cerebral venous thrombosis or the source of intracerebral hemorrhage such as an aneurysm or an arteriovenous malformation (AVM). Such a study result can help explain the mechanism of stroke and can affect therapy. It must be kept in mind that this is an invasive vascular procedure and it is not without risk of a significant complication.

The fact that routine cerebral angiography is not without risk has led to the development of noninvasive tests of the extracranial, and recently the intracranial, circulation. These studies include direct visualization of the carotid bifurcation (termed *direct tests*) and monitors of the more distal internal carotid artery circulation (termed *indirect tests*). The categorization of the most commonly performed of these studies is outlined in Table 5-3. Carotid ultrasound is performed by way of B-mode or Doppler technique. The B-mode scan gives information primarily about the vessel wall, whereas the Doppler study primarily analyzes the moving column of blood. These studies have been combined in the so-called *duplex carotid scan*. Despite its potential, the ability of the carotid scan to evaluate the initial 2 cm of the internal carotid artery, which is the region of the vessel most commonly affected by atherosclerosis, is subject to certain limitations. These limitations make the combination of direct and indirect tests, the so-called *carotid noninvasive battery*, mandatory in order to achieve an optimal degree of accuracy.

The most common indirect tests include oculoplethysmography and ophthalmodynamometry (which measure retinal pressure), periorbital Doppler ultrasound (which measures anterograde and retrograde flow characteristics of the periorbital arteries), and thermography (which correlates facial temperature with extracranial vessel perfusion). The distal effect of internal carotid artery stenosis can also be detected with transcranial Doppler ultrasonography (TCD) of the middle cerebral artery. This is a noninvasive means of using an ultrasound probe to penetrate the skull, allowing measurement of the flow velocity of the intracranial vessels. These tests are important from a clinical standpoint because they become abnormal as in-

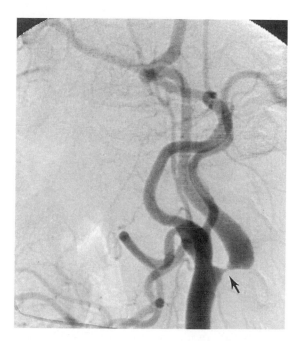

FIG. 5-3. Cerebral arteriogram which demonstrates a high-grade internal carotid artery stenosis (*arrow*).

TABLE 5-3. Noninvasive Tests of the Carotid Circulation

DIRECT TESTS	INDIRECT TESTS
Doppler ultrasonography	Oculoplethysmography
B mode ultrasound	Transcranial Doppler ultrasound
Duplex (Doppler combined with B-mode) ultrasound	Periorbital Doppler ultrasound
Bruit analysis	Thermography
	Opthalmodynamometry

ternal carotid stenosis becomes hemodynamically significant.

Digital intravenous subtraction angiography (DISA) represents a contrast study designed to visualize the extracranial and intracranial circulation by way of intravenous injection. This test was initially thought to have great potential to obviate the need for both other carotid noninvasive studies and routine angiography. Unfortunately, it is not completely noninvasive and has been associated with severe complications, including death. Furthermore, its accuracy in assessing the carotid bifurcation is similar to that of carotid ultrasound, and it is often limited in its ability to assess the intracranial circulation as well as the vertebrobasilar circulation. Digital subtraction techniques can also be applied to intra-arterial studies. This allows less contrast agent to be injected, but the views can be limited and the information derived incomplete. Carotid noninvasive studies do not necessarily obviate the need for cerebral angiography but they can help guide the clinician in selecting which patients are best suited for arteriographic evaluation.

Electroencephalography (EEG) is not routinely indicated in stroke disease. It can be useful in distinguishing focal seizure activity from fluctuating symptoms of stroke or TIA. The absence of an abnormality by EEG, in a patient with motor or sensory deficit secondary to stroke without accompanying cortical impairment, supports a subcortical location for the stroke; this is seen most commonly in lacunar-type stroke.

Lumbar puncture is also not routinely indicated in stroke disease. Evidence of mass effect secondary to stroke clearly contraindicates its performance. There are several clear-cut indications for lumbar puncture, if it can be performed safely, including positive syphilis serology, an unexplained fever or evidence of meningeal irritation, or the presence of atypical features such as relatively young age. It is important to remember that a lumbar puncture should not be performed in patients on anticoagulant therapy. Furthermore, the use of a high-resolution CT brain scan usually allows an adequate evaluation of a possible hemorrhagic lesion that would contraindicate anticoagulants. On the other hand, the sensitivity of CT scan in evaluating possible SAH is 89% according to one study. Thus, a lumbar puncture becomes mandatory if there is clinical suspicion of SAH even if the CT scan is negative.

Other studies that are useful in selected instances include serum lipid profile, blood cultures if there is a fever or other reason to suspect bacterial endocarditis, platelet function studies, and a connective tissue screen especially if vasculitis is suspected. In addition, a lupus anticoagulant assay, anticardiolipin antibody titers, protein C level, protein S level, and antithrombin III level should be obtained if a prothrombotic state is being considered. These studies may be especially pertinent in a relatively young patient with symptoms of stroke or TIA or in older individuals who have no known risk factors for cerebrovascular disease.

Magnetic resonance imaging (MR) brain scans appear to be more sensitive than CT scan for detecting cerebral infarction, especially in the region of the posterior fossa. An example of a midbrain infarct which was demonstrated by MR brain scan, when the CT brain scan was negative, is illustrated in Figure 5-4. CT scan has a sensitivity of approximately 70% in the detection of ischemic stroke, and it often takes several days for the infarct to be demonstrated by CT. On the other hand, CT is useful for immediately distinguishing an ischemic stroke

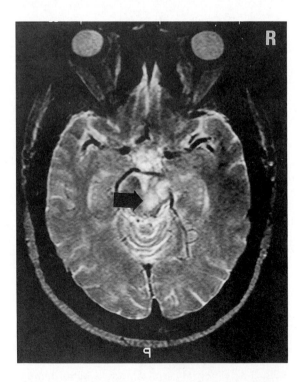

FIG. 5-4. MR brain scan which demonstrates an extensive infarction of the right midbrain (*arrow*).

from a hemorrhagic stroke. This is its primary purpose, from a clinical standpoint, because localization can usually be ascertained on the basis of signs and symptoms. The ability of MR to distinguish hemorrhagic from ischemic lesions has not been clearly delineated; therefore, a CT scan remains the preferred initial neuroimaging procedure in dealing with an acute stroke.

ISCHEMIC STROKE AND TRANSIENT ISCHEMIC ATTACK

PRESENTATION AND LOCALIZATION

Clinically, it does not usually take a great deal of acumen to diagnose a stroke. The patient presents typically with the sudden onset of a neurologic deficit referable to the central nervous system (CNS). Hemispheric events can be associated with headache; alteration of consciousness; speech disturbance including aphasia or dysarthria; homonymous hemi field visual deficits; cognitive impairment that might include apraxia or agnosia; and also contralateral motor or sensory dysfunction. Symptoms and signs referable to the brain stem or cerebellum include dysarthria, dysphagia, ataxia, diplopia, vertigo, nausea, various forms of nystagmus, drop attack, and various "crossed" impairments in sensory and motor function such as numbness on one side of the face and the opposite side of the body.

Certain clinical features are useful for cerebral localization. Infarcts involving the middle cerebral artery distribution typically result in aphasia, if the dominant hemisphere is affected, as well as contralateral motor weakness in which the face and arm are significantly weaker than the leg. Infarcts involving the anterior cerebral artery distribution typically cause significantly greater weakness in the contralateral leg than in the arm or face. An isolated homonymous hemianopia is usually localized to the contralateral posterior cerebral artery distribution.

A paresis which equally affects the face, arm, and leg, with no evidence of sensory loss or cortical dysfunction, is characteristic of lacunar infarct. This stroke syndrome, termed *pure motor stroke*, is usually attributable to a small infarct of the posterior limb of the internal capsule. The most common lacunar syndromes and their most likely anatomic correlates are outlined in Table 5-4.

Brain-stem syndromes often involve "crossed" findings such as numbness on one side of the face and the contralateral body or bilateral weakness.

TABLE 5-4. Most Common Lacunar-Type Stroke Syndromes and Associated Area of Involvement

LACUNAR SYNDROME	ANATOMIC LOCALIZATION
Pure motor	Posterior limb of the contralateral internal capsule or basis pontis
Pure sensory	Thalamus or parietal white matter
Sensorimotor	Posterior limb of the contralateral internal capsule
Clumsy hand-dysarthria	Basis pontis
Hemiparesis, hemiataxia	Midbrain or internal capsule

Since the extraocular movements are controlled, at the nuclear level, within the brain stem, visual manifestations such as diplopia and nystagmus are not uncommon. Dysarthria is more commonly seen with brain-stem stroke but can also be seen with hemispheric stroke. Bilateral visual loss suggests ischemia involving the vertebrobasilar system since the posterior cerebral arteries, which supply the occipital (visual) cortex, usually receive their primary blood supply by way of the vertebrobasilar system.

It is important to be able to distinguish carotid distribution TIAs from vertebrobasilar distribution TIAs. The internal carotid artery arises at the bifurcation of the common carotid artery within the neck. The internal carotid artery gives rise to the anterior and middle cerebral arteries. The circle of Willis is located at the base of the brain, at the origin of the vessels. The anterior cerebral arteries are connected by way of the anterior communicating artery, and the posterior communicating arteries serve as conduits between each internal carotid artery and the ipsilateral posterior cerebral artery. The external carotid artery is not usually clinically significant for cerebral blood supply unless there is significant stenosis or total occlusion of the ipsilateral internal carotid artery. In such a circumstance, the external carotid artery can become an important supplier of intracranial blood flow by way of collateralization through the ophthalmic artery. Such a phenomenon serves as the basis for performing periorbital Doppler ultrasound.

The vertebral arteries join at the mid-pons level to form the basilar artery. This artery then ascends along the ventral surface of the brain stem and terminates at the base of the brain, giving rise to the posterior cerebral arteries. The vertebrobasilar arterial system also supplies the entire brain stem and the cerebellum. It has been reported that the vertebrobasilar system is more susceptible to hypotension than the carotid system. Furthermore, vertebrobasilar TIAs appear to be more common than those affecting the carotid circulation.

The manifestations of carotid *vs* vertebrobasilar TIA are summarized in Table 5-5. It can be difficult to distinguish the two types, and it is not uncommon to see patients with symptoms referable to both carotid and vertebrobasilar distribution. Transient monocular blindness, or amaurosis fugax, always points to the carotid system as the involved distribution, whereas bilateral visual loss suggests the vertebrobasilar system. Transient aphasia is also a good indicator of carotid involvement, while it can be difficult to sort out the distribution when the signs are primarily motor or sensory. Perioral numbness typically represents brain-stem ischemia, and this is an important distinguishing characteristic. Many older people suffer from episodic vertigo. It is usually wise to attribute vertigo to vertebrobasilar insufficiency only if other symptoms of brain-stem dysfunction are present. Syncope can be seen secondary to vertebrobasilar ischemia; however, isolated syncope is much more commonly seen secondary to vasovagal phenomenon or to primary cardiac disease. Syncope is unlikely to be related to brain-stem ischemia unless other signs are associated with it, such as the sudden onset of vertigo and quadriparesis followed by a transient loss of consciousness.

PATHOGENESIS AND TREATMENT

A mechanistic approach should be adopted toward cerebral ischemia. An accurate evaluation of the mechanism of the ischemic stroke or TIA will certainly affect possible therapy. It is especially pertinent to recognize that TIA or minor stroke is a common harbinger of a major stroke. Typical lacunar-type stroke usually represents a thrombosis of a small, penetrating intracerebral artery. It is most commonly associated with hypertension or diabetes mellitus, and it is not believed to be related to embolic disease in most cases. Lacunar stroke is usually diagnosed on the basis of clinical features and by CT scan, which usually either shows a small (1 cm or less) area of infarction in a subcortical location or is negative. Lacunar strokes tend typically to have a good prognosis for functional recovery. One would not expect that an extensive cardiac or extracranial vascular work-up is necessary. Furthermore, there is little, if any, need to consider possible anticoagulant therapy. The major therapeutic approach should be toward optimal antihypertensive or diabetic management and intensive rehabilitative therapy.

It is important to try to distinguish cerebral embolus from large-artery thrombosis as accurately as possible, mainly because most recent studies support the efficacy of immediate use of anticoagulant therapy in preventing recurrent cerebral embolus. The most important indicator of cerebral embolus is the documentation of a cardiogenic source of embolus in a patient with an ischemic stroke. Other

TABLE 5-5. **Manifestations of Transient Ischemic Attack**

CAROTID DISTRIBUTION	VERTEBROBASILAR DISTRIBUTION
Aphasia	Bilateral visual loss
Transient monocular blindness (amaurosis fugax)	Ataxia
	Quadriparesis
Hemiparesis	Perioral numbness
Hemisensory deficit	"Crossed" sensory or motor deficits
Homonymous hemianopsia in combination with motor or sensory deficit	Combination of two or more of the following:
	Vertigo
	Syncope
	Dysarthria
	Diplopia
	Nausea
	Dysphagia
	Drop attack especially when seen in association with a motor or sensory deficit

features that help to support cerebral embolus as the most likely mechanism include multiple vascular territory involvement, conversion of an initially ischemic to hemorrhagic infarct, sudden onset of maximal neurologic deficit without premonitory TIA, and evidence of embolic involvement of other organs. Large-artery thrombotic stroke is often preceded by TIAs, and the location of the ischemia does not tend to follow a specific vascular territory as it does with cerebral embolism. For example, a branch occlusion of the inferior division of a middle cerebral artery would most likely be embolic in origin.

The therapy for ischemic stroke remains controversial; however, the following general principles can never be overemphasized:

1. Early mobilization of the patient, as tolerated, to prevent complications of bed confinement
2. Proper bowel program consisting of stool softener with bulk agent and cathartic, as needed
3. Consultation with the appropriate rehabilitative services that may include speech therapy, occupational therapy, and physical therapy
4. Consultation with social services to assess possible placement in a rehabilitative facility or nursing home or to aid in the evaluation of home care needs
5. Emotional support that might include the judicious use of antidepressant therapy and referral to support groups such as stroke clubs
6. Long-term management of risk factors for ischemic stroke such as optimal antihypertensive therapy and proper diet

Optimal control of hypertension in acute ischemic stroke does not need to be immediately achieved, and overly aggressive blood pressure control can be deleterious. Hypotension can impair cerebral perfusion in acute stroke as cerebral autoregulation (the maintenance of CBF despite blood pressure fluctuations) is disrupted. Therefore, gradual lowering of an elevated blood pressure is recommended in acute ischemic stroke unless, of course, the patient is in hypertensive crisis.

Anticoagulant therapy is the most efficacious in preventing stroke when there is a definite cardiogenic source of embolus. In the Stroke Prevention in Atrial Fibrillation Study, treatment was far superior to placebo in the prevention of stroke in patients with nonvalvular atrial fibrillation. The risk reduction for embolic events was 67% for warfarin and 42% for aspirin at a dose of 325 mg per day. This study is proceeding to answer which is the optimal agent from a risks vs benefits standpoint. It is important to recognize that anticoagulants are definitely contraindicated if there is evidence of cerebral hemorrhage by CT scan or if the patient has a bleeding diathesis or another medical condition that prevents the use of anticoagulants. A major concern is the potential for anticoagulants to convert an initially ischemic stroke to a hemorrhagic infarct. Factors that appear to increase the likelihood of this occurring include too long a prolongation of the coagulation parameters, large infarction, advanced age, and poorly controlled blood pressure. The use of long-term anticoagulation therapy also requires that the patient be compliant.

Anticoagulant therapy is also used for a progressive stroke, especially in the vertebrobasilar territory, and for the acute management of TIA. The efficacy of anticoagulants in these circumstances remains a moot point; however, they tend to be used regularly in selected patients by clinicians with considerable experience in ischemic stroke.

Several therapeutic modalities have gained attention as having the capability to reduce infarct size. These therapies include calcium channel-blocking agents, agents which serve as free radical scavengers, tissue plasminogen activator, and GM1-ganglioside. Their possible efficacy has not yet been established, however, as we await the results of ongoing clinical trials.

The Canadian Cooperative Study reported that aspirin, at dosage of 325 mg four times per day, reduced the risk of stroke and sudden death in men who had TIA by approximately 50%. Unfortunately, no benefit was seen in women. A further study, performed in Britain, found that 300 mg of aspirin per day was of equal efficacy to 1300 mg per day. A recent study found a benefit with 75 mg per day. The European Stroke Prevention Study found that the combination of aspirin, at a dose of 330 mg t.i.d., with dipyridamole, at a dose of 75 mg t.i.d., was superior to placebo and reduced the risk of stroke in both men and women. The agent ticlopidine, which is a nonsteroidal anti-inflammatory drug, has antiplatelet activity. In one study of subjects with TIA or minor stroke, there was a 21% reduction in stroke in patients receiving ticlopidine, 250 mg b.i.d., compared with those receiving aspirin, 1300 mg per day; the effect was even greater in women than in men. In another trial, there was a 30% reduction in stroke, heart attack, or vascular death compared with aspirin. The side effects, especially the small but real risk of neutropenia and thrombocytopenia, as well as cost, have limited the use of ticlopidine to date.

There have been three recent studies which have demonstrated that carotid endarterectomy is superior to medical therapy in subjects with symptomatic internal carotid artery stenosis of 70% to 99%. These studies were based on medically stable patients and the performance of the cerebral arteriogram and the surgical procedure at medical centers where the complication rate was exceptionally low. These studies are continuing to address the issue of the best therapy for subjects with 30% to 69% stenosis.

INTRACEREBRAL HEMORRHAGE

CLINICAL APPROACH

A number of possible etiologies exist for ICH (Table 5-6). The most common mechanism is hypertensive intracerebral hemorrhage. This type of bleeding is related to the presence of microaneurysms that form as a sequela of chronic hypertension. These are termed *Charcot–Bouchard aneurysms*, and their location corresponds to the most frequent sites of hypertensive intracerebral hemorrhage: the basal ganglia, thalamus, pons, and cerebellum. The most common site of occurrence is in the lenticulostriate artery territory, with at least half of all hypertensive bleeds occurring in the region of the basal ganglia. For all intents and purposes, a patient presenting with a basal ganglionic or thalamic hematoma who is also hypertensive has hypertension as the mechanism, and it is highly unlikely that another etiology

TABLE 5-6. Causes of Spontaneous Intracerebral Hemorrhage

1. Hypertension
2. Intracranial aneurysm
3. Arteriovenous malformation
4. Bleeding diathesis
5. Anticoagulant therapy
6. Illicit drugs (*e.g.*, cocaine)
7. Mycotic aneurysm
8. Hemorrhagic metastasis
9. Bleed into a primary brain tumor
10. Bleed into a brain abscess
11. Arteritis secondary to connective tissue disease
12. Amyloid angiopathy
13. Hemorrhagic leukoencephalopathy
14. Idiopathic? cryptic arteriovenous malformation

such as an AVM needs to be considered. On the other hand, only about 50% of lobar hemorrhages are hypertensive in mechanism, and other diagnoses need to be excluded.

The patients should be examined for evidence of head trauma, especially if no history is available, and all patients with ICH should be screened for a bleeding diathesis. In addition, a previous history of malignancy, especially lung cancer, breast cancer, renal cell carcinoma, melanoma, and thyroid carcinoma, should raise the suspicion of a hemorrhagic metastasis. Multiple lobar hemorrhages in an elderly patient, especially if there is a history of dementia, should raise the question of amyloid angiopathy.

It can be difficult to distinguish a patient with ICH from a patient with an ischemic infarct on clinical grounds. Certain features, however, help in making this distinction. An intracerebral bleed tends to be a precipitous event with no premonitory symptoms except, perhaps, for a headache. If hypertension is the mechanism, one usually finds an impressively elevated blood pressure on presentation and there is often a history of poor compliance with antihypertensive therapy. The bleeding tends to spontaneously subside, in patients who survive, within about 4 to 5 hours. During this interval, however, the patient's neurologic status may progressively deteriorate.

Signs of increased intracranial pressure are often found in a patient with ICH. These signs might include severe headache, alteration of consciousness, papilledema, pupillary asymmetry, and posturing of the extremities. It is not uncommon for the event to be catastrophic, and patients may often present in a moribund condition with little to be offered from a medical standpoint. The mortality rate approaches 50% within 30 days.

The CT brain scan is the definitive study in most patients with ICH. An area (or areas) of increased attenuation is typically apparent within the parenchyma (Fig. 5-5). This study also reveals whether or not there is an intraventricular extension, which, if present, is associated with a worse prognosis. This finding reflects the fact that larger hemorrhages are more likely to have an extension within the ventricular system. Larger hematomas, greater than 3 cm, are associated with a significantly worse prognosis than smaller hematomas. The prognosis depends not only on the size and the presence of intraventricular extension but also on the location of the hematoma. A large hemorrhage, for example, is not required to cause devastating results when the area of involvement is the pons.

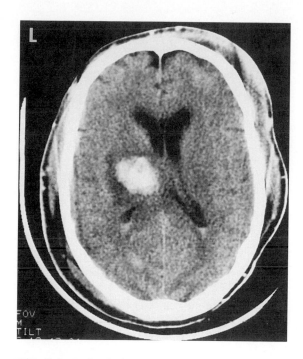

FIG. 5-5. Left thalamic hematoma, as demonstrated by CT brain scan, in a patient with long-standing hypertension.

Atypical location, lack of a definite history of hypertension, relatively young age, or CT scan findings suggestive of a vascular anomaly or tumor may lead to angiographic investigation. This procedure is often best delayed until the hemorrhage has reabsorbed and the mass effect has resolved; this will allow better visualization of the vessels in the area of the bleed so that a possible vascular anomaly such as an AVM or aneurysm can be excluded. The complete reabsorption of the hematoma by CT scan usually occurs in 6 to 8 weeks. It is important to keep in mind that arteritis secondary to systemic lupus erythematosus or polyarteritis nodosa can result in intracranial hemorrhage.

MANAGEMENT

The guidelines outlined for routine care of patients with ischemic stroke also apply to patients with hemorrhagic stroke. The major aspects of therapy for ICH concern the treatment of increased intracranial pressure, aggressive control of elevated

blood pressure, protection of the airway, and evacuation of the hematoma in selected cases. A significant number of patients have a limited neurologic deficit, and they can be expected to have a very good outcome. These patients primarily require optimal blood pressure control, if hypertensive, and an evaluation by the rehabilitative service if appropriate.

Patients presenting in a stuporous or semi-comatose state may still have a reasonably good prognosis if they are medically stable and relatively young, and if they do not have progression of the neurologic deficit. Surgical evacuation of an intracerebral hematoma, in selected cases, may possibly result in a dramatic improvement. This is especially important in patients with cerebellar hematoma *prior* to the development of long tract signs or respiratory compromise.

The management of significantly increased intracranial pressure is an emergent problem and requires aggressive management. The primary methods are to use a combination of hyperventilation (to lower CBF) and either mannitol or glycerol to combat cerebral edema. Corticosteroids were not found to be beneficial in one recently published series. A significant component of vasogenic edema is often associated with intracerebral hemorrhage, which makes at least part of the mass effect amenable to antiedema therapy. This acute management must be tempered by prognostic implications. A moribund patient will usually not have a significant response to such therapy, but this type of management may allow time to establish the diagnosis, to evaluate for possible surgical intervention, and to give the family more time to prepare for the imminent death of a loved one.

The presence of intraventricular extension is usually associated with a poor prognosis. Blood within the ventricles can promote an inflammatory reaction, a ventriculitis, that can lead to a communicating hydrocephalus. Such patients should be monitored for this development, because they may show progressive neurologic deterioration and may require ventricular shunting.

SUBARACHNOID HEMORRHAGE

The two most likely causes of spontaneous (*i.e.*, nontraumatic) SAH are rupture of an intracranial aneurysm and bleeding associated with an AVM.

These possibilities must be considered in any patient presenting with a severe headache. This is especially pertinent if coexistent meningeal irritation is evident.

INTRACRANIAL ANEURYSM

An aneurysm represents a localized outpouching of an artery and is often described as *berry* or *saccular*. Most intracerebral aneurysms (approximately 85%) are found at the base of the brain, specifically at vessel bifurcations. Intracerebral aneurysms are usually congenital in origin and are related to a defect within the vessel wall. Hemodynamic factors, such as hypertension or a coexistent AVM, may promote the enlargement or rupture of an aneurysm.

The typical presentation of a ruptured berry aneurysm is a severe headache secondary to extravasation of blood into the subarachnoid space. The headache is often accompanied by meningeal irritation and focal neurologic deficit. One clinical syndrome is the presence of a third cranial nerve palsy accompanied by a severe headache. This is related to the relatively common occurrence of an aneurysm at the junction of the internal carotid artery and posterior communicating artery in the vicinity of the third cranial nerve as it traverses from the midbrain (Fig. 5-6).

A large intracerebral aneurysm can be demonstrated by CT scan; however, confirmation generally requires cerebral angiography. These techniques are capable of allowing the incidental detection of an unruptured aneurysm. A study performed to evaluate the natural history of unruptured aneurysms led to the finding that no patient with an aneurysm less than 1 cm in diameter suffered a rupture during the follow-up. On the other hand, 38% of patients with an aneurysm 1 cm or greater in diameter had an eventful rupture. One may conclude from this study that incidental aneurysms, 1 cm or greater in diameter, are at such a significant risk for eventual rupture that surgical clipping of the aneurysm in selected individuals may be indicated.

The mortality and major morbidity associated with aneursymal rupture are greatest within the first 2 weeks of onset. For patients who survive the initial bleed, a significant rate of complications including rebleeding, vasospasm with secondary ischemic infarction, and the development of hydrocephalus may occur. According to one series, the mortality rate at 8 months was approximately 50%,

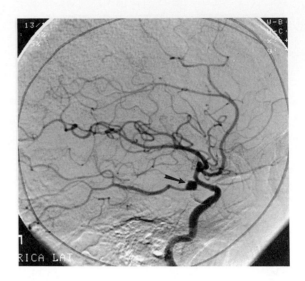

FIG. 5-6. Cerebral arteriogram which demonstrates an aneurysm of the right posterior communicating artery (*arrow*).

with one-quarter of the patients being able to return to work and one-quarter being significantly disabled. The outcome appears to be improved by effective surgical clipping of the aneurysm. The major goals of therapy are to stabilize the patient medically, and neurologically, so that surgery can be performed safely. This goal depends greatly on the prevention of rebleeding and vasospasm.

Approximately 20% to 30% of patients with aneurysmal rupture will rebleed within the first 2 weeks, and the result will be fatal in about 75% of instances. The risk of vasospasm with secondary ischemic infarction appears related to the amount of subarachnoid blood. An accurate estimate of the incidence of vasospasm is difficult to determine because it depends on several factors, including the length of survival, the timing of surgery, and the criteria for what constitutes vasospasm.

The natural history of a ruptured intracerebral aneurysm is improved by surgical clipping of the aneurysm, assuming that the patient is medically and neurologically stable, and that the neurosurgeon has exceptional skill and experience. The most opportune time to operate remains controversial, although many neurosurgeons now advocate early surgery (*i.e.*, within the first 2 or 3 days) if the patient has only headache and/or minor neurologic deficit. Beyond the first few days, the risk of vasospasm precludes surgery for approximately 2 weeks. Most studies appear to support the use of antifibrinolytic therapy in preventing recurrent bleeding, especially if surgery is delayed. The most commonly used agent, epsilon aminocaproic acid, has been reported to reduce the risk of rebleeding by approximately 50%. Despite this, its use has been tempered by recent reports that suggest that this agent does not have a convincing salubrious effect on outcome. Various therapies have been used to prevent vasospasm. Nimodipine, a calcium channel-blocking agent, is now available for the prevention of aneurysmal rupture—mediated vasospasm. The recommended oral dosage is 60 mg every 4 hours for 21 consecutive days.

ARTERIOVENOUS MALFORMATION

AVM is an anomaly of embryonal development in which a tangle of arteries and veins is associated with a tendency to bleed suddenly. Aneurysms are generally the most common cause of SAH in persons between the ages of 20 and 70 years, whereas AVMs are second in order of frequency and usually present by 40 years of age. The vascular anomaly is present from birth, and the lesion usually manifests itself between the ages of 10 and 30. The reason why AVMs are twice as common in men as in women is unknown. The prevalence of AVM in the general population is estimated at 0.14%; fortunately, most AVMs remain clinically silent throughout life.

Approximately 50% of patients who are symptomatic from an AVM have either ICH or SAH. Another 30% of patients present with seizure; the remaining 20% of patients present with headache, focal neurologic deficit, or dementia. Of patients presenting with ICH, one-quarter to one-half suffer serious consequences, including death. In addition, the recurrence rate of hemorrhage is 7% within the first year. Of patients with AVM who present with seizure, 1% will suffer ICH within 1 year. Due to such statistics, physicians have searched for a therapeutic intervention that might reduce the risk of ICH.

The optimal therapy is total surgical resection of the AVM if this can be performed safely with minimal neurologic sequelae. There has been considerable interest in embolization of nonsurgically accessible AVMs; however, at least one study has found no significant reduction in the recurrence rate for hemorrhage with this modality. Conventional radiation therapy has been tried in an effort to encase the AVM with scar tissue to prevent rebleeding, but no benefit was found. The use of proton-beam therapy, although not routinely available, has been found to reduce the risk of rebleeding especially after the first 12 months post-therapy. Reduction in the size of an AVM can also be seen with gamma radiation, the so-called gamma knife, but this therapy is reserved for inoperable AVMs. An improvement in neurologic status has been reported with both proton-beam and gamma-knife radiation. This therapy, which holds considerable promise, is designed to reduce the lumen diameter of the involved vessels and to thicken the surrounding wall of the AVM. One can see total obliteration of the AVM in selected cases.

QUESTIONS AND DISCUSSION

1. A 65-year-old man presents with the recent onset of right hemiparesis that equally involves his face, arm, and leg. No headache, speech disturbance, sensory loss, or other neurologic deficit is noted. Past medical history is pertinent for long-standing hypertension. There is no history of heart disease, and an electrocardiogram reveals normal sinus rhythm and left ventricular hypertrophy. The serum VDRL and FTA-ABS are both nonreactive. What diagnostic studies appear to be definitely indicated in this patient?

   A. Echocardiogram
   B. Lumbar puncture
   C. Cerebral angiography
   D. EEG
   E. None of the above

This patient has a pure motor stroke with no evidence of cortical involvement clinically. This finding, in association with long-standing hypertension, strongly supports the diagnosis of a left lacunar infarction that most likely involves the posterior limb of the internal capsule. The pathogenesis involves a small-artery thrombotic occlusion, and the patient does not require an extensive work-up for an embolic source such as echocardiography or cerebral angiography. The lumbar puncture is also not definitely indicated since the syphilis serology is nonreactive and meningeal irritation is not evident from a clinical standpoint. The electroencephalogram, if it is completely normal, might help to confirm the presence of a subcortical process but, based on the clinical features, it becomes a superfluous study. Thus, the correct answer is (E). If, on the other hand, there were atypical features, such as the absence of hypertension or the presence of atrial fibrillation, then a follow-up CT scan might be in order in an effort to corroborate the presence of a lacune in the capsular region and thus further support the diagnostic approach as outline above.

2. A 47-year-old male patient is found in his home in an unresponsive condition. On admission to the emergency room, he is noted to have labored respirations, his blood pressure is 220/140, he has asymmetric pupils and early papilledema, and he postures his right side when stimulated. The proper diagnostic approach to this patient would be:

    A. Emergency lumbar puncture to rule out meningitis
    B. Careful examination for evidence of head trauma
    C. Stat blood work including CBC, prothrombin time or partial thromboplastin time, platelet count, and arterial blood gas
    D. Stabilization of the patient medically, including blood pressure control and possible intubation
    E. B, C, and D

This patient most likely has a large intracerebral hematoma, based on clinical features described previously, that is probably hypertensive in mechanism. His prognosis does not appear to be good but, given his young age and the fact that a diagnosis has not yet been established, it is important to stabilize him medically, to examine him for head trauma to evaluate the possibility of subdural or epidural hematoma, and to perform diagnostic studies including CT brain scan and the blood work previously listed. The answer is (E). A lumbar puncture is certainly not indicated in light of the evidence of increased intracranial pressure.

3. A 73-year-old woman is admitted with the new onset of right-sided weakness and nonfluent aphasia. Her weakness primarily involves the face and right upper extremity. She is found to have atrial fibrillation on electrocardiography, and a CT scan reveals an early left middle cerebral artery distribution ischemic infarct and an old right middle cerebral artery infarct. The most likely mechanism of her stroke is:

A. Cerebral large-artery thrombosis
B. Cerebral embolus
C. Lacune

The answer is (B). The fact that this is associated with cortical deficit (aphasia) rules out the possibility of lacune, and the CT scan is not compatible with this diagnosis. This could possibly represent a large-artery thrombosis; however, the presence of a definite cardiogenic source of embolus (atrial fibrillation) and multiple vascular territory involvement makes cerebral embolus the most likely mechanism.

4. A 36-year-old right-handed male patient has been having recurrent right-sided headache for several years. This has been attributed to migraine. The patient is examined in the emergency room for new onset of right (focal) seizures. A CT brain scan is performed with contrast, and it reveals a large left cerebral hemispheric contrast enhancing lesion that has characteristics of an AVM. This diagnosis is confirmed by cerebral angiography. A therapeutic approach that would seem appropriate in this patient would include:

    A. Surgical resection of the AVM
    B. Initiation of anticonvulsant therapy
    C. A course of routine radiation therapy
    D. Embolic therapy of the AVM

This AVM is large and presumably involves the dominant cerebral hemisphere. Therefore, resection of the AVM would not be indicated because it might well leave the patient with a significant neurologic deficit. As discussed in the chapter, routine radiation therapy has not been found to be protective in preventing complications from an AVM, although proton-beam therapy and the gamma knife both appear to show considerable promise. Embolization therapy, although an attractive concept, has not been established as providing significant benefit in such patients. The correct answer is (B), because this patient has developed focal epilepsy as a complication of his AVM.

SUGGESTED READING

Allen GS, Ahn HS, Preziosi TJ, et al: Cerebral arterial spasm—a controlled trial of nimodipine in patients with subarachnoid hemorrhage. N Engl J Med 308:619, 1983

Bloomfield P, Wheatley DJ, Prescott RJ, et al: Twelve-year comparison of a Bjork-Shiley mechanical heart valve with porcine prosthesis. N Engl J Med 324:573, 1991

Broderick JP, Brott T, Tomsick T, et al: The risk of subarachnoid and intracerebral hemorrhage in blacks as compared with whites. N Engl J Med 326:733, 1992

Canadian Cooperative Study Group: A randomized trial of aspirin and sulfinpyrazone in threatened stroke. N Engl J Med 299:53, 1978

Dyken ML, Wolf PA, Barnett HJM, et al: Risk factors in stroke. Stroke 15:1105, 1984

Easton JD, Sherman DG: Management of cerebral embolism of cardiac origin. Stroke 11:433, 1980

Gant M, Blakely JA, Easton DJ, Ellis DJ: The Canadian–American ticlopidine study (CATS) in thromboembolic stroke. Lancet 1:1260, 1989

Hass WK, Easton DJ, Adams HP, Pryse-Phillips W: A randomized trial comparing ticlopidine hydrochloride with aspirin for the prevention of stroke in high-risk patients. N Engl J Med 321:501, 1989

Kelley RE, Kovacs AG: Mechanism of in-hospital ischemia. Stroke 17:430, 1986

Kjellberg RN, Hanamura T, Davis KR, et al: Bragg-peak proton beam therapy for arteriovenous malformations of the brain. N Engl J Med 309:269, 1983

Levine M, Hirsh J: Hemorrhagic complications of long-term anticoagulant therapy for ischemic cerebral vascular disease. Stroke 17:111, 1986

Mohr JP, Caplan LR, Melski JW, et al: The Harvard Cooperative Stroke Registry: A prospective registry. Neurology 28:754, 1978

North American Symptomatic Carotid Endarterectomy Trial Collaborators: Beneficial effects of carotid endarterectomy in symptomatic patients with high grade stenosis. N Engl J Med 325:445, 1991

Poungvarin N, Bhoopat W, Viriyavejakul A, et al: Effects of dexamethasone in primary supratentorial intracerebral hemorrhage. N Engl J Med 316:1229, 1987

Sivenius J, Laakso M, Penttila IM, et al: The European Stroke Prevention Study: Results according to sex. Neurology 41:1189, 1991

SPAF Investigators: Preliminary report of the Stroke Prevention in Atrial Fibrillation Study. N Engl J Med 322:863, 1990

Chronic Headache: Current Concepts in Diagnosis and Treatment

Joel R. Saper

Perspectives on migraine are changing rapidly. With these changes comes a reconsideration of fundamental attitudes toward the headache problem, among which are who suffers from headache, why, when, and how should it be treated.

During the past several years, the emphasis on peripheral phenomena (blood vessels and muscles) and separateness between migraine and tension headache disorders has been challenged, and this challenge is reflected in a reappraisal of the treatment of headache. Several authors have cited data supporting the view that migraine and tension headache are physiologically related entities, with a varied symptomatic expression reflecting a central or central–peripheral disturbance of neuroreceptor and neurovascular function.

The central hypothesis is supported by physiologic events that are purported to occur during headache, the symptom overlap between migraine and tension headache, the general acknowledgment that clinical phenomena including pain cannot be satisfactorily or entirely explained by disturbances of the vascular or muscular structures alone, conflicting vascular flow studies that appear to challenge traditional views on the order of events in migraine, and therapeutic considerations that raise doubts as to the presumed mechanism of well-known headache therapies. Drugs initially believed useful for migraine or muscle contraction headache appear valuable in both disorders. In fact, the wide-ranging pharmacologic actions of drugs found useful in chronic headache disorders appear to share an influence on central brain mechanisms more than a specific vascular or muscular influence.

EPIDEMIOLOGY OF HEADACHE

Seventy-six percent of women and 57% of men report at least one significant headache per month, and over 90% have experienced a headache in their lifetime (CDC, 1991). Headache prevalence in children increases from 39% at age 6 to 70% by age 15. Moreover, it is estimated that 1 million days of missed school and over 150 million days of lost work per year are attributable to headache. Lost-productivity estimates for the United States work force per year range from $6.5 to $17.2 billion.

Among migraine sufferers, 86% of females and 82% of males report some disability with each attack. Thirty-one percent of persons with headache have regular, periodic functional impairment. Despite the painful and disabling impact of headache, many such patients do not seek medical care. Sixty percent of females and 70% of males with typical migraine have never been properly diagnosed.

In a recent report from the Centers for Disease Control (1990), a 60% increase in the prevalence of migraine during the years 1980–1989 was noted. Eight percent of sufferers are hospitalized at least

William J. Weiner and Christopher G. Goetz, eds. *Neurology for the Non-Neurologist*, Third Edition. Copyright © 1994, 1989 by J. B. Lippincott Company. Copyright © 1981 by Harper and Row Publishers, Inc.

once yearly, and 4% of men and 3% of women have a persistently impaired existence.

Independent of quality-of-life considerations, it is estimated that the annual cost of a migraine sufferer to an employer is from $5256 to $6864 per man and $3168 to $3600 per woman.

CLASSIFICATION of HEADACHE

The *primary headaches*, that is, migraine and cluster headaches, are those in which no consistently identified organic cause can be determined. *Secondary headaches* are those associated with a variety of organic etiologies. Until recently, the primary classification of headache was based upon the Ad Hoc Committee Report, published in 1962. Following an international effort engineered by Professor Jes Olesen of Copenhagen, the International Headache Society (IHS) has proposed a new classification of headache, informally known as the International Classification. This comprehensive document attempts to reconcile the many and complex aspects of headache into a usable system. Its ultimate acceptance and usability remain to be defined, but it has, if nothing else, organized headache comprehensively for the first time.

The new classification of headache gives more precision to the diagnosis of headache in general, and migraine specifically. Common migraine is now called *migraine without aura* and is defined in terms of duration, quality, and associated symptoms accompanying each attack.

Classic migraine is now called *migraine with aura*, and the features of the aura are delineated in greater detail.

Tension-type headache is the new term for what has previously been called tension headache, muscle contraction headache, stress headache, and ordinary headache. The classification distinguishes between patients with episodic (acute) tension-type headaches and chronic tension-type headaches, with subclassifications based upon the presence of absence of increased tenderness of the pericranial muscles or increased electromyographic (EMG) activity.

Cluster headache and chronic paroxysmal hemicrania are also classified, as are a variety of miscellaneous conditions and headache phenomena. Thirteen categories of headache are subdivided into 129 different subtypes.

TRADITIONAL CONCEPTS in HEADACHE PATHOGENESIS

THE "MUSCLE THEORY"

The muscular concept of headache states that tension-type headaches are secondary to increased muscle contraction in the pericranial and cervical musculature. Studies, however, do not support this mechanism as a primary cause of pain. In fact, more muscle contraction is present in migraineurs than in tension headache patients!

THE "VASCULAR THEORY" OF MIGRAINE

This concept is fundamentally committed to the belief that migraine aura is primarily due to cerebral ischemia from vasoconstriction as the initial event and that the headache itself is the result of reactive vasodilation. Pain is thought to be enhanced by vasoactive polypeptides in the tissues surrounding the external carotid artery.

However, cerebral blood flow (CBF) studies do not support the traditional vascular theory. A decrease in CBF does occur during migraine with aura but not in migraine without aura. However, *the changes in migraine with aura are neither sufficient nor anatomically consistent to explain the neurologic events.*

In migraine with aura, a wave of reduced blood flow (oligemia) spreads forward from the occipital area and precedes the aura. It persists into the headache phase.

Historically important work by Leao demonstrated that electrically stimulated rabbit cortex exhibited a wave of spreading electrical depression that moved over the cortex at a rate of 2 to 3 mm/minute. This rate of spreading depression is similar to the spread of oligemia in patients with migraine with aura. Lashley, a researcher who himself suffered migraine with aura, mapped out the rate of progression of his own scintillating scotoma across his visual field. He calculated that it corresponded to a rate over his occipital cortex of 2 to 3 mm/minute. Thus, the rates of development of the scotomata, spreading oligemia, and spreading electrical depression are approximately the same. Many authorities now believe that the oligemia is secondary to a primary neurogenic event.

THE NEUROGENIC CONCEPTS

The neurogenic theory of migraine suggests that migraine is caused by a primary disturbance of brain function. CBF studies in migraine with aura are most consistent with a primary neuronal event producing secondary vascular changes. Magnetoencephalographic studies of the brain during a migraine attack support the concept of spreading depression in migraine, as described earlier.

In favor of the neurogenic concept of migraine are the following:

The presence of premonitory symptoms suggestive of hypothalamic origin;

The visual aura that crosses vascular territories (due to spreading depression?);

Associated symptoms, such as nausea/vomiting and hypersensitivity to sensory stimuli;

Magnetoencephalographic findings confirming spreading depression; and

Magnetic resonance spectroscopy showing increased high-energy phosphate consumption and low intracellular magnesium.

These studies and the data described later in the text suggest that the brain of migraineurs, even between attacks, is physiologically abnormal (see Welch, 1990).

Thus, while the traditional view of headache pathogenesis relies upon explanations involving vasoconstriction, vasodilation, and muscle contraction, increasing data support the view that neurogenic concepts are of primary importance. Moreover, most drugs that control migraine preventively, and perhaps symptomatically as well, appear to do so via a mechanism involving serotonin or serotonin receptor dynamics.

DIAGNOSTIC EVALUATION OF HEADACHE DISORDERS

Over 300 causes of headache are established and, to some extent, each general category of disease must be considered in the evaluation of a headache patient. A thorough and complete history with emphasis on onset, quality, and quantity of pain; frequency; and provoking influences must be determined. A complete physical examination with appropriate emphasis on neurologic, otologic, and general physical considerations is likewise necessary. Psychological factors must be considered, but premature emphasis should be avoided, since most authorities now believe that psychological factors are not the likely cause of headache except in a very small group of patients.

A complete set of blood studies (looking for metabolic, infectious, autoimmune, and endocrinologic disturbances), electroencephalogram (EEG), and computed tomography (CT) scan or magnetic resonance imaging (MR) are indicated in most patients with chronic, persistent headache or those associated with neurologic, mental, or behavioral disturbances. Specific tests evaluating carotid flow, cardiac function, serum catecholamines, specific otologic functions, temporomandibular joint (TMJ), and others are appropriate when indicated by the nature of the history and physical examination.

GENERAL TREATMENT CONSIDERATIONS

A global assessment of the patient's life-style, emotional needs, and physiologic vulnerabilities is essential. The traditional focus of physicians on symptoms must make way for an emphasis on the individual primarily and the symptom secondarily.

The successful preventive as well as symptomatic treatment of migraine requires patience and innovativeness. Therapy in all cases must be modeled to meet individual differences in general health, psychological makeup, headache pattern, and patient compliance.

MIGRAINE

A more detailed description of treatment of headache can be found in the *Handbook of Headache Management*. Migraine can be classified as either *migraine with aura*, formerly called classic migraine, or *migraine without aura*, formerly called common migraine. Migraine with aura is the most well known of the two subtypes but accounts for less than 20% of all migraine attacks. Despite this disproportion, a large number of physicians incorrectly employ the features of migraine with aura as the diagnostic criteria for all migraine attacks.

Migraine with aura is a biphasic event in which a prodromal phase (aura) is followed by a headache phase. This preheadache phase is typically characterized by one or more physiologic events, usually of a neurologic nature *e.g.*, transient visual, motor, or sensory phenomena).

The headache phase of a migraine with aura usually begins at about the time that the prodromal symptoms fade. It is frequently characterized by unilateral, but sometimes bilateral, pulsating pain that lasts for hours to a day or longer. The pain is usually moderate to intense in severity, but may be mild. Although the prodromal symptoms generally precede the headache in a migraine with aura attack, neurologic or ophthalmologic symptoms may develop during or even after the onset of the headache.

Hemiplegic, aphasic, and *hemisensory migraine* are terms applied to a subgroup of migraine with aura; they refer to the nature of the premonitory signs and symptoms, reflecting sharply focal disturbances involving the cerebral hemispheres. *Vertebral basilar migraine* (VBM) is yet another variant. The preheadache phase of VBM reflects disturbances in the brain stem and hypothalamic, thalamic, occipital, and posterior cerebral regions, all of which are fed by branches of the vertebrobasilar arterial system. Thus, ataxia, ophthalmoplegia, loss of consciousness, dysarthria, vertigo, or sensory, autonomic, and bilateral visual disturbances can occur.

When the neurologic deficits in migraine with aura are intense or prolonged, the term *complicated migraine* may be used. The neurologic symptoms of migraine with aura may not terminate, occasionally resulting in permanent residual deficits.

By contrast, migraine without aura has a less sharply defined onset and is not heralded by a distinct prodromal event, although vague and widely varied constitutional, psychic, gastrointestinal, and autonomic disturbances may precede the headache by several hours or days. The headache may be unilateral or bilateral; it is usually intense in severity; and it commonly affects the eyes, frontal regions, temples, vertex, and occiput. The headache often lasts for a day or longer, sometimes lasting up to a week.

Migraine may actually have at least four, or perhaps even five, phases. Well before the first sign of the neurologic events in migraine with aura, or the headache in migraine without aura, many patients will experience changes in mood, appetite, sleep, fluid and electrolyte balance, or bowel function. Changes in appetite may take the form of food cravings, and disturbances of mood may take the form of euphoria, lethargy, or depression. These phenomena give way over several hours to days to the aura in migraine with aura or to the headache in migraine without aura. Following the attack of head pain, patients generally feel fatigued and lethargic, and they may rarely feel confused for a day or longer, thus providing the basis for a *postictal* phase.

Most but not all attacks of migraine are accompanied by head pain. The pain is commonly uni-lateral but may be bilateral in one-third or more of the cases. Although the pain is frequently throbbing, as the attack evolves a dull aching, nonthrobbing discomfort may prevail. Pain may be located anywhere about the head or neck and may actually begin with a throbbing or tightness in the neck area. Pain may vary from mild to annoying, to severe and incapacitating.

It must be emphasized that migraine is a generalized disorder, simultaneously affecting many systems throughout the body. Anorexia, abdominal cramping, nausea, vomiting, diarrhea, and other gastrointestinal disturbances are frequently present and are thought to arise on a cerebral level. Visual symptoms are wide and varied, ranging from photophobia and blurred vision to major scotomata or hemianoptic disruptions. Autonomic disturbances including lassitude, mental cloudiness, and irritability may precede, accompany, or follow both migraine with aura and migraine without aura types of attack. Confusion, difficulty in speaking, and disorientation have all been reported in children and may occur as a component of the VBM form.

The term *migraine equivalents* describes various autonomic symptoms such as abdominal pain, nausea, vomiting, tachycardia, vertigo, cyclic edema, and chest, thoracic, and pelvic pain that are all thought to be caused by the same pathophysiologic event of migraine, only without head pain accompaniments. Migraine equivalents frequently occur in children who have a predisposition to migraine and who may experience, among other symptoms, gastrointestinal disturbances in a moment of excitement and proneness to motion sickness. These are thought to represent early manifestations of the physiologic overactivity.

The pattern of each migraine attack may vary or may be remarkably similar. Only 20% of patients will consistently experience pain on the same side. The attack may begin at any time of the day or night, and nocturnal awakening with pain is common. The frequency of attacks varies throughout the lifetime of the patient; it ranges from only one or two attacks over the years to almost daily attacks, particularly with overuse of analgesics or ergotamine tartrate. Some patients will report a clustering of their attacks, whereas others will experience a randomized pattern. Headaches occurring during the premenstrual period (particularly during the premenstrual days) are common in women with migraine.

Migraine is a genetically determined disorder, but the exact mode of inheritance remains uncertain. Both dominant and recessive patterns are believed to be present. In our studies, 70% to 90% of patients with chronic headache have a family history. Migraine might begin at any time in life, but most often it begins in childhood, adolescence, or during the early twenties. Migraine in children may take the form of either the migraine with aura or migraine without aura type, or it may be manifest by migraine equivalents. Childhood migraine may terminate before adulthood or may continue with the same or altered pattern throughout the adult years. Migraine tends to lessen after middle age, but many patients continue to experience it well into later life.

Menopause often brings some relief; however, in postmenopausal women who take exogenous estrogens, the migraine predisposition continues until the estrogens are reduced. Late-onset migraine after 40 years of age is not unusual, although cerebrovascular disease must be considered before the diagnosis of migraine is established.

Studies in children show that the male–female ratio before the age of 12 appears to be approximately equivalent, with the same percentage of boys as girls experiencing headache. However, by age 21 or older approximately 80% of all migraine sufferers are women. This finding appears to reflect the important estrogenic influence on the migraine predisposition.

PATHOGENESIS

During the past several years, increasing attention has been paid to the term *daily chronic headache* or *chronic daily headache*. This term embodies a daily or almost daily headache pattern which frequently, but not always, evolves from a more typical, intermittent migraine form. It is now recognized that intermittent, occasional migraine may progress to a daily or almost daily form, frequently exhibiting features which have traditionally been referred to as *tension headache*. Though the topic is controversial, many of the leading experts in head pain now believe that the traditional concept of tension headache, currently being referred to as *tension-type headache*, is really a variant form of migraine.

Daily chronic headache, therefore, is often used synonymously with *transformational migraine*, suggesting that intermittent migraine has progressed to its daily form. Clinically, patients experience daily or almost daily mild to moderate neck or head pain, and superimposed upon this pattern is a periodic attack of rather typical migraine, occurring anywhere from once or twice per week to less often. Many cases of transformational migraine appear to have been provoked by excessive use of analgesics or ergotamine tartrate. The use of symptomatic medications for migraine more than 2 days per week for a period of time may result in the increase of headache frequency and intensity, a concept referred to as *rebound*. Many cases of transformational migraine appear to have been provoked to the progressive form by the excessive use of symptomatic treatments.

Additional clinical accompaniments to daily chronic headache are depression and anxiety states, sleep disturbance, and excessive symptomatic medication usage. Treatment requires addressing all of these factors and particularly the elimination of frequent use of symptomatic medications. Inpatient-level care is often required for the most severe cases.

Migraine can be treated in nonpharmacologic and pharmacologic ways. Pharmacologic treatment can be either symptomatic (rescue, abortive) or preventive.

NONPHARMACOLOGIC TREATMENT OF MIGRAINE

The nonpharmacologic treatment of migraine emphasizes a variety of interventions, including biofeedback and stress management training and avoidance of provoking influences ranging from dietary considerations to changing sleep time and awakening time. Biofeedback and stress management have well-established track records in many patients with chronic recurring headache. The mechanism by which these interventions work is not established, but it is the general consensus among headache authorities that they are worthwhile in a large number of patients with recurring benign headache.

Linkage of certain foods to the onset of headache has not been satisfactorily established, but anecdotally it is noted that many patients will regularly or periodically be sensitive to certain food components, including tyramine, monosodium glutamate, and many other additives and food ingredients.

More recently, emphasis has been placed on the chronobiologic relationships in migraine. Migraine is a periodic illness, and many factors related to headache appear linked to circadian or other hypothalamic rhythms. Migraine-prone patients seem to fare better once they establish regular patterns in primary life functions. Awakening at the same time each day (delayed awakening on weekends is often headache-provoking) and maintaining regular bedtime hours; avoiding missed meals and significant delays in food intake from expected times; avoiding major changes in eating or activity patterns on holidays, weekends, and vacations; and establishing "sameness" from day to day can be significantly helpful in avoiding headache onsets.

PHARMACOLOGIC TREATMENT OF MIGRAINE

SYMPTOMATIC (RESCUE) TREATMENT

The pharmacologic, symptomatic treatment of migraine should be considered when headaches occur infrequently and medications used for this approach are clinically acceptable. The route of administration for symptomatic treatment may be as critical as the choice of medication.

Ergotamine Tartrate and Other Alkaloids

Ergot alkaloids are effective within the first 1 to 2 hours in an estimated 90% of patients who are administered the drug parenterally; in 80% of patients who receive the rectal form; and in up to 50% of patients who receive the oral form. The effects of ergotamine have been traditionally assumed to be via an arterial vasoconstrictive influence. More recently, a central (brain) effect has been considered, as well as influence on neurogenic inflammation.

The dose required to alleviate an evolving migraine is variable and depends in part on the method of delivery. Parenteral treatment with dihydroergotamine (0.5 ml to 1.0 ml intravenously [IV] or intramuscularly [IM]) is usually effective. (Dihydroergotamine-45 is currently the only available parenteral form of ergot alkaloid.) The effective dose for ergotamine tartrate (*e.g.*, Cafergot) is usually 1 mg to 2 mg rectally or 2 mg to 6 mg orally.

Ergotism is a serious and well-known consequence of ergotamine overuse. Susceptibility to ergotism is variable. Recently, dependency on ergotamine tartrate has been reported in patients taking ergotamine as infrequently as three times per week, with the development of "rebound" or "ergotamine withdrawal headache" as a consequence. Ergotamine tartrate should be used no more than 2 days per week, since greater frequency of usage can lead to dependency and increasing headaches.

Isometheptene Mucate (Midrin)

Isometheptene mucate is a sympathomimetic agent which in a combined form (Midrin) exerts a beneficial effect on the acute attack of migraine. Although the general contraindications to the use of Midrin are the same as those for ergotamine, a lesser likelihood of adverse responses exists with this agent. Mild sedation and gastrointestinal distress occur in some but not most patients. Generally the drug is well tolerated.

Nonsteroidal Anti-inflammatory Drugs

The nonsteroidal anti-inflammatory drugs (NSAIDs) have symptomatic as well as preventive value. A large number of agents are available. Naproxen sodium (Anaprox) has been most widely evaluated. The dose of naproxen is 275 mg, 1 to 2 tablets, to be taken at the onset of headache. Other NSAIDs include meclofenamate sodium (Meclomen) at 100 mg to 200 mg, indomethacin (Indocin) at 25 mg to 50 mg, and ibuprofen (Motrin) at 400 mg to 800 mg; all agents should be taken at the onset of the attack.

Indomethacin suppositories (50 mg) are particularly valuable for patients with nausea and vomiting during attacks. Parenteral ketorolac (Toradol) at a dose of 30 mg to 60 mg may be of benefit when parenteral treatment is required.

The NSAIDs have well-known contraindications, which include gastrointestinal and renal disease, and side effects which include the aforementioned and also dermatologic disturbances.

Analgesics

Although analgesics (narcotic and non-narcotic) may benefit some patients during an acute migraine attack, the potential for overuse is sufficiently serious to make their routine use inappropriate for frequent headaches. These agents are appropriate in periodic attacks that occur no more than two times per week and in patients without patterns of compulsive drug taking or addictive behavior (including past and family history). The mixed analgesics, such as those containing barbiturate, aspirin, and caffeine (*e.g.*, Fiorinal) or barbiturate, acetaminophen, and caffeine (*e.g.*, Fioricet), are available with and without codeine. These agents remain particularly popular but must be used with restraint and with limited prescription amounts to avoid excessive usage and the development of rebound (see later text).

Phenothiazines, Other Antiemetics, and Related Medications

The phenothiazines may be effective as antiemetics and may also have some pain-relieving benefit. These and related substances can be administered in conjunction with symptomatic drugs and are most effective when given by the parenteral or suppository route.

The dose of chlorpromazine (Thorazine) is 25 mg to 50 mg IM, rectally, or in tablet form. Promethazine (Phenergan) is administered in a dose of 25 mg IM or rectally, or 50 mg orally. Prochlorperazine (Compazine) has a higher incidence of acute dystonic reactions associated with its use when compared with other agents such as chlorpromazine.

Metoclopramide hydrochloride (Reglan) in dosages of 10 mg orally three times a day or in intravenous form can provide antiemetic effects and also may be of value in enhancing oral absorption. Hydroxyzine (Vistaril) in doses of 50 mg to 100 mg orally or 75 mg IM may likewise be effective as an antiemetic and may enhance the benefit of other agents used to treat an attack. Hydroxyzine may also have primary analgesic effects.

The symptomatic usefulness of steroids should be noted. Prolonged refractory attacks may benefit from steroidal therapy. Prednisone in doses of 40 mg to 60 mg administered orally for 3 to 5 days or 8 mg to 16 mg of dexamethasone given by intramuscular administration may be used. Recently, an increased concern for the development of avascular necrosis of bone in patients using periodic steroids has been raised. It is advisable to avoid steroid use on a routine basis. They should be reserved for patients in whom less troublesome agents have failed to bring adequate relief and even then should be used selectively and infrequently, with short-term trials advisable.

Sumatriptan

Sumatriptan is a selective 5-HT agonist, and preliminary studies demonstrate its usefulness for the symptomatic treatment of acute migraine and cluster headache. It is generally considered safe. The side effects are generally mild, and it has the advantage of controlling nausea as well as headache. The drug will be available in self-inject syringes as well as in an oral form. Its mechanism appears to be the control of neurogenic inflammation, but there is speculation that it works centrally as well.

PREVENTIVE PHARMACOLOGIC AGENTS

The preventive medical management of migraine employs the daily use of a medication or a combination of medications presumed to block the biologic events leading to migraine. Such a program should be considered when the frequency of migraine attacks exceeds the safety limitations for the use of symptomatic medications or concurrent medical conditions contraindicate the use of medications employed to abort headaches. Generally, a frequency of more than four major attacks per month justifies consideration of a preventive program. Preventive treatment should be employed for a term of 3 to 6 months followed by a gradual reduction of medication, since natural remissions of headache may not be recognized when preventive medication therapy is maintained.

For most patients, combined preventive and symptomatic treatment is justified, since even under the best of preventive circumstances, periodic attacks will occur and require acute intervention.

Beta-Adrenergic Blockers

Beta-adrenergic blockers represent the treatment of first choice for migraine prophylaxis, unless contraindicated or unwise in a particular clinical circumstance. Among the beta-blocking agents that are useful in the prevention of migraine are the nonselective blocking agents propranolol (Inderal) and nadolol (Corgard), which impose a competitive blockade in both $beta_1$- and $beta_2$-adrenergic receptors. Selective beta blockers, including metoprolol (Lopressor) and atenolol (Tenormin), which selectively block $beta_1$-adrenergic receptors, may be of equal value, although anecdotally the nonselective blockers have been considered more effective. Many clinicians now believe that influences other than beta blockade are responsible for the antimigraine effects of these agents, and an effect on the central nervous system is considered likely by some.

Therapy with the beta-blocking drugs requires individual dose determination. One agent may be more effective for a particular patient than another similar medication. Nadolol is started at a dose of 20 mg twice a day and increased to tolerance or efficacy, occasionally up to 120 mg to 160 mg twice a day (240 mg to 320 mg total dose). Nadolol can be effective in some patients in a once-a-day dose regimen. It may produce fewer "central" effects than propranolol.

Propranolol is available in two forms, a short-acting form and the newer long-acting form (Inderal LA). With the short-acting form, treatment may begin at doses between 20 mg and 40 mg given three to four times a day and increased to a total dose of 400 mg per day, in three to four divided doses. Inderal LA is best employed in a twice-per-day regimen, beginning at 80 mg once or twice per day and increasing to 160 mg twice per day as tolerated.

Higher-dose regimens of beta-blocking agents may be of value in some cases, but if some efficacy is not demonstrated at moderate doses, higher dose regimens are usually of little value. After prolonged usage, slowly discontinuing the medication over several weeks is advisable. Approximately 24 to 48 hours are required for complete dissipation of its effects after the final dose.

Calcium Antagonists
(Calcium Channel Blockers)

Increasing attention has focused on calcium antagonists in treatment of various headache conditions. Their mechanism of effectiveness is unknown but may not be directly related to effects on blood vessels, since central effects are present. Of the available calcium antagonists, verapamil (Isoptin, Calan) is considered the agent of choice for headache. It is usually administered beginning at 80 mg two to three times per day and is increased to approximately 160 mg three to four times per day.

The calcium antagonists are of special benefit in patients who suffer from migraine and simultaneous vasoconstrictive tendencies such as Raynaud's phenomenon/disease and asthma. Beta-blocking agents aggravate these conditions. Calcium antagonists are also more appropriate than beta blockers in the presence of bradycardia. Among their side effects are headache (particularly with nifedipine), depression, vasomotor changes, tremor, gastrointestinal distress, dizziness, pedal edema, orthostatic hypotension, and bradycardia.

Antidepressants

The tricyclic antidepressants (TCAs), particularly amitriptyline (Endep and Elavil), nortriptyline (Aventyl), doxepin (Sinequan, Adapin), and others, have been reported as effective in migraine prevention, although their value in the treatment of daily chronic pain and tension-type headache is better established. The usual dose of amitriptyline and doxepin ranges from 25 mg to 150 mg a day, often given in a single bedtime dose. Nortriptyline doses range from 25 mg to 75 mg. Common side effects include sedation, dry mouth, urinary retention, constipation, blurred vision, intense dreaming with nightmares, weight gain, and hypotension. Contraindications include cardiac arrhythmias, narrow angle glaucoma, myocardial infarction, severe prostatism, and uncontrolled seizures.

Monoamine oxidase–inhibiting antidepressants (MAOIs), particularly phenelzine (Nardil), can be quite effective in the prevention of migraine. MAOIs influence the extracellular metabolism of biogenic amines, and disturbances of this system have been proposed in migraine. The usual dose of phenelzine is 15 mg three to four times per day; usually it is given in divided dosages beginning with 15 mg per day for several days, with a gradual increase in dose until benefit is achieved or safety limitations are reached.

Traditional concern over MAOIs has waned during the past several years, since it has been recognized that their use may be much safer and less restrictive than previously believed. Moreover, combinations of an MAOI and amitriptyline have been reported efficacious in the treatment of pain as well as depression disorders.

Simultaneous use of MAOIs with beta blockers and calcium channel blockers must be carried out with extreme caution, since severe orthostatic hypotension with syncope is frequently encountered.

Fluoxetine is an atypical, nontricyclic antidepressant with potent 5-HT reuptake inhibitory properties. It has fewer anticholinergic effects than the TCAs, has arguably fewer cardiovascular effects, and may cause weight loss. It may be used in combination with the TCAs, but combination use results in enhanced blood levels of fluoxetine and the other agent. Toxic responses and side effects include headache, nausea, and vomiting, all more likely to occur at higher dosages.

Fluoxetine has not been firmly established as an agent valuable in the treatment of migraine, but preliminary data suggest that it might be. Unlike the other agents which generally aid in sleep when given at night, fluoxetine generally interferes with sleep, even when given earlier in the day.

Fluoxetine cannot be combined with MAOIs and must be discontinued 5 weeks before an MAOI is added to a treatment program. Conversely, MAOIs must be discontinued 3 weeks before fluoxetine is added to a treatment program.

Generally the dose begins at 20 mg per day and may increase to 40 mg to 60 mg per day in patients who tolerate the treatment. Adverse behavioral disturbances, including suicidal compulsions, have occurred in patients taking fluoxetine. The direct relationship to the drug or its extent remains to be determined.

Nonsteroidal Anti-inflammatory Agents

The NSAIDs are useful in both symptomatic and preventive treatment of migraine. Naproxen sodium (Anaprox) has been most successfully established as an effective preventive agent. Indomethacin (Indocin) has shown its greatest value in the prevention of variants of cluster headache. The dose of naproxen sodium for migraine prevention is one to two 275-mg tablets twice a day. Gastrointestinal effects and long-term effects on renal function must be considered, and the drug should not be used in the presence of contraindications. The presumed mechanism is an influence on prostaglandin and platelet metabolism.

Ergot Derivatives (Methysergide, Methylergonovine)

Methysergide (Sansert) is an effective preventive medication for migraine, with a beneficial response demonstrated in up to 50% to 65% of patients. The usual dose of methysergide is 2.0 mg once or twice per day up to a maximum of 8.0 mg per day in four divided doses. It should not be used in patients with peripheral vascular disease, coronary artery disease, hypertension, serious gastrointestinal distress, or pregnancy. Activation of peptic ulcer disease is possibly related to the drug's enhancement of gastric acid secretion.

Methysergide should not be administered for more than 5 to 6 months without interruption of therapy for at least 1 to 2 months, because of the potential development of fibrosis in the retroperitoneal region, lungs, and heart valves. The risk is now considered idiosyncratic (not related to duration of use or dose) and occurs in 1/2000 patients taking methysergide. Although these changes tend to regress after discontinuance, they may not. A peripheral vascular occlusive reaction similar to Leriche's syndrome has been reported, and aggravation of pre-existing angina pectoris is common.

Periodic review in patients taking methysergide or methylergonovine consists of CT scan of the abdomen with contrast (for fibrotic lesions), a chest x-ray (to evaluate for pleuropulmonary fibrosis), and a cardiac examination (to rule out valvular fibrosis). These are recommended after 6 months of continuous therapy.

Mild to moderate adverse reactions occur frequently and thus limit the overall usefulness of methysergide. The most common untoward reactions include transient muscle aching, abdominal distress, hallucinations, and a sense of swelling of face or throat.

Methylergonovine, a derivative of methysergide, appears less likely to cause arterial constriction and has a greater venoconstrictive effect. It has been recently used for the prophylaxis of migraine. Dosage is 0.2 mg to 0.4 mg t.i.d. The same restrictions that apply to methysergide are present, and every 6 months a review for fibrotic lesions is recommended, though there is no evidence that methylergonovine produces the fibrotic condition.

Cyproheptadine

Although cyproheptadine (Periactin) has been used alone with occasional success in the prevention of migraine in adults, it is considered the treatment of choice for prevention of childhood migraine. Dosages range from 4 mg to 8 mg three to four times per day for adults and 4 mg two to three times per day in children.

Anticonvulsants

Occasionally, patients with intermittent migraine or mixed syndromes will benefit from anticonvulsants or antineuralgic agents, including carbamazepine (Tegretol), phenytoin (Dilantin), and baclofen (Lioresal). The mechanisms by which these agents help "non-neuralgic" syndromes is yet to be determined.

Valproate, well known for its anticonvulsant effects, has recently been shown to be effective in both migraine and daily headache syndromes. Long-term control studies are under way. The usual dose of valproate (Depakote) is 1000 mg to 2000 mg per day in three to four divided doses. This drug, like the other anticonvulsants, is potentially teratogenic, although unlike carbamazepine and phenytoin it does not interfere with the efficacy of oral contraceptives, an important warning in fertile women who must take the anticonvulsants.

TENSION-TYPE HEADACHE, CHRONIC DAILY HEADACHE, COMBINED HEADACHES, TRANSFORMATIONAL MIGRAINE

Tension headache is defined by the Ad Hoc Committee as:

Ache or sensations of tightness, pressure, or constriction, widely varied in intensity, frequency, and duration; long-lasting and commonly suboccipital, associated with sustained contraction of skeletal muscles, usually as part of the individual's reaction during life stress.

Combined headaches (vascular and muscle contraction) are:

Combinations of vascular headache of the migraine type and muscle contraction headache prominently coexisting in an attack.

Historically, clinicians have used the term *tension headache* to characterize a daily or almost daily chronic headache disorder without vascular-type features that is likely but not necessarily associated with provocation by stress or emotional factors. Traditionally, migraine and muscle contraction headaches have been considered distinct entities. Studies over the past several years have raised serious challenges to traditional positions. A serious reappraisal of our attitudes concerning this headache entity is under way. Attention to the transformation from intermittent migraine to daily chronic headache and to central elements purported to be involved in this process is growing and is considered the basis for the clinical events and treatment approaches.

The concept of transformational migraine includes a syndrome which is characterized by intermittent, periodic migraine in the first 10 to 20 years of life, followed by the gradual evolution or transformation to a daily tension-type headache with periodic acute attacks of migraine headache superimposed. Symptoms include head and neck pain, sleep disturbance, depression, anxiety and panic phenomena, and analgesic or ergot overuse syndromes. Many clinicians consider this a variant form of migraine or a progressive, pernicious form. Many believe that this form of migraine is the most likely refractory syndrome that requires the aggressive treatment of headache experts and centers. It is also the most likely to be associated with analgesic rebound and ergotamine dependency syndromes. It is unclear whether excessive use of analgesics or ergotamine tartrate promotes the transformational phenomena (likely in many cases) or whether there is a spontaneous intrinsic progressive process (also likely in many instances).

TREATMENT FOR CHRONIC DAILY HEADACHE

SYMPTOMATIC TREATMENT

For acute muscular pain, simple analgesics, NSAIDs, and TCAs are useful. For acute periodic migraine superimposed upon the daily "muscle-like" phenomena, simple analgesics, NSAIDs, ergotamine tartrate, Midrin, or other drugs mentioned earlier are appropriate.

PREVENTIVE TREATMENT

Because chronic headache forms frequently result in daily or almost daily headache, preventive treatment is advisable. The TCAs (see migraine prophylaxis) are used on a daily basis. In addition to their value in daily pain states, these medications are particularly valuable in controlling accompanying depression and sleep disturbance, which are frequently encountered in this population. Dosages range from 25 mg to 150 mg at bedtime if tolerated. Pain treatment response may have little to do with existing depression or its elimination.

Antidepressants can be combined with beta-blocking agents and calcium antagonists, and in this regard nadolol and verapamil have been found most useful.

This population of patients is very complex. Analgesic overuse, psychological distress, and family and other complicating problems frequently render even the most appropriate pharmacotherapeutic intervention ineffective. In my experience, a comprehensive treatment program, including inpatient-level care, psychotherapy, family involvement in treatment programs, dietary modification, biofeedback, and several other interventions, is frequently necessary to bring about satisfactory control of this difficult headache process.

HEADACHES IN CHILDREN

Unlike adults, children with migraine will frequently experience a variety of nonheadache symptomatology, including episodic vertigo, abdominal pain, light sensitivity, mood change, and gastrointestinal distress. It is generally believed that these physiologic phenomena reflect the primary mechanism of the migraine syndrome, those factors that produce headache. Many affected children will experience more typical headaches during the course of their lifetimes.

The pharmacologic treatment of headache in children does not differ appreciably from that in adults. Cyproheptadine (Periactin) may be the treatment of choice for the prevention of childhood migraine. Children appear to tolerate both preventive and symptomatic agents quite well.

Biofeedback, dietary restriction, and behavioral treatment may be the most important and even the critical therapeutic intervention in children with recurring headache.

CLUSTER HEADACHE AND CHRONIC PAROXYSMAL HEMICRANIA

Perhaps the most intense headache pain is seen in patients with cluster headache. The cluster headache is a vascular headache with many similarities to migraine, and it appears to be caused by an autonomic dysfunction with secondary blood flow disturbances. The mechanism is not well understood, but a current hypothesis is that it is a manifestation of hypothalamic disturbances occurring in a rhythmic fashion.

The term *cluster headache* comes from the tendency for the attacks to "cluster" in bouts of individual, short-duration headaches. The bouts may last for several weeks or months, followed by a period of remission lasting months to years. Cluster headaches occur most often in men after age 20, whereas migraine, a related "vascular" headache syndrome, is more frequently seen in women. The cluster headache is most commonly found in men who have a rugged, masculine appearance with leonine facies, hazel or blue eyes, and heavy smoking and drinking habits, and who appear to have a higher-than-average risk for heart attacks early in life.

Although cluster headache generally tends to "cluster," the *chronic cluster headache* is a form of cluster headache that is not intermittent. This chronic cluster variant frequently evolves from a more typical, episodic pattern. The attacks of pain in chronic cluster headache are identical to those of the classic variety, but the bouts of pain have no remission for years at a time.

Each cluster attack is characterized by a distinct episode of pain lasting 30 minutes to 2 hours. The pain is always unilateral, usually in or around the eye, accompanied by ipsilateral lacrimation, nasal congestion and rhinorrhea, and radiation of pain to the neck or jaw on the same side. The face on the side of pain is often reddened, the conjunctivae are injected, and not uncommonly the patient will pace, scream, cry, or pound his hand or head against something during the intense attacks of pain. Generally, the pain builds to a peak and then falls rapidly. Patients sometimes describe a sustained milder discomfort for hours subsequent to the peak attack. The headache may occur at any time of the day or night, and multiple attacks are likely over a 24-hour period. The attacks occur not infrequently during sleep time, and occasionally two to three attacks are experienced throughout the night.

Like other vascular headaches, cluster headache can be provoked by certain foods, changes in temperature, and other "migraine" triggers, but the most reliable and consistent triggers are alcohol and sleep. Although many patients with cluster headache overuse alcohol, most are forced to give it up during the cluster period. Alcohol may be consumed without aggravation to the headache during remission, but during the cluster period even the smell of alcohol may serve to trigger the attacks. Likewise, a night's sleep or simple nap in the afternoon may precipitate a headache during a cluster period.

Although no one fully understands the nature of this process, clustering may reflect the biologic cycle that, during certain phases, renders the individual responsive to the triggering events. This process may involve hypothalamic chronobiologic rhythms.

Chronic paroxysmal hemicrania (CPH) possesses significant similarities to cluster headache and may be a variation of it. In contrast to cluster headache, CPH most commonly occurs in young women, sometimes before the age of 10. The frequency of the attacks can be up to ten times a day. CPH is distinguished by its remarkable sensitivity to the drug indomethacin but not to the medications generally useful for cluster headaches.

TREATMENT OF CLUSTER HEADACHE

The symptomatic treatment of cluster headache involves the use of oxygen (100% O_2 via a mask at 7 liters/min for 10 to 15 min), ergotamine tartrate in rectal form, or parenteral DHE. Because of the repetitive nature of cluster headache, symptomatic treatments must be used in conjunction with preventive agents.

Preventive therapy for cluster headache primarily rests on the use of verapamil in a dose of 120 mg to 160 mg t.i.d. to q.i.d., lithium 300 mg t.i.d., ergot derivatives (methysergide or methylergonovine), or valproate. Steroids are reliably effective in preventing attacks in 80% to 90% of patients. Because of the adverse consequences associated with their use, short-term trials of steroids should be used in a limited way. Seven- to 10-day treatments with prednisone at a dose of 60 mg a day for the first 5 days and then tapered are recommended for acute attacks that break through preventive treatment, as an "insurance agent" when patients are traveling or at the onset of treatment to bring immediate relief before preventive agents can become effective.

Because cluster headache produces desperate behaviors and excruciating pain, admission to the hospital for parenteral dihydroergotamine-related therapies is recommended in refractory cases.

SPECIAL TREATMENT STRATEGIES

ELIMINATION OF DAILY ANALGESICS OR FREQUENT USE OF ERGOTAMINE TARTRATE

During the past several years, numerous reports have emphasized the importance of eliminating daily analgesics or frequent use of ergotamine tartrate as an essential element to bring headaches under control. The *rebound phenomenon* is defined as a clinical condition by which the daily or almost daily use of a symptomatic agent enhances and worsens the frequency of headache. This problem may represent the single most important factor contributing to treatment refractoriness in patients with long-standing headache.

Ergotamine tartrate or analgesics used more than 2 days per week on a regular basis may bring about this phenomenon in patients with migraine or migraine-like headache. Though more frequent use is acceptable on a once-a-month basis, such as around the menstrual period, the regular use of symptomatic agents such as these more than 2 days per week on a regular basis appears to be a serious problem.

Thus, an initial step in the treatment of patients with chronic recurring headache is detoxification and removal of offending agents from treatment regimens. The process is often difficult and may require hospitalization. Patients fear the elimination of analgesics or ergot prior to the establishment of an effective preventive treatment program and thus resist the discontinuance of symptomatic drugs prior to efficacious prevention. However, effective prevention is generally not possible untildetoxification and removal of analgesics have occurred.

Psychological factors, as well as obsessive drug-taking behaviors, must be confronted, and a broad medical and behavioral approach may be required.

SPECIAL DRUG TECHNIQUES

The pharmacologic treatment of patients with chronic headache must be individually determined. Persistent and innovative attempts to develop appropriate treatment protocols are frequently necessary to bring about recognizable improvement.

Raskin has recently described a program of intravenous administration of dihydroergotamine in dosages ranging from 0.5 mg to 1.0 mg every 8 hours over a period of 3 to 5 days (see *Handbook of Headache Management*, 1991). This treatment can bring important control over even the most refractory cases of headache, including those caused by substance withdrawal. Personal experience with this therapy supports Raskin's contention of efficacy, although the extent and applicability of this treatment remain to be determined. Intravenous dihydroergotamine therapy is best carried out in an inpatient setting and should be reserved for those patients in whom standard interventions are of little value.

Parenteral therapies for acute or protracted headache beyond dihydroergotamine include phenothiazine regimens, hydrocortisone, and Ketorolac. For further details, see *Handbook of Headache Management*, 1991.)

The MAOIs have proved useful in some cases of refractory headache. Although caution and special instructions to the patient are necessary, most patients can use these drugs without serious ill effects or undue risk.

In the symptomatic treatment of migraine, absorption from the gastrointestinal tract can be the determining factor in establishing effectiveness. The use of metoclopramide (Reglan) 10 mg one to three times per day may enhance the effectiveness of any of the oral preparations. Treatment with metoclopramide can precede the use of any of the oral agents by 10 to 15 minutes and can be helpful in avoiding some of the nausea that frequently occurs with the use of ergotamine tartrate or as part of the headache itself. Rectal forms of medicines are likewise useful in overcoming the gastrointestinal factors accompanying attacks.

MENSTRUAL MIGRAINE

Menstrual migraine represents a most difficult variation of migraine. Many women will experience their most severe headache at this time of the month, and frequently it is superimposed on other changes that occur as part of the menses. Ergotamine tartrate is probably the most effective agent for the reversal of this headache, and preventive therapy, which might include NSAIDs, beta blockers, and other agents, may be necessary. Special techniques are available (see *Handbook of Headache Management*, 1991).

It is particularly important when using combinations of medication to exercise appropriate caution, periodic educational review, and diagnostic monitoring. Laboratory studies to monitor biochemical parameters, electrocardiographic evaluation to assess QRS intervals and conduction disturbances, and blood drug level assessments are strongly recommended.

Despite the apparent reliability of an individual patient, intentional or inadvertent noncompliance is common. Periodic review of treatment regimens and appropriate counseling are likewise worthwhile and add measurably to the likelihood of treatment efficacy.

TREATING THE EMOTIONAL PROBLEMS ASSOCIATED WITH PATIENTS WITH HEADACHES

There is little doubt that emotional factors contribute to headache frequency and refractoriness in some, but not necessarily most, patients with headaches. At times, dealing with these factors may be essential, and the nature of the approach may determine the success or failure of treatment. Patients are increasingly unwilling to accept explanations that suggest emotional factors as the primary cause of recurring headaches. In my experience, many individuals who require psychological intervention will accept help as long as it represents a component of a broader treatment program, not the only form of therapy advised by the physician. Psychotherapy in its traditional form or as biofeedback or stress management programs can be important adjunctive treatments for patients with difficult headache problems. It is my opinion that psychological distress is not the common denominator that distinguishes patients with headaches from those who do not suffer from them. A biologic vulnerability, perhaps aggravated in some patients by emotional and other factors, seems a more reasonable explanation.

INPATIENT UNITS

In 1979, this author and associates established the first inpatient program directed to the treatment of headache. Over the course of the past few years, several other units have been developed. The inpatient treatment program provides a comprehensive intervention that includes detoxification from overuse of symptomatic medications, aggressive pharmacotherapy, milieu treatment, dietary modification, identification and restriction of aggravating influences, psychological and family intervention, and educational programs. Chronic illnesses such as headache frequently require this degree of intervention for treatment success.

Prospectively evaluated outcome studies from our unit demonstrate that over 75% of patients receive prolonged benefit from aggressive inpatient stays in a comprehensive facility. Duration of treatment in the hospital unit is between 7 and 10 days for most patients. A marked reduction in symptomatic drug use, emergency service utilization, work absences, and reduced productivity is noted.

QUESTIONS AND DISCUSSION

CASE 1

RT, a 37-year-old nurse at a psychiatric hospital, experienced daily headaches of a constant type for the past 10 years. For this she has taken four Cafergot suppositories P.B./day for the past 6 years and prior to that she had been taking daily methysergide. Her headaches are described as constant, nonthrobbing, and occurring "from the neck up to the eyes." The pain usually responds for 2 hours to the Cafergot suppositories.

During the past month, the patient was admitted to a major hospital for the treatment of head pain. During the period of hospitalization she was treated with various symptomatic as well as preventive medications, including meperidine hydrochloride (Demerol), acetaminophen with codeine, propranolol, clonidine, and high doses of amitriptyline. No improvement was noted. During the last days of hospitalization, she was given Bellergal twice daily in addition to the four ergotamine suppositories.

Soon after the Bellergal was instituted, the patient began to experience burning sensations down her right forearm and hand along with weakness. She reported this symptom to her physicians who told her she had an "ulnar neuropathy," and she was discharged on her Cafergot and Bellergal. Two weeks after discharge the patient sought another medical opinion.

Her general physical examination was completely normal including her blood pressure. Her general neurologic examination was entirely normal except for findings restricted to the right upper extremity. Her skin was cool and dry from the elbow down. There was a distinct pallor noted on the right as opposed to the left side, and peripheral pulses in the radial and ulnar regions could not be palpated. The skin was hyperesthetic to light touch and pin prick, but vibratory and position sensations were intact. Graphesthesia was impaired. Strength was normal, as were reflexes in the brachioradialis, biceps, and triceps regions.

1. A more appropriate therapy while the patient was at the "major" hospital would have been to:

    A. Increase the patient's daily use of ergotamine suppositories.
    B. Send the patient to a psychiatrist.
    C. Administer biofeedback.
    D. None of the above

2. The symptoms in this patient's right arm are attributable to:

    A. Compression neuropathy
    B. Cerebral ischemia
    C. Ischemic neuropathy
    D. Multiple sclerosis

The patient was hospitalized and all ergotamine was reduced. Within 3 days the patient's right arm was almost normal except for some mild hyperesthesia. The headaches improved after a period of initial intensification, and control was maintained on a regimen of propranolol and amitriptyline.

This patient was experiencing ergotamine dependency with a "rebound" medication–headache cycle at the time she entered the major hospital. Acute signs of ergotism were not present until Bellergal, which contains small amounts of ergotamine tartrate, was administered in addition to the 8 mg ergotamine that she was taking in the form of rectal suppositories.

In the first question, only (D) represents a logical alternative, since her doctor should have recognized the dangerous level of ergotamine being taken and the likelihood of the rebound syndrome. The tingling in RT's arm (the second question) was due to ischemic neuropathy, a component of the generalized ischemia occurring as part of ergotism, which apparently was incited by the additional amounts of ergotamine contained in the Bellergal.

CASE 2

JP is a 45-year-old physician (pediatrician) who has suffered from daily headaches for the past 10 years. His headaches are described as unilateral, occurring on either the right or left side, usually in the temporal region. Occasionally, there is a throbbing discomfort in an orbit and a coexistent neck pain. The headaches come on between 3 AM and 7 AM. The attacks can be easily aborted within approximately 1 hr by two tablets of Cafergot. The attacks are unassociated with any neurologic symptoms. Mild hypersensitivity to light, occasional nausea, and scalp tenderness are sometimes present.

For this headache Dr. JP has tried various preventive measures including methysergide 2 mg four times daily, propranolol up to 320 mg/day, amitriptyline 100 mg on retiring, secobarbital (Seconal) 100 mg on retiring, lithium carbonate 300 mg four times daily, Bellergal Space Tabs twice daily, and clonidine. These medications failed to alter the frequency or intensity of the attacks; however, methysergide did tend to delay the time of onset, pushing it toward 7 AM to 9 AM rather than during the sleeping hours.

Dr. JP's past health has been normal, and a full medical as well as neurologic examination was normal. No reduction of peripheral pulses, cardiac abnormalities, mental changes, or reflex abnormalities were noted.

1. The best diagnosis in this patient is the following:

    A. Daily muscle contraction headaches
    B. Mixed headache syndrome
    C. Cluster headaches
    D. Ergotamine rebound headaches

2. The single most appropriate first therapeutic effort would be to:

    A. Obtain psychiatric consultation.
    B. Provide biofeedback.
    C. Administer TCAs.
    D. Remove ergotamine tartrate.

The answers are 1 (D) and 2 (D).

Once again we see the pattern of daily ergotamine use along with daily recurring vascular headaches even though typical migraine should not be occurring on a daily basis. When all ergot was removed in this patient and propranolol administered, improvement occurred. Although a second headache type, probably muscle contraction headaches, seemed to emerge subsequently, the patient is doing better on a program of propranolol and amitriptyline.

CASE 3

RS is a 37-year-old assembly line worker who has had daily headaches for the past 10 years. His headaches are of two types and occur in two separate patterns.

The first type occurs daily and affects the occipital regions, with radiation usually in a bilateral manner to both temporal regions. There is often frontal tightness associated with this headache. The intensity of this headache varies throughout the day but is usually present upon rising in the morning and retiring in the evening. The headache is described as deep and nonthrobbing with some sharp and "burning" elements to it. Associated symptoms do not exist.

The second headache occurs much less frequently, occurring six to ten times a month. This headache is distinctively more intense, with a throbbing nature to it. It is usually located in an eye, temple, or across the vertex. It is more often unilateral but may be bilateral and usually lasts 10 to 48 hours. This headache is unassociated with any pre-headache phase but is usually accompanied by intense photosensitivity, nausea, vomiting, pallor, peripheral vasoconstriction, hyperacusis, stiff neck, general malaise, and 12 hours of fatigue following the remission of the pain.

This patient has had numerous diagnostic studies, of both invasive and noninvasive type, which are all reported as normal. He has been treated without success with propranolol, methysergide, Fiorinal, acetaminophen, clonidine, Bellergal, and amitriptyline. Currently the patient takes 12 aspirin, 6 Excedrin, and 2 Fiorinal a day for his constant pain, and on the days of his intense attacks takes additionally 4 to 6 propoxyphene hydrochloride (Darvon). His headaches respond only minimally to these regimens, but he believes that they are more effective than those administered by his physicians.

His general medical health is good except for epigastric distress between meals.

General, physical, and neurologic examinations were entirely within normal limits except for some mild epigastric pain on deep palpation.

1.   The best diagnosis in this patient is:

   A. Intractable migraine
   B. Tension-type headache
   C. Trigeminal neuralgia
   D. Transformational migraine

2.   Since propranolol and amitriptyline were used previously without success in this patient, the best explanation for the current success is:

   A. Placebo response
   B. A change in headache pattern
   C. A reduction of analgesics
   D. Other

The answers are 1 (D) and 2 (C).

All analgesics were slowly removed, resulting in some withdrawal discomfort and increased headaches. Subsequently, propranolol and amitriptyline were administered and the daily headaches improved dramatically.

This patient appears to have been experiencing transformational migraine. Current work among authorities suggests that daily use of analgesics may impose a refractoriness to therapy and create an "analgesic rebound" cycle similar to that seen with ergotamine overuse.

CASE 4

JD is a 50-year-old man who works as a designer. He has had headaches since 30 years of age. His headaches are described as occurring daily at this time, but previously occurred less frequently. His headaches occur four to five times a day and last for 1 to 2 hours. They usually begin in the occipital region but quickly radiate to the right or left orbit. The pain is described as intense and has at times caused him to consider suicide. Associated with the pain is intense lacrimation of the involved eye and nasal discharge. The involved side of his face becomes erythematous. The attacks can be brought on by alcohol and are thought to be worsened by sandwich meats.

For this headache, the patient has been receiving injections from his wife, a nurse, of 75 mg Demerol twice daily for the past 3 years. In addition, the patient takes six Cafergot suppositories a week, eight Darvon, and handfuls of aspirin a day. He also takes at least one box of Alka-Seltzer every 2 days. He is otherwise healthy but complains of epigastric distress.

1.   The best diagnosis for this headache syndrome is:

   A. Cluster headache
   B. Migraine
   C. Tension-type headaches
   D. Sinus headaches

2.   Appropriate means to begin treatment would include the following:

   A. Removing analgesics slowly
   B. Administering lithium
   C. Administering a "steroid burst"
   D. Trying oxygen inhalation symptomatically

This patient is experiencing cluster headaches of a chronic type (answer 1A). Appropriate therapy would include all of the choices of the second question because B, C, and D are among the acceptable modes of treatment for cluster headaches.

CASE 5

A 34-year-old woman has had a history of headaches for approximately, 15 years. Her headache patterns began somewhat sporadically, but during her early twenties manifested as a "mild headache" daily and intense headache periodically. This intense headache occurred approximately one time a month and was associated with nausea, vomiting, and photosensitivity. The headaches frequently occurred during her menstrual period and would last for approximately 2 to 3 days. The location of the pain was occipital, with some radiation to her eyes and frontalis region. The mild daily headache was bitemporal in location and not associated with any additional complaints.

During the past several years, this patient has had an intensification of her headache process, and she has found it necessary to use ergotamine tartrate (2 mg suppository) once or twice daily. As long as she takes the ergotamine, she experiences little, if any, head pain, but without the ergotamine her head would "explode." Currently, she experiences no nausea or vomiting, photosensitivity, or obvious triggering events as long as she takes her egotamine. This is in contrast to her initial intense headache, which was triggered by menstrual periods, alcohol, and stress.

There is a family history of headaches in an aunt and younger sister.

The past medical history was found to be noncontributory.

The physical examination revealed normal mental status and normal general as well as neurologic findings, except for tender and tense cervical muscles and the presence of cold lower extremities with faintly present dorsalis pedis pulses bilaterally.

1. Early on, this woman's headache pattern seems most likely to represent:

    A. Cluster headaches
    B. Chronic paroxysmal hemicrania
    C. Transformational migraine
    D. All of the above
    E. None of the above

2. Currently, this patient's problem seems most likely to be related to:

    A. Intensification of classic migraine (migraine with aura)
    B. Intensification of common migraine (migraine without aura)

C. Evolution to cluster headache
D. Ergotamine rebound headache
E. Both A and B

3. The intense headache during her early twenties and its association with menstrual periods suggest:

    A. Tension-type headache with periodic depression
    B. Cluster headaches
    C. Sinus headaches
    D. Classic migraine (migraine with aura)
    E. None of the above

The correct answers are 1 (C); 2 (D); and 3 (E).

SUGGESTED READING

CDC. Prevalence of chronic migraine headaches—United States, 1980–1989. Morbidity and Mortality Weekly Report 40:331–338, 1991

Lance JW: Mechanism and Management of Headache, 4th ed. London, Butterworth Scientific, 1982

Markus DA: Migraine and tension-type headaches: The questionable validity of current classification systems. Clin J Pain 8:28, 1992

Olesen J: Classification and diagnostic criteria for headache disorders, cranial neuralgias, and headache pain. Cephalalgia 8(Suppl 7):1, 1988

Olesen J, Edvinson L (eds): Basic Mechanisms of Headache. Amsterdam, Elsevier Science Publishers, 1988

Rapoport A, Weeks RE, Sheftell SD et al: The "analgesic washout period": A critical variable in the evaluation of headache treatment efficacy. Neurology (Suppl)36:100, 1986

Raskin NH: Headache, 2nd ed. New York, Churchill Livingstone, 1988

Rose FC (ed): Handbook of Clinical Neurology. Amsterdam, Elsevier Science Publishers, 1986

Saper JR: Changing perspectives on chronic headache. Clin J Pain 2:19, 1986

Saper JR, Silberstein SD, Gordon CD et al: Handbook of Headache Management. Baltimore, Williams & Wilkins, 1991

Silberstein SD (ed): Intractable headache: Inpatient and outpatient treatment strategies. Neurology (Suppl 2) 42, March 1992

Mathew NT (ed): Headache. Neurologic Clinics 8 (November 1990):781–992

Epilepsy

Donna C. Bergen

What is a seizure, and who can have one? A convulsive seizure is one of the most dramatic occurrences in medical practice and in everyday life. Although the physical characteristics and the electroencephalographic phenomena of convulsions are well known, the pathophysiology of seizures is still being investigated. No one really knows why an individual attack starts precisely when it does, or even why it finally comes to an end. Certainly, any human being can and will have a generalized (or tonic-clonic) convulsive seizure in appropriate circumstances (*i.e.*, brain hemorrhage, severe hypocalcemia, certain drug intoxications). The vexing question considered here, however, is why and how some people have seizures that occur unpredictably and recurrently, without an acute cause. This disorder is called *epilepsy*.

Although not all aspects of seizures are understood, seizures occur when groups of cerebral neurons behave abnormally. Different types of seizures probably have different neuronal mechanisms. The most closely studied seizure type is the *focal cortical seizure*. The production of focal epilepsy requires the occurrence of certain types of brain injury such as penetrating head trauma, cerebral infarction, or brain tumor. The cause of epilepsy is obscure in many cases.

Brain injury and subsequent gliosis (scarring) alter the electrical properties of certain neurons, changing both their electrical firing properties and their ability to recruit and synchronize other neuro-

nal activity. The basic cellular abnormality underlying these changes is not clear but may involve increased membrane permeability to sodium and calcium, selective loss of vital inhibitory neuronal input, and/or functionally disruptive distortions of neuronal and glial anatomy.

The pathophysiology of nonfocal seizures is even more obscure than that of focal epilepsy. In these disorders the entire cerebral cortex appears to participate in the generation of convulsive "grand mal" attacks as well as in the brief losses of consciousness called *petit mal seizures*. In the latter case, widespread, congenital abnormalities in neuronal connections or excitability are thought to underlie the disease.

A clear perception of the varied types of epilepsy is necessary not only to understand its pathophysiology but also to be able to diagnose and treat the disorder accurately and successfully.

Some definitions of a few rather loosely used terms may help at this point (Table 7-1). *Grand mal* is used to designate tonic-clonic, generalized, convulsive seizures. Such attacks may begin *de novo*, without focal onset, in patients with primary generalized epilepsy. They may also result from the spread of localized seizure discharges from a cortical focus. Except for the onset of the attack, such secondary convulsions may look like those of primary generalized epilepsy.

An *absence attack* refers to an episode of loss of awareness, usually due to a petit mal seizure. The

William J. Weiner and Christopher G. Goetz, eds. *Neurology for the Non-Neurologist*, Third Edition. Copyright © 1994, 1989 by J. B. Lippincott Company. Copyright © 1981 by Harper and Row Publishers, Inc.

TABLE 7-1. Simple Classification of Seizure Disorders

I. Primary generalized epilepsy (grand mal, petit mal, myoclonic seizures)
II. Focal epilepsy (with or without secondarily generalized seizures)
III. Multifocal epilepsy (multiple seizure types; akinetic, tonic, atypical absences seizures)

term is occasionally wrongly applied to the psychomotor seizure, a focal seizure usually arising from the temporal lobe, described in the section on focal epilepsy.

Although somewhat mysterious in etiologic terms, perhaps the easiest type of epilepsy to deal with clinically is *primary generalized epilepsy* (see Table 7-1). The disorder is a genetic one, probably transmitted as an autosomal dominant gene with relatively low penetrance. The typical patient often has a first-degree relative with one or more parts of the syndrome (including febrile seizures). The type of seizure seen in this syndrome varies, and includes generalized tonic-clonic convulsions, petit mal attacks, and myoclonic seizures. Petit mal seizures are typically brief; they last less than 15 seconds; they occur without warning or aura; and they consist mainly of an arrest of behavior and a loss of responsiveness and awareness. Automatisms are sparse, often limited to rhythmic blinking. The patient may not be aware of the attack, and the spells often occur in clusters or many times throughout the day.

Myoclonic seizures are also brief, although often more dramatic. They range in intensity from a few brief bilaterally synchronous jerks of the arms or head nods, to more violent muscular contractions that may cause the patient to fall. The patient is often unaware of an attack (myoclonic petit mal seizure) and is unable to describe it. Both myoclonic and petit mal seizures are often called *minor motor seizures*, because of their relatively unalarming appearance. They are clearly related pathophysiologically, usually responding to the same anticonvulsants.

Generalized tonic-clonic seizures are the type of seizure best known by the layperson. In primary generalized epilepsy an attack begins with a sudden loss of consciousness, sometimes with a loud cry and stiffening of the limbs and trunk, the tonic phase of the seizure. The patient is apneic and is usually cyanotic. After 15 to 30 seconds this posture begins to be interrupted by short, rhythmic, bilaterally synchronous jerks of the arms and legs; breathing remains ineffectual. After 30 to 45 seconds these clonic movements slow and then stop. The muscles are then flaccid, respirations are deep, rapid, and often stertorous, and consciousness slowly returns. After a single convulsion, most patients are awake in 10 to 15 minutes, but postictal confusion may persist much longer. Such an attack is without an aura or any focal neurologic sign such as strong adversive head and eye movements or postictal hemiparesis. Obvious physical stresses and physiologic abnormalities accompany these attacks, including hypoxemia, acidosis, and autonomic disruptions such as cardiac arrhythmias and hypertension. Pulmonary edema can occur, and it may play a role in the syndrome of sudden death that occurs occasionally even in young, otherwise healthy patients with epilepsy.

Patients with primary generalized epilepsy have normal neurologic examinations; they are of normal intelligence; and they give no history suggesting prior brain injury. The electroencephalogram (EEG) shows normal background activity, often interrupted by bursts of generalized spike and wave discharges. The condition usually becomes symptomatic in midchildhood or adolescence, or occasionally earlier in the guise of febrile convulsions of infancy. Pharmacologic control is usually successful, and the eventual remission rate is high, probably approaching 80%. Primary generalized epilepsy is not a common form of seizure disorder in adults, accounting for about 10% of patients in large epilepsy clinics.

Although it may present in a similar fashion, the pathophysiology and clinical implications of focal (partial) epilepsy are profoundly different than those of the genetic disorder. First, the occurrence of focal seizures almost always implies the existence of focal brain disease. Second, an almost unlimited variety of focal seizure types may be seen, depending on the site of brain injury. As in the diagnosis of all forms of epilepsy, taking a meticulous history not only from the patient but also from witnesses to the seizures is essential, because it is the precise sequence of events making up the attacks that reveals the site of seizure onset in the brain, and the route and extent of seizure propagation through the brain.

For example, a patient with a meningioma growing over the right brain may present with focal motor seizures of the left leg due to irritation of nearby cerebral motor cortex by the tumor. Such an attack may spread down along the precentral (motor) gyrus, involving the homolateral arm before stopping in 1 or 2 minutes. If intrinsic cerebral inhibitory mechanisms or appropriate pharmacology fail, such a seizure may spread suddenly into thalamic and other brain structures with strong, widespread axonal projections, and a generalized convulsion ensues. Unless the clinician obtains the history of focal onset of such an attack, a mistaken diagnosis of primary generalized epilepsy may be made and a search for localized brain disease may be left undone.

A completely different symptom complex may be reported by the patient with temporal lobe injury, such as that following head trauma, anoxia, or complicated febrile convulsions. A temporal lobe (psychomotor, complex partial, limbic) seizure often begins with a subjective experience such as a sudden feeling of strangeness, a hallucination of an unpleasant odor or taste, or an abrupt sensation of nausea that appears to move upward from the epigastrium. If the seizure discharges remain confined to a small area of the temporal lobe, the attack may not proceed further and may end in 30 to 60 seconds. If it spreads throughout both sides of the limbic system, consciousness may be lost. The patient may stare vacantly or may appear to look about, is usually unresponsive, and often makes simple movements (automatisms) such as lip smacking, grimacing, or hand wringing. He or she may stand or sit still or may walk about aimlessly. Because of the intimate relationship of limbic cortical structures with the hypothalamus, autonomic signs are common in complex partial seizures; flushing, piloerection, gastric rumbling, and sweating are examples. Should the seizure stop at that point, the ictal phenomena also stop abruptly, but the patient may remain confused for several minutes or longer, and if the seizure has started in the speech-dominant hemisphere, language function may be temporarily impaired postictally. On the other hand, if the ictal activity spreads even further, or generalizes, a full-fledged tonic–clonic seizure occurs. Patients may be able to describe vividly the aura (onset) of such attacks, but many temporal lobe seizures give no recalled warning before a loss of consciousness occurs, and the physician must rely on witnesses for a full description of the episodes.

Focal epilepsy, with or without secondary generalization of the attacks, is by far the most common form of seizure disorder seen by the primary care physician and by most neurologists. Within that category, complex partial seizures are the most prevalent type. Many patients with partial seizures find complete relief from attacks with medication, but another large group continues to have some seizures even with competent medical advice and optimal therapy.

The clinical picture becomes even more complex in the patient with multifocal or diffuse brain injury. Such a person may be subject to two, three, or sometimes even more seizure types. Generalized motor convulsions, focal seizures of any type, or absence attacks may all occur chronically. Additional patterns may also be present, often as fragments (tonic seizures) or distinctive types of episodes such as sudden losses of muscle tone with falling (akinetic seizures). Such patients often bear other stigmata of cerebral injury such as mental retardation or cerebral palsy. In these cases, seizures are usually difficult if not impossible to control with drugs and are almost always lifelong.

Epilepsy is thus a chronic if not permanent condition for most patients, demanding daily anticonvulsant therapy for years, and the toll taken on many aspects of patients' lives is high. Epilepsy carries a stain of fear and shame for many of their friends, colleagues, and even family members. Although this attitude is gradually softening, epilepsy is still a condition to be hidden from those outside the family (and sometimes from those inside as well). When the condition is poorly controlled, it can dominate and define relationships between parents and children, spouses, and siblings. Children are often sheltered excessively by parents and teachers, and social maturation is delayed or prevented. Marriage and parenting rates for those with epilepsy, even those with no other evidence of neurologic disease, are below normal. Suicide rates are above average.

The employability of those with epilepsy is also reduced. Some employers are reluctant to have a person with seizures on the premises, fearing injury and liability. Others worry over potentially higher medical costs for the employee. Even obtaining medical insurance may be difficult.

Difficulty with driving makes appropriate employment even more elusive. State regulations vary, but usually the seizure patient who cannot demonstrate complete, long-term control of the attacks is prohibited from driving. Public transport and carpools are often inadequate resources, and this problem alone makes working a major challenge for many people who have epilepsy. A diagnosis of epilepsy thus has far-reaching implications for the life of the patient. It is, therefore, essential that the diagnosis be neither missed nor misapplied.

Epilepsy is diagnosed by the patient's history and not by head scanning, EEG, or neurologic examination. In cases where a seizure disorder is seriously suspected, the physician must spend adequate time with the patient and others, to acquire a clear impression of the nature of the attacks.

First, simply asking what the attacks are like often produces a vague description as the patient produces a composite picture of his experiences. Asking for an account of the last episode, or of the last one the patient recalls well, will more often evoke precise details and a coherent impression. The physician should ask what the patient was doing when he had the attack. He should inquire about the first thing that occurred when the attack started and what happened next. He should also ask how the patient felt after the episode ended, and if any focal weakness or speech difficulty was present.

Second, the physician should also ask if all the attacks were similar or if and how they varied. Seizures are highly stereotyped events, like broken records. Unless there is more than one seizure type, each type with its own stereotypy, significant variation in the pattern of attacks argues against epilepsy.

Third, the physician should ask if anything tended to bring on an episode. Aside from some unusual cases of "reflex epilepsy," in which specific physical stimuli reliably provoke seizures, epileptic attacks characteristically occur without warning, one of their most frightening aspects. The attack that always begins during an argument with a girlfriend, or exclusively at home and never at work, may represent emotional symptoms rather than epilepsy.

Fourth, the duration of each attack should be appropriate. Except for brief minor motor attacks, most seizures last only 30 seconds to 3 minutes, with additional postictal periods depending on the type of seizure. Episodes that last many minutes to hours are usually not epileptic.

Fifth, what do witnesses see and how does the attack begin? Patients with clear auras at the start of a seizure ("Oh, there's that nasty smell again . . . ") may sometimes have postictal amnesia for a focal onset that was obvious to onlookers. The physician should inquire if the patient was fully or partially responsive during an attack.

The unwitnessed attack of "simple" loss of consciousness may not be as simple when carefully scrutinized. A diagnosis of vasovagal syncope should not be missed, since the typical prodrome is almost always remembered vividly by the patient. Giddiness, weakness, sweating, nausea, and fading or graying-out of vision are highly suggestive of true syncope. Witnesses report the unsupported victim of syncope as crumpling or sliding to the ground, whereas the patient with convulsions usually falls stiffly. The diagnosis may be made more difficult by the helpful bystander who immediately sits or stands up the fainting victim, prolonging the period of cerebral hypoxia and the faint, sometimes to the point of producing myoclonic jerks and cyanosis that are later reported as seizure activity (socalled *convulsive syncope*). Urinary incontinence is not rare in syncope but tongue biting is, so that this sign usually implies a convulsion.

Stokes–Adams attacks must be differentiated from seizures. The usual attack of unconsciousness has no warning. Again, the patient is seen to fall suddenly and limply to the ground. A witness is vital, since the movements of a generalized convulsion are unknown to the patient but are easily described by onlookers. Syncope from cardiac arrhythmias rarely causes incontinence or tongue biting. The attacks are usually short, and consciousness is regained quickly and completely.

Discriminating between petit mal and complex partial seizures may also be a diagnostic hurdle, but one that is easily cleared. The former is probably overdiagnosed and is much rarer than the latter. Even patients often name their seizures incorrectly: most patients presenting to an epilepsy clinic with self-proclaimed "petit mal" attacks in fact have complex partial seizures. Making the correct diagnosis is important, because only one of the two seizure types implies the presence of focal brain disease, and the therapy for the two types is completely different.

If a reliable witness can be found, the duration of the attacks can accurately discriminate between the two seizure types. Almost all petit mal seizures last less than 15 seconds, and many are briefer. On the other hand most complex partial seizures continue over 30 seconds, with many lasting a minute or two.

The patient often reports an aura for complex partial seizures, although this is not always the case. There is never an aura in petit mal epilepsy, and often the attacks are so subtle that the family usually reports many more seizures than the patient notices.

The petit mal seizure has no aftereffects, whereas several minutes or more of confusion often follow a complex partial seizure. In the latter, postictal language difficulty or other focal neurologic signs may be reported.

If confusion still exists after these points have been checked, the EEG may help. Three per second spike and wave activity is seen in over 80% of untreated petit mal patients, especially if hyperventilation is performed. Focal temporal spikes may be seen in complex partial seizures, but there is a dismaying 70% false-negative rate in a single EEG in patients with the disorder.

PSEUDOSEIZURES

Sometimes the most difficult differential diagnosis is between a seizure disorder and pseudoseizures, or seizure-like episodes of psychogenic origin. Like organic seizures, pseudoseizures vary tremendously in presentation, from convulsive-like episodes to transient alterations in consciousness or sensation. Faced with this diversity, one must fall back on the general rules previously discussed. Attacks that do not follow the usual "rules of behavior" of epilepsy should not be labeled as a seizure.

Episodes tightly related to stress or personal events and circumstances should be particularly scrutinized. Patients with epilepsy also often relate a correlation between seizures and stress, but the relationship is a loose one. The immediate triggering of an attack by an argument, for example, is typical of pseudoseizures.

After applying these general guides, a meticulous comparison between the pseudoseizure and the specific type of epileptic attack mimicked can further solidify the diagnosis. For example, the person with pseudoepileptic "grand mal" seizures may report an awareness of his or her surroundings during the throes of the attacks, which is an impossibility for a person in a convulsion. Full consciousness and accurate orientation may be regained instantly after the "seizure," which does not occur in genuine grand mal epilepsy.

Ancillary signs may not be of much diagnostic help. Urinary incontinence and even bodily injury occur with surprising frequency in pseudoseizures. Tongue biting is unusual but not unheard of.

A witness can sometimes provide small but highly suggestive clues. The pseudo–grand mal attack, for example, may include such atypical motor features as head shaking from side to side, or alternating (not synchronous) extension and flexion of the arms.

Even ictal and psychotic or functional hallucinations can usually be distinguished from one another. Psychotic hallucinations are usually complex and highly meaningful, often including auditory commands to do specific things. Likewise, functional "hallucinatory" experiences are colorful and varied, whereas the ictal experience is stereotyped, is not usually emotionally charged or significant, and is relatively brief.

The most elusive diagnosis often involves the pseudo complex partial seizure. Here the physician must rely on the monotonously repetitive nature of the true complex partial seizure. The onset of the true complex partial seizure, for example, may include distortions of reality or psychic perceptions that are impossible for the patient to describe satisfactorily. Nevertheless, the patient will usually admit that the experience is always the same from episode to episode, and that once an attack starts, it proceeds in a predictable manner. On the contrary, the pseudoseizure is typically varied from attack to attack, one time including "déjà vu," another time including numbness of the hands, another time nausea and dizziness, and so on. In general, the more varied, elaborate, and colorful the events of the episodes, the less likely they are to be epileptic.

If an attack occurs in the hospital or office, drawing a serum prolactin level within 30 minutes, and another 2 hours later, may clinch the diagnosis. Virtually all patients having a grand mal seizure are found to have greatly elevated serum prolactin levels immediately after the episode. (The 2-hour specimen is used as a *post hoc* "baseline" value.) Many, but not all, complex partial seizures also cause such elevations, so that a positive prolactin test is a reliable sign of epileptic activity, but a negative test is not helpful.

Occasionally, the only accurate way to distinguish seizures from pseudoseizures is to record an attack on EEG. This is often done with simultaneous video recording, so that the electrophysiologic and clinical characteristics of an episode may be defined and preserved for review. Importantly, however, patients with pseudoseizures may also have real seizures.

TREATMENT OF EPILEPSY

Medical therapy is begun once a diagnosis of seizures has been firmly established. There are two major reasons to treat seizures; first, in order to prevent potential harm from the single attack, and second, to maximize the chances of eventual seizure control and remission of the disorder.

Patients sometimes question or even reject adequate medical treatment of "mild" seizures, for example, the occasional brief complex partial or focal sensory attack. Since the drugs themselves have certain undesirable side effects and risks, both the physician and the patient must be convinced that therapy is worthwhile. The answer to the dilemma must be found in the observation of the natural history of seizure disorders as a group. Many observations have shown the same thing: the natural history of most untreated seizure disorders is to get worse with time, and the remission rate for epilepsy is higher with early medical treatment. In addition, a commonly observed progression is the initial occurrence of short, relatively unobtrusive focal seizures that are followed later by convulsions. Every patient with focal seizures must be regarded as being at risk for convulsions.

The treatment of a single, apparently nonfocal grand mal convulsion is a debated therapeutic issue. Those who believe that no treatment is indicated unless a second seizure occurs point to repeated studies showing "only" a 30% to 35% recurrence rate after a single attack in some studies. Those who recommend treatment point to other studies with more rigorous patient selection criteria and longer follow-up, with rates up to 70%.

Once a decision for therapy has been made and the reason for the seizures elucidated and treated if necessary, the physician must choose the drug that he or she feels will give the highest chance of successful seizure control at the lowest risk. That drug is then started in an appropriate manner and is increased slowly to the point at which the seizures are satisfactorily controlled, or at which the patient suffers unacceptable dose-related side effects. If the latter occurs, the drug has failed and another drug should be chosen and started. The first drug should eventually be withdrawn after the second drug has reached therapeutic levels, the goal being monotherapy if possible and appropriate for seizure type.

The patient should be instructed to keep an accurate calendar of any attacks, including the time of day and circumstances in which they occur. Reports by memory are inaccurate and are subject to distortion by expectation as well as by the memory-blurring effect of anticonvulsants.

Anticonvulsant blood level monitoring has proved to be valuable in seizure management. It can aid decision making when a patient taking more than one drug becomes toxic. In addition, although the slavish pursuit of the usual "therapeutic level" may not always be sensible, such guides may be helpful in managing convulsive epilepsy, when the only alternative is dosage guess-work and waiting to see if an attack will occur. Drug levels are also beneficial in judging patient compliance. When drawn at the same time of day at the same laboratory, and without interference from other medications or illness, anticonvulsant blood levels are remarkably stable from sample to sample.

The initial choice of anticonvulsant must be guided by the seizure(s) under consideration. Primary generalized epilepsy may have several manifestations: petit mal, grand mal, or myoclonic seizures, or combinations of these seizure types. Minor motor attacks usually respond readily to valproate, ethosuximide, and clonazepam. The grand mal seizures of primary generalized epilepsy are also usually well controlled by valproate, so that there is even a rationale for monotherapy in this condition. If ethosuximide or clonazepam is used for the minor attacks, however, a second antiepileptic drug such as diphenylhydantoin or carbamazepine must be added if grand mal seizures are present.

Focal or grand mal attacks are an indication for one of the "big three" antiepileptic agents, carbamazepine, diphenylhydantoin, or primidone. Although the reasons are obscure, it has been repeatedly observed that failure of seizure control with one of these three drugs does not ensure failure with the others, so that if unacceptable side effects, allergy, or ineffectiveness calls for the rejection of one drug, the others should be tried (Table 7-2).

Occasionally, the use of carbamazepine or diphenylhydantoin in patients with focal epilepsy with generalization produces a phenomenon that reminds us that the mechanisms of action of anticonvulsants differ from drug to drug. The medication may prevent the generalized attacks but may allow the focal seizures to occur. In such cases, phenobarbital (starting at small doses and increasing if necessary) sometimes "finishes off" the partial seizures.

Treatment of the retarded or otherwise brain-injured patient with multiple seizure types or akinetic seizures is beyond the scope of this chapter

TABLE 7-2. Major Antiepileptic Drugs

Phenobarbital*
Diphenylhydantoin (Dilantin)*
Ethosuximide (Zarontin)
Primidone (Mysoline)*
Carbamazepine (Tegretol)*
Divalproex sodium (Depakote)*
Valproic acid (Depakene)

* Available as generics.

and is usually challenging enough to require the assistance of a neurologist or epileptologist.

Although some general principles govern their use, the antiepileptic drugs vary enough in their metabolism, side effects, and interactions with other drugs as to require separate comment.

Starting with the oldest antiepileptic drug in common use, phenobarbital has only a limited place in therapy (see Table 7-2). It is occasionally helpful in focal seizures, especially those originating outside the temporal lobe. The sedative effect of phenobarbital that has caused it to be superseded by other anticonvulsants in adults is often reversed in children, in whom the drug may cause hyperactivity. Allergic reactions from maculopapular rash (common) to toxic hepatitis (unusual) may also be a problem. The very long half-life of phenobarbital, often more than 30 hours, makes induction of therapy a slow process, and the results of any dosage manipulations are very delayed. A consequent advantage, however, is that the drug need not be taken more than once a day, usually at bedtime.

Primidone has some of the same drawbacks as phenobarbital, since at least part of its effect derives from its prompt conversion to phenobarbital in the body. Primidone's side effects also include occasional depression and impotence. The half-life of primidone itself, and probably of some of its other effective metabolites, is short, and thus it should be given in three divided daily doses. The drug must be started slowly to avoid producing nausea.

Diphenylhydantoin avoids the sedative side effects of the barbiturates but brings problems of its own. Chronic but usually harmless laboratory abnormalities such as macrocytosis and elevated alkaline phosphatase are common. Allergic skin reactions from the common maculopapular eruption to the rare but devastating Stevens–Johnson syndrome may occur. Dose-related side effects are predictable and characteristic, consisting of nystagmus at low doses and ataxia at higher ones. Long-term side effects have been well cataloged and include gingival hyperplasia, hirsutism, osteoporosis, and particularly in children, facial coarsening. Therapy is easily induced, and most people tolerate the immediate use of full doses. The half-life of about 24 hours allows single-dose daily use.

For most epileptologists carbamazepine is the preferred drug for complex partial or grand mal seizures. It is generally well tolerated by patients but requires initial slow titration of dose to avoid complaints of light-headedness. Blood level measurements are essential with carbamazepine, because the same levels can be achieved by doses which vary three-fold in different people. Dose-related side effects are easily monitored, consisting of blurred or double vision in most people. Many patients show a transient, usually mild, leukopenia on induction, and severe leukopenia is a rare cause for stopping the drug. Serious side effects are no more frequent than with diphenylhydantoin or phenobarbital, most commonly toxic hepatitis.

Valproic acid is used mainly for minor motor attacks for which it is often effective even at low doses and is also useful in some grand mal epilepsies. It is generally tolerated well, but idiosyncratic side effects such as weight gain, reversible alopecia, and tremor can present a problem. The use of an enterically stable form (divalproex sodium) generally obviates the nausea and vomiting caused by the earlier version of the drug. Fatal toxic hepatitis has been reported, mainly in young children on polytherapy during the first 6 months of use. Blood levels of valproic acid tend to vary more than they do with other anticonvulsants, and they are less useful.

Clonazepam is often helpful in minor motor seizures. It produces the sedation characteristic of all the benzodiazepines. Dosage decrements must be done particularly slowly to avoid withdrawal seizures.

The behavioral changes induced by antiepileptic drugs are a subject of lively debate. The sedating effects of the barbiturates are obvious. Careful cognitive function testing, however, reveals that most antiepileptic drugs, at the usual therapeutic doses, cause measurable impairment of reaction time, memory, and concentration. Of the major anticonvulsants, carbamazepine is probably least likely to offend in this way.

Surprisingly, the effects of anticonvulsants on the maturing brain are almost entirely unknown, but animal experiments suggest that they may cause significant reduction in the development of normal neuronal complexity. Considering the well-demonstrated immediate and long-term harm of repeated seizures, however, their continued use in children is not questioned.

The point at which antiepileptic drugs may be safely stopped in a well-controlled patient is debatable. A time span of 3 to 5 years without any seizure or aura is cited by most experts as a reasonable time at which to consider a trial without drugs. The subject is complex, however, and the reader is referred to the Suggested Reading list for more information.

Although most patients with epilepsy are helped to achieve substantial control of seizures, many patients on optimal drug therapy continue to have seizures serious or frequent enough to cause major disruptions to life. Such patients are sometimes referred to specialized treatment centers for investigation into possible surgical treatment. If seizures can be demonstrated to emanate from a surgically accessible focus that can be removed without the possibility of neurologic injury, significant relief or cure may be achieved.

QUESTIONS AND DISCUSSION

1. Patients with primary generalized epilepsy may have which of the following types of seizures?

   A. Petit mal
   B. Myoclonic
   C. Grand mal
   D. All of the above
   E. None of the above

The answer is (D). Patients may have any combination of these seizures. Sometimes grand mal attacks are preceded or led into by clusters of petit mal or myoclonic spells.

2. The physiologic substrate of clinical seizure activity is:

   A. Abnormal neuronal discharge
   B. Hyperactive glial potentials
   C. Repeated disturbances in cerebral blood flow
   D. Autoimmune mechanisms

The answer is (A). In focal epilepsy, groups of hyperirritable neurons, perhaps released by loss of inhibitory input and affected by anatomic distortions, overact and are able to hypersynchronize the activity of other neuronal populations. This activity spreads and causes focal or even generalized seizures.

3. Some relatively common causes of new epilepsy after adolescence are:

   A. Brain tumor
   B. Penetrating head injury
   C. Cerebral infection
   D. B and C
   E. A, B, and C

The answer is (E). New onset of seizure disorder in adulthood demands a full investigation into the cause. Epilepsy is thus better regarded as a symptom rather than as a disease.

4. High blood levels of diphenylhydantoin are usually accompanied by:

   A. Somnolence
   B. Hair loss
   C. Ataxia
   D. Pulmonary edema
   E. Weakness

The answer is (C). Ataxia is much commoner than somnolence. Sedation is caused by diphenylhydantoin only at extremely high levels, as would be caused by deliberate overdosing. Hair loss may occur with valproate, but not with diphenylhydantoin. Neither pulmonary edema nor muscle weakness is typical of diphenylhydantoin effect. Ataxia is seen in most patients with blood levels above 30 mg/dl.

SUGGESTED READING

Aird RB, Masland RL, Woodbury DM: The Epilepsies: A Critical Review. New York, Raven Press, 1984

Annegers JF, Shirts SB, Hauser WA et al: Risk of recurrence after an initial unprovoked seizure. Epilepsia 27:43, 1986

Chadwick D: The discontinuation of antiepileptic therapy. In Pedley TA, Meldrum BS (eds): Recent Advances in Epilepsy, Vol 2. Edinburgh, Churchill Livingstone, 1985

Dodrill C, Batzel LW: Interictal behavioral features of patients with epilepsy. Epilepsia (Suppl 2)27: 564–576, 1986

Fish DR, Smith SJ, Quesney LF et al: Surgical treatment of children with medically intractable frontal or temporal lobe epilepsy: Results and highlights of 40 years' experience. Epilepsia 34:244, 1993

King DW, Flanigin HF, Gallagher BB et al: Temporal lobectomy for partial complex seizures: Evaluation, results, and 1-year follow-up. Neurology 36:334, 1986

Laidlaw J, Richens A: A Textbook of Epilepsy, 2nd ed. Edinburgh, Churchill Livingstone, 1982

Leppik IE, Goldensohn ES, Hauser WA et al: Epilepsy through life: Recent advances in understanding and treating epilepsy during pregnancy, childhood, adulthood, and old age. Epilepsia (Suppl 4)33:S1, 1992

Morselli PL, Pippenger CE, Penry JK: Antiepileptic Drug Therapy in Pediatrics. New York, Raven Press, 1983

Prince DA: Mechanisms of epileptogenesis in brainslice model systems. In Ward AA, Penry JK, Purpura D (eds): Epilepsy. New York, Raven Press, 1983

Resor SR Jr, Kutt H (eds): The Medical Treatment of Epilepsy. New York: Marcel Dekker, 1992

Reynolds EH: Mental effects of antiepileptic medication: A review. Epilepsia (Suppl 2)24:S24, 1983

Theodore WH, Porter RJ, Penry JK: Complex partial seizures: Clinical characteristics and differential diagnosis. Neurology 33:1115, 1983

Wyllie E: The Treatment of Epilepsy: Principles and Practice. Philadelphia: Lea & Febiger, 1993

CHAPTER 8

Multiple Sclerosis

William A. Sheremata
Lawrence Honig

Multiple sclerosis (MS) is a disease characterized by the appearance of neurologic deficits in multiple areas of the central nervous system (CNS) over time. While the cause is unknown, the dominant pathology is in the CNS white matter: major immune-mediated destruction of myelin sheathing is evident, although nerve axon fibers themselves are preserved. MS is almost twice as common in women as in men and occurs predominantly in young adults. In the United States, peak incidence occurs at about age 24. MS is more common in northern regions of Europe and the United States, where the prevalence may exceed 1/1000 population; in these areas it is the most frequent cause of chronic disability in the young and middle-aged population. Certain clinical presentations appear commonly, but there also is a panorama of less common symptoms and signs.

Epidemiologic studies have long suggested that risk of MS in part related to geographic location in temperate zones during childhood years: individuals born or migrating to warmer climates before the age of 15 appeared to have reduced risk. However, recent evidence makes it likely that much of the geographic distribution of the disease is related more to genetic predispositions of certain peoples than to the latitude of their residence. Other evidence has delineated epidemics of MS in the Faroe Islands, Iceland, and Sardinia, raising the possibility that young adults might carry the risk of MS to disease-free populations. These findings suggest a

viral etiology in the initiation of illness. Prior investigations of causative factors of MS have consisted of numerous "false starts," most notably with a variety of viral or nutritional hypotheses. The possibility of retroviral involvement in MS has in recent years been brought to the fore by the finding that human retroviruses HIV and HTLV-I, a human lentivirus and oncovirus, respectively, both may cause demyelinating CNS disease. Additional support for such a possibility comes from the fact that naturally occurring animal retro-lentiviruses produce neurologic disease, with visna-maedi causing an immune-mediated demyelinating condition in sheep, similar to MS.

DIAGNOSTIC CRITERIA

MS remains a clinically diagnosed disorder, despite marked technical advances in laboratory support. When evaluating a particular clinical presentation, a set of the minimum criteria for the diagnosis of MS should be borne in mind.

Schumacher and colleagues, in 1965, outlined criteria for two types of disease—*relapsing–remitting* and *chronic progressive myelopathy*—and outlined minimum criteria for diagnosis. *Definite MS* was diagnosed in patients where other diseases had been eliminated with reasonable certainly *and* (1) the patient had two attacks of CNS disease lasting

William J. Weiner and Christopher G. Goetz, eds. *Neurology for the Non-Neurologist*, Third Edition. Copyright
© 1994, 1989 by J. B. Lippincott Company. Copyright © 1981 by Harper and Row Publishers, Inc.

24 hours or more when clinical evidence indicated involvement of two separate areas of the nervous system *or* (2) the patient had a minimum of 3 months of progressive spinal cord involvement.

The 1983 Workshop on the Diagnosis of MS has broadened these criteria to include supporting laboratory data. Because of their increasing acceptance and their importance in clinical practice and clinical investigation, they are reprinted in Table 8-1. These criteria supplement earlier definitions by allowing "paraclinical" tests such as evoked potentials, urodynamic and neuroimaging studies as well as cerebrospinal fluid (CSF) examination to support the clinical criteria elicited from history and neurologic examination. These are strict criteria, and many patients can be recognized as having MS by experienced physicians before they meet these criteria.

CLINICAL PRESENTATION

Charcot originally described MS over a century ago, recognizing three types of disease: disseminated, brain-stem, and spinal. The "spinal" form was least common, occurring in about one of ten patients. Presently, it is recognized that the majority of the symptoms and signs of MS are attributable to spinal cord and brain-stem involvement. In particular, motor and sensory signs in the limbs derive preponderantly from spinal cord lesions. Cognitive problems are common, although they are less easily recognized.

ONSET

While early sensory symptoms are a hallmark of MS, initial clinical presentation commonly is that of a young person who complains of being unable to walk on a street without tripping over the curb or uneven sections of pavement. Alternatively, the patient may complain that one or both legs are heavy or numb. Objective signs of decreased motor strength vary greatly but occasionally may be severe. Also variable is the rate of progression of debility after first awareness of difficulty. Interpretation of onset complaints such as unexplained falling depends in large part on the findings of neurologic examination. Some patients may not have complaints referable to the lower extremities, yet examination may reveal weakness and evidence of spasticity. Conversely, other patients who present

TABLE 8-1. Criteria for the Diagnosis of Multiple Sclerosis

CLINICALLY DEFINITE MULTIPLE SCLEROSIS

Two attacks and clinical evidence of two separate lesions.

or

Two attacks; clinical evidence of one lesion and paraclinical evidence* of another separate lesion. The two attacks must involve different parts of the central nervous system (CNS), must be separated by a period of at least 1 month, and must each last a minimum of 24 hours. However, certain historical information may be substituted for clinical evidence of one of the two lesions.

LABORATORY SUPPORTED DEFINITE MULTIPLE SCLEROSIS

Two attacks; either clinical or paraclinical evidence* of one lesion, and cerebrospinal fluid (CSF) oligoclonal bands and/or increased CSF IgG

or

One attack; clinical evidence of two separate lesions; and CSF oligoclonal bands and/or increased CSF IgG

or

One attack; clinical evidence of one lesion and paraclinical evidence* of another, separate lesion and CSF oligoclonal bands and/or increased CSF IgG

CLINICALLY PROBABLE MULTIPLE SCLEROSIS

Two attacks and clinical evidence of one lesion

or

One attack and clinical evidence of two separate lesions

or

One attack; clinical evidence of one lesion and paraclinical evidence* of another, separate lesion

LABORATORY SUPPORTED PROBABLE MULTIPLE SCLEROSIS

Two attacks and CSF oligoclonal bands and/or increased CSF IgG

CLINICALLY POSSIBLE MULTIPLE SCLEROSIS†

---

* *Definition of Paraclinical Evidence of a Lesion:* "The demonstration by means of various tests and procedures of the existence of a lesion of the central nervous system (CNS) which has not produced signs of neurological dysfunction but which may or may not have caused symptoms in the past. Such tests and procedures include the hot bath test, evoked response studies, tissue imaging procedures (including CT and MRI of the brain and spinal cord) and reliable expert urological assessment, provided that these tests and procedures follow the guidelines and are interpreted according to the newly established criteria." (Poser et al., 1983)
† Clinically possible MS, although included originally, is no longer a diagnostic category.

primarily with sensory complaints and decreased well-being may initially lack objective findings.

Several studies have attempted categorical surveys of symptoms and signs occurring with the first attack of MS (Table 8-2). The findings of Kurtzke represent a cross section of experience in the United States and Canada. Symptoms attributed to corticospinal tract lesions were found in 64% of patients, and sensory disturbances were present in 42%. Incoordination was recorded in 43% and an internuclear ophthalmoplegia in 13%. Complaints related to other brain-stem signs were present in 40%.

Only one-third of patients who present with a single symptom have neurologic findings limited solely to that symptom. For example, in patients with retrobulbar neuritis almost half exhibit signs attributable to spinal cord and/or brain-stem lesions. Similarly, "la belle indifference," emphasized by Charcot, is often noted in early MS. Rather than euphoria, this sign is evidence of an inappropriate emotional response to what should be a traumatic emotional experience. Blunted affect or inappropriate response to affliction can reflect denial of illness or depression but also can be an important, although subtle, manifestation of other nervous system disease such as frontal lobe dysfunction. These and other subtle observations often pass undetected, but when noted can be helpful in reaching a correct diagnosis.

MOTOR AND SENSORY SPINAL CORD SYMPTOMS

Motor and sensory signs of CNS involvement in MS result primarily from spinal cord involvement (Fig. 8-1). The lower extremities are more often affected than the upper extremities and often show early and symmetrical involvement. Predilection for the lower extremities may be understood as a consequence of greater risk of disease in the longest fibers running from frontal motor cortex to anterior horns: longer axons are likely to be more involved if lesions occur randomly throughout the neuraxis. In a study of early MS, we found that among patients examined within their first 3 years of illness, only half of those with clinically definite MS had brain lesions evident by magnetic resonance imaging (MR). Many of these patients did, however, have recognizable lesions of the spinal cord, despite the considerable technical limitations of spinal cord MR.

Motor symptoms referable to the corticospinal tract are described by patients as heaviness, weakness, stiffness, failure of a body part to respond to command, or even "numbness." Findings on examination include decreased strength, increased tone, hyperreflexia, clonus, and Babinski signs. Motor difficulties may often be relatively mild and are usually described in the context of walking. However, problems in gait may in part be related to visual and cerebellar difficulty. It is important to examine all the muscle groups in both upper and lower extremities to detect changes in tone and strength. Amyotrophy is uncommonly recognized clinically, although it is seen in about half of cases at death. When present it is a sign of root entry zone involvement by demyelinative lesions. It rarely poses a problem in the differential diagnosis of motor neuron disease. Radicular pain is probably a more common manifestation resulting from root entry zone lesions. It should be remembered that motor signs not infrequently may be present without any complaints.

Sensory symptoms may be prominent without consistent objective findings on examination. Com-

TABLE 8-2. Findings in the Original Attack of Multiple Sclerosis in Three Reports

WILSON (100 CASES) (% OF CASES)	
Motor	46
Sensory (paresthesias)	23
Cerebellar	10
Sphincter disturbances	9
Seizures	1

MCALPINE (REVIEW OF PUBLISHED REPORTS) (% OF CASES)	
Motor	40
Optic neuritis	22
Sensory (paresthesias)	21
Diplopia	12
Vertigo	5
Bladder dysfunction	5

KURTZKE (% OF CASES)	
Motor (corticospinal)	64
Cerebellar (incoordination)	43
Sensory	42
Brain stem	40
Visual	24
Internuclear opthalmoplegia	13

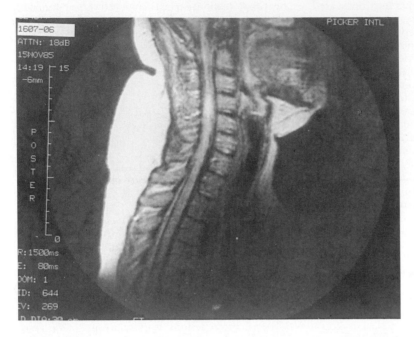

FIG. 8-1. Magnetic resonance imaging of the cervical spinal cord from a 35-year-old woman with acute onset of quadriplegia after a 6-month history of multiple sclerosis. There is an area of marked "increase in signal" in the middle portion of the cervical cord associated with cord swelling.

plaints of glove and stocking distributions of sensory deficits are common. Findings are much less frequent than are complaints. However, suspended sensory loss can be an important finding. Such relative decreases in pain and temperature sensation can be found in the mid to lower thoracic dermatomes by careful examination in a substantial number of cases. Patients may report Lhermitte's phenomenon, consisting of an electric shock sensation, a vibration, or dysesthetic pain radiating down the back and often into the arms or legs, usually occurring on neck flexion. It is an important symptom, although nonspecific, since it occurs in many myelopathies including that of cervical spondylosis. Lhermitte's sign can often be elicited on examination and is thought to reflect the presence of posterior column plaques. Proprioceptive difficulty may be difficult to detect even when clinically significant; however, careful examination can often document this difficulty.

OPTIC AND RETROBULBAR NEURITIS

Optic neuritis is associated with a typical group of visual symptoms, including blurring, darkening, scotomas, decreased color perception, and occasionally flashes, as well as pain, which may be exacerbated upon movement of the affected eye. The pain may be described as a dull ache, or as a sharp jab with eye movement, and may precede or accompany the appearance of visual loss, often calling attention to visual difficulty. Descriptions of visual aberrations vary among patients, with common descriptions including "a curtain coming down" as well as "blurring." A small proportion of patients will proceed to "black out" or "white out" of vision, with somewhat poorer prognosis for recovery of good vision. Objectively large central scotomas may occur but are more commonly the residium of an attack involving an optic nerve. When severe optic nerve involvement is combined with marked deficit from a spinal cord lesion the combination has been termed *Devic's syndrome* or *neuromyelitis optica*. It is uncertain if this syndrome has any special significance; it has been found with the same or greater frequency even in areas where MS is rare, such as in parts of Asia. The exact relationship of either isolated optic neuritis or transverse myelitis to MS is not known. As many as 50% to 80% of cases of retrobular neuritis may ultimately progress to clinically obvious MS, with a great risk in women, whereas only about one in five cases of transverse myelitis is subsequently diagnosed as MS.

Swelling of the optic disc, or papillitis, may be evident on careful inspection of the nerve head during the acute presentation. When the patient is seen in consultation by a neurologist, without the benefit of a full ophthalmologic examination, this will often be designated as retrobulbar neuritis. Recent MR studies have shown great variability in the location of the lesion causing visual symptoms. A small scotoma is frequently detectable in the visual field even after recovery of good vision. Color desaturation is usually demonstrable, although Ishihara color plates may not be sufficiently sensitive. Paroxysmal retrobulbar neuritis may also occur, with repeated, yet only momentary, blurring or obscurations of vision. The recurrent visual difficulty may occur many times a day or only occasionally. However, the whole period of disturbed vision usually lasts 3 to 8 weeks, the approximate length of an exacerbation of MS.

CEREBELLAR, BRAIN-STEM, AND SPECIAL SENSORY LESIONS

Cerebellar lesions are common in MS, with signs occurring in approximately half of patients. Action (or kinetic) tremor is common, and although severe resting or postural tremor is infrequent, it may if present be totally disabling. The affected individual may exist in a totally dependent state, constituting a major nursing problem (1% of our experience). In many patients, mild hand tremor is present and may compound other motor problems. Cerebellar gait disorders, often with titubation of the trunk and/or head, are common. Scanning dysarthric speech may result from bilateral cerebellar involvement. Charcot's original triad of MS consisted of nystagmus, scanning speech, and upper extremity tremor, although few patients show this exact clinical complex.

Brain-stem or cranial nerve lesions occur with almost equal frequency as cerebellar signs, and include extraocular muscle abnormalities (diplopia, internuclear ophthalmoplegia [INO], nerve or gaze palsies, or nystagmus), trigeminal neuralgia, facial palsies and myokymia, hearing and vestibular deficits (vertigo), and rarely glossopharyngeal neuralgia (Fig. 8-2).

Diplopia occurs in 12% to 22% of patients and is secondary to demyelinative plaques involving the intramedullary portions of the sixth and third nerves or the medial longitudinal fasciculus (MLF).

INO occurs in about 13% of patients as a result of lesions affecting the MLF. Bilateral INO is a patho-

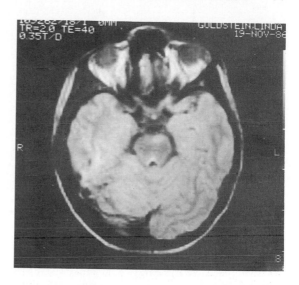

FIG. 8-2. Magnetic resonance imaging of the brain stem showing the presence of a prominent lesion in the pons. The patient has prominent facial myokymia related to this lesion.

gnomonic sign of MS (although unilateral INO is frequently a sign of brain-stem infarction). An incomplete bilateral INO is easily missed. The essential clinical finding is bilateral abducting nystagmus with adduction weakness. This may be asymptomatic or may be associated with transient diplopia or vertigo upon movement of the head or eyes.

Nystagmus is an important finding in MS. The majority of patients exhibit nystagmus, although it may not be obvious early in the clinical course. Eye movements may seem to be jerky, especially when visualized under a fluorescent light. As the examiner becomes presbyopic, care must be exercised not to miss this important sign, as the absence of nystagmus mitigates against the diagnosis of MS.

Trigeminal neuralgia (tic douloureux) occurs in about 1% of MS patients. Severe momentary lancinating jabs of pain in the distribution of the maxillary or mandibular divisions of cranial nerve V are the only symptom. The pain may prevent eating, since contact with trigger zones may predictably produce pain. The pain usually responds well to carbamazepine but subsequently may be refractory to this agent.

Facial myokymia involving the lower face is an important, although not common (1% to 5%), finding of MS. These adventitious movements are most often unilateral but may be difficult to see. Their presence may require some patience to detect, but they argue strongly for a diagnosis of MS.

Hearing loss of some degree is more common among MS patients than in the general population. Severe hearing loss is rare, although it can occur at any time in the clinical course. Earlier literature suggested that losses were irreversible, but significant improvement often occurs on long-term follow-up of those with sudden severe onset of deafness.

Vertigo is a frequent symptom (10% to 15%) among patients and may be symptomatically associated with diplopia. Severe vertigo occurs in approximately 5% of patients, often noted early in the clinical course. Recovery after several weeks is usual.

Olfactory abnormalities have been reported in MS, including in early drawings of olfactory lesions by Charcot. However, they have been less frequently reported in recent literature, and their explanation is not obvious. Some difficulty likely owes to technical problems in assessing smell and the widespread prevalence of decreased smell in the general population. Nevertheless, recent investigations using standardized test procedures have documented olfactory dysfunction in a large proportion of patients.

GENITOURINARY SYMPTOMS

Urinary retention, urgency, frequency, and stress or overflow incontinence are frequent in MS and may be acutely presenting signs of the disorder. Bladder symptoms are more common in women. Retention is usually secondary to a hypotonic (hyporeflexic) bladder. While it may occur transiently early in the clinical course of MS, late in the illness it is usually permanent, requiring catheterization because it is refractory to medical measures. Frequency and incontinence are more commonly associated with detrusor hyperreflexia and sphincter dyssynergia. Careful urodynamic studies may establish the type of bladder dysfunction, but these neurogenic bladders are often managed empirically, albeit frequently with only partial relief of symptoms. The end result of hyperreflexic bladder often is a small contracted organ associated with incessant urinary frequency, repeated secondary injections, and stone formation owing to excessive fluid restriction by the patient. In years past, urinary tract infection accounted for the majority of deaths in MS.

Sexual impotence is reported in as many as 30% of male MS patients. Etiologic factors include upper motor neuron and sensory spinal lesions, as well as secondary effects of bladder dysfunction, pharmacologic therapy, depression, and anxiety. When first recognized it may be transitory and may exhibit apparent response to various proffered therapies; however, it usually becomes refractory to medical treatment. Surgical management through implantation of a penile prosthesis frequently provides satisfactory results.

COGNITIVE DYSFUNCTION AND EMOTIONAL ASPECTS

Cognitive symptoms may arise in as many as 50% of MS patients. The cognitive changes may be categorized as those of subcortical dementia, with signs of slowed processing and memory retrieval, decreased motivation, and disturbed executive function, rather than frank amnesia, apraxia, or aphasia as seen in cortical dementias. Cognitive dysfunction becomes more prominent in chronic progressive disease and in other patients with longer duration of disease, and seems to correlate with increased degree of cerebral white matter disease rather than with clinical disability. Electroencephalography may show mild background slowing. Long-latency evoked potentials, such as the auditory P30, show prolongation. Severe dementia is uncommon (5%). But it is not infrequent that high-functioning executives or professionals with only relatively minor gait, sensory, or visual problems are unable to continue in their employment. Whether cognitive deficits or affective components are responsible for such problems is unclear.

Depression is documented in 60% or more of patients and indubitably contributes to disruption of personal and family life in addition to employment difficulties. Denial of illness, frustration, and anxiety may be compounded by fatigue. Many patients report major social difficulties following false reassurances that early symptoms are emotionally based. Not only do patients experience personal frustration and side effects from sedative drugs, but family members and friends may reject patients' pleas for help. Thus it is often more appropriate for the diagnostician to admit inability to provide or exclude a diagnosis on the basis of subjective complaints, and recommend careful follow-up, than to provide diagnoses of "hysteria" or functional illness. Psychological counseling may also be better accepted in this context.

PAROXYSMAL SYMPTOMS

Symptoms which may last only seconds to hours occur in the course of MS. Such symptoms are not commonly recognized and may be ascribed to "hysteria." They probably occur considerably more commonly than in the 3% to 4% of patients documented to experience them. Paroxysmal symptoms include both sensory symptoms (visual blurring, trigeminal pain, paresthesias, Lhermitte's phenomenon, body pain) and motor symptoms (dysarthria, dystonia ["tonic seizures or spasms"], choreoathetosis, ataxia, falling, and akinesia). Paroxysmal falling is unexplained by ataxia, motor phenomena, or epileptic seizures, and is often not recognized as such. The majority of these paroxysmal conditions respond well to carbamazepine. In some cases phenytoin and acetazolamide have proved useful. These transient symptoms of MS are often the source of diagnostic confusion, due to their misinterpretation as transient ischemic attacks, epileptic seizures, cataplexy, convulsive syncope, or hysteria.

Epileptic seizures have been reported to occur in as many as 10% of MS patients with long-term follow-up, which approximates the frequency of seizures following other kinds of cerebral insults. However the prevalence of epileptic seizures in the patient pool at any given time is actually much lower (1% to 2%), and it is likely that some reported "seizures" represent nonepileptic convulsions. When epileptic seizures do appear early in the clinical course, it is a poor prognostic sign, especially if status epilepticus occurs.

PAIN

Pain is not uncommon in MS. Usually it is of neurogenic origin rather than of a secondary musculoskeletal nature. Paroxysmal pains include those of tonic spasms and trigeminal neuralgia. The most common chronic pain is a dull tingling sensation, or painful paresthesia. Acute spinal exacerbations are often accompanied by a band-like body-encircling pain or by back pain, reflecting the level of the spinal cord lesion. High cervical plaques may acutely cause head pain. These spinal symptoms are likely due in part to root entry zone involvement and usually respond promptly to steroid treatment.

NATURAL HISTORY

Multiple sclerosis in most patients is characterized by the appearance of symptoms of CNS deficit over hours to days. New symptoms and most recurrent symptoms last from days to months. If symptoms persist a day or longer they probably indicate the appearance of new loci of white matter disease. Evanescent symptoms are difficult to evaluate. They may indicate the presence of new pathologic lesions but in many instances are more likely to reflect adverse effects of physiologic changes on central conduction. Increased temperature is a well-known factor in exacerbating MS symptoms, but changes in blood ionic composition (pH, $[Ca^{++}]$, $[HCO_3]$) and other physiologic parameters can show pronounced effects upon conduction in demyelinated fibers. This resulting paroxysmal phenomena may be due to ephaptic transmission (cross talk) or to ectopic generation of spontaneous potentials as through mechanical deformation of damaged nerves.

The natural course of the relapsing–remitting form of the disease is part of a wide and unpredictable spectrum. Relapses may occur one or more times per year, or even monthly. On the other hand, some patients may have only one or a handful of attacks in a lifetime. Some people do not have symptoms their entire life, despite the pathology of MS being found at autopsy. In younger patients early in their disease, increased frequency and severity of attacks is often seen, sometimes later "burning out." Recovery from an exacerbation usually occurs over days to weeks, and occasionally continues over a period of months. Upon resolution of an exacerbation, neurologic signs may disappear completely, although meticulous examination usually will detect some residua. Subsequent exacerbations are sometimes more difficult to recognize, in part because the patient is less alarmed by them and because new deficits can be more difficult to detect when superimposed on prior multifocal neurologic impairment. MS, usually defined as chronic disease at this stage, takes on a waxing–waning character, although deficits tend to accumulate, with many patients exhibiting progressively more disability.

Chronic progressive disease may be the presenting form of MS or may occur subsequent to varying durations of relapsing–remitting disease. It is relatively more common among men. About 10% to 20% of patients under the age of 30 at onset show a chronic progressive course. In older patients, chronic progressive disease at onset of MS is more common. Conversion to a rapidly progressive course carries a bad prognosis for life as well as function. Patients with this "malignant" or life-threatening form of illness (also called *acute multiple sclerosis*) may die of brain-stem disease or status epilepticus. This course is a reflection of widely disseminated lesions. Improved management of these patients is resulting in a better prognosis. In addition, as patients with milder illness are recognized, the proportion of patients with a malignant presentation has statistically declined to about 5% of the total. Slowly progressive forms of illness may appear to plateau or "burn out," although slow progression may be continuing, with the changes too gradual for easy recognition by the patient or physician.

McAlpine found that after 10 years of disease 80% of MS patients with relapsing–remitting disease had "unrestricted" neurologic function. Of these, 85% continued without severe disability for a further 10 years. More recent studies also show that life-span expectancy is only slightly reduced in MS patients, representing at most a 7-year difference in younger patients compared with their non-MS cohort and even less difference in older patients. Newer techniques are allowing diagnosis of increasing numbers of patients with benign disease who might otherwise have gone undiagnosed—as well as arriving at different diagnoses for some patients with more severe diseases that otherwise might have been labeled MS. The net result of these forces is that inclusion and exclusion, respectively, of these individuals yield an overall "better" prognosis for the MS population.

CONTRIBUTORY FACTORS IN THE NATURAL HISTORY OF MS

Infections of the respiratory tract, particularly influenza, have been shown to increase the risk of exacerbation in MS. However, it has also been noted that MS patients have relatively fewer respiratory infections. Mechanisms accounting for reduced risk (of infection) are unknown, but it might be related to immune activation. Urinary tract infections or other intercurrent illnesses also can both cause temporary worsening of chronic symptoms and be associated with lengthy exacerbations.

Pregnancy itself appears to be associated with decreased MS disease activity, although the puerperium seems to be accompanied by increased risk of exacerbation, particularly the months immediately following delivery. However, not all reports are consistent in this regard.

Clinically, trauma or surgery, even minor, appears to be associated with an increased risk of exacerbation in MS. However, a number of studies have not come to this conclusion about this association. An increased risk of exacerbation has been noted within the month following spinal anesthesia (but not after lumbar puncture alone).

Emotional stress may antedate MS exacerbations. Recent well-designed studies have come to strong, statistically supported conclusions supporting this observation. The relationship of stress and immune-mediated tissue responses has spawned a new field of investigation: psychoneuroimmunology. Few findings directly applicable to MS and other human illness have come forth as of yet. However, immune responses have been shown to reduce brain-stem noradrenaline in experimental animals. It is possible that depression, known to be associated with altered control of CNS monoamines, may in MS be related to such changes.

VARIANTS OF MULTIPLE SCLEROSIS

Transverse myelitis may subsequently evolve into MS, but 80% or so of cases do not. Some cases will have disseminated involvement limited to the optic nerve (Devic's disease). Finding subclinical brain-stem or optic nerve involvement makes a diagnosis of MS likely.

Neuromyelitis optica (Devic's disease) is a syndrome consisting of optic nerve and spinal cord demyelination. It may represent a related but separate entity from MS since it occurs with similar or increased frequencies in Asia and South America, areas where MS is otherwise infrequently recognized. Moreover, disease onset occurs over a much wider age range than in MS. Recent MR findings may serve to differentiate both transverse myelitis and Devic's disease from MS.

Acute (malignant) MS occurs predictably when MS is associated with histocompatibility haplotypes HLA B7 and DR2 as well as in a few other patients. The prognosis of this grave type of presentation appears to improve with aggressive immunosuppression. Death occurs within weeks to months but may be avertable by aggressive measures.

Concentric sclerosis of Balo is a very rare disease (only about 40 cases have been described pathologically) which clinically follows a fulminant monophasic course compatible with acute MS, with death in weeks to months, but is pathologically distinguished by concentric lamellar demyelinating lesions in the white matter.

Diffuse sclerosis of Schilder is an extremely rare chronic or subacute myelinoclastic disorder which can be separated from adrenocorticoleukodystrophy (ADL) by careful pathologic studies. Patients show one or two large demyelinative plaques characteristic of MS in the cerebral hemispheres.

MS with demyelinative peripheral neuropathy is an uncommon clinical disorder. While morphometric and neurophysiologic abnormalities may occur in MS, they do not appear to have any clinical relevance. Severe demyelinative attack on cranial nerve or spinal root entry or exit zones can result in apparent peripheral symptomatology. Cases of combined peripheral and CNS disease in MS must be clearly differentiated from adult-onset leukodystrophies (such as metachromatic leukodystrophy) where such combined involvement is characteristic.

PATHOLOGY

MS is an inflammatory disease affecting CNS white matter. Lymphocytes, both CD4 and CD8 subsets, and monocytes are found penetrating the white matter surrounding small blood vessels, destroying myelin but usually sparing axons. Individual lesions are termed *plaques* and vary greatly in size. With time perivenular lesions may coalesce, forming plaques several centimeters in size. Plaques are distributed throughout the neuraxis and can be demonstrated radiologically, as well as pathologically. They tend to be conspicuous in the periventricular white matter, particularly adjacent to the frontal and/or occipital horns of the ventricular system (Fig. 8-3). Spinal cord involvement is cardinal, with the cervical cord having a particular predisposition. Optic nerves, chiasm, periaqueductal gray matter, and corpus callosum are also prominently affected.

Microscopically active plaques are less clearly circumscribed and very intensely cellular, particularly along the margin of active demyelination. While there is no agreement as to the subsets of lymphocytes predominating in lesions, electron microscopic studies show that myelin is actively destroyed by the invading macrophages. These changes are associated with interstitial edema and swelling of astrocytic foot processes. Inactive (old) plaques are relatively acellular and often are intensely gliotic. The traversing axons are reduced in number and may disappear completely. These plaques are sharply demarcated from normal tissue. Areas of incomplete myelination referred to as *shadow plaques* are thin myelin sheaths and are now known to be areas of *remyelination*. They are more typically located in more superficial white matter at the gray–white junction.

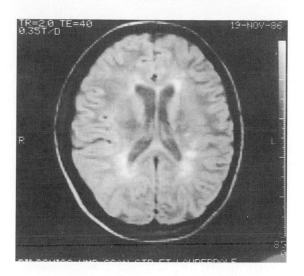

FIG. 8-3. Magnetic resonance imaging of the brain of a 30-year-old woman with multiple sclerosis of 6-year duration. This scan shows a typical prominent periventricular "increase in signal" indicative of the presence of demyelinating lesions.

PATHOPHYSIOLOGY

Experimental demyelination produces conduction delays, or blocks, and dispersion of impulses. This may impair normal physiologic responses. In acute lesions, the inflammatory reaction itself impairs axonal function. Function may resume when the inflammation subsides. But the axon, while regaining ability to conduct under optimal conditions, becomes hyperexcitable and prone to spontaneous discharge. Cross talk (ephaptic transmission) and hyperexcitability may explain paroxysmal phenomena. The susceptibility of demyelinated axons to total conduction block with increased temperature or physiologic alterations satisfactorily explains the effects of heat, fever, and illness resulting in the reappearance or aggravation of symptoms in MS.

IMMUNE RESPONSE

Altered immune responses have been detected in numerous studies. Lymphocytes are often present in modestly increased numbers in the CSF. In pathologic specimens of plaques, there are both helper (CD4) and suppressor–cytotoxic (CD8) T cells present, as well as macrophages that primarily have direct responsibility for myelin damage. In addition to these cell types not normally represented in brain, MS plaques show a variety of cell surface molecules (histocompatibility antigens, T-cell receptors), adhesion factors (integrins), and soluble cytokines (IFN, interleukins IL-1, IL-2, TNF, TFGB). Immunoglobulin IgG is increased in the CSF of MS patients and frequently shows oligoclonal bands, with reactivity to myelin proteins. The increased IgG apparently is mostly due to intrathecal synthesis, with occasional contribution of breakdown of the blood–brain barrier. Thus, findings have not implicated a particular single type of immune response, nor necessarily a single antigen in the nervous system that might serve as a specific target, although increasing attention is focused on myelin basic protein.

While considerable data suggest prominent involvement of an abnormal immune response in MS, the factors responsible for this are unknown. Viruses or other microorganisms have been considered responsible in part for provoking autoimmunity, without any conclusive evidence. Genetic background also seems important. Two hypothetical mechanisms that might explain the apparent autoimmunity of MS are that myelin might be damaged either as a consequence of "molecular mimicry" or simply as an "innocent bystander." Mimicry implies that myelin has structural similarity to some exogenous virus or substance, and thus is attacked as an unfortunate side effect of the body's response to this outside insult. In the bystander model, an outside virus or factor causes CNS destruction and exposure, thus prompting an anti-self response.

GENETIC FACTORS

Histocompatibility antigens (HLAs) have been extensively studied in MS. In Northern European populations there is significant over-representation of HLA haplotypes A3, B7, and DR2 (which are in linkage disequilibrium) among MS patients. In the Shetland and Orkney Islands the entire populations exhibit A3 and B7. The presence of B7 and DR2 together increases the likelihood of a malignant course for affected individuals. Other recent studies have confirmed that there is a 10 to 20 times increased risk for siblings of MS patients, apparently greatest for identical twins, lending credence to a role of genetic factors in the etiopathogenesis of the disease.

LABORATORY DATA

CEREBROSPINAL FLUID EXAMINATION

Examination of CSF obtained by lumbar puncture is important in the evaluation of patients. Cell counts reveal small numbers of mononuclear cells (lymphocytes), generally fewer than 100/mm^3. Total protein content is often normal but may be mildly elevated, although rarely greater than 100 mg/dl. IgG is very often elevated ($>$10.5% of total CSF protein). Increased IgG synthesis rate calculated from CSF and serum concentrations of albumin and IgG can be found in about 70% of patients. An increase in CSF IgG with normal CSF protein or albumin always indicates the presence of increased IgG synthesis. Oligoclonal IgG bands can be demonstrated by properly performed CSF agarose gel electrophoresis in 90% to 100% of MS patients at some point in their illness. Bands are not specific for MS, as they may be found in various infectious or inflammatory disorders of the CNS. Myelin basic protein (a structural protein of myelin) is increased in the CSF of virtually all MS patients during acute exacerbations, although it is technically difficult to detect due to problems with specimen handling and assay problems. All fluid should be promptly frozen for storage and shipping prior to any testing.

EVOKED RESPONSES

Visual evoked responses are tested optimally by performance of a light and dark checkerboard pattern reversal stimulus. Computer averaging of occipital scalp electrode potentials normally shows a major positive wave (P100) with a latency of about 100 msec, which varies somewhat with age and the stimulus parameters (frequency, check size, total subtended visual field, contrast ratios, and luminances) used by the laboratory. Prolonged latencies of the P100 wave are abnormal and, if monocular, specifically reflect prechiasmal disease. Abnormal findings are more prevalent with increased duration of disease, and ultimately may be present in more than 75% of patients.

Brain-stem auditory evoked responses (BAERs) are obtained using auditory click stimuli. Seven waves can often be discerned, although only waves I through V are clinically useful. Normal results are specific to each laboratory because of dependence on parameters such as stimulus polarity, rate, intensity, and electrode placement. Increased latencies between waves I and V are seen in about 75% of patients with brain-stem signs. Although increasing duration of illness makes abnormal BAERs more likely, these are the least sensitive evoked potentials for MS.

Somatosensory evoked responses are obtained by stimulating sensory or mixed nerves of an extremity (median, ulnar, posterior tibial, or peroneal). Short-latency (<50 msec) scalp potentials reflect conduction in the dorsal column–medial lemniscal somatosensory system. Abnormalities in the response are sensitive for dysfunction of this system, although the studies and their interpretation can be technically difficult.

NEUROIMAGING STUDIES

X-ray computed tomography (CT) may reveal white matter lucencies and ventriculomegaly. Active lesions often show contrast enhancement, particularly with administration of "double contrast." However, MR is so superior for visualizing plaques of MS that CT is not indicated except for the occasional acute attack in which other processes such as an intracranial bleed needs to be ruled out. Nevertheless, ventricular enlargement can be found in more than 30% of MS patients.

MR is remarkably sensitive in visualizing cerebral lesions in MS, although the findings are not specific for MS and over-reliance on brain images should be avoided. MR images bear a striking resemblance to gross sections of brain in their representation of normal anatomy and plaques; MR is actually more sensitive than inspection of brain sections in its ability to reveal the presence and location of demyelinative lesions. The lesions of MS are best visualized with a moderately T2-weighted MR pulse sequence. Demyelinating plaques appear as areas of increased T2 signal (increased brightness in the recorded image), due to their increased water content. They are most commonly seen in the peri- and supraventricular white matter but can be present as single or multiple lesions of varying size anywhere in the white matter of the cerebral hemispheres, cerebellum, or brain stem with no obvious relationship to the ventricular system. Many patients scanned within 3 years of the onset of MS do not show cerebral lesions by MR. A number of these patients do show MR-demonstrable lesions in the spinal cord.

Serial scanning of MS patients at intervals of weeks to months reveals that many cerebral white matter lesions of MS are stable, but some come and go without accompanying clinical symptomatology. Contrast enhancement following injection of a Gadolinium chelate is valuable in plaque identification in their active phase and is especially useful in identifying brain-stem and spinal cord plaques.

DIFFERENTIAL DIAGNOSIS

Dissemination of lesions in the nervous system over protracted periods of time is infrequently seen in other disorders. Rare cases of vascular disorders (principally systemic lupus erythematosus and vascular malformations) and neoplastic disease may occasionally resemble MS. Diagnosis of MS is most difficult early in the clinical course. If only one CNS lesion is demonstrated clinically and radiologically, a diagnosis of MS cannot be established. Other paraclinical tests such as CSF analysis and evoked potentials may be useful in confirming a laboratory-supported diagnosis of MS, and tests such as nerve conduction velocity may help lead one to other diagnoses.

Disseminated encephalomyelitis and viral (or postinfectious) encephalomyelitis are acute illnesses with disseminated central demyelination and MR findings like those of MS. It is a monophasic illness. If relapsing or progressive signs occur, the diagnosis of MS is likely.

Optic or *retrobulbar neuritis* may also result from inherited, nutritional, vasculitic, and ischemic syndromes. In young individuals these latter include systemic lupus and syphilis. In such individuals scotomas are often small and multiple in number. In addition, there is little subsequent change in these visual field abnormalities. Prognosis of isolated idiopathic optic neuritis is currently being prospectively studied in Europe. Preliminary results suggest that a large proportion of affected individuals, especially women, eventually qualify for the diagnosis of MS. In addition, MR reveals multiple brain lesions characteristic of MS in many otherwise asymptomatic patients with retrobulbar neuritis.

Brain-system signs such as bilateral INO are virtually pathognomonic of MS but may be mimicked by the ocular muscle weakness of myasthenia gravis and by the ocular ataxia of fixed cerebellar lesions. Pontine gliomas may rarely be associated with an INO. Diabetes can produce isolated ocular palsies but rarely creates a problem in differential diagnosis. Trigeminal neuralgia, in combination with other brain-stem signs, may be a manifestation of pontine gliomas and posterior fossa invasion by pharyngeal tumors. In these latter disorders, the corneal reflex is often diminished, an extremely rare finding in MS.

Familial spinocerebellar degenerations can occasionally be difficult to distinguish from MS early in its presentation, especially when family history is withheld. These disorders are much rarer than MS. Friedreich's ataxia typically begins at an early age and has peripheral nerve involvement. Spastic ataxia is dominantly inherited, and onset also occurs early in life. Olivopontocerebellar degeneration is usually recognized by its dominant pattern of inheritance and rather stereotypic presentation within a family. CSF and visual evoked responses are usually normal in these disorders.

Compressive myelopathy has always been a major consideration in the differential diagnosis of patients with progressive myelopathies. The advent of MR has eased the task of ruling out clinically significant intervertebral disc herniations/protrusions (cervical spondylosis), syringomyelia, spinal canal tumors, and intraparenchymal neoplasms. However, spinal cord lesions having increased T2 signal, with or without contrast enhancement, must not be assumed to represent spinal cord tumors as they may represent demyelinating lesions with edema. Retaking a complete history and performing other paraclinical tests in a search for evidence of disseminated disease is most helpful. Follow-up MR examinations can reveal changes in spinal cord size and signal characteristics.

Transverse myelopathy is a term describing a spinal cord disorder appearing to involve a single level. Transverse myelitis typically presents with subacute onset of weakness and numbness and progression to paraplegia within days to weeks. Subsequent partial or complete recovery suggests that the process is primarily demyelinative. Ischemic spinal cord disease can be associated with systemic lupus erythematosus, vasculitides, or disease of the radicular arteries. Transverse myelitis may rarely be a manifestation of a paraneoplastic process. Acute spinal cord infarction usually has onset over minutes to hours and involves the lower thoracic dermatomes. It may be seen in those with diabetes, atheromatous vascular disease, aortic aneurysms, or after aortic surgery. Because infarction usually involves only the anterior two-thirds of the cord, these individuals have clear motor and sensory levels, with sparing of proprioception.

Tropical spastic paraplegia ("Jamaican neuropathy") was first described during the past century but has recently been shown to be due, in a large proportion of cases, to infection by the human adult T-cell leukemia virus HTLV-I. This disorder shows a wide distribution, with prevalence in the Caribbean region, tropical Central and South America, Japan, and Africa. It occurs, albeit uncommonly, in U.S. natives. Clinically it usually appears as an indolent progressive myelopathy with bladder and sexual dysfunction (in men) with a spastic paraparesis. Onset in the third or fourth decade of life and the chronic progressive nature of the illness are similar to MS. Although optic neuritis has been noted in some cases, prominent brain-stem signs are infrequent. In addition, peripheral neuropathy is common. Serum testing reveals antibody to HTLV-I. Only a small proportion ($<1\%$) of seropositive individuals have neurologic disease; infection is endemic among certain populations, with transmission modes similar to that for HIV (blood transfusions, intravenous drug use, sexual, maternofetal). Recently, we and others have recognized an ataxic syndrome associated with a second human retrovirus, HTLV-II. This probably is the basis of "ataxic neuropathy," which was also described in Jamaica when Jamaican neuropathy was first recognized.

Vitamin B$_{12}$ deficiency may cause subacute combined degeneration (SCD) of the spinal cord. The symptoms of dorsal column sensory involvement and lateral column upper motor neuron dysfunction can resemble MS. However, SCD usually occurs later in life and is rare in the younger age-groups in which MS commonly has onset. B$_{12}$ deficiency may result from partial gastrectomy or tropical sprue, and should always be ruled out by serum studies. Some MS patients may have moderately low B$_{12}$ levels. However, it is not difficult to make the distinction between MS, in which brain-stem and optic nerve involvements occur, and B$_{12}$ deficiency, which features peripheral neuropathy, dementia (with psychosis), and megaloblastic anemia. An increased incidence of B$_{12}$ deficiency in MS has recently been reported.

Vitamin E deficiency is a rare cause of myelopathy, typically in children with a malabsorption syndrome. Since animal fat is the major source of this essential vitamin, dietary elimination of animal fat has been utilized to produce experimental models in primates. Demyelination as well as motor neuron damage have been demonstrated. Serum tocopherol levels may help in clinical diagnosis.

Sjögren's syndrome has been reported to include some patients with progressive or relapsing CNS symptoms and brain MR findings resembling MS. Sjögren's syndrome is a chronic inflammatory autoimmune disorder whose cardinal features are keratoconjunctivitis sicca (dry eyes) and xerostomia (dry mouth). Salivary gland biopsy is useful in revealing lymphocytic infiltration, and autoantibodies SS-A and SS-B (also known as anti-Ro and La) are usually present. Peripheral neuropathy, and especially sensory neuronopathy, may be associated with Sjögren's syndrome. However, examination of the MS patient population shows that while up to one-third may indeed have dry mouth and/or dry eyes, only a few have low titers of various autoantibodies, and only extremely few (<1% to 3%) meet diagnostic criteria for Sjögren's syndrome. In these few cases it is likely a concomitant rather than an etiologically significant diagnosis.

Lyme disease and neurosyphilis are infectious diseases that cause serial multifocal nervous system disease and thus can appear similar to MS. Both disorders may be associated with dermatopathy and arthropathy during their course. Lyme manifestations include cranial neuritis, radiculoneuritis, (peripheral neuropathy, and mild cognitive symptoms. Typically there is a pronounced chronic lymphocytic meningitis, with cell counts often higher than in MS. In rare cases there is a chronic progressive clinical encephalomyelitis with sensory and motor abnormalities and brain MR foci of increased T2 signal predominantly in white matter. Such cases have led to concern over diagnostic confusion of this treatable infectious disease with MS. However, even in Lyme seropositive patients the two diseases may be distinguished by clinical course as well as by CSF antibody studies. Syphilis may manifest a meningovascular picture or tabes dorsalis with prominent dorsal column signs. Exposure to the pathogenetic spirochetal organisms *Borrelia burgdorferi* for Lyme and *Treponema pallidum* for syphilis can be ascertained by use of specific serum (Western blot) and CSF antibody tests. However, positive antibody tests do not indicate that a patient's symptom complex results from this exposure. Despite considerable interest in overlap of Lyme disease symptoms with those of MS, it is now clear that the Lyme organism is only very rarely the cause of an MS-like clinical presentation.

TREATMENT AND THERAPY

Treatment can be divided into disease-modifying and symptomatic categories. The former includes various therapies designed to modulate or suppress the immune response or its inflammatory end result. The latter includes a large armamentarium of neuropharmacologic agents that ameliorate dysfunction of different parts of the nervous system.

Anti-inflammatory therapy with steroids (methylprednisolone or prednisone) or adrenocorticotropic hormone (ACTH) have been the mainstays of treatment of acute exacerbations of MS. Exacerbations are significantly shortened, but the extent of ultimate recovery is not altered. The most common treatment presently used is intravenous administration of methylprednisolone (Solu-Medrol) in doses of 500 mg to 1000 mg (or 10 to 15 mg/kg) daily for 5 days. This may be accomplished on an inpatient or outpatient basis. Some neurologists have favored oral prednisone courses (0.5 to 1 mg/kg/day with taper over 2 to 4 weeks) as a substitute for intravenous administration, although *such regimens have now been shown to produce an unfavorable outcome in the treatment of optic neuritis in patients with isolated disease or occurring during the course of MS.* In the view of the medical advisory board of the National Multiple Sclerosis Society and in the opinion of the authors, *prednisone is contraindicated in MS.* Other regimens include use of ACTH given by intravenous or intramuscular injection, 80 units daily, for 1 to 4 weeks. During prolonged administration of steroids or ACTH there frequently is mood alteration. Euphoria may be more prominent among those patients with extensive brain involvement and can often be controlled by prescription of lithium carbonate.

Immunosuppressive regimens have been employed in a number of recent trials. The pharmacologic agents azathioprine (Imuran) and cyclophosphamide (Cytoxan) have been used individually or in combination with steroids or ACTH for the prevention of exacerbations or progression of disability and have shown some efficacy in a number of studies. Other immunosuppressive therapies that have been investigated and found to be either without efficacy or with modest benefits outweighed by morbidity include plasma exchange in combination with cyclophosphamide, cyclosporine (Sandimmune), and chlorambucil. A number of other immunomodulatory therapies are still under investigation, including total lymphoid irradiation, oral methotrexate, FK-506, intravenous immunoglobulin, oral copolymer-1, oral myelin basic protein, and intravenous monoclonal antibodies to CD3 or CD4 markers. More specific experimental therapies that have been proposed include other monoclonal antibodies, including some against cell adhesion molecules, and vaccination against specific T-cell receptor V regions. All immunosuppressive therapies carry some risk, particularly with regard to infection in MS patients who often already have compromised genitourinary and pulmonary systems. Patients with rapidly progressive disease should generally be referred to specialized centers.

Antiviral therapy with interferons may be administered via intrathecal, intramuscular, or subcutaneous routes. Human alpha and beta interferons have shown beneficial effects in decreasing frequency of MS exacerbations. Approval of recombinant beta interferon for treatment of the relapsing and remitting of MS is widely anticipated but has not been given. However, human gamma interferon has been convincingly shown to *cause* MS exacerbations. Investigations with alpha and beta interferons are continuing; appropriate dosage and duration of therapy have not been determined, and side effects and cost of therapy may be limiting factors. Interferons may act through their immunomodulatory effects or through antiviral action. Other antiviral therapies have not yet been tested in MS.

Physical and emotional rest have always been emphasized in the management of MS. Stress of any kind may increase the symptoms of the illness and may be associated with exacerbations; conversely, rest tends to ameliorate them. Apart from maintaining good health, patients should be encouraged to work within their physical limitations. Frustration may require psychological counseling, although psychoanalytic therapy has not been productive in our patients.

Spasticity is a major unremitting problem in many patients, and while physical therapy can be helpful, pharmacologic intervention is of much benefit. Diazepam (Valium) in 2.5-mg to 5-mg doses can prevent spasms in the lower extremities at night. Similar small doses can also alleviate stiffness and spasms in the morning. Baclofen (Lioresal) may also be used and should be initiated in 5-mg doses and slowly increased. Care should be exercised in prescribing even small doses of diazepam or baclofen since replacement of spasticity by weakness can result in a greater handicap. Dantrolene (Dantrium) is occasionally helpful but may produce a loss of well-being in some patients. Some patients find that carbamazepine alleviates paroxysmal leg spasms. Other drugs such as cyclobenzaprine (Flexeril) and other "muscle relaxants" are not especially helpful in the management of upper motor neuron spasticity.

Bladder dysfunction is very common. Acute urinary retention in the young patient often responds to sporadic catheterization as needed. However, appropriate urologic care and follow-up are impor-

tant. Hyper-reflexic bladders are much more common. Propantheline is helpful in controlling nocturia but somewhat less so in the management of daytime urinary frequency. Dyssynergia occurs in the majority of patients and often is manifested as incomplete emptying. Failure to empty the bladder leads to increased risk of urinary infections and the risk of pyelonephritis. Timed voiding and fluid restriction are occasionally sufficient to achieve better emptying. Failing this, intermittent catheterization is always preferable to placement of an indwelling catheter because of the risks of infection. Urinary prophylaxis with antibiotic therapy is controversial. Many physicians avoid such suppressive therapy, even in the case of an indwelling catheter, because of the risk of selection of resistant bacteria, particularly *Pseudomonas* species, although nitrofurantoin or trimethoprim and sulfamethoxazole (Septra) is used by some patients with benefit. Acidification of the urine by ascorbic acid (2g to 4g orally per day) with or without mandelic acid may be helpful without introducing the risk of resistant bacteria.

Sexual dysfunction in men is often the product of spinal cord disease, but psychological factors are equally important. If appropriate urologic and sleep studies documenting the absence of morning erections suggest a neurourologic etiology, penile prostheses may provide satisfactory results.

Physical therapy can improve gait and general level of function. Regular range-of-motion exercises can prevent contractures and maintain purposeful function in the upper extremities, especially during lengthy disability. Long-term maintenance therapy may be helpful in preventing patients from premature reliance on wheelchairs. Lightweight ankle–foot orthoses may be prescribed for drop foot and can greatly assist in achieving a near-normal gait. Personal contact with the therapist may also be crucial in psychological support of the patient. Recent experience with body cooling suggests this approach may be helpful in increasing exercise tolerance in MS.

QUESTIONS AND DISCUSSION

1. How is the diagnosis of MS made?

    A. Clinical history and neurologic findings
    B. CT examinations of the head
    C. CSF examination
    D. MR of the brain
    E. All of the above

The answer is (A). The diagnosis is always clinical. CSF and MR are especially helpful procedures but do not replace history taking and neurologic examination.

2. Major disability in MS is usually due to

   A. Optic nerve involvement
   B. Cerebral hemispheric lesions
   C. Brain-stem involvement
   D. Spinal cord disease
   E. All of the above

The answer is (D). Spinal cord lesions account for the majority of the disabling motor and sensory symptoms of MS. Brain-stem and optic nerve deficits also figure importantly, with cerebral white matter involvement being less commonly symptomatic.

3. The three most useful laboratory tests in supporting the diagnosis of MS are

   A. MR of the brain
   B. CSF cell count
   C. CSF immunoglobulin analysis
   D. Visual evoked responses
   E. Somatosensory evoked responses

The answers are (A), (C), and (D).

4. Trigeminal neuralgia

   A. Never occurs in young adults
   B. Occurs in young adults only with pontine gliomas
   C. Responds to most sedative drugs
   D. Is only treated surgically
   E. Usually responds well to carbamazepine

The answer is (E). While carbamazepine (Tegretol) is first-line treatment, phenytoin (Dilantin) and baclofen (Lioresal) are also useful in treatment. Surgery is a last resort.

5. Urinary frequency in MS

   A. Is rarely a significant problem
   B. Is always a sign of injection
   C. Predictably responds to propantheline (anticholinergics)
   D. Requires careful evaluation and management
   E. Should be disregarded

The answer is (D). Consultation and management by a urologist supplement the care by the attending physician. The major goal is to avoid damage to ureters and kidneys (hydronephrosis).

6. Treatment of MS

   A. Is a waste of time
   B. Always requires the use of ACTH
   C. Should take into consideration the patient's clinical activity and disability
   D. Should be limited to ACTH and physical therapy
   E. Is limited to a low-fat diet

The answer is (C). Management of the patient's psychological reaction, clinical status, and disabilities must always be taken into consideration. Sometimes the patient's most obvious disability is of least concern to him or her.

7. The risk of MS in the sister of a patient

   A. Is about 100/100,000
   B. Is increased significantly
   C. Is significantly decreased
   D. Is increased only if HLA B7 is present
   E. Is about the same as in any other community member

The answer is (B). Several studies have shown that the risk of MS is several times higher than chance in a sibling.

8. Chronic progressive MS

   A. Has a good prognosis
   B. May occur at any point in the illness but is more common after age 30
   C. Is ten times more common in women than in men
   D. Most frequently arises at age 20 to 30
   E. All of the above

The answer is (B). Chronic progressive disease becomes more and more likely with age of onset after 30. It is also more common among men.

9. Which of the following statements concerning lumbar puncture are true?

   A. It can cause exacerbations of MS.
   B. When performed for spinal anesthesia it may cause exacerbation.
   C. It is helpful in establishing a diagnosis when oligoclonal bands are present.
   D. It is helpful in establishing a diagnosis when IgG synthesis is increased.

E. It should not be performed because it is too risky.

The answers are (B), (C), and (D). Lumbar puncture, properly performed, is a safe diagnostic procedure. Risks of spinal anesthesia should be weighed carefully. CSF electrophoresis and immunoglobulin quantitation are helpful.

SUGGESTED READING

Adams CW: Color Atlas of Multiple Sclerosis and Other Myelin Disorders. Dobbs Ferry, NY, Sheridan Medical Books, 1989

Antel J (ed): Multiple Sclerosis. Neurologic Clinics. Vol 1, No 3. Philadelphia, WB Saunders, 1983

Cook D, Dowling PC: Multiple sclerosis and viruses: An overview. Neurology 20:80, 1980

Hallpike JF, Adams CW, Tourtellotte WW (eds): Multiple Sclerosis: Pathology, Diagnosis and Management. Baltimore, Williams & Wilkins, 1983

Honig LS, Ramsay RE, Sheremata WA: Event-related potential P300 in multiple sclerosis: Relation to MRI and cognitive impairment. Arch Neurol 49:44, 1992

Koprowski H, Defreitas E, Sandberg–Wohlheim M et al: Retroviruses and multiple sclerosis. Nature 318:154, 1985

Kurtzke JF, Beebe GW, Nagler B, et al: Studies on natural history of multiple sclerosis 4: Clinical features of the onset bout. Acta Neurol Scand 44:467–499, 1968

Lauer K: On the diagnostic value of different CSF investigations in multiple sclerosis. J Neurol 231:130, 1984

McAlpine D, Lumsden CF, Acheson ED. Multiple Sclerosis, A Reappraisal, 2nd ed. Edinburgh, Churchill Livingstone, 1972

McDonald WI, Barnes D: Lessons from magnetic resonance imaging in multiple sclerosis. Trends Neurosci 12:376, 1989

Matthews WB: McAlpine's Multiple Sclerosis, 2nd ed. Edinburgh, Churchill Livingstone, 1991

Poser CM, Paty DW, Scheinberg L et al: New diagnostic criteria for multiple sclerosis: Guidelines for research protocols. Ann Neurol 13:227, 1983

Rao SM (ed): Neurobehavioral Aspects of Multiple Sclerosis. New York, Oxford University Press, 1990

Rudick RA, Goodkin DE (eds): Treatment of Multiple Sclerosis: Trial Design, Results, and Future Perspectives. London, Springer–Verlag, 1992

Schumacher GA, Beebe G, Kibler RF et al: Problems of experimental trials of therapy in multiple sclerosis: Report by the panel on the evaluation of experimental trials of therapy in multiple sclerosis. Ann NY Acad Sci 122:552, 1965

Wilson SAK. Neurology. London, Edward Arnold, 1940

Parkinson's Disease

William J. Weiner

Parkinson's disease is the most common akinetic rigid syndrome and the most frequently encountered extrapyramidal movement disorder. It is a neurodegenerative disease of unknown etiology that most often begins at 58 to 60 years of age. Approximately 10% to 15% of patients will have disease onset before age 50. As the population of the United States ages, the number of people who will be at risk for the development of Parkinson's disease increases. Diagnostic and therapeutic knowledge is important not only because of the prevalence of the disorder but also because the pharmacology of Parkinson's disease has led to fundamental changes in the way investigators and physicians view central nervous system neurotransmitter function.

CLINICAL FEATURES

Parkinson's disease is characterized by a typical history of progressive neurologic disability and the following four major neurologic signs: resting tremor, cogwheel rigidity, bradykinesia, and impaired postural reflexes. It is often observed that by the time a patient presents to a physician for evaluation of this problem, the syndrome has been present for 1 to 2 years. Unilateral tremor involving a single limb is the most common presenting symptom and sign. However, careful history taking often reveals that difficulty buttoning shirts or blouses, fastening snaps, cutting food with the proper utensils, alterations in handwriting (Fig. 9-1), a feeling of stiffness, or a general feeling of overall slowness may have been noted up to 12 to 24 months earlier, and that these symptoms have gradually become worse. In addition, a patient may note that chewing food has become slow and laborious and that his voice fluctuates and seems to intermittently lose volume. Additional questions that help to illustrate the clinical problems in a patient with bradykinesia and impaired postural reflexes include inquiring whether or not the patient has difficulty rising from low, soft chairs or sofas, has difficulty entering and leaving an automobile, has difficulty turning from his back to his stomach or *vice versa* while lying in bed, or has difficulty maintaining balance in a crowd. The patient may have noticed that occasionally he is unable to stop walking forward (propulsion) or backward (retropulsion). Family members may also report that the patient's face has changed and that he does not smile as much (masked facies; Fig. 9-2), that he seems to stare all the time (reptilian stare), that his posture has become stooped and flexed (simian posture; Fig. 9-3), and that he has become exasperatingly slow. It may take 30 to 90 minutes to dress in the morning and even longer to disrobe in the evening.

The elucidation of this history may make the diagnosis of parkinsonism evident. It is apparent

William J. Weiner and Christopher G. Goetz, eds. *Neurology for the Non-Neurologist*, Third Edition. Copyright © 1994, 1989 by J. B. Lippincott Company. Copyright © 1981 by Harper and Row Publishers, Inc.

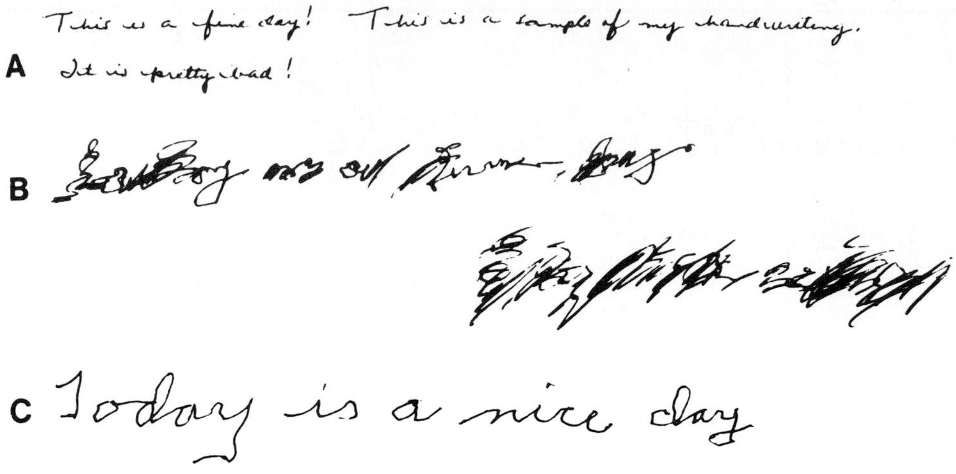

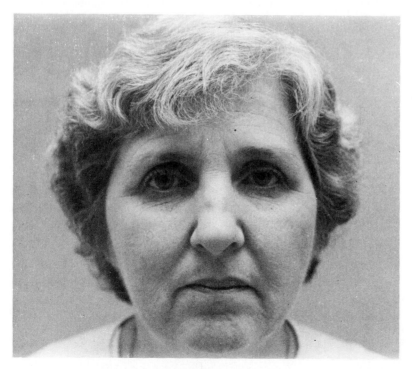

A *This is a fine day!   This is a sample of my handwriting.*
It is pretty bad !

B *[handwriting sample]*

[handwriting sample]

C *Today is a nice day*

FIG. 9-1. (*A*) This handwriting sample is from a 55-year-old patient with untreated Parkinson's disease. It is a good example of the typical micrographic handwriting that is often characteristic of this condition. (*B*) The handwriting samples shown in *B* and *C* are from the same patient with essential tremor. Handwriting sample *B* is prior to treatment with propranolol and is typified by the large, sloppy script. (*C*) This is the handwriting sample from the patient with essential tremor while being treated with propranolol (160 mg/day). The improvement in the handwriting is obvious. Changes in written script can provide excellent clues to the type of movement disorder that is present (see Chap. 10).

FIG. 9-2. Typical masked facies in a patient with Parkinson's disease.

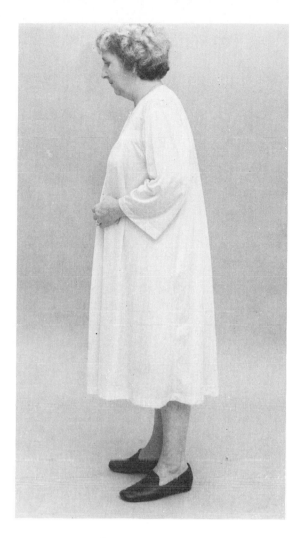

FIG. 9-3. Mild simian posture in a patient with Parkinson's disease. Note the flexion of the upper extremity and the slight flexion of the upper trunk and the head.

history of encephalitis, or exposure to various toxins including the use of street drugs.

Resting tremor is the most frequent presenting sign in these patients. The appearance of this tremor often precipitates the patient's visit to the doctor. The tremor is highly characteristic and consists of a low- to medium-amplitude five to seven cycles/second alternating movement. *Tremor* is defined as the involuntary rhythmic oscillatory sinusoidal movement that results from the alternating or synchronous contractions of reciprocally innervated antagonistic muscles. Resting tremor has been described as "pill rolling" because of the movement of the fingers and thumb. The tremor, however, may begin in the hands, legs, or face and most often appears unilaterally in a single limb. It will often progress to involve the second limb of the same side before becoming bilateral. With the exception of impaired postural reflexes, the major signs of parkinsonism appear most often as unilateral manifestations, often confusing the unfamiliar and raising inappropriate diagnostic categories. Careful observation of the tremor will reveal that it is a resting tremor that tends to be ameliorated when a purposeful movement is undertaken. A simple, quick way of assessing whether a tremor is primarily a resting or kinetic tremor is to have the patient perform a finger-to-finger and finger-to-nose maneuver and to observe the affected limb when it is posturally supported in a resting position. The patient with a resting tremor will perform these maneuvers and a marked amelioration of tremor will be observed during this time. The patient with kinetic tremor will be observed to have no tremor at rest but will develop typical dysmetric movements as the hand reaches the target object. When the limbs are observed in a totally supported and at-rest position, the patient with resting tremor will be seen to have the tremor, whereas those patients with kinetic tremor will not.

Cogwheel rigidity is a sign that can be present in a unilateral or bilateral distribution depending on the stage of illness. The patient does not complain of "cogwheeling." This sign is elicited by passive movement of the limb and neck through a full range of motion. When present, this sign is particularly elicitable when the neck is flexed and extended and when the elbow and wrist are fully flexed and extended. There is, in addition to increased tone, a characteristic ratchet-like sensation felt with passive movement. This can often be observed but is more easily palpated by the examiner as the limb is flexed and extended. There are some

that not all patients will present with all of these symptoms and that a patient will occasionally present with only a single symptom and yet will have parkinsonism. Additional questions that may help determine the etiology of the syndrome are directed at whether or not there is a family history of neurologic syndromes, concurrent drug use, past patients in whom the initial symptomatology is cervical or low back discomfort, and the question of whether or not increased muscle tone is responsible for this symptom has been raised.

Bradykinesia is an additional characteristic sign that is certainly responsible for a great deal of the disability associated with parkinsonism. Slowness of voluntary movement is characteristic of this syndrome and accounts for the difficulty in such diverse activities as turning over in bed, rising from chairs, chewing food, dressing, walking, and numerous other activities of daily living. Some of these difficulties can be easily observed during an examination by watching the patient rise from a chair, walk to the examining room, and undress. Observe the general slowness with which the simplest maneuvers are undertaken. Again, this can initially be seen as a unilateral finding.

A final important sign in these patients is impaired *postural reflexes*. Postural reflexes refer to the ability of the patient to right himself and keep from losing his balance when sustaining minor postural perturbations (*e.g.*, being jostled in a crowd). In addition, these reflexes also encompass the ability of patients to turn around and change directions while walking without losing their balance and falling. These reflexes can be simply and effectively evaluated by observing the patient walk 10 to 15 steps and turn around. A patient with normal postural reflexes should be able to pivot and turn without taking extra steps. In parkinsonism one will often observe that it takes the patient 3 to 5 steps to change direction. The second office test of postural reflexes includes a mild thrust to the chest wall with the admonition to the patient that he is not to step backward. The examiner must position himself, or have someone else positioned behind the patient during this maneuver, since the response may be 0 to 1 steps backward, 7 to 8 steps backward (retropulsion), or no step backward but complete loss of balance and falling (Fig. 9-4). Impaired postural reflexes with frequent falls are a source of severe disability in fully advanced parkinsonism because of associated morbidity (subdural hematomas and fractures of the hips or wrists). This is frequently overlooked in discussions of parkinsonian symptomatology, and it is most important to remember because this sign, just as any other major sign, may be seen in relative isolation. It is rare but possible to see elderly patients with Parkinson's disease whose main manifestation of the disease is impaired postural reflexes. These patients may have as their presenting complaint frequent falls without loss of

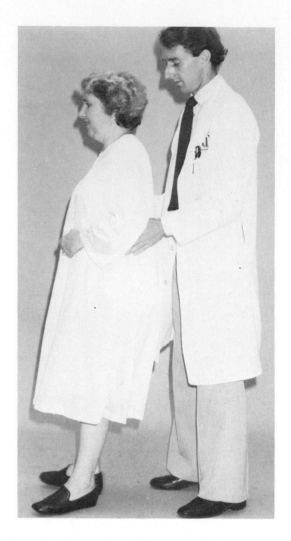

FIG. 9-4. This picture illustrates the loss of postural reflexes often seen in patients with Parkinson's disease. The examiner has just finished administering a backward thrust to the patient's chest and has instructed the patient to maintain her posture. However, it can be seen that the patient's postural response is quite poor and that rather than maintaining a fixed posture response to the thrust or taking one to two steps backward, the patient appears to have lost her balance entirely and requires the assistance of the examiner to prevent her from falling to the ground.

consciousness. These people have often undergone extensive diagnostic work-ups to evaluate the falling episodes, including 24-hour cardiac monitoring, electroencephalograms (EEGs), 5-hour glucose tolerance tests and other systemic blood work, and occasionally even cerebral angiography. These tests will have been performed despite the fact that routine outpatient evaluation will often reveal that the primary neurologic abnormality in these patients is impaired postural reflexes, which suggests the correct diagnosis.

This discussion of the symptoms and signs of parkinsonism should serve to remind the examining physician that there is no single pathognomonic sign of the disorder and that it is a constellation of symptomatology and signs that results in this clinical diagnosis. There is no known biologic marker of Parkinson's disease, and therefore there is no definitive laboratory or imaging study that confirms the diagnosis. The diagnosis is clinical and is dependent on the interpretation of the patient's history and neurologic examination. The diagnosis of parkinsonism does not necessarily mean that the patient has Parkinson's disease.

Parkinson's disease is characterized by a specific neuropathology. The substantia nigra (a pigmented midbrain nucleus) bears the brunt of the pathologic changes, with depigmentation, neuronal loss, and the presence of intracytoplasmic inclusion bodies (Lewy bodies). Patients who present with tremor, rigidity, bradykinesia, and impaired postural reflexes but who do not have this specific neuropathology are diagnosed as having an akinetic rigid syndrome or parkinsonism but not Parkinson's disease.

PHARMACOLOGY

Early studies demonstrated that there were regional concentration differences in dopamine in different areas of the brain. The corpus striatum (a basal ganglia nuclear group) was determined to have a high concentration of dopamine. Neurochemical investigation of the brains of patients who died with Parkinson's disease were conducted, and the corpus striatum concentration of dopamine was low compared with the dopamine concentration in nonparkinsonian corpus striatum. This finding was the first definitive biochemical lesion in an adult-onset degenerative disorder of the extrapyramidal system. Parkinson's disease could now be defined by loss of dopamine in the corpus striatum and degen-

eration of the substantia nigra. Further study revealed that the high concentration of dopamine in the corpus striatum was not located in the neurons of the striatum but was anatomically situated in the terminals of neurons whose origin was the substantia nigra. In other words, there exists an anatomic pathway between the substantia nigra and the corpus striatum. The nigrostriatal pathway utilizes dopamine as its neurotransmitter, and it became clear that the progressive loss of substantia nigra neurons was accompanied by a progressive loss of dopamine in the striatum. Since the projection pathway was degenerating and the dopamine is anatomically located within the projection pathway, it is not surprising that dopamine was progressively lost in this disorder.

The series of discoveries that led to the knowledge that Parkinson's disease was associated with the loss of a specific regionally located neurotransmitter (dopamine) was a remarkable advance in our understanding of adult-onset neurodegenerative disorders. In 1967 enormous quantities of levodopa (4 g to 8 g/day) were administered to Parkinson's disease patients and the remarkable therapeutic response was observed. In order for levodopa to have a therapeutic effect, it must cross the blood–brain barrier and be decarboxylated to dopamine. The enzyme that decarboxylates dopa to dopamine is ubiquitous and also decarboxylates several other aromatic amino acids. This enzyme, termed *aromatic amino acid decarboxylase* or *dopa decarboxylase*, is found in several extracerebral locations, including the gastrointestinal tract, liver, and kidney. When orally administered levodopa is absorbed, it is acted on by the extracerebral, decarboxylase and is converted to dopamine, which cannot cross the blood–brain barrier. If levodopa is administered alone, enormous quantities are required to overcome the peripheral decarboxylase systems and achieve a therapeutic benefit. The use of a peripheral decarboxylase inhibitor (carbidopa) with levodopa results in a much lower dose of levodopa being administered to achieve a central effect. Since the replenishment of the neurotransmitter dopamine in the striatum results in remarkable clinical improvement in patients with Parkinson's disease, it is implied that the neural substrate that dopamine acts on (the striatal dopamine receptors) is essentially intact in this disorder.

TREATMENT

All medications currently used to treat Parkinson's disease provide symptomatic relief only and do not alter the underlying pathogenesis of the disorder; in other words, the natural progression of Parkinson's disease continues despite current treatment. The treatment of each patient with Parkinson's disease should be highly individualized to provide acceptable symptomatic relief. Early Parkinson's disease in which patients exhibit only mild resting tremor can often be treated effectively with anticholinergics (e.g., trihexyphenidyl, benztropine). The anticholinergics are useful because the striatum contains high levels of both dopamine and acetylcholine and the dopamine deficiency state in the striatum of patients with Parkinson's disease produces a relative cholinergic hyperactivity. Anticholinergics exert their beneficial effect by partially correcting this apparent cholinergic excess.

Amantadine is also useful in the treatment of early Parkinson's disease and can be helpful for early bradykinesia. Amantadine has both anticholinergic activity and mild dopaminergic activity. The latter may be related to the drug's ability to alter dopamine uptake or release. Combined treatment with anticholinergics and amantadine may provide symptomatic relief for 6 to 18 months. The progression of the disease process will eventually result in the need for more powerful dopaminergic stimulation.

The use of levodopa as a precursor loading strategy to increase central dopamine and to ameliorate Parkinson's disease has been one of the remarkable therapeutic advances in neurology. However, high-dose levodopa administration produces anorexia, nausea, and vomiting. These symptoms occur because of the high levels of circulating peripheral dopamine that are present as a result of extensive extracerebral decarboxylation and that result in the stimulation of the area postrema, the emesis center. The development of peripheral dopa decarboxylase inhibitors in large part ameliorated these problems and led to the development of combination therapy with levodopa and carbidopa (the peripheral decarboxylase inhibitor). This drug is available in a fixed ratio of 10:100, 25:250, and 25:100, with the numerator indicating the milligram dose of carbidopa and the denominator, the milligram dose of levodopa. The single and most important advantage of this drug is the ability to administer less levodopa to obtain the same central effect. This results in a reduction of nausea and vomiting. In fact, the ease of administration of carbidopa–levodopa (Sinemet, Atamat) therapy for both the patient and the treating physician has resulted in its almost exclusive use in the treatment of patients with Parkinson's disease who require levodopa.

Bromocriptine (Parlodel) and pergolide (Permax) are additional dopaminergic agents to treat Parkinson's disease. Bromocriptine and pergolide are direct-acting dopamine receptor agonists that have been demonstrated to be effective in the treatment of Parkinson's disease. Since dopamine receptor agonists exert their effect on the striatal dopamine receptors (which presumably are not involved in the substantia nigra degenerative process), it was felt that they would perhaps be effective when carbidopa–levodopa fails and that they might not produce the same toxic effects as carbidopa–levodopa. Clinical experience with bromocriptine and pergolide has shown that they are effective not only in the treatment of Parkinson's disease but also in ameliorating motor fluctuations in patients treated with carbidopa–levodopa. Bromocriptine and pergolide are most often used in practice when patients have developed complications of carbidopa–levodopa treatment. Although there have been attempts to use dopamine receptor agonists as monotherapy to treat early Parkinson's disease, these agents have not been useful in this situation. They are not as effective in providing symptomatic relief as carbidopa–levodopa, and they are not as well tolerated.

Selegiline hydrochloride (Eldepryl), a monoamine oxidase B inhibitor, has also been used to treat motor fluctuations in moderate to advanced Parkinson's disease. This drug inhibits the catabolism of dopamine and promotes dopaminergic activity. Selegiline Hcl has also been used in early Parkinson's disease and has been shown to delay the need for carbidopa–therapy. There has been considerable discussion as to whether or not this effect in early Parkinson's disease is "neuroprotective" or simply symptomatic. The evidence suggests that the effect of selegiline Hcl in this situation is symptomatic.

COMPLICATIONS

Although there is no question that carbidopa–levodopa is the mainstay of therapy in this disorder, numerous problems are associated with its use (Table 9-1). However, it should be recognized that several long-term follow-up studies of patients with Parkinson's disease who were treated with these agents showed that at the end of 5 and 6 years of treatment most patients were either no worse than

TABLE 9-1. Toxicity Associated with Chronic Levodopa Therapy

Central toxicity	Dyskinesias
	Motor fluctuations
	"On–off" phenomenon
	Loss of drug efficacy
	Psychiatric disturbance
	Sleep disturbance
Peripheral toxicity	Nausea and vomiting
	Cardiac arrhythmias
Mixed central and peripheral toxicity	Orthostatic hypotension

prior to treatment or better than before they were treated. This finding is extraordinary because prior to levodopa treatment the prognostic outlook in Parkinson's disease was dismal. Several major side effects are associated with the use of levodopa and carbidopa–levodopa, including drug-induced dyskinesias, drug-induced psychiatric problems, and motor fluctuations.

Levodopa- and carbidopa–levodopa–induced *dyskinesias* are striking long-term complications of this type of therapy. The dyskinesias are most often choreic. Chorea consists of irregular, unpredictable, brief, jerky movements that flit from one body part to another in a continuous random sequence. Occasionally carbidopa–levodopa–induced dyskinesias are dystonic in quality. Dystonia describes movements that are dominated by sustained muscle contraction, frequently resulting in twisting repetitive movements and abnormal postures. The dyskinesia may involve the lingual, facial, and buccal regions, the limbs, and the axial musculature. It is dramatic to see patients with this drug-related disorder because these patients were always characterized by their slowness and poverty of movement. The chorea seen in this setting is quite similar to that seen in Huntington's disease or tardive dyskinesia.

Levodopa-induced dyskinesias are quite frequent and are seen in more than half the patients at the end of 5 years of carbidopa–levodopa treatment. The severity of the chorea may increase with continued treatment, and the dose of levodopa required to elicit chorea may decrease with time. Conversely, a reduction in dosage will invariably ameliorate this drug-induced movement disorder. Although the chorea may be severe, the parkinsonian patient rarely complains, and the family or the physician is usually the first to notice the chorea and become concerned about it. This common response

to the movement disorder is probably best explained by the fact that often while patients are choreatic they are still able to voluntarily move around with relative ease, and given their choice all parkinsonian patients would rather be choreatic and mobile than bradykinetic. Levodopa-induced dyskinesia can, in some patients, be as disabling as bradykinesia.

The *psychiatric side effects* of long-term dopaminergic therapy include altered sleep patterns, vivid nightmares, auditory and visual hallucinations, paranoia, and frank psychosis. While there may be a continuum in the expression of these side effects, with the increasing severity of each complication being related to dose and treatment duration, there are also reports that such a continuum does not represent an individual patient response. Whether or not single patients display the entire spectrum of psychiatric complications or the spectrum represents a wide range of response to chronic dopaminergic treatment, it is certain that the following complications are drug-related and are frequently seen. These complications, which include alterations in sleep patterns beginning with increasing insomnia, day–night reversal, vivid nightmares, visual hallucinations, increasing paranoia, and paranoid psychosis, can be ameliorated by dosage reduction. A new approach to the treatment of visual hallucinations and paranoia in these patients is the use of clozapine (Clozaril), an atypical neuroleptic that does not produce motor side effects.

Fluctuations in motor performance are an additional complication of chronic carbidopa–levodopa therapy. After a variable period of treatment, patients note that the beneficial effects of the drug begin to wear off before they are due to take their next dose ("wearing off" or end-of-dose akinesia) and that they may be very akinetic in the morning before the first dose of medication (morning akinesia). One or more doses often do not seem to work. Later, particularly in patients on multiple overlapping doses of carbidopa–levodopa the fluctuations from a mobile state, or "on," to obvious parkinsonism, or "off," may appear random, with no obvious relation to dosage timing. The transition between relatively normal function to complete re-emergence of the parkinsonian state can occur in several minutes and can persist for up to 3 to 4 hours. Sudden, rapid, unpredictable fluctuations between these two extremes have been termed the *on–off phenomenon*. Clinically, these fluctuations can be striking, and the dramatic nature of these transitions can occasionally be observed during an office evaluation. A patient may be seen in a severely parkinsonian state ("off") with marked cogwheel rigidity, resting tremor, severe akinesia to the degree that the patient is unable to rise from a chair, and impaired postural reflexes to the point of falling or being unable to stand. During 5 to 6 minutes, the same patient may turn "on" and be observed to be able to stand and sit without any difficulty, to be without cogwheeling, to have no tremor, and to be able to walk relatively normally and not look at all parkinsonian. The observer who is unfamiliar with these rapid transitions is astounded by these fluctuations, and the uninformed observer may believe that the severe parkinsonian state, or "off," may reflect a nonorganic problem of an emotional nature.

This is a perplexing problem that seems to be related to alterations in central dopamine receptor site responsiveness and to fluctuating levels of available neurotransmitter. Attempts have been made to alter this phenomenon by the administration of multiple doses of the drug during the day, but these efforts have not been effective.

The recent introduction of a controlled-release formulation of carbidopa–levodopa (Sinemet CR) has been very useful to many patients with end-of-dose wearing off and early morning akinesia. In addition, Sinemet CR at bedtime may alleviate nighttime freezing, painful dystonia, and nocturnal tremor, all of which may make it extremely difficult for the parkinsonian patient to sleep. Sinemet CR is formulated as a 50:200 carbidopa–levodopa preparation. This drug is not entirely absorbed, and the amount of Sinemet CR which is biologically equivalent to standard carbidopa–levodopa is variable. It usually requires administration of approximately 30% more Sinemet CR in total mg/day dosage.

Additional therapeutic maneuvers to alleviate motor fluctuations include the use of dopaminergic receptor agonists and restricted-protein diets. Bromocriptine and pergolide can also provide relief to the patient who is experiencing motor fluctuations. When these drugs are used in this situation they should be tried one at a time and should be administered beginning with a very low initial dose with a gradual upward titration schedule. Each individual agonist may ameliorate symptoms for months to years. The restricted-protein diet is particularly effective in those patients who report a relatively dramatic effect of diet on their response to carbidopa–levodopa. Levodopa shares the same gastrointestinal transport system as other amino acids, and high-protein meals result in greater competi-

tion for the uptake system and lower the amount of levodopa available to the central nervous system. In patients who note loss of efficiency of carbidopa–levodopa when administered with a protein meal, the restricted-protein diet may provide smoother motor response throughout the day.

Gradual loss of responsiveness to levodopa has been noted in patients on long-term treatment. Whether this represents a true loss of efficacy of the drug or is another reflection of the progressive nature of this disorder is unknown. Although carbidopa–levodopa is the mainstay of therapy in these patients, it should be used cautiously and only when needed. Carbidopa–levodopa is associated with severe side effects, and in a large Parkinson's disease clinic most of the time is usually spent in the management of drug-related side effects. The introduction of this agent should be delayed until the patient's symptoms justify its use. However, carbidopa–levodopa treatment should be implemented whenever the patient's ability to perform adequately in his occupation, household work, or recreational activities is impaired. There is no need to withhold treatment until full disability ensues. When the initial diagnosis of Parkinson's disease is made, the symptoms may be mild and may be perfectly well controlled with a combination of anticholinergic medication and amantadine.

These problems associated with chronic dopaminergic agonist therapy in Parkinson's disease have led to the therapeutic recommendations already discussed. However, there are many patients who require long-term carbidopa–levodopa treatment and who also have these severe side effects. At the present time the therapeutic decisions involve balancing drug-related side effects against drug-induced improvement. However, this approach eventually leads to the double-bind situation in which the patient requires increased levodopa to improve his parkinsonism but decreased levodopa to decrease his dopaminergic toxicity syndrome. The introduction of bromocriptine or pergolide can often be useful in this situation. Bromocriptine or pergolide administration provides dopaminergic stimulation of the postsynaptic striatal dopamine receptor and also allows a reduction in carbidopa–levodopa dose. In some patients, this titration of doses up and down, respectively, will provide relief from drug-induced side effects and will provide continued motor improvement.

A *drug holiday* is a therapeutic measure in which all dopaminergic treatment is withdrawn for 5 to 7 days and is then reinstituted. In the specific situation in which patients have persistent psychiatric or motor side effects from their drugs and yet become too parkinsonian whenever the drug dose is reduced, a drug holiday is a therapeutic option that has been associated with improved function lasting weeks to months. However, the withdrawal of dopaminergic treatment will result in the appearance of a severe parkinsonian state. The patient may become totally dependent for all activities of daily living and must be hospitalized to receive total care. Complications that may occur secondary to the patient being so severely parkinsonian include deep venous thrombosis, pulmonary emboli, aspiration, and compressive neuropathies. If a drug holiday is employed, it should only be undertaken in an institution familiar with this procedure.

DRUG-INDUCED PARKINSONISM

Drug-induced parkinsonism can be precipitated by any drug that decreases central dopaminergic response. Drugs that block the dopamine receptor (*e.g.*, neuroleptics, metoclopramide) or deplete central dopamine (*e.g.*, reserpine) often result in parkinsonian symptomatology. Parkinsonism induced by drugs can mimic all of the features seen in idiopathic Parkinson's disease. Akinesia is usually the most common sign, and resting tremor is seen less often. Other features that may help distinguish drug-induced parkinsonism from Parkinson's disease include a clear history of drug ingestion of a compound known to interfere with central dopamine activity, a relatively short duration of parkinsonian symptoms to significant disability (1 to 2 months *vs* 6 to 12 months), bilateral instead of unilateral presentation of symptoms and signs, and the presence of other drug-related motor abnormalities (*e.g.*, tardive dyskinesia; see Chap. 10).

The diagnosis of drug-induced parkinsonism requires a high index of suspicion. Once the diagnosis is made, treatment should be directed to stopping the offending drug. In almost all patients with this syndrome the parkinsonism will resolve. Active treatment, if required, may be with anticholinergics, amantadine, or carbidopa–levodopa, all of which have been successfully used. In patients in whom drug-induced parkinsonism does not resolve, idiopathic Parkinson's disease may have been unmasked.

FURTHER CONSIDERATIONS

Although the etiology of Parkinson's disease remains unknown, there have been recent attempts to alter the progression of this disorder. This approach to treatment, sometimes referred to as "neuroprotective," has been based on interfering with both exogenous and endogenous oxidative processes in the parkinsonian brain with the antioxidant vitamin E and selegiline Hcl. These oxidative processes may contribute to dopaminergic cell death, and these drugs, through different mechanisms, may slow the process. A very large, well-controlled study indicated that vitamin E (2000 units/day) did not slow progression of Parkinson's disease. This same study demonstrated that selegiline Hcl had mild symptomatic effects in Parkinson's disease, and this confounded the issue of whether or not the effect of selegiline Hcl in early Parkinson's disease was neuroprotective or symptomatic. At the present time there is no proof that a "neuroprotective" therapy exists for Parkinson's disease. Research in this area continues, and it is hoped that it will be successful.

There has been considerable interest in the role of fetal tissue (mesencephalon) implants in the treatment of Parkinson's disease. The concept involves the transplantation of the dopaminergic cell area from aborted fetal brain into the brain of the patient with Parkinson's disease. Although there have been reports that some Parkinson's disease patients who have received fetal tissue implants have improved, no investigations have claimed that the procedure has become a standard therapy. In fact, there is a great deal of confusion about whether or not the procedure actually works. Considerable research is required to clarify a myriad of issues including what age fetal brain to use, which anatomic area within the brain of the Parkinson's disease patient should receive the implant, how many fetal brains per Parkinson's disease patient are required, which Parkinson's disease patients should receive the implant, and whether the disease process will affect the transplanted dopaminergic cells.

The levodopa treatment era in Parkinson's disease has also led to broadening the scope of what is considered to be the central nervous system dysfunction seen in this disorder. Although James Parkinson did not originally describe mental deterioration as part of the illness, it has become increasingly apparent that dementia is often associated with Parkinson's disease. There is evidence from the prelevodopa era to suggest that 25% to 30% of patients with Parkinson's disease were eventually institutionalized because of dementia and not because of incapacitating motor performance. However, the increased longevity and maintenance of communicative abilities in patients with Parkinson's disease have led to the observation that dementia is often seen as Parkinson's disease progresses. Recent studies confirm earlier observations that as many as 25% of patients with Parkinson's disease may develop dementia. Dementia must be differentiated from drug-induced altered mental states, since the former is not amenable to treatment but the latter are.

Any drug or degenerative process that interferes with central dopaminergic activity can lead to parkinsonism. The dysfunction of the dopamine system may involve the nigral (presynaptic) neuron or the striatal dopamine receptor (postsynaptic).

Drugs or degenerative processes that affect not the presynaptic nigrostriatal dopaminergic pathway but the striatal dopamine receptors may result in the same clinical signs. The latter situation is sometimes referred to as *postsynaptic parkinsonism*. Examples of postsynaptic parkinsonism include drug-induced states and metabolic disturbances that result in calcification of the basal ganglia (often not seen on skull films but visible on computed tomography [CT] or magnetic resonance imaging [MR]) and familial striatonigral degeneration. Since the pathology in these syndromes is located primarily within the striatum and involves the dopamine receptors, it should not be surprising that carbidopa–levodopa therapy has less effect in these disorders. Several additional syndromes that may have elements of both pre- and postsynaptic dopaminergic dysfunction include olivopontocerebellar (OPC) degeneration, progressive supranuclear palsy (PSP), and the Shy–Drager syndrome. Clinical clues to the diagnosis of the latter syndromes, in addition to the variable response of the parkinsonian features to levodopa, include the presence of a marked intention tremor (OPC), the failure of voluntary conjugate gaze (PSP), and the presence of severe orthostatic hypotension (Shy–Drager).

QUESTIONS AND DISCUSSION

1. A 62-year-old right-handed man went to his physician with the following problems. He has noticed for the last 6 months that his handwriting has been changing and that it appears small and cramped. In addition, he has the feeling that his right hand is not as strong as it used to be, and he notices occasionally that he has to struggle to button his shirt. The week prior to his visit, his wife noticed that his right hand appeared to be shaking when he was resting quietly in an easy chair.

The most likely diagnosis in this patient based on history alone is:

A. Parkinson's disease
B. Wilson's disease
C. Huntington's disease
D. Dystonia

Neurologic findings present on examination might include which of the following?

A. Bilateral limb chorea, linguofaciobuccal dyskinesias
B. Resting tremor of the right hand, cogwheel rigidity of the right upper extremity
C. Fixed dystonic posturing of the right hand
D. Kinetic tremor of the right hand
E. Three-step retropulsion, two to three extra steps in turning maneuvers

The correct answer to the first question is (A), and the correct answers to the second question are (B) and (E). This is a typical history of Parkinson's disease characterized by slow progression of the disability and a predominantly unilateral presentation of the symptoms and signs. In addition, the handwriting is described as cramped and small (micrographic). The feeling of weakness in an involved extremity is a common complaint, although often there are no objective signs of weakness. The presence of unilateral signs of tremor and cogwheel rigidity is typical. The additional finding on examination that the postural reflexes are also impaired (retropulsion is present, and there are increased steps on turning maneuvers) is an indication that a thorough examination will often reveal additional signs of neurologic dysfunction.

2. A 59-year-old right-handed woman has a 5-year history of left upper extremity resting tremor. She has been treated with carbidopa–levodopa for the last 4 years. Although she states that originally her tremor was much improved, she has been having difficulty with increasing involuntary, wild, "dancelike," gyrating, nonpurposeful movements of the left upper and lower extremities. In addition, her husband relates that occasionally the patient remarks that there are visitors in the house when no one is visiting. Closer questioning of the patient about this reveals that she often sees

people who are not really there. She speaks lucidly about this and recognizes that they are not real. The correct diagnosis in this patient would be:

A. Dystonic posturing of the left upper extremities
B. Tardive dyskinesia
C. Parkinson's disease and dopaminergic toxicity
D. Wilson's disease and dopaminergic toxicity

The correct answer is (C). The patient's initial presenting complaint is the spontaneous appearance of a unilateral resting tremor that is relieved by dopaminergic agents. This is a characteristic early presentation of unilateral Parkinson's disease, and the additional information that dopaminergic therapy ameliorated the symptoms suggests the diagnosis of Parkinson's disease. The patient's present complaints can be diagnosed as part of the chronic dopaminergic toxicity syndrome and in particular as dopaminergic-induced chorea and hallucinations. Choreiform movements that are induced by dopaminergic therapy in patients with Parkinson's disease are not phenomenologically distinguishable from the chorea seen in many other choreatic states. The hallucinations reported by this patient are also typical, since the most common hallucinosis seen in this setting involves nonthreatening visual hallucinations.

(A) is incorrect because dystonic postures and movements are not wildly gyrating. (B) is incorrect because there is no drug history of neuroleptic medication, and tardive dyskinesia is by definition secondary to chronic neuroleptic ingestion. (D) is incorrect because Wilson's disease does not produce initial onset of neurologic symptoms so late in life. Wilson's disease presenting with neurologic symptomatology has its average age of onset at 19 years.

The most appropriate therapy in this patients would be:

A. Addition of a neuroleptic (a dopamine receptor antagonist)
B. Raising the dose of carbidopa–levodopa
C. Addition of an anticholinergic
D. Reduction in the dose of carbidopa–levodopa

The correct answer is (D). The patient's current problem of dyskinesias and hallucinations is secondary to chronic dopaminergic agonism, and the most appropriate therapy would be to reduce the

dose of this drug. In all instances, these two drug-induced effects will be ameliorated when the dose is reduced. When the dose of the dopaminergic agents is reduced or the agents are discontinued, the patient's parkinsonian features will re-emerge. In this case, if the patient's only symptom is resting unilateral tremor or mild parkinsonism, it would be wise to alter pharmacologic therapy to the anticholinergic agents and carbidopa–levodopa if needed.

(A) is incorrect, even though the addition of neuroleptic would result in decreased chorea and decreased hallucinations. These drug-induced effects are thought to be related to altered sensitivity of central dopamine receptor sites. Any therapy that interferes with dopaminergic activity will tend to ease the symptoms (this is the basis for dose reduction ameliorating dopaminergic toxicity) so that the dopamine receptor site antagonism produced by the neuroleptics would also ameliorate the symptoms. However, in the treatment of dose-related side effects there would be no reason in this instance to mask the toxic symptoms with the addition of another potent centrally active drug. In addition, the antidopaminergic action of the neuroleptics will eventually result in markedly increased parkinsonian symptomatology. (B) is incorrect because this is a drug-induced syndrome and raising the dose of the drug will not ameliorate the problem but will exacerbate it. (C) is incorrect because anticholinergics will not improve chorea, and there is even some clinical evidence that anticholinergics will exacerbate chorea.

3. A 65-year-old right-handed man presents with difficulty seeing the food on his plate. His family says that his problem has been getting worse for the last 12 months and that the patient also has difficulty walking up stairs. In addition, he describes difficulty buttoning his shirt, rising from a chair, and turning over in bed. The family also reports that his facial expression has changed (does not smile as much) and that a tremor of his left hand is occasionally noted. Examination reveals a resting tremor of the left hand, cogwheel rigidity in the left upper extremity, and mildly impaired postural reflexes. Additional findings include increased extensor tone in the neck and marked impairment of voluntary conjugate gaze. The patient is unable to look down voluntarily, and there is also moderate impairment of upward gaze. In addition, right and left lateral gaze are not normal. The correct diagnosis in this patient would be:

A. Wilson's disease
B. Huntington's disease
C. Parkinson's disease
D. Progressive supranuclear palsy (PSP)
E. Shy–Drager syndrome

The correct answer is (D). PSP is an idiopathic midbrain and brain-stem degenerative disorder that is characterized by parkinsonian features and progressively impaired voluntary conjugate gaze. This patient is described as having parkinsonian features (resting tremor, cogwheel rigidity, impaired postural reflexes, and mild bradykinesia) and also has markedly impaired conjugate gaze. A useful office maneuver to distinguish whether the gaze dysfunction is supranuclear or nuclear is the doll's head procedure. In this maneuver, the head is passively flexed and extended, and in a separate maneuver it is rotated to the right and to the left while the passive motion of the eyes is observed. In a patient with a supranuclear gaze dysfunction, the eyes will move reflexly and conjugately in an appropriate direction. This maneuver and its physiology are discussed in greater detail in the chapter on the examination of the comatose patient.

(A) is incorrect because of the late onset of neurologic symptoms and the type of eye movements observed. (B) is incorrect because of the late onset of neurologic symptoms and because the movement disorder is not that seen in adult-onset Huntington's disease. Although definite parkinsonian features are present, (C) is incorrect because of the additional findings of disturbed volitional gaze. (E) is incorrect because the syndrome, although often having parkinsonian features, is characterized by the presence of severe orthostatic hypotension.

4. The degenerative cellular pathology seen in Parkinson's disease is localized primarily in the:

A. Cerebral cortex
B. Thalamus
C. Cerebellum
D. Substantia nigra
E. Corpus striatum

The loss of cell bodies and their projection systems in the correct answer to the first part of this question results in what biochemical lesions?

A. Loss of acetylcholine in the striatum
B. Loss of dopamine in the striatum
C. Loss of dopamine in the cerebral cortex
D. Loss of acetylcholine in the cerebellum

The correct answer to the first part of the question is (D), and the correct answer to the second part of the question is (B). Parkinson's disease is pathologically characterized by depigmentation Lewy bodies and cell loss in the substantia nigra. The destruction of the nigral striatal projection system results in the loss of dopamine in the striatum. Dopamine is the neurotransmitter used by this system, and the dopamine within the striatum is primarily contained within the axonal terminations of the nigral neurons. These are not seen well histologically, and hence the striatum does not show major pathologic changes in parkinsonism.

SUGGESTED READING

Barbeau A: Six years of high level levodopa therapy in severely akinetic parkinsonian patients. Arch Neurol 33:333, 1976

Cotzias GC, Van Woert MH, Schiffer LM: Aromatic amino acids and modification of parkinsonism. N Engl J Med 276:374, 1967

Hohen MM, Yahr MD: Parkinsonism: Onset, progression, and mortality. Neurology 17:427, 1967

Jenner P, Shapira AHV, Marsden CD: New insights into the cause of Parkinson's disease. Neurology 42:2241, 1992

Koller WC (ed): *Handbook of Parkinson's Disease*, 2nd ed. New York, Marcel Dekker, 1992

Lang AE, Weiner WJ (eds): *Drug-Induced Movement Disorders*. Mt. Kisco, NY, Futura Publishing Co., 1992

The Parkinson Study Group: Effect of deprenyl on the progression of disability in early Parkinson's disease. N Engl J Med 321:1364, 1989

Weiner WJ, Lang AE: Parkinson's disease. In *Movement Disorders: A Comprehensive Survey*. Mt. Kisco, NY, Futura Publishing Co., 1989

Hyperkinetic Movement Disorders

Stewart A. Factor
William J. Weiner

Strange, abnormal involuntary movements are the hallmarks of a number of neurologic diseases that are collectively termed *hyperkinetic movement disorders*. In such conditions, the movements are easily visible, and intelligent observation allows the clinician, in most instances, to suggest the proper diagnosis or class of disorders. The characteristic tremor of Parkinson's disease, which is present at rest but lacking during volitional movements, is such an example (see Chap. 9). In this chapter, six other neurologic diseases will be described. All are visually dramatic because bizarre and abnormal involuntary movements are their major descriptive feature. The non-neurologist will certainly encounter these patients in an office practice and will also identify them in the community, in parks, buses, or supermarkets. The disorders discussed are idiopathic torsion dystonia, essential tremor, Huntington's disease, Wilson's disease, Gilles de la Tourette's syndrome, and tardive dyskinesia.

DEFINITION OF TERMS

Dystonia: Involuntary muscle contractions producing twisting movements that are repetitive and often result in abnormal postures. They vary in speed from more rapid to slow, with sustained muscle contractions lasting seconds to hours.

Tremor: Involuntary rhythmic oscillating movement that results from the alternating or synchronous contraction of reciprocally innervated antagonist muscles. Tremor may be characterized by its prominence only during certain activities.

Chorea: Excessive, spontaneous movements, irregularly timed, nonrepetitive, randomly distributed, and often with a flowing "dance-like" quality that involves multiple body parts.

Tics: Repetitive, brief, rapid, involuntary, purposeless, stereotyped movements that involve single or multiple muscle groups. The tic can be a patterned sequence of coordinated movements that may be complex or simple.

Myoclonus: Rapid, shock-like, arrhythmic (usually), and often repetitive involuntary movements.

IDIOPATHIC TORSION DYSTONIA

Dystonia has a number of unusual but characteristic features. Onset of the movements may occur in association with specific voluntary actions of the involved muscle groups (*e.g.,* writer's cramp) or with any movement of these muscle groups (action-induced dystonia). Dystonia may be caused in one body part by movement of another (overflow dystonia). In addition, dystonia may occur at rest. Dys-

William J. Weiner and Christopher G. Goetz, eds. *Neurology for the Non-Neurologist*, Third Edition. Copyright © 1994, 1989 by J. B. Lippincott Company. Copyright © 1981 by Harper and Row Publishers, Inc.

tonic movements typically worsen with anxiety, heightened emotions, and fatigue, while they decrease with relaxation and disappear during sleep. There may be diurnal fluctuations in the dystonia that manifest as little or no involuntary movement in the morning followed by severe disabling dystonia in the afternoon and evening. One particular form of idiopathic dystonia with onset in childhood is characterized by this feature and its response to levodopa (dopa-responsive or Segawa's dystonia).

Dystonia may involve a variety of muscle groups. When the upper face and eyelids are involved and the eyes are involuntarily kept closed, the patient has blepharospasm. When the lower face, lips, and jaw are involved and the patient presents with involuntary opening or closing of the jaw, retraction or puckering of the lips, and repetitive contractions of the platysma, the patient has oromandibular dystonia. Pharyngeal dystonia is associated with dysphagia, dysphonia, or dysarthria and is typically action-induced. Lingual dystonia may occur at rest, presenting as sustained or repetitive protrusion of the tongue or upward deflection of the tongue against the hard palate, or it may be action-induced with speaking or eating. Laryngeal dystonia causes spasmodic dysphonia in which the speech is tight, constricted, and forced. The smooth flow of speech is lost, and certain sounds are held longer and overemphasized. Spasmodic dysphonia is typically action-induced by speech.

Dystonic contractions of the neck muscles are manifested as torticollis, retrocollis, anterocollis, or laterocollis. In spasmodic torticollis rapid jerking and twisting neck movements may accompany sustained posturing of the neck. Some patients may appear to have a fixed abnormal neck posture without the spasmodic movements. Dystonic movements of the arms (brachial dystonia) most commonly present as pronation of the arm, often behind the back. The movements are often action-induced as in writing (writer's cramp), manipulating a musical instrument (musician's cramp), and other occupational maneuvers. Truncal dystonia manifests as lordosis, scoliosis, kyphosis, tortipelvis, or opisthotonos. Dystonic movement of the legs (crural dystonia) may occur with action or at rest and presents most commonly with equinovarus posturing of the foot while walking, twisting of the foot, or increased elevation of the leg when walking. The knee usually maintains a hyperextended position with crural dystonia. Some patients are able to walk backward or run without incident, but when they attempt to walk normally the dystonia recurs.

Patients with dystonic disorders often discover ways to suppress or hide the movements using an interesting array of "sensory tricks," usually consisting of postural alterations or counterpressure maneuvers. There are, however, some bizarre tricks that have been observed, including singing in patients with blepharospasm or oromandibular dystonia and dancing in patients with cervical or truncal dystonia. Typically, these tricks lose their effectiveness as the disease progresses. The mechanism by which these maneuvers work is unknown.

Dystonia is often misdiagnosed as hysterical or psychiatric in origin. The misdiagnosis occurs because of the varied, often bizarre, movements and postures, the occurrence of action-induced dystonia, the worsening of dystonia with stress and improvement with relaxation, diurnal fluctuations, and the effectiveness of various sensory tricks. Knowledge of the unusual characteristics of dystonic disorders will be helpful in avoiding a misdiagnosis.

CLASSIFICATION

Classification of dystonia frequently utilizes age of onset, mode of inheritance, distribution of movements, and diagnosis. The age-of-onset classification separates patients into four subgroups: infantile (under 2 years of age), childhood (2 to 12 years), juvenile (12 to 20 years), and adult (older than 20). Childhood-onset dystonia carries a worse prognosis than dystonia that first occurs at later ages.

Dystonia may be inherited or sporadic. There has been an important recent discovery in relation to the heredity of dystonia. Genetic studies in Ashkenazi Jewish and non-Jewish families with dystonia have indicated that an autosomal dominant pattern with reduced penetrance exists. Linkage analysis studies have located the gene in both types of families on chromosome 9. In addition, segregation analysis of adult-onset focal dystonia suggests dominant inheritance as well. An X-linked form of dystonia has also been described in the Philippines.

The distribution of dystonia is categorized as either focal, multifocal, hemidystonia, or generalized. Focal dystonia refers to dystonia in a single body part. Multifocal dystonia includes dystonic movements in more than one body part. Segmental dystonia is a form of multifocal dystonia in which contiguous body parts are affected. Hemidystonia refers to an arm and a leg on the same side being involved. Finally, generalized dystonia refers to the presence of dystonia, in at least one leg and the trunk, as well as in an additional body part (cranial, cervical, brachial), or in both legs and the trunk. This classification is important in formulating a proper diagnosis; for example, hemidystonia almost always is the result of an infarction or space-occupying lesion, while generalized dystonia is more than likely idiopathic. Generalized dystonia clearly has a worse prognosis than focal dystonia or hemidystonia.

The last classification scheme is by diagnosis, with patients designated as having either primary or secondary dystonic disorders. The primary dystonias include those that are inherited and idiopathic, whereas the secondary dystonias have a known cause, such as stroke or neoplasm.

PRIMARY DYSTONIA

Dystonia is typically the only neurologic abnormality in patients with primary dystonia, and any distribution of abnormal involuntary movements may be observed. The primary dystonias have an insidious onset and may be progressive in nature. Initially the movements are often action-induced.

Five criteria for the diagnosis of *idiopathic torsion dystonia* (ITD) were established by Herz in 1944 and are still applicable today. These include the following: (1) the patient exhibits dystonic movements or postures; (2) the patient must have a normal perinatal and developmental history; (3) there should be no precipitating illnesses or exposure to drugs known to cause dystonia; (4) there is no evidence of intellectual, pyramidal, cerebellar, or sensory deficits; and (5) investigation for secondary causes of dystonia (particularly Wilson's disease) is negative.

Two factors are indicators of a poor prognosis in ITD—onset in childhood and onset in a crural distribution. Poor prognosis in ITD refers to an increased disability since life span is not shortened. A majority of crural dystonia patients have onset of disease in childhood. Childhood-onset patients differ from those with adult onset in relation to prognosis, presentation, and distribution. For this reason, ITD patients are categorized as adult onset and childhood onset. There is a definite overlap between the two groups, and variable ages of onset in individual families and dominant mode of inheritance suggest that the two categories represent variable presentations of the same disorder.

CHILDHOOD-ONSET DYSTONIA

ITD usually begins between 6 and 12 years of age. Typically, the initial presentation is that of a gait disorder (crural dystonia). The foot is often twisted and plantar flexed during ambulation, and patients usually toe walk. The dystonia is action-induced (walking) in the early stages and disappears at rest. As the disorder progresses, this pattern changes and dystonia may be present at rest, often with frequent sustained postures. Marsden and Harrison found that 79% of these patients progress relentlessly over a period of 5 to 10 years and 50% become either bedridden or wheelchair-bound. In adult life, the patient often stabilizes and may even improve to some degree, but the disorder does not spontaneously remit. Transient remissions may occur early in the disorder, and these may last hours to years. In those children with onset other than in the leg and without crural involvement the prognosis is better. Fewer of these patients become totally incapacitated. In a majority of childhood-onset dystonias a clear family history is documented.

ADULT-ONSET DYSTONIA

Adult-onset ITD presents more commonly with brachial, truncal, and craniocervical dystonia and only rarely with crural dystonia. Only 18% of these patients progress to generalized dystonia, with an even smaller percentage becoming wheelchair-bound or bedridden. The dystonia usually remains in the body part where it presented as a focal dystonia; however, it may spread to a contiguous body part, on rare occasions becoming segmental in distribution. The course is typically benign, and remissions occur in approximately 20% of patients. In these patients, family history is less obvious.

CRANIOFACIAL DYSTONIA

Blepharospasm—oromandibular dystonia syndrome was first described by Henry Meige in 1910 and is often referred to as *Meige's syndrome*. Blepharospasm and oromandibular dystonia may also be accompanied by pharyngeal, laryngeal, or cervical dystonia. Blepharospasm, in isolation (referred to as *essential blepharospasm*), is more common than oromandibular dystonia. Blepharospasm is often preceded by eye irritation, photophobia, and increased blinking. It may start in one eye and spread to the other, or it may start in both. Approximately 12% of these patients are functionally blind due to the inability to voluntarily open the eyes. Features that aggravate blepharospasm include looking upward, stress, fatigue, watching television, walking, driving, talking, and even yawning. Sensory tricks utilized by patients to open the eyes include forced raising of the eyelids, pressure on the superior orbital ridges, and rubbing the eyelids. In addition, some find that forced jaw opening, neck movements, and wearing dark glasses are helpful. Oromandibular dystonia is frequently accompanied by tongue protrusion, soft palate dystonia, and nasal flaring. It may be aggravated by talking, chewing, or swallowing. Sensory tricks utilized include pressing on the lips or teeth with the fingers or pressing on the hard palate with the tongue. Meige's syndrome typically affects women more commonly than men and presents in the sixth decade of life. The onset of the disorder often begins with blepharospasm, which is later followed by oromandibular dystonia and pharyngeal dystonia. Other dystonic movements in other body parts may occur in some patients, and essential tremor may also be an associated problem. The severity of the dystonia fluctuates from day to day and disappears with sleep. Spontaneous remissions have been observed but are rare.

SPASMODIC TORTICOLLIS

Spasmodic torticollis is the most common focal dystonia (Fig. 10-1). The age of onset is in the fourth or fifth decade, and women are more frequently affected than men. The disorder is characterized by abnormal involuntary movements and typical postures of the neck and shoulders, which are often painful. Initially, the patient may not perceive the abnormal movements or postures, which may be brought to his attention by others. This suggests a problem with perception of head position. The movements are only intermittent at first and associated with specific actions. Most patients deteriorate during the initial 5 years and symptoms then stabilize. The condition is ultimately characterized by fixed dystonic postures that are present at rest, worsen with action, and improve in sleep. Spontaneous remissions occur in 10% to 30% of patients, most commonly in the first year. All patients eventually relapse.

Rotation of the neck (torticollis) is the most common posture seen, with lateral flexion (laterocollis), flexion (anterocollis), and extension (retrocollis) also occurring in various combinations. Factors that may exacerbate torticollis include emotional stress, fatigue, walking, working with the hands, and attempting to look in the opposite direction of the dystonic contractions. Sensory tricks have involved the use of a light touch or pressure to the chin or cheek with fingers or other objects such as a pen or eyeglasses. This will lessen the head tilt for a variable duration of time. Spasmodic torticollis may be associated with Meige's syndrome, writer's cramp, and essential tremor and has also been observed in patients with generalized dystonia. Complications

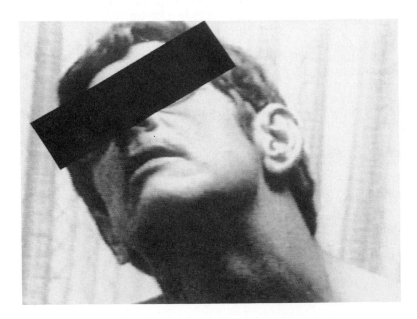

FIG. 10-1. Spasmodic torticollis resulting in a fixed cervical posture with extension, lateral flexion, and rotation to the right.

of prolonged torticollis occur in one-third to one-half of patients and include degenerative osteoarthritis of the cervical spine and hypertrophy of the sternocleidomastoid muscle.

WRITER'S CRAMP

Writer's cramp (Fig. 10-2) is a dystonic spasm that is induced by a specific task (action-induced dystonia). These patients present with a change in their handwriting, which becomes sloppy and illegible. Some patients squeeze the pen tightly and press down hard on the writing surface, resulting in a jerky writing motion and tearing of the paper. In others the fingers splay and pull away from the pen involuntarily. Initially, the dystonic contraction occurs with persistence of task but, as the disorder progresses, it occurs with initiation of the task. Other tasks performed with the same hand are normal. The disorder is usually asymmetrical at first; however, in those patients who learn to write with the opposite hand the disorder may become bilateral. Writer's cramp is often associated with essential tremor. Some other occupational cramps that have been reported include pianist's and violinist's palsy, golfer's palsy, and dart thrower's palsy. The common factor in all of these disorders is the occurrence during the performance of a well-learned motor (manual) task.

SECONDARY DYSTONIA

In order to make a diagnosis of ITD, known causes of dystonia, that is, secondary or symptomatic dystonias (Table 10-1), must be excluded. Clues to the diagnosis of a secondary dystonia can be uncovered by a thorough history and physical exam, as well as by radiologic and laboratory testing. Usually there are examination findings suggestive of dysfunction of other parts of the central nervous system, including the cranial nerves, pyramidal system, cerebellar system, and higher cortical function tasks, in addition to the dystonia. There is usually an obvious onset to the dystonia, and dystonia is present at rest from the start. The presence of hemidystonia suggests a focal lesion such as a tumor, infarction, abscess, or arteriovenous malformation in the basal ganglia. In those patients with a single nonprogressive event such as an infarction or trauma, the dystonia will usually stabilize and not be progressive. The examiner should be cautious, however, because secondary dystonia may mimic idiopathic dystonia quite closely. An important feature of secondary dystonia, which examiners must be aware of, is that dystonia may have a delayed onset after a cerebral insult. In adults the most frequent cause of delayed-onset dystonia is cerebral infarction. Delay durations have varied from weeks to years and are often associated with an improvement of the original

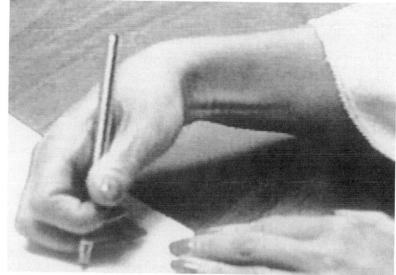

FIG. 10-2. Writer's cramp is an action-induced dystonic spasm resulting, in this patient, in wrist flexion, metacarpophalangeal joint extension, extension of the thumb, and flexion of the distal interphalangeal joints, leaving the patient with an inability to continue writing.

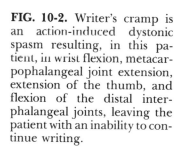

TABLE 10-1. Secondary Causes of Dystonia

I. Degenerative disorders
  1. Parkinson's disease
  2. Huntington's disease
  3. Progressive supranuclear palsy
  4. Hallervorden–Spatz disease
  5. Olivopontocerebellar atrophies
II. Metabolic disorders
  1. Wilson's disease
  2. Leigh's disease
  3. GM_1 and GM_2 gangliosidoses
  4. Hexosaminidase deficiency
III. Drugs
  1. Dopamine antagonists (*e.g.*, haloperidol, thioridazine, prochlorperazine)
  2. Dopamine agonists (*e.g.*, levodopa, bromocriptine)
IV. Vascular disease
  1. Basal ganglia infarction
  2. Basal ganglia hemorrhage
  3. Arteriovenous malformation
V. Neoplasms
  1. Astrocytoma or glioma of the basal ganglia
  2. Metastatic neoplasm
  3. Cervical spinal cord tumor
VI. Other
  1. Head trauma
  2. Thalamotomy
  3. Anoxia (in adulthood or perinatal)
  4. Meningitis (fungal or tuberculosis)
  5. Syringomyelia
  6. Colloid cyst of the third ventricle
  7. Munchausen's syndrome
  8. Toxoplasmosis abscess of basal ganglia (in AIDS patients)

neurologic deficit. In children the most frequent cause of delayed-onset dystonia is perinatal trauma or hypoxia. The reason for the delay is unclear. A history of perinatal difficulties must be excluded if a diagnosis of ITD is to be made.

PATHOLOGY AND NEUROCHEMISTRY

Dystonia is considered to be the result of basal ganglia dysfunction. Since there have been only a few cases of ITD reported with autopsy results (and most of them were without abnormality), the pathologic–anatomic basis of this movement disorder has been related almost exclusively to cases of second-ary dystonia. Anatomic abnormalities in published cases of secondary dystonia have most commonly involved the putamen and, to a lesser extent, the caudate nucleus and the thalamus. These findings have been supported by radiologic studies. In those rare cases of ITD with pathologic abnormalities, the microscopic changes were observed in the brain stem. In one case of generalized dystonia, neurofibrillary tangles were found in the locus ceruleus and other brain-stem nuclei. In one case of Meige's syndrome, neuronal loss was observed in multiple brain-stem nuclei. Whether these abnormalities relate directly to the clinical syndrome remains to be proved.

The neurochemical basis of dystonia is even less clear. It has been suggested that the abnormality in this disorder is in the dopamine and acetylcholine systems. Clinical evidence to support these hypotheses includes the onset of dystonia after treatment with dopamine receptor antagonists and the response of dystonia to anticholinergic medications. Recently, a noradrenergic imbalance in the lower portion of the brain stem involving the lateral tegmentum of the medulla oblongata and locus ceruleus has been hypothesized. In some areas, norepinephrine is elevated, while in others the levels are diminished. Other theories have included alterations in gamma-aminobutyric acid (GABA) or cerebral somatostatin.

TREATMENT

In the absence of a clear understanding of the etiology and neurochemistry of dystonia, medical treatment has been less than satisfactory. A number of therapeutic modalities have been tested, and varied responses have been observed. The most widely used medications in the treatment of dystonia are the anticholinergics. Fahn, in an open-label trial, found high doses of either trihexyphenidyl or ethopropazine (no longer available in the United States) to be beneficial in ITD. Twenty-three children and 52 adults were treated, and doses were gradually increased until a favorable response was observed or side effects occurred. Significant improvement was seen in 61% of children and 38% of adults. The average daily dose of trihexyphenidyl in children and adults was 41 mg and 24 mg, respectively. Adults were less tolerant of the anticholinergic side effects than the children. Side effects included blurred vision, dry mouth, urinary difficulties, sleep pattern alteration, forgetfulness, weight loss, and personality changes. The longest duration of efficacy in children and adults was 13 years and 7 years, respectively. Severity of disease was not a good predictor of response to the anticholinergics, but patients with hemidystonia did not respond well. This result was later confirmed by a double-blind study with trihexyphenidyl.

Tetrabenazine and reserpine, dopamine-depleting agents, have been reported to be effective in some patients with Meige's syndrome. The effectiveness of dopamine antagonists such as haloperidol has been inconsistent, and studies utilizing these drugs have been inconclusive. Because of the threat of tardive dyskinesia, these drugs should be avoided. Mixed therapeutic results with baclofen, carbamazepine, and the benzodiazepines have been observed.

Numerous surgical techniques have been utilized with less than adequate results. Stereotaxic thalamotomy with the ventral tier of the thalamus as the target is the most commonly utilized surgical technique in generalized dystonia. Bilateral procedures of this type can result in pseudobulbar palsy. Stimulation of the cervical spinal cord by extradural electrodes has not been helpful. In blepharospasm and Meige's syndrome myectomy has been tried. This procedure consists of the extirpation of the lid protractors and strengthening of the lid retractors. Recurrence of blepharospasm weeks to months after this procedure is not unusual. In spasmodic torticollis, selective peripheral denervation is a new technique under investigation in a number of institutions. Results have been promising.

The biggest recent advance in the treatment of dystonia is the use of botulinum toxin, one of the most lethal toxins known. Botulinum toxin A (Botox) has been utilized therapeutically since 1980. In 1990, Botox was approved by the Food and Drug Administration for treatment of blepharospasm, strabismus, and hemifacial spasm secondary to cranial nerve VII compression. Its use is now more widespread, and it is routinely utilized to treat all types of focal dystonia.

Botox acts presynaptically at the cholinergic neuromuscular junction. It is endocytosed into the nerve terminal and then blocks the release of acetycholine from vesicles. Its blockade of the neuromuscular junction results in weakness of the muscle and a decrease in muscle spasms. Botox is administered by direct intramuscular injection. All side effects are local, secondary to its primary effect of weakening muscles.

In blepharospasm, Botox is injected into the orbicularis oculi with two injections in the upper lid and one injection in the canthus and lower lid. In addition, one or two injections are given in the frontalis muscle in the forehead, if necessary. The total dose is 15 to 30 units per eye. Improvement is seen after 3 to 7 days, with moderate to marked functional improvement in 70% to 90% of patients. The response lasts 2 to 4 months so that treatment is needed three or four times per year. Side effects include ptosis, diplopia, and increased tearing, all of which are transient.

Spasmodic torticollis is probably the most common disorder treated with Botox at this time. Multiple studies have shown significant improvement in 60% to 90% of patients treated. Treatment requires an average of about 250 units per treatment; response occurs in 3 to 7 days and lasts 3 to 4 months. Thus, patients require two to four treatments per year. Neck muscles to be injected are chosen based on the presence of hypertrophy and spasm, pain, and in relation to the posture itself. Side effects are transient and include neck weakness, dysphagia, and a "flu-like" syndrome.

Spasmodic dysphonia of the adductor type, previously poorly responsive to any therapy, responds dramatically to Botox. The thyroarytenoid muscles are approached through the neck with electromyographic guidance. The only adverse effect is a breathy, whispery voice, which improves over days to weeks. Injection is required two to four times per year.

Other forms of focal dystonia are currently under investigation with regard to Botox therapy. Treatment of oromandibular dystonia and limb dystonias (writer's cramp) has shown promise. Most neurologists feel that Botox is the treatment of choice for the majority of focal dystonias because of its greater efficacy than standard medical therapies and fewer side effects.

Physicians administering Botox should be very familiar with the disorders treated, the mechanism of action and effective doses of Botox in each disorder, and the anatomy of the area injected. It is expected that the disorders treated with Botox will expand beyond dystonia.

ESSENTIAL TREMOR

Tremor may be the sole manifestation of a disorder or part of a syndrome. Tremor can be classified by its anatomic location, frequency, and relation to rest, posture, and movement. *Resting tremor* refers to tremor while the body part is at rest, *postural tremor* refers to tremor occurring while the body part is maintaining posture against gravity, and *kinetic tremor* refers to tremor during goal-directed movements.

Essential tremor (ET) is a monosymptomatic, familial disorder of the nervous system. It has been referred to as a benign disorder because it does not effect life span; however, this can be misleading since ET may be quite disabling. It occurs in a sporadic form, a familial form with a dominant inheritance, and a senile form in those with onset after age 65 and no family history. ET is characterized by a postural tremor that is most evident in the upper extremities. The tremor may have a kinetic component as seen in finger-to-nose testing, although it is often not as dramatic as in cerebellar disorders. Resting tremor, as seen in Parkinson's disease, does not occur. The frequency ranges from 4 Hz to 12 Hz. A maneuver to potentiate tremor during physical exam involves having patients hold their two index fingers close together without touching while having the elbows held out like wings.

The onset of ET is variable, but there appear to be two incidence peaks, in the second and sixth decades. Onset may be in the elderly (senile tremor), but tremor is not considered a sign of old age. The fingers and hands are affected first, then the tremor moves proximally. Tremor may occur in the left and right hands simultaneously or in one hand at a time; when bilateral, it may be symmetrical or asymmetrical. Though hemitremor has been observed, it is rare. When tremor is asymmetrical, it usually is worse in the dominant hand. Tremor may spread to the head and neck. Approximately 60% of patients with ET have head involvement, and in some instances head tremor is the sole manifestation. Head tremor may present as a vertical nod (yes–yes) or as a horizontal nod (no–no). Voice tremor occurs in approximately 24% of patients with ET. The voice is characterized by rhythmic alteration in intensity, with the same frequency as the hand tremor. Less often, tremor occurs in the jaw, face (lips, tongue), trunk (if present while standing only, this is referred to as *orthostatic tremor*), and legs. There are also task-specific tremors, such as primary writing tremor.

ET is a slowly progressive disorder. In some patients it remains stable for prolonged periods of time before progression is noticed. It is not unusual for patients to seek medical advice after having the tremor disorder for one or two decades. Initiation of a specific posture may aggravate the tremor early in the course. Later it is aggravated by many different movements or postures. The tremor disappears during sleep and worsens with anxiety, fatigue, temperature changes, local pain, aminophylline, and possibly hunger. Alcohol improves the tremor, but despite this phenomenon there is not an increased incidence of alcoholism in this patient population. ET is a clinically heterogeneous disorder that may go unnoticed by the patient, may simply be an embarrassment, or may actually be disabling, leading to difficulties with writing, drinking, and using kitchen utensils. The fact that ET may be disabling suggests that it is more than just a "constitutional peculiarity."

A number of attempts at classifying ET exist. One approach is to divide ET into four subtypes based on clinical, pharmacologic, and physiologic features. The first group has enhanced physiologic tremor (frequency 6 Hz to 12 Hz). The second group includes those patients with benign ET that is familial and decreased by alcohol and beta-blocking agents (frequency 5 Hz to 7 Hz). The third subtype occurs in those patients with a severe disabling ET that is sporadic and not decreased by alcohol and beta blockers (frequency 4 Hz to 6 Hz). Finally, the fourth group includes patients with tremor associated with other neurologic conditions. Questions regarding the validity of this classification have been raised.

ET is an autosomal dominant disorder with 100% penetrance. Family history can be identified in 50% to 75% of patients. ET is the most common movement disorder, with at least 5 million people in the United States having been diagnosed. However, there are many more people with this problem who have not sought a diagnosis.

PATHOLOGY AND PATHOPHYSIOLOGY

Since ET is neither life threatening nor life shortening, the opportunity to examine the central nervous system post mortem is not frequent. In those cases that have been examined pathologically, there is no distinctive central nervous system pathology. In fact, only six reported pathologic examinations have been published, and the consensus is that there is no discernible pathology in the cerebellar or extrapyramidal systems.

The pathophysiology of ET remains unknown. Both central and peripheral mechanisms have been suggested, and evidence exists supporting both. At present, a central mechanism is considered most likely. The most tantalizing evidence presented has been with positron emission tomography. In four patients with ET, enhanced cerebral blood flow was observed in both cerebellar hemispheres in relation to postural tremor.

An interesting pathophysiologic postulate is that ET represents an exaggeration of physiologic tremor, a normal phenomenon that can be recorded in all people by the use of an accelerometer and can be observed clinically in some normal individuals (8 Hz to 12 Hz). Physiologic tremor can be seen in almost everyone when the hands are held out and a sheet of paper is placed over the fingers. The tremor starts at a frequency of 6 Hz and increases to a frequency of 8 Hz to 12 Hz in childhood. It then decreases with age. Possible physiologic mechanisms include inherent properties of motor neuron firing, oscillations in the stretch reflex causing synchronization of motor neuron discharges, or a supraspinal rhythmic input to the motor neurons. This tremor is known to be exacerbated by anxiety, emotional stress, thyrotoxicosis, caffeine, and other stimulants. Evidence suggesting that physiologic tremor may be a forme fruste of ET and that both originate from the same neuronal oscillators has been presented. In this view, ET begins as enhanced physiologic tremor and then progresses in severity over time. This theory has been challenged. Others have presented evidence that physiologic tremor and ET are two distinctive tremors with different frequencies.

ASSOCIATED DISORDERS

ET has occasionally been assumed to be a forme fruste of the presenile olivopontocerebellar atrophies or to be linked to idiopathic Parkinson's disease. Though no evidence has been found to support the former, some evidence is available suggesting a linkage between ET and Parkinson's disease. It has been observed that in patients with ET, Parkinson's disease occurs more frequently. On the other hand, at least four studies have demonstrated no clear link. Patients with Parkinson's disease have a postural tremor that is clinically similar to that of ET, and this may be a reason for the variations in reports. It is possible that, since ET and Parkinson's disease are both very common movement disorders, overlap of the two may simply represent coincidence.

Other disorders that have been associated with ET include Charcot–Marie–Tooth hereditary neuropathy (Roussy–Lévy syndrome), focal dystonias, and myoclonus. Postural tremor is frequently pres-

ent in patients with ITD. This tremor can be indistinguishable from ET. It is particularly frequent in patients with spasmodic torticollis and Meige's syndrome. A family history of ET is not uncommon in these disorders. A definite link between these disorders has not been proved.

The most important disorder in the differential diagnosis of ET is Parkinson's disease. Although many patients with ET are misdiagnosed as having Parkinson's disease, the two disorders can usually be differentiated by history and physical exam. Parkinson's disease presents at an older age than ET, and the tremor of parkinsonism occurs at rest, whereas that of ET is a postural and kinetic tremor. Patients with parkinsonism have rigidity, bradykinesia, micrographia, and postural difficulties; ET is associated with none of these. The handwriting of a patient with ET is usually large and tremulous. Sometimes a handwriting sample alone can lead to the correct diagnosis (see Fig. 9-1). Postural and kinetic tremor secondary to cerebellar lesions can be differentiated from ET because of the presence of other signs of cerebellar dysfunction.

TREATMENT

The usefulness of the beta receptor antagonist propranolol in ET is well known. It plays an important role in the treatment of this disorder. It is particularly useful in controlling postural and kinetic tremor in the upper extremities and may make a significant difference to the patient in terms of being able to feed himself or write legibly. This may be true even though propranolol may not abolish the tremor but may only markedly decrease its amplitude, having little or no effect on frequency.

Although propranolol is the treatment of choice in ET, there are often markedly inconsistent therapeutic results. From 50% to 70% of patients treated with propranolol show a decrease in amplitude of tremor. There does not appear to be a correlation between plasma concentration of propranolol or its metabolites and a reduction in tremor. There are no apparent features that separate responders and nonresponders, but some have found that tremors with lower amplitude and higher frequency respond less well.

The dosage of propranolol may range from 60 mg to 320 mg/day; it begins to exert its effect in 2 to 6 hours after a single dose and may last as long as 8 hours. Withdrawal from propranolol may result in a rebound increase in amplitude of the tremor, which may last longer than a week. Recently a long-acting propranolol has been found to be effective in ET. Once-a-day administration leads to better response secondary to better compliance. The site of action of propranolol, whether central or peripheral, has not been fully established.

There are certain groups of patients with ET in whom the use of propranolol is contraindicated. They include patients with chronic obstructive lung disease, asthma, and congestive heart failure. In these instances the substitution of a different beta antagonist, such as metoprolol, may result in amelioration of the tremor and no bronchospastic symptoms. Metoprolol is a beta receptor antagonist that is relatively selective in its action; however, patients who do not respond to metoprolol also do not respond to propranolol. It has been suggested that the selectivity of this agent is lost when higher doses are used, and at higher doses bronchospastic symptoms may re-emerge. Acute side effects of beta blockers include bradycardia and syncope, while chronic problems include fatigue, depression, and impotence.

Primidone, an anticonvulsant, has recently been studied and found to be as effective as, if not superior to, propranolol in reducing amplitude of tremor in 60% to 70% of patients. The major problem has been acute adverse effects, which are frequent (30%) and include vertigo, a general ill feeling, unsteadiness, nausea, ataxia, and confusion. These side effects clear spontaneously within 1 to 4 days, and patients should be encouraged to stick with the drug during this time. In this treatment situation primidone is used in lower doses (50 mg to 250 mg/day). As with propranolol, response has varied from patient to patient, and the reason for this is unknown. Plasma levels of primidone and its metabolites do not correlate with responsiveness. Although one metabolite of primidone, phenobarbital, has been shown to have efficacy in ET, it is not as effective as primidone. It has been shown that improvement of ET with primidone is not related to the action of phenobarbital. It is likely that a combination of primidone and propranolol will be more effective than each drug used alone. There are no well-defined factors which are predictive of response to primidone or propranolol.

One of the features of the clinical history which an adult with ET will often give is the salutary effect of alcohol on the tremor. In fact, alcohol may be the most effective agent, with 75% of patients responding quickly and dramatically. The occasional use of alcohol (particularly prior to dinner) in patients with ET is a reasonable recommendation.

Benzodiazepines are another group of medications that may be successful in treating ET. Alprazolam was evaluated in 24 subjects in a placebo-controlled double-blind trial, and significant improvement was observed utilizing maximum doses of 3 mg/day. Clonazepam has also been examined, but to treat a subgroup of patients with kinetic predominant tremor. In an open trial, 14 patients were treated with a maximal dose of 2.2 mg/day and had a 70% improvement. Clonezepam was more effective for this variant than propranolol. A major side effect of this class of medications is sedation.

A new treatment under investigation for ET is the use of botulinum toxin A (Botox). Pilot studies have been completed in patients with head, hand, and voice tremors with moderate to marked functional improvement and tremor reduction in approximately 70% of patients. Larger studies are currently under way.

Finally, it is felt by many that surgery is under-utilized in ET, especially in those patients with severe disability. Stereotaxic thalamotomy of the ventral intermediate nucleus can be a very effective and long-term treatment. Treatment with this technique should be reserved for patients with severe unilateral or symmetrical tremor, severe functional disability, and poor response to medical therapy. Bilateral surgery often results in severe dysarthria. Recently, chronic stimulation of the ventral intermediate thalamic nucleus has been evaluated in treating tremors. Chronic stimulating electrodes are implanted and connected to a pulse generator. Almost 90% of patients improve markedly, with many having complete relief of tremor. This strategy is felt to be superior to thalamotomy, especially when treatment is required bilaterally.

HUNTINGTON'S DISEASE

Huntington's disease (HD) is a chronic degenerative disorder of the central nervous system characterized by choreiform movements and progressive mental deterioration. It is inherited in an autosomal dominant pattern and commonly presents in adult life. The word *chorea* is derived from the Greek word for dance (*choreia*) and was originally used to describe the dance-like gait and continual limb movements of infectious forms of chorea (Sydenham's chorea or St. Vitus' dance). The term *chorea* now is applied to a class of abnormal involuntary movements as defined at the beginning of this chapter. Choreiform movements disappear during sleep and are often exacerbated by nervousness and emotional distress. A patient with HD may manifest his disease initially with chorea or mental deterioration, although eventually both abnormalities are seen.

HD may begin any time from the first to the seventh decade but most commonly presents between the ages of 35 and 42. The onset of chorea is almost always insidious, with a few irregular movements of the face and limbs. The typical history includes slight clumsiness or restlessness that progresses to "piano-playing" movements of the fingers and facial grimacing. Family members notice a peculiar gait associated with irregular involuntary hand movements. The patient may try to mask the involuntary facial movements by chewing gum. The muscles remain strong and the ability to initiate movements remains preserved, but the carrying out of a continuous movement is frequently impeded by the superimposition of the chorea. The reflexes are frequently brisk, but patients rarely have Babinski signs until the final stages of the disease. The voice is often affected by this condition, and abnormalities of respiratory and articulatory muscles may lead to dysarthria and erratic, sometimes explosive speech. As the disorder progresses, the chorea may diminish, and rigidity and dystonia may ensue. Occasionally, these other movement disorders, including dystonia, parkinsonism, and myoclonus, may dominate the picture instead of chorea. Approximately 5% to 15% of patients have onset in childhood. Sixty percent of these patients have parkinsonian features, not chorea. This has been referred to as the *Westphal variant*. There is an increased incidence of seizures in children with HD. These patients progress more rapidly than adults and die on average in 9 years. For unknown reasons, childhood-onset patients more frequently inherit the disease from their fathers.

Progressive intellectual deterioration may manifest itself as personality change, depression, or dementia. Some patients show more emotional than intellectual decline, becoming irritable, excitable, and even apathetic. Inattention, poor concentration and judgment, and eventual memory loss progress until the patient is overtly demented. Voluntary movement difficulties include abnormal ocular motor function, gait difficulties, and loss of finger and hand dexterity. The ocular motor difficulties include impairment of fixation, increased ocular reaction time, loss of smooth pursuit movements, and an inability to look toward an object without accompanying head movements and blinking. These findings are frequently observed early in the course of the disease. The gait abnormality is not due solely to the choreiform movements. The gait has characteristics of both basal ganglia and cerebellar dysfunction: a wide-based stance, swaying motions, spontaneous knee flexion, and a variable cadence. This abnormal gait also has a stuttering and dancing character. Many patients with HD are unable to maintain tongue protrusion.

Adult-onset Huntington's patients live 10 to 30 years (average 17) with the disease and usually die of pulmonary causes (aspiration pneumonia), cardiac disease (ischemic heart disease), trauma-related injuries (subdural hematoma) from multiple falls, or nutritional deficiencies. Slower progression of disease is associated with older age of onset and heavier weight at onset. Patients inheriting the disease from their mothers also tend to have slower progression. The final stages of the disease include loss of ambulatory function, severe dysarthria, dysphagia, and dementia. The loss of functional capacity and rate of progression can be correlated in some patients with the degree of caudate nucleus atrophy seen on computed tomography (CT) or magnetic resonance imaging (MR) scan and caudate nucleus hypometabolism measured on positron emission tomography.

The clinical picture of HD is variable, and some patients have more chorea than mental changes; however, the reverse is also possible. This can lead to difficulties with diagnosis. Since HD is an inherited, progressive, debilitating disorder with no cure, accurate diagnosis is of the utmost importance. In the patient with adult-onset chorea, dementia, and a positive family history, the diagnosis can be easily made. However, in patients with chorea and even dementia who have no family history, the diagnosis of HD cannot be made with complete assurance. If a patient has chorea but a definite lack of family history, the chorea may be due to another etiology. Often, family members are protective of the involved person or the spouse may not be informed of the presence of HD in the family so that a family history will be impossible to obtain. Failure to obtain accurate family history is the biggest source of diagnostic error. Dementia and emotional symptoms are not essential for the diagnosis and are not considered sufficient evidence of HD in a family. However, a history of family members having been hospitalized for these reasons in middle age or because of neurologic problems helps to raise the index of suspicion in patients with typical choreiform movements. A recent follow-up study of 49 patients suspected to have HD on clinical grounds but without family history revealed that 75% did indeed have the disease. Final diagnosis in this study was based on pathology or the onset of other cases within the family over time. Nonpaternity and mild, late onset of disease are the most likely explanations for apparently sporadic cases. There are a number of other disorders that present with chorea (Table 10-2).

GENETICS

HD is inherited as an autosomal dominant disorder with 100% penetrance. Children of an affected parent have a 50% risk of developing the disease. The emotional impact of the disease on such children is profound. Children must watch as a parent deteriorates slowly and inexorably, while also facing the prospect of inheriting the same disorder. Enormous advances have been made in the last decade regarding the genetics of HD. In 1983, the discovery of a DNA marker (polymorphism) linked to the HD gene on the short arm of chromosome 4 raised the possibility of presymptomatic and prenatal testing. Since that time the addition of other markers closer to the gene has increased accuracy to 99%. Because these are linked markers and not the actual gene, the testing could not result in 100% accuracy, thus leaving a 1% chance of a crossover event separating the marker and the gene and therefore a 1% chance of error.

Recombinant testing for at-risk individuals utilizing these markers is currently being performed in a number of centers around the world. The availability of such a test at this time raises a number of ethical questions, most fundamental of which is why predictive testing should be performed for an ill-

TABLE 10-2. Differential Diagnosis for Adult-Onset Chorea

1. Benign hereditary chorea
2. Senile chorea
3. Familial Alzheimer's disease with myoclonus
4. Creutzfeldt–Jakob disease
5. Wilson's disease
6. Neuroacanthocytosis
7. Tardive dyskinesia
8. Basal ganglia infarction
9. Parkinson's disease patients treated with levodopa
10. Inherited cerebellar ataxia

ness without a cure or an effective means of therapy. The impact of revealing to a young healthy person the rather bleak future of HD may be devastating. The results could be marital difficulties leading to disruption of the family and divorce, loss of employment, and even suicide. Recent experience has demonstrated the common occurrence of severe depression in individuals who test positive. On the other hand, some individuals would rather have the opportunity to learn to cope with the future illness and prepare and plan for themselves and their families instead of leading a life of uncertainty from day to day. Finally, many people have realistic hopes that future research will lead to useful therapies and possibly a cure. There are also legal and social issues related to predictive testing that need to be addressed. Early studies showed that approximately 75% of at-risk patients would be interested in participating in predictive testing; however, with the advent of such testing the number of at-risk individuals who wished to participate was far lower.

Linkage analysis (recombinant) testing is not for diagnostic purposes in symptomatic individuals. The purpose is to learn whether an asymptomatic individual in a family with HD is a carrier. The test is quite complicated, comparing the genetic markers (DNA polymorphisms) in affected and unaffected family members. Thus, blood samples are required from many relatives with and without the disease. The testing involves careful evaluation of the family history, neurologic examination, and post-test follow-up. A team of geneticists, psychiatrists, neurologists, social workers, and representatives from Huntington's lay support groups is usually involved. A series of visits is arranged for these evaluations, and the test is not performed until a later (fourth or fifth) visit. Even if testing is not currently desired, it has been recommended that blood be drawn from affected members and stored at the Huntington's disease DNA bank in Indiana for future generations.

Most recently, the HD collaborative research group reported the discovery of the actual HD gene on chromosome 4 and the genetic abnormality within it. The gene is called IT15 (IT = interesting transcription) and the gene product has been named "Huntington." The abnormality is a polymorphic trinucleotide repeat sequence ((CAG)n) that is expandable and unstable. In normal individuals this sequence repeats 11 to 34 times, but in HD there are 42 to 66 copies. Longer segments appear in juvenile cases, suggesting that there is a correlation between length and age of onset of symptoms. The trinucleotide repeat sequence also appears to expand with each additional generation.

This discovery will likely revolutionize preclinical testing, eliminating complex linkage analysis and the need for involvement of many family members, and will result in 100% accuracy. As of the time of this writing, such testing has not been initiated. The gene could also be utilized for prognostic testing if the information about sequence length and age of onset is correct. Finally, with the discovery of the normal function and distribution of the Huntington protein, a better understanding of the neurobiology and pathogenesis of HD could unfold. The ultimate result would be a rational therapeutic intervention. These are the challenges of the next decade.

PATHOLOGY, NEUROCHEMISTRY, PATHOGENESIS

Postmortem examination of brain tissue from patients with HD reveals characteristic pathologic abnormalities. Grossly, the caudate nucleus and cerebral cortex are atrophied. On microscopic examination there is severe neuronal loss and gliosis in the striatum, with the caudate nucleus being more affected than the putamen. Neuronal loss and gliosis may be seen in a wider distribution, and in advanced cases brain weight may decrease as much as 30%. Occasionally patients come to postmortem examinations with well-documented chorea and no pathologic changes.

Postmortem studies have also revealed that levels of many transmitters, biosynthetic enzymes, and receptor binding sites are abnormal. Those that appear to have the most significance as far as pathophysiology is concerned will be discussed. GABA levels have been found to be diminished in the striatum and globus pallidus, and the levels of glutamic acid decarboxylase (GAD), the synthetic enzyme of GABA, have also been found to be reduced in the same areas; levels of both are normal in other parts of the brain. GABA is an inhibitory transmitter that is released by the striatonigral pathways to modulate the outflow of dopamine from the nigrostriatal pathway. The result of the diminished GABA levels is an increase in dopamine activity. GABA is also the transmitter in neurons projecting from striatum to the globus pallidus. There are actually two projections, one to the external segment and the other to the internal segment. Recent studies have shown that the projection to the exter-

nal segment (also containing enkephalins) is the first to degenerate. The depletion of GABA is probably a secondary result of a yet-unknown pathogenic mechanism.

Somatostatin, a neuropeptide that has been studied in HD, is known to be widely distributed throughout the brain, including the basal ganglia and cerebral cortex. A three- to five-fold increase in somatostatin levels has been discovered in the caudate, putamen, and globus pallidus in HD patients as compared with controls. Investigations suggest that somatostatin enhances release and action of dopamine and may therefore contribute to the functional dopamine excess and symptomatology in HD. It appears that somatostatin-producing neurons in the basal ganglia are selectively spared, thus suggesting that cell death is selective in terms of both regions and cell type. Striatal cholinergic interneurons also appear to be spared.

Numerous other neurochemical abnormalities have been discovered in HD patients. These include diminished levels of substance P, cholecystokinin, met-enkephalin, and angiotensin-converting enzyme, plus an increase in neuropeptide Y. All these abnormalities are seen in the basal ganglia. The significance of these neurochemical changes is unclear at this time.

The pathogenesis of HD is unknown. However, the demonstration that toxic amounts of excitatory amino acids (excitotoxins) cause biochemical and morphologic changes in animal models similar to those seen in HD suggests that these toxins may play an important role. Glutamate is the major neurotransmitter of the corticostriatal projections. It has been suggested that this excitatory amino acid or some other candidate (quinolinic acid, a metabolite of tryptophan) acts as a toxin while overstimulating its natural target cells in the caudate and putamen. The toxicity may be related to excessive amounts of the neurotransmitter, prolonged stimulation of the receptors, or altered sensitivity of receptors. Cell death is related to a secondary influx of calcium ions into the cells.

TREATMENT

DOPAMINERGIC ANTAGONISTS

Since the basic pathophysiology in this disorder is related to relative striatal dopaminergic overactivity, the mainstay of therapy remains dopamine receptor site antagonists. Phenothiazines (*e.g.*, chlorpromazine) and the butyrophenones (*e.g.*, haloperidol) share the property of dopaminergic receptor blockade and are the accepted mode of therapy in HD for those patients requiring symptomatic relief of chorea. The amelioration of chorea is felt to relate to blockade of striatal dopamine receptors, whereas amelioration of the often severe psychotic behavior may relate to dopamine receptor antagonism in the limbic system. Treatment with these agents should be limited to patients with disabling chorea and/or psychosis and even in these cases should be used as sparingly as possible. Therapy with these agents commonly results in sedation, lethargy, and depression. Also, it has been observed that a decrease in chorea secondary to neuroleptics does not significantly improve the patient's total functional capacity. Some patients actually have reported an overall improvement with discontinuation of these medications.

Other agents that decrease striatal dopaminergic activity include reserpine and alpha-methylparatyrosine. Historically, reserpine was the first agent reported to be of use in the treatment of chorea. A rauwolfia alkaloid, reserpine acts to block intravesicular neurotransmitter reuptake and thereby depletes the brain of dopamine. Because it also acts to deplete central norepinephrine and serotonin stores, reserpine's activity is not specific, but it is still used in the treatment of HD because it has a less severe side effect profile. Alpha-methylparatyrosine inhibits tyrosine hydroxylase and thereby prevents the synthesis of dopamine and norepinephrine. Amelioration of choreatic movements in patients with HD has been noted after intravenous administration of this agent.

CHOLINERGIC AGONISTS

In the striatum, a balance exists between two major neurotransmitters, dopamine and acetylcholine. Viewed from the perspective of this chemical balance, Parkinson's disease and HD have opposite pathophysiologies. In parkinsonism, a decreased influence of the dopaminergic system is the primary pathophysiologic lesion, so there is a functional predominance of cholinergic activity. Therapy is aimed at increasing dopaminergic and decreasing cholinergic influences. In contrast, in HD the primary pathophysiologic lesion appears to relate to a functional predominance of the dopaminergic system. Anticholinergic agents, therapeutic in Parkinson's disease, might be expected to aggravate HD, and in some patients this has been demonstrated. Cholinergic agents, contraindicated in parkinsonism, might be therapeutic in the treatment of HD. Physostigmine and other centrally active cholinesterase inhibitors have been shown to ameliorate the choreatic movements of patients with HD. Because of their rapid metabolism, however, these agents are therapeutically impractical. Choline chloride, the dietary precursor of central acetylcholine, has been administered to choreatic patients without effect.

GABA AGONISTS

Replacement therapy with GABA and GABA analogues has been attempted. Sodium valproate, which inhibits GABA transaminase and raises central GABA concentration, has been tried alone and with GABA agonist supplementation, and no amelioration of chorea was noted. Isoniazid when given with pyridoxine also acts as a GABA transaminase inhibitor and in preliminary studies has been reported to lessen involuntary movements in a few patients with HD. This has not been confirmed in other studies. Although GABA levels are decreased in the basal ganglia of patients with HD, therapeutic maneuvers to address this transmitter change have not been successful.

EXCITOTOXIN ANTAGONISTS

In the only study based on the excitotoxin hypothesis, a large, long-term, controlled trial was performed utilizing baclofen. Baclofen inhibits release of glutamate and aspartate and exerts a protective effect against potent excitotoxins in animal models. It was hypothesized that baclofen might slow the progression of HD; however, results did not bear this out. There are a number of glutamate-receptor antagonists available experimentally, but trials have been withheld because of toxicity.

PSYCHIATRIC THERAPY

Although the foundation of therapy in HD remains pharmacologic, psychiatric research has yielded a number of therapeutically pertinent observations. Psychiatric care is important to the management of behavioral problems implicit in the disease, whether they are related to psychotic or demented behavior. The management of these problems, from a behavioral viewpoint, is not specific to HD, and the same environmental restrictions and general supportive care administered to other psychotic and demented patients are required.

Aspects of HD that present unique psychological dilemmas appear to stem from the special genetic character of the disorder. The disease affects at least 50% of family offspring but does not manifest itself until middle age. These facts mean that all medically aware members of a given family must spend their childhood, adolescence, and early adulthood under the stress of possibly developing this devastating condition. Investigation of the off-spring of parents with HD with attention to emotional attitudes and family planning revealed a seeming paradox that even with well-educated adults and sound counseling regarding the genetic consequences of bearing children, the fertility rate remained 2.15 per person at risk. The emotional evolution of these adults provides insight into their psychological dilemma and allows for earlier intervention in anticipated psychiatric complications. The investigator cited four states encountered by at-risk adults: (1) shocked disbelief, a brief reaction occurring when confronted with the genetic reality of HD; (2) a stage of depression merging into (3) an angry stage, which can be handled with a variety of psychological adjustments ranging from sublimation to projection; and (4) denial, when the patient may intellectually still recognize the disorder but emotionally dissociates himself from it. With the disease psychologically compartmentalized, child-bearing and future planning become issues emotionally unrelated to the disease. Whether these stages are unique to HD has not been confirmed. The dynamics, however, may serve the physician in anticipating possible dilemmas in patients at risk and in attempting to intervene with a reasonable perspective. It is important to realize that the necessary supportive intervention may additionally involve relatives, spouses, and neighbors of the nuclear family.

WILSON'S DISEASE

Wilson's disease (WD), or hepatolenticular degeneration, is an autosomal recessive disorder of copper metabolism. The gene locus has been located on chromosome 13. Accumulation of copper causes signs and symptoms that are neurologic, psychiatric, hepatic, and/or ocular in nature; however, they may be quite variable, making WD a difficult disorder to recognize. The importance of recognizing WD cannot be overstated because it is a treatable and often reversible disorder that, if not diagnosed, inevitably results in death. There is no question that the only way to make the diagnosis is "always" to keep it in mind. Approximately 75% of deaths due to WD today result from lack of proper diagnosis.

CLINICAL MANIFESTATIONS

The most common neurologic presentation of WD is a speech disorder or extrapyramidal disorder beginning at 18 to 20 years of age. WD has a slowly progressive course, often with a single symptom predominating for months or even years before other manifestations appear. However, there may be a sudden dramatic worsening of what appears to be a stable neurologic deficit. Incoordination involving fine finger movements such as handwriting and typing is frequently an early manifestation. It may be subtle at first but worsens as the disorder progresses. Tremor is also a common early manifestation. It may occur at rest so that when associated with rigidity, bradykinesia, and/or gait difficulty, WD may mimic Parkinson's disease. The tremor may also be postural or kinetic in nature. When severe it takes on a flapping quality at the wrist with high-amplitude oscillations and "wing-beating" appearance at the shoulder often resulting in significant disability. Focal or generalized dystonia is also a common and predominant symptom of WD. Chorea is rare but may result in movements and a gait disorder which resembles Huntington's disease. Dysarthria is a consistent feature of WD. It is sometimes associated with dysphagia, and frequently patients show frustration due to difficulty in communicating. Often patients develop fixity of facial muscles, with retraction of the upper lip, the mouth constantly agape, and upper teeth protruding; this gives the patient the highly characteristic appearance of grinning or having a "vacuous smile." Approximately 6% of patients have had generalized seizures, although seizures are not an early feature. Most patients have seizures after the initiation of penicillamine, possibly related to copper mobilization. Seizures also could be a prelude to death if they go untreated with standard anticonvulsant therapy.

A majority of the symptoms are exacerbated by emotional stress and ameliorated by calm and sleep. There is also an acute dystonic form of WD in which patients appear ill and have a high fever, significant muscle rigidity, rapid emaciation, and confusion. This picture can be confused with neuroleptic malignant syndrome. This acute presentation could be a preterminal event, so proper diagnosis is of utmost importance. Because of the protean nature of WD, it is very important to consider this diagnosis in all patients presenting with movement disorders under the age of 40.

Approximately 25% of WD patients are first seen by psychiatrists for a wide range of emotional difficulties. At least 50% have early psychiatric manifestations, although there are no psychiatric manifestations that are specific for WD, and diagnoses may range from adolescent adjustment reactions to depression and schizophrenia. The most common features include abnormal behavior, such as irritability, incongruous behavior, aggression, and personality change. Depression and cognitive impairment are also common, but schizophreniform psychosis is rare. Psychiatric problems may be seen in a pure form without neurologic deficits, making differentiation from the primary psychiatric disorders quite difficult. However, there frequently are neurologic findings in association with the psychiatric symptoms, and this clinical situation should raise the index of suspicion that WD may be the etiology of the patient's problem. In fact, psychiatric symptoms are more closely related to the presence of neurologic than hepatic features. In one study, personality change and irritability appeared to be more frequent in patients with bulbar and dystonic features. With neuropsychological testing, asymptomatic patients appear to be normal, whereas neurologically impaired patients have clear changes. In order to diagnose this treatable illness, some have advocated that all patients admitted to psychiatric wards under the age of 30 should be screened for WD.

Hepatic disease may be superimposed on neurologic manifestations or, as in 50% of patients, may be the presenting problem. Hepatic disease usually presents at an earlier age than the neurologic symptomatology of WD. There are four different presentations for hepatic WD. First, there may be a transient acute hepatitis that resolves spontaneously. This is often misdiagnosed as infectious mononucleosis or viral hepatitis because patients present with the typical hepatic symptoms and signs such as jaundice, malaise, and anorexia. The second presentation is that of a fulminant hepatitis, which is seen in adolescents and which presents with sudden onset of jaundice and ascites progressing relentlessly to hepatic failure and death. A history of fulminant hepatitis in a sibling of a patient suspected of having WD is significant. Third, and most common, is a chronic active hepatitis that presents with weakness, anorexia, jaundice, malaise, and abnormal liver function tests. Finally, patients may present with cirrhosis. A family history of cirrhosis may be an important diagnostic point. Hepatic WD patients may be psychologically and neurologically normal.

All patients with WD and neurologic symptoms exhibit a Kayser–Fleischer (KF) ring in the cornea.

This is a golden or greenish brown ring that represents copper deposition in the Descemet's membrane. The ring is seen easily around the limbus in patients with light-colored or blue eyes but may be quite difficult to see in those with brown eyes. A slit lamp examination should be performed by an experienced ophthalmologist in order to accurately diagnose a KF ring in all those suspected of WD. Although a KF ring is not pathognomonic, its presence is important in the diagnosis of WD. The KF ring fades with adequate chelation therapy. Another unusual ocular manifestation of WD is the sunflower cataract, a disk-shaped opacity with frond-like radiations that is often described as a "cataract like the rays of the sun."

NEUROPATHOLOGY

The lenticular nuclei are involved bilaterally and symmetrically in WD. The lesions vary from softening and discoloration to frank cavitation. Other areas less significantly involved include the subcortical white matter, cerebellum (most commonly the dentate nucleus), and other nuclei that make up the basal ganglia. Excess copper is distributed throughout the central nervous system. Neuronal loss is observed in the basal ganglia and, to a lesser extent, in the cerebral cortex.

PATHOGENESIS

Excessive accumulation of copper leads to organ system dysfunction and clinical stigmata of WD. Ceruloplasmin, a copper-containing polypeptide, is deficient in 95% of patients with WD. The relationship between deficient ceruloplasmin and the pathogenesis of WD is unknown. Ceruloplasmin has a number of specific activities at a cellular level; however, the loss of these actions does not appear to be related to the pathogenesis of the disorder. Treatment with ceruloplasmin is not effective, and during chelation therapy the ceruloplasmin level may rise, fall, or remain the same and is, therefore, of no value in following treatment adequacy.

Biliary excretion of copper in WD is impaired and copper accumulates in the liver, binding to thiol and carboxyl groups on copper storage proteins. The copper binding alters both structure and function of storage proteins, disrupting normal cellular activity in a variety of ways. When storage reaches capacity, excess copper begins to move into extrahepatic storage sites. This explains why KF rings may not be seen in hepatic WD.

DIAGNOSIS

A high index of suspicion is very important in making the diagnosis of WD. This is especially true when evaluating patients 40 years or younger who present with extrapyramidal disorders, psychiatric disorders (especially when associated with neurologic signs and symptoms), and hepatic disease. In addition, a family history of WD or hepatic disease at a young age should alert the physician to a possible diagnosis of WD. Once suspected, the diagnosis of WD can be confirmed using four tests: (1) a slit lamp examination for KF rings; (2) a serum ceruloplasmin level (usually low in WD); (3) 24-hour urinary copper excretion (usually elevated in WD); and (4) a liver biopsy with quantitation of copper concentration, which is the most definitive of all tests. Clinical evaluation and tests 1, 2, and 3 are usually sufficient to make the diagnosis of WD in symptomatic patients, while liver biopsy is generally not required. In a patient with a neuropsychological presentation, absence of a KF ring probably indicates that the patient does not have WD. If ceruloplasmin level is low, examination for a KF ring must be performed. If ceruloplasmin is normal and a KF ring is present, a liver biopsy should be performed to make the diagnosis. Hepatic WD is the most difficult presentation to diagnose because ceruloplasmin may be falsely elevated or normal in WD hepatitis and a KF ring may be absent. If confusion remains after serum ceruloplasmin levels, slit lamp exam, and 24-hour urinary copper concentration, then liver biopsy is required.

WD is inherited as an autosomal recessive disorder, which means that each sibling of a WD patient has a 25% chance of having the disease. All siblings of WD patients should be screened. If they have WD, treatment will prevent the onset of clinical stigmata. These at-risk siblings should have slit lamp examination and ceruloplasmin determination along with physical and neurologic exam at regular intervals. If a KF ring is present, ceruloplasmin level is low, and urinary excretion of copper is elevated, the diagnosis of WD is clear and liver biopsy is not required. However, if the serum ceruloplasmin level is low but a KF ring is absent, the patient may be a heterozygote for WD and a liver biopsy will be necessary to make a definitive diagnosis. From 10% to 20% of heterozygotes have low serum ceruloplasmin levels, but these patients do not require treatment. In the near future, presymptomatic diagnosis will be possible utilizing genetic linkage analysis. With the recent discovery of multiple markers close to the gene on chromosome 13, multilocus linkage analysis could make possible accurate and informative testing of potential carriers in families with WD. Advantages of this technique include its noninvasive nature and early (possibly prenatal) diagnosis. Neuroimaging techniques are not diagnostic in WD, but typical lesions can be observed. On CT scanning, atrophy of the head of the caudate and putamen is seen early and cavitation of the putamen is seen late. On MR scanning, hypointense lesions are observed in the lenticular nucleus, thalamus, and caudate nucleus on T1-weighted images and hyperintensity on T2.

TREATMENT

Once the diagnosis of WD is confirmed, treatment should be instituted without delay. D-penicillamine, a chelating agent with thiol groups to bind copper and remove it from organ systems, is the treatment of choice: 1 g to 2 g given in four divided doses on an empty stomach to assure maximal absorption. Pyridoxine, 25 mg/day, should be added because of an antipyridoxine effect of penicillamine. Improvement occurs from 2 weeks to 1 year after the institution of therapy. The variation in response is due to the size of the abnormal body pool of copper, size of the initial penicillamine dose, patient compliance, and variation in strength of copper binding from patient to patient. There is no set pattern as to which symptoms clear first; however, dystonia tends to be more resistant than tremor and dysarthria. The characteristic smile typically remains. Improvement of psychiatric manifestations is unpredictable. Sequelae resulting from irreversible structural damage to the liver or brain will remain unchanged. Between 75% and 80% of WD patients will respond successfully to penicillamine. In the first 2 months of therapy complete blood count, urinalysis, and liver enzyme levels should be examined frequently. Some WD patients initially worsen with penicillamine therapy during the first 2 weeks to 2 months. The actual frequency of this occurrence is unknown. In addition, a small percentage of WD patients continues to progress and will die despite treatment. The reason for this is unknown.

Adverse effects of penicillamine occur both early and late. Early adverse effects include hypersensitivity reactions, fever, rash, adenopathy, leukopenia, thrombocytopenia, collagen vascular disorders, and bone marrow suppression. If any of these reactions are severe, therapy should be interrupted until symptoms subside. Then prednisone should be given followed by the reinstitution of penicillamine. Late adverse effects occurring after a year of therapy include nephrotic syndrome, agranulocytosis, thrombocytopenia, Goodpasture's syndrome, pemphigus, myasthenia gravis, elastosis perforans serpiginosa, and dermopathy. Serious intolerance to penicillamine occurs in only 3% to 5% of patients, and these patients require alternative therapy. Trientine which, like penicillamine, is a copper chelating agent, is the alternative therapy of choice at a dosage of 1 g to 1.5 g/day. Adverse effects include collagen vascular disorders and iron deficiency anemia. British anti-Lewisite (BAL) is another chelating agent utilized in WD; however, its use is limited by severe toxic effects and the fact that it is available only for intramuscular injection. Two newer therapies have been reported in the literature. The first, zinc sulfate, induces excretion of copper by way of the gastrointestinal tract. Doses utilized range from 300 mg to 1200 mg/day. Zinc is less toxic than penicillamine and does not cause an initial worsening of symptoms. It has been used successfully as both initial treatment and maintenance. A problem with using zinc as initial therapy relates to its slowness to act and its apparently only modest effect on negative copper balance. The second new treatment is tetrathyromolybdate, a compound that prevents absorption of copper in the gastrointestinal tract and removes serum copper from the toxic pools by forming complexes with copper and albumin. Pilot studies with this agent are under way. Copper-rich foods should be avoided, including shellfish, chocolate, nuts, mushrooms, and liver.

Frequently, patients who are stable or, more commonly, asymptomatic will be tempted to stop their chronic medication, perhaps because it may be difficult for asymptomatic patients to connect their good health to their medication. Discontinuing chelation therapy invariably results in disaster; many patients who do so will die of fulminant hepatitis within 3 years. It is the physician's job to reinforce the need for medication and to inform these patients of the disastrous results that lie ahead should the medication be stopped.

GILLES DE LA TOURETTE'S SYNDROME

Gilles de la Tourette's syndrome (GTS) is a disorder dominated by tics and behavioral abnormalities.

Tics are classified according to whether they are motor or vocal, simple or complex. Simple motor tics are abrupt, brief, isolated movements involving individual muscle groups. Examples of simple motor tics are eye blinks, head jerks, and shoulder shrugs. Complex motor tics are more coordinated, sequential, and complicated movements that may appear purposeful (resembling normal acts) but are inappropriately intense and timed. Examples of complex motor tics include eye deviation, facial grimacing, hand shaking, touching, jumping, hitting, kicking, squatting, copropraxia (obscene gestures), and echopraxia (mimicking the movements of others). Sometimes a cluster of simple tics will appear to be complex. Simple vocal tics are a variety of inarticulate noises and sounds. Examples include snickering, snorting, barking, throat clearing, or grunting. Complex vocal tics are actually linguistically meaningful utterances. They can include the utilization of words ("no-no"), phrases ("oh boy"), or even sentences. Classic forms of complex vocal tics include palilalia (involuntary repetition of words or sentences), echolalia (involuntary repetition of words or sentences just spoken by another person), and coprolalia (involuntary utterances of curse words). Vocal tics in general tend to occur at phrase junctions in speech and can cause blockage or hesitation of speech patterns.

Other forms of tics have recently been defined. Generally, tics are clonic or rapid in nature. When they are slow, twisting, and result in brief sustained postures (resembling dystonia), they have been referred to as *dystonic tics*. *Sensory tics* are patterns of somatic sensations that have been variously described as a pressure, tickle, temperature change, or uncomfortable feeling localized to specific body regions and resulting in dysphoric feelings. These uncomfortable sensations may provoke a motor or a vocal tic. This indicates that the tic itself may actually be a voluntary movement. The uncomfortable sensation is usually relieved by this movement, but relief is only temporary. As such, these movements are often repeated. An example of a sensory tic is a burning sensation or pain behind the eye, leading to an eye blink or an eye deviation.

Tics have a number of characteristic features that help to differentiate them from other movement disorders. They are usually suppressible. Often when patients with GTS come into the physician's office their history of tics is a better indication than just observation because patients can suppress tics in the office. In addition, tics tend to wax and wane, so they vary in intensity over time. Tics also tend to change location over time. More frequently tics begin in the eyes with eye blinking and then move so that there are neck movements or shoulder shrugs or other types of movements. This suggests a tendency to migrate in a rostral caudal fashion. Patients will often describe an inner tension that is relieved by the tic itself. When patients suppress tics, the inner tension grows and they will often experience a flurry of tics once the suppression is released. Patients will often give a history of having few tics during work but having a flurry when they return home at the end of the day. Tics, in general, increase with stress, anger, and excitement and decrease with relaxation and sleep.

CLINICAL SPECTRUM OF TIC DISORDERS

Tic disorders represent a continuum from a mild, transient form to a potentially devastating neurobehavioral disorder. Studies of large families have indicated that various types of tic disorders occur in individual families and that they all appear to represent varied severity of a single disease. Transient tic disorder, probably the most common and mildest form, is defined by a duration of less than 12 months; as such, the diagnosis is often retrospective. In these patients tics are usually of the simple motor type. Chronic multiple tic (CMT) disorder is a more severe form than transient tic disorder. In CMT, patients have multiple motor or vocal tics but not both; multiple motor tics are much more common. The duration of CMT is greater than 1 year. GTS represents the full expression of the disorder. Diagnostic criteria for GTS (DSMIIIR) include the presence of multiple motor tics, at least one vocal tic, onset before the age of 21, and duration of disease greater than 1 year. CMT disorder and transient tic disorder most likely represent mild forms of GTS and thus represent partial expression of the disorder. In its most severe form GTS is a chronic, complex, fluctuating disorder. Although coprolalia, echolalia, intellectual dysfunction, and psychopathology are common manifestations of the disorder, they are not required for diagnosis. Although coprolalia is probably responsible for the notoriety of GTS, it is rare. It is distinguished from emotion-driven swearing by its cadence, volume, and context, and it can be mild and transient. GTS is more common in males than females (3:1 ratio) and has an age of onset between 3 and 21 (average of about 6). It is often sudden in onset. Estimates of the prevalence of this disorder are probably significantly lower than actual prevalence because, in the

milder cases, many individuals are unaware that they have a tic disorder; in many the tics are not bothersome, so they do not seek medical assistance. Spontaneous remissions are rare but do occur. GTS is usually a chronic, lifelong disorder. The natural history of the disease is that it reaches its maximum level of disability in adolescence and then in adulthood it tends to diminish in severity. Despite the continued presence of tics, adult tics are often mild and inconsequential. The severity of tics in childhood has no bearing on the severity in adulthood, as even the most severe tics can improve or even disappear. Moderate to severe tics in late adolescence, however, can be an indication that patients will have more severe tics in adulthood. In general, despite difficulties in school at young ages, most patients are employed or go on for further education as young adults and become very well adjusted. The need for treatment also diminishes in adulthood.

ASSOCIATED BEHAVIORAL DISTURBANCES

Obsessive–compulsive disorder (OCD) is present in as many as 70% of GTS patients. This behavioral disorder is the only one that is clearly linked genetically to GTS and may, in fact, represent an alternate expression of this disorder. Symptoms can result in significant stress and disability. Examples of compulsive symptoms include ordered arranging habits, rituals of decontamination including repeated hand washing, checking rituals (locks on doors or cars and stove switches), and ritualistic counting. Obsessive thoughts can often intrude on conscious thoughts and interrupt daily routine. Examples include fears and images of injuries to loved ones, fear of contamination with germs or dirt, feelings of responsibility for misfortune of others, and feelings of doubt that one has performed tasks that are already completed. Obsessive thoughts and compulsive symptoms often go together. Compulsive behavior and tics, particularly complex ones, can overlap, and it may be difficult to differentiate them. OCD symptoms wax and wane and increase with stress.

Another common behavioral disturbance is attention deficit hyperactivity disorder (ADHD). In these patients, the disorder can result in a short attention span, restlessness, poor concentration, diminished impulse control, and hyperactivity. It may be present in up to 60% of children with Tourette's syndrome, and it is not uncommon for ADHD to precede the onset of tics. ADHD seems to be more common in those patients with severe tic disorder. Stimulant medications that are generally utilized for primary ADHD may actually provoke or exacerbate tics. In these cases it is difficult to know whether the tic is primarily due to the drug or whether the patient has GTS.

Other behavioral abnormalities include learning disabilities, aggressiveness, anxiety, panic disorder, depression, mania, conduct disorders, phobias, dyslexia, and stuttering. These disorders have been found to be 5 to 20 times more common in those with GTS than in the general population. Finally, sleep disorders are present in about half of the GTS patients. Problems include somnambulism, night terrors, nightmares, sleep initiation, and maintenance.

DIAGNOSIS

The diagnosis of GTS is based on clinical symptoms; there are no tests that are diagnostic. Because the features can be so varied, there is often a delay in diagnosis, perhaps as long as 12 years. Many patients diagnose themselves. In the last few years there have been a number of television shows that have either discussed the disorder itself or had a person with the disorder as a character. Often patients with the symptoms will see these shows and make an appointment with a physician, seeking confirmation of their diagnosis.

There are several other diseases that cause tics, which have been seen in patients with stroke, tumor, head trauma, encephalitis (and postencephalitic syndrome of encephalitis lethargica), and carbon monoxide poisoning. Location of lesions from these disorders has been the frontal lobe, temporal lobe, and basal ganglia. The most common cause of tics occurs with chronic use of neuroleptic medications (tardive tics). These patients usually have onset in adulthood and have a clear history of neuroleptic exposure prior to the onset of the disorder. Finally, tics can be a manifestation of a chronic neurodegenerative disorder such as neuroacanthocytosis.

GENETICS AND PATHOPHYSIOLOGY

Segregation analysis of multiple large families has indicated that GTS is an autosomal dominant disorder with variable expressivity—as transient tic disorder, CMT disorder, GTS, or OCD. It also is sex-influenced, with males affected more than females. These studies have been supported by twin studies. Despite clear genetic influences, there appear to be nongenetic factors that influence the form and severity of the disorder. Such factors may include maternal life stresses during pregnancy, gender of the child, severe nausea and/or vomiting in the first trimester, and birthweight. To this point, genetic linkage analysis has not led to a specific chromosome containing this autosomal dominant gene.

The neuroanatomic location of the abnormality resulting in GTS is unknown. It is suspected from cases of secondary tic disorders and positron emission tomography studies that the basal ganglia and the frontal and temporal lobes may be involved. Postmortem studies have not resulted in any specific findings.

The biochemical basis of GTS is also not clearly understood. However, there is evidence to suggest that increase in activity of the dopamine system is involved. This evidence includes (1) response to dopamine antagonist medications, (2) response to dopamine-depleting medications (reserpine, tetrabenazine), (3) exacerbation of tics with levodopa and stimulants (pemoline, amphetamine, methylphenidate), (4) the occurrence of tardive tics, and (5) the presence of alterations in dopamine metabolites in the cerebrospinal fluid of patients with GTS. Two hypotheses related to this increase in dopamine stimulation have been suggested. The first is that there is dopamine receptor supersensitivity in the basal ganglia. The second is the possibility that there is an increase in dopamine input to the striatum. There have been evaluations of a number of other neurotransmitter systems. Of most interest in the recent literature is alteration in the opiate system.

TREATMENT

Effective pharmacologic treatment is available for GTS and its many behavioral manifestations. Patients should be evaluated by a team of specialists who can approach the disorder in a multifaceted way. This team should include a neurologist, psychiatrist, and social worker. It may be found that many patients with this disorder do not need treatment at all as their symptoms may be mild. If the symptoms are not disruptive or disabling, then patients should be treated supportively. Some patients may do well with some behavioral therapy such as relaxation training and self-monitoring. Pharmacologic treatment should be utilized only in those patients who are disabled by their symptomatology. The team approach to evaluating patients can dictate which group of symptoms requires treatment (*e.g.*, tics or the behavioral disorder). Treatment should be directed toward those specific symptoms that are most disabling.

With regard to tics, dopamine receptor antagonists (neuroleptics) are the most effective drugs available. Doses of haloperidol ranging from .25 mg to 2.5 mg/day at bedtime can be effective in up to 80% of patients. Side effects, however, can limit its usefulness. These include sedation, dysphoria, weight gain, tardive dyskinesia, acute movement disorders (akathisia, acute dystonia, parkinsonism), depression, poor school performance, and school phobias. Other neuroleptic medications with fewer side effects are now available for use. Pimozide can be utilized at a dose of 1.5 mg to 10 mg/day. This drug can cause prolongation of the QT interval, which ultimately can lead to cardiac dysrhythmias. Electrocardiogram is required at baseline and should be monitored. Fluphenazine, trifluoperazine, and thioridazine are other neuroleptics that can be utilized.

Clonidine, an alpha$_2$-adrenergic agonist, has been utilized in GTS. Studies have found that it can be useful in tics but more so for behavioral aspects of the disorder. Its efficacy in tics is controversial. Daily doses range from .15 mg to .5 mg. Side effects of this medication include sedation and low blood pressure. Other agents utilized with some success, which have not been studied in controlled trials, include clonazepam, reserpine, tetrabenazine, calcium channel blockers, and opiate antagonists.

When treating OCD, behavioral modification techniques can be useful; however, pharmacologic intervention is usually necessary. Recently it has been found that fluoxetine, an antidepressant that blocks serotonin uptake, can be extremely useful at doses of 20 mg to 60 mg/day. Clomipramine, another serotonin uptake inhibitor, has also been utilized in primary OCD with favorable results and may be useful in GTS.

ADHD can be disabling in GTS. The standard therapies for primary ADHD, stimulant medications such as methylphenidate, dextroamphetamine, and pemoline, can intensify tics and are relatively contraindicated in these patients. It is recommended that behavioral therapy and educational approaches be utilized first. If pharmacologic therapy is needed, the first drug to be utilized should be clonidine, which can be helpful for behavioral abnormalities. Another drug that has recently been recommended for this problem is desipramine, a tricyclic antidepressant. If these medications are ineffective in controlling these symptoms and if the ADHD is more disabling than the tics, then stimulant medications can be utilized. The patients should be informed that the tics may intensify with this treatment. Escalations in doses of stimulants should be cautious.

TARDIVE DYSKINESIA

Tardive dyskinesia (TD) is an iatrogenic movement disorder related to treatment with dopamine receptor antagonists (neuroleptics and antiemetics). The term *tardive* refers to the fact that this movement disorder occurs after chronic therapy with these drugs. However, in recent years the chronic exposure requirement has been questioned, since some cases have occurred shortly after initiation of therapy.

Over the last decade, it has become increasingly clear that a number of variants of TD exist. The most common is the classic TD syndrome characterized by choreiform movements. Patients with TD may exhibit multiple abnormal movements at the same time, and the variants are named for the movement abnormality that dominates the clinical picture, such as tardive dystonia, tardive tics, or tardive myoclonus. There are clear differences beyond clinical phenomenology, and separation of these syndromes is important from a practical standpoint. This section will discuss only the classic TD syndrome, since most of our knowledge of TD is related to this particular disorder.

Classic TD is characterized by orobuccolingual (OBL) chewing-type movements or dyskinesias. The tongue often exhibits a writhing-type movement that will result in pushing out the cheeks (bonbon sign); it may also exhibit repetitive protrusions (flycatcher's tongue). These movements vary in severity from extremely mild, where the patient may be totally unaware, to severe enough to cause dysarthria and dysphagia. On examination the tongue movements tend to decrease with protrusion. In addition, patients can have jaw movements (opening, closing, deviations), facial grimacing, blepharospasm, cheek retraction and puffing, pouting, puckering, and lip smacking. Chorea can also be present in the limbs (piano-playing movements of the fingers) and in the axial regions (dance-like movements). Involvement of intercostal and diaphragm musculature results in respiratory dyskinesia. These patients have grunting, sighing, air gasping, and belching sounds as part of their picture and may become short of breath. If severe, mechanical ventilation may rarely be necessary. Chorea may also result in pelvic thrusting and twisting movements. When two or more choreic movements occur in succession, more complex movement patterns may be observed. The movement may be increased or brought out by activating tasks such as testing dexterity maneuvers (finger or toe tapping, rapid alternating movements) or by walking. Anxiety and fatigue also increase the movements.

There is no way of predicting which patients may be predisposed to the development of TD; therefore, the best policy is to limit the administration of neuroleptic medication to those who have psychotic disturbances. In some patients with choreiform movements the continued administration of neuroleptics will result in a progressive movement disorder. In these patients OBL dyskinesias may spread to involve the axial and limb musculature. Another example of progression might be an increase in the severity and amplitude of the individual choreiform movements. It is for this reason that the use of a neuroleptic to treat TD is unwarranted. The use of the etiologic agent as the therapy is reserved for only the most extreme clinical situations (*e.g.*, life-threatening respiratory dyskinesias).

Early descriptions of patients who might be predisposed to the development of TD define those patients as being female, chronically institutionalized, brain damaged, and psychotic. Many of these preconditions thought necessary for the development of TD have been abandoned. The most important of these notions to be abandoned was the concept that pre-existent major psychiatric disease had to be present in order for a patient to develop TD. Unfortunately, it has been repeatedly demonstrated that after chronic administration of neuroleptics, patients with normal psychiatric histories and patients with normal neurologic histories can and do develop TD. TD is different from most drug-induced disorders because the discontinuation of the causative agent (the neuroleptic) in many instances does not result in the amelioration of the movement disorder. In fact, as many as 50% of patients with TD may have an irreversible neurologic syndrome. The fact that a large percentage of patients who develop this syndrome have an irreversible problem is an indication of the serious nature of this disorder.

PATHOPHYSIOLOGY

Multiple pharmacologic conditions can result in the clinical manifestations of chorea. The most important mechanism involves alterations in striatal dopaminergic activity. It has been proposed that the chronic administration of neuroleptics results in a chronic blockade of striatal dopamine receptor sites

and that this chronic blockade of these receptor sites ultimately induces alterations in the sensitivity of dopamine receptors. Animal models have confirmed this.

In the most simple conceptual terms, TD has been proposed to be a chemical denervation supersensitivity. Although choreiform movements may begin when the neuroleptic is chronically administered without a change in dosage, the most common clinical setting in which the movement disorder begins is after the neuroleptic dosage is lowered or discontinued. This latter setting is in keeping with the postulate of lowering the pharmacologic blockade of the dopamine receptor and allowing normal dopaminergic mechanisms to resume their interaction with the sensitized receptor. Although there is evidence in both animal models and human studies to support this notion, there have been inconsistencies. For this reason, evaluation of other neurotransmitter abnormalities and mechanisms in the presence of TD has been carried out. The findings in some of these studies have led to pharmacologic trials with various agents.

Neurotransmitter abnormalities that have been suggested in TD include a decrease in GABA activity in the basal ganglia. Both animal and human studies have indicated that this is a possibility. Some studies have indicated that an overactivity of norepinephrine is present and that decreased activity of serotonin may also occur. Finally, there has been some suggestion that a decrease in acetylcholine activity in the striatum might play a role. Another possible mechanism to explain TD relates to direct neurotoxicity by neuroleptic medications. It has been theorized that the blockade of dopamine receptors results in an increase in dopamine turnover. This, in turn, results in the formation of increased free oxyradicals that ultimately damage striatal neurons.

PREVENTION

As in all iatrogenic disorders, prevention is preferable to treatment. This is especially true in the case of TD, in which the syndrome itself may be irreversible. There are a series of simple steps that may help to limit the development of TD in the general population.

First of all, the number of subjects at risk should be limited. This implies that these agents (neuroleptics) should be employed only in major psychiatric illness, in which they are indicated. These agents should not be used for minor episodes of anxiety, restlessness, insomnia, or other minor psychiatric disturbances. The development of TD does not depend on any pre-existent brain damage or psychiatric history, and patients who are normal psychiatrically can develop TD if exposed to neuroleptic agents. A second and a third means of decreasing the incidence of TD would be to limit the dose of neuroleptic employed and to limit the duration of neuroleptic treatment. Both of these are common-sense approaches to the problem and seem realistic, although there is little clinical information in the literature to confirm these concepts. After all, if TD develops as a result of chronic neuroleptic blockade of the dopamine receptor, limiting the dose of neuroleptics employed, and therefore limiting the amount of blockade, may well be a contributing factor to the prevention of TD. In the same manner, limiting the duration of blockade by limiting the duration of treatment with neuroleptics may also decrease the incidence of tardive dyskinesia. It is always wise clinically to limit the dose of a pharmacologic agent to the symptoms one is trying to treat or control. Neuroleptic administration is no exception, and the dose of neuroleptic administered should be tailored to each patient. When neuroleptics are totally withdrawn from patients with relapsing psychosis the relapse rate is significant. However, an initial episode of psychotic behavior does not necessitate the chronic lifelong administration of neuroleptics.

The concomitant use of anticholinergics and neuroleptics on a long-term basis may be a risk factor for TD. The only reason for the concomitant use of anticholinergics and neuroleptics is to treat drug-induced parkinsonism, a transient phenomenon usually resolving within 3 months. If the patient develops drug-induced parkinsonism and is treated with anticholinergics, at the end of 3 months the anticholinergic should be slowly withdrawn to assess whether or not continued antiparkinsonian therapy is required. If the drug-induced parkinsonism has abated, there is no point in administering a pharmacologic agent that is no longer indicated. Since the use of anticholinergics is directed toward the treatment of drug-induced parkinsonism, and since drug-induced parkinsonism in most cases is transient and reversible, it seems unwise to chronically administer an anticholinergic with a neuroleptic, even if the concomitant use of these drugs represents only a small increase in the risk factor for the development of TD.

An additional approach that may help limit the development of TD is the early recognition of the syndrome and discontinuation of all neuroleptics, if psychiatrically possible, when the first abnormal movements are detected. The chronic continued administration of neuroleptic in the face of developing choreiform movement disorder may result in exacerbation of the chorea in both severity of the movements themselves and spread their to other body areas. The best chance of both stopping the progression of the movements and reversing the movements resides in early detection of abnormal movements.

A final approach to the prevention of TD relates to the use of antipsychotic agents that do not cause this syndrome. Presently, only one such agent exists, clozapine. Clozapine appears to have less effect on the dopaminergic nigrostriatal pathway and has a preference for D1 rather than D2 receptors. Typical neuroleptics have preference to blockade D2 receptors, and it is alterations in these receptors that are thought to be important in the development of TD. So far there have been no cases of new-onset TD reported with treatment with clozapine. Clozapine has been approved for use in patients who have psychosis that does not respond to typical neuroleptics and in cases where typical neuroleptics are contraindicated. The presence of TD represents such a contraindication. There are serious side effects associated with this medication, the most important of which is agranulocytosis. For this reason, a weekly white blood count is required when patients receive this drug. This ultimately leads to great expense. With more experience this restriction may be altered and the cost diminished. It is anticipated that in the future other agents with a similar pharmacology will become available, at which time the incidence of TD could diminish significantly.

TREATMENT

The management of a patient who has already developed TD is a difficult clinical problem. Medical therapies are frequently inadequate.

The first approach to these patients should be careful review of whether or not neuroleptics had been or still are psychiatrically indicated. In many instances, there is no major psychiatric indication for the use of these agents. If this is true, these neuroleptic agents should be discontinued. In many patients, the choreiform movement disorder becomes worse when the neuroleptics are discontinued. This should not be surprising because TD is related to increased dopamine receptor site sensitivity secondary to chronic neuroleptic blockade, and if the patient is having movements (indicating alteration in dopamine receptor site sensitivity) while on the neuroleptics, and the drug is discontinued and the blockade is abolished, the abnormally sensitive dopamine receptor would be exposed to normal dopaminergic physiology. This time period is often difficult to manage because the patients often do become worse. This should not be confused with worsening of the disease process itself, and generally speaking this rebound TD on withdrawal of the neuroleptic persists for only 2 to 6 weeks. At the end of this withdrawal period an assessment of the extent of the baseline disorder is possible. The chronic syndrome has been reported to be irreversible in 30% to 50% of cases, depending on the age of the patient.

Pharmacologic intervention in this choreiform movement disorder is based on the pathophysiologic mechanisms. The pharmacology of chorea is such that agents that decrease dopaminergic activity within the brain will decrease chorea. Consequently, agents like reserpine or tetrabenazine, which deplete the brain of dopamine, will ameliorate the chorea seen in TD. Side effects of these agents are of concern and include orthostatic hypotension, parkinsonism, depression, and gastrointestinal problems.

The other drugs that interfere with dopaminergic activity include neuroleptics. Despite the fact that an increased neuroleptic dosage can ameliorate the chorea in TD, this is an incorrect approach because it will place the treating physician in a position of using the causative agent to treat the disorder. This situation should be avoided.

Use of the newly available atypical antipsychotic medication clozapine has actually been associated with improvement of TD symptoms. It is unclear whether the clozapine itself improves the disorder or if the disorder reverses because the causative neuroleptic has been removed and replaced by clozapine.

Other pharmacologic approaches to the treatment of TD are based on manipulation of other neurotransmitter systems that may be abnormal in TD. Increasing cholinergic activity will decrease chorea, and interfering with cholinergic activity (anticholinergics) may increase chorea. Anticholinergic medications have no role in the treatment of TD. Conversely, there has been interest in the use of cholinergic agents in the treatment of chorea. Several attempts at precursor loading strategy have been made using drugs such as choline and lecithin. These agents have not provided effective therapies. The use of a variety of GABA agonists, including valproate, diazepam, clonazepam, and baclofen, has also been disappointing, but some patients do respond. Noradrenergic antagonists such as propranolol and clonidine have been successful in some patients. These drugs, however, are safe and are reasonable choices in the treatment of TD. Finally, recent studies have indicated that vitamin E, an antioxident, may improve TD symptoms. Vitamin E may be helpful by blocking free oxyradical damage to neurons.

TD can remain refractory to treatment in many instances, and it is far better to prevent the development of TD than to have to manage and treat it.

QUESTIONS AND DISCUSSION

1. Match the neurologic term with the appropriate description:

   A. Tremor
   B. Chorea
   C. Dystonia

   1. Excessive, spontaneous movements irregularly timed, nonrepetitive, randomly distributed, and "dance-like"
   2. An abnormal sustained posture
   3. Involuntary rhythmic oscillating movement resulting from alternating or synchronous contraction of reciprocally innervated antagonist muscles

   The correct answers are (A) and (3), (B) and (1), and (C) and (2).

2. A patient presents with sustained involuntary eye closure and forced involuntary mouth opening. Which diagnoses are to be considered?

   A. Meige's syndrome
   B. Adverse effect of neuroleptic medication
   C. Wilson's disease
   D. All of the above

   The answer is (D). The description is that of blepharospasm and oromandibular dystonia. This may be Meige's syndrome or an adverse effect of neuroleptics. Orofacial dystonia may also be a manifestation of Wilson's disease, and this diagnosis should be considered if the patient is less than 40 years old when the syndrome begins.

3. A 19-year-old patient complains of the recent onset of shaking which occurs when the patient lifts a cup to drink or tries to retrieve food with a fork. When his index fingers are approximated the tremor worsens. A sister has a history of liver disease. This description suggests:

A. Essential tremor
B. Huntington's disease
C. Wilson's disease
D. Parkinson's disease

(A) and (C) are correct. The description is that of a postural and kinetic tremor. This may be seen in essential tremor, which may be familial or sporadic and frequently occurs in adolescence or early adult life. Wilson's disease must also be considered in all patients under the age of 40 with the occurrence of any movement disorder and particularly if there is a family history of liver disease.

4. Drugs which might be effective in ameliorating essential tremor include:

A. Alcohol
B. Acetazolamide
C. Amphetamine
D. Propranolol
E. Primidone

(A), (B), (D), and (E) are correct. The latter two are frequently used treatments for essential tremor. Amphetamine may induce a tremor similar to essential tremor or worsen an already present tremor.

5. A patient presents with a generalized choreiform disorder which began at the age of 40. He denies any neurologic or psychiatric problems prior to the onset of his current problem, and he never received neuroleptic medications. He denies a family history of any similar movement disorder; however, his mother was institutionalized at the age of 55 for psychiatric reasons. What is this patient's possible diagnosis?

A. Huntington's disease
B. Parkinson's disease
C. Essential tremor
D. Idiopathic torsion dystonia

(A) is the correct answer. Huntington's disease is an autosomal dominant disorder with onset in middle life. Although psychiatric symptoms are insufficient to make a diagnosis of Huntington's disease, a family history of a parent with psychiatric disease in a patient with a choreiform disorder is very suggestive.

6. Which of the following is not inherited in an autosomal dominant fashion?

A. Idiopathic torsion dystonia
B. Huntington's disease
C. Essential tremor
D. Wilson's disease
E. Tourette syndrome

The correct answer is (D). Wilson's disease is inherited as an autosomal recessive disorder.

7. Botulinum toxin is utilized in therapy for all except:

A. Spasmodic torticollis
B. Tics
C. Blepharospasm
D. Tremor

The answer is (B). Tics are not treated with this drug. Botulinum toxin therapy is accepted as safe and effective in focal dystonia. Recent studies suggest that it is also useful in tremor.

SUGGESTED READING

Dening TR, Berrios GE: Wilson's disease: Psychiatric symptoms in 195 cases. Arch Psychiatry 46:1126, 1989

Fahn S: High dosage anticholinergic therapy in dystonia. Neurology 33:1255, 1983

Jahanshahi M, Marion M, Marsden CD: Natural history of adult onset idiopathic torticollis. Arch Neurol 40:548, 1990

Jankovic J, Brin MF: Therapeutic uses of botulinum toxin. N Engl J Med 324:1186, 1991

Kurlan R: Tourette's syndrome: Current concepts. Neurology 39:1625, 1989

Lang AE, Weiner WJ: Drug-Induced Movement Disorders. Mt. Kisco, NY, Futura Publishing Co., 1992

Marsden CD, Harrison MJG: Idiopathic torsion dystonia (dystonia musculorum deformans): A review of 42 patients. Brain 97:793, 1974

Singer HS, Walkup JT: Tourette syndrome and other tic disorders: Diagnosis, pathophysiology, and treatment. Medicine 70:15, 1991

Weiner WJ, Lang AE: Movement Disorders: A Comprehensive Survey. Mt. Kisco NY, Futura Publishing Co., 1989

C H A P T E R 1 1

Neurologic Complications of Alcoholism

Bernard B. Megaffin
William C. Koller

Although alcohol is able to alter almost every organ system, its effects upon the nervous system are of particular importance because of the diverse and severe neurologic complications that are common to alcoholics. These disorders have been previously grouped by Victor into the following five categories. In this review, they will be discussed according to this classification.

Alcohol intoxication
  Drunkenness
  Coma
  Pathologic intoxication
Withdrawal syndrome
  Tremulousness
  Hallucinosis
  Seizures
  Delirium tremens
Nutritional disease secondary to alcoholism
  Wernicke-Korsakoff syndrome
  Polyneuropathy
  Optic neuropathy
  Pellagra
Disease of uncertain pathogenesis associated with alcoholism
  Cerebellar degeneration
  Marchiafava–Bignami disease
  Central pontine myelinolysis
  Cerebral atrophy and dementia
  Myopathy

Neurologic disorders associated with cirrhosis
  Hepatic stupor and coma
  Chronic hepatocerebral degeneration

ALCOHOL INTOXICATION

The manifestations of acute alcohol intoxication are easily recognizable. Although the depressant effects upon the central nervous system (CNS) predominate at higher blood levels, excitation and uninhibited behavior are frequently observed as early signs. Speech may be increased and slurred, the gait ataxic, and cognition impaired. With further drunkenness, drowsiness, stupor, and coma may result. It should be stressed that alcohol intoxication, especially at blood levels greater than 500 mg/dl, may cause coma resulting in death.

In a certain population of patients, alcohol has an even more excitatory effect. This reaction has been variously labeled as *pathologic intoxication* or *acute alcoholic paranoid state*. Although this state is not well studied, it is said to consist of irrational and destructive behavior that may follow the ingestion of only small amounts of alcohol. The patient usually has no recollection of the episode. The mechanism underlying this paradoxical reaction is unknown.

Most symptoms of alcohol intoxication are related to its depressive action. Recent studies indicate the intoxicating effect of alcohol appears to be

146

through potentiation of the inhibitory effects of cerebral cortical neurons by the primary inhibitory neurotransmitter of the brain, gamma-amino-butyric acid (GABA).

The usual manifestations of intoxication require no specific therapy. Coma caused by alcohol requires the maintenance of airway, breathing, and circulation, with consideration of endotracheal intubation to prevent aspiration. The supportive care is no different from that required in coma from other causes (*e.g.*, hypoglycemia, meningitis, subdural hematoma, hepatic encephalopathy). These other causes should be considered because of their prevalence in the alcoholic, especially if the blood level is not consistent with the patient's level of obtundation. Pathologic intoxication may require the use of restraints and the parenteral administration of sedatives (*e.g.*, benzodiazepines).

ALCOHOL WITHDRAWAL SYNDROME

A variety of neurologic symptoms may occur in the chronic drinker after a period of relative or absolute abstinence from alcohol, termed the *abstinence* or *withdrawal syndrome*. The most common manifestation of the withdrawal syndrome is *tremulousness*, or "*the shakes.*" This occurs after several days of drinking and frequently appears in the morning after an abstinence as short as 6 to 8 hours of sleep. Associated symptoms consist of general irritability, mild autonomic hyperactivity, anorexia, nausea, and vomiting. Patients have clear mentation, but they tend to be inattentive, with poor recollection of past events. The tremor is generalized and of fast frequency, and increases in severity with activity and emotional stress. It may decrease in a quiet environment. The tremor, increased arousal, and autonomic instability may last for several days.

A second major manifestation of the withdrawal syndrome is *disordered perception* and *hallucinosis*, with an incidence of 10% to 25%. Initially, there may be nightmares and disturbances of sleep. Tactile, visual, and auditory inputs may become distorted and misinterpreted. True hallucinations may be visual or auditory or a combination of the two, and occasionally tactile (*e.g.*, the feeling that bugs are crawling on oneself [formications]) or olfactory. Visual hallucinations most often take the form of human, animal, or insect life. Auditory hallucinations may be either acute or chronic and are usually vocal in nature, with God or friends

often speaking directly to the person. The voices are most often maligning and reproachful and may disturb and threaten the individual. Suicide may even be attempted to escape the verbal abuse. Hallucinations usually begin during the first day after the cessation of drinking and may last as long as a week. Initially, most patients do not recognize that they are hallucinating, and it is only when the hallucinations cease that they acknowledge their occurrence.

Chronic auditory hallucinosis presents a unique feature of this condition. In a small number of patients, the auditory hallucinations continue for weeks to months, and a schizophreniform personality evolves, characterized by paranoid ideations and disordered thoughts. It has been suggested that repeated attacks of acute auditory hallucinosis may lead to a chronic, unremitting form.

A third major manifestation of the abstinence syndrome is *withdrawal seizures*. The majority of these seizures, or "rum fits," occur within 8 to 48 hours following the cessation of drinking, with a peak incidence between 12 and 24 hours. Most often the seizures are single, but several may occur consecutively. They are usually generalized with loss of consciousness. Rarely, status epilepticus may occur. In the alcoholic, a focal seizure, evidence of trauma, more than six seizures, seizures continuing longer than 6 hours, or a prolonged postictal confusional state should institute a search for a structural (*i.e.*, space-occupying) brain lesion such as subdural hematoma. Persons with a seizure tendency may have their seizures potentiated by a short abstinence (*e.g.*, overnight) after drinking. During the period of high-risk seizure activity the electroencephalogram (EEG) may be transiently abnormal. The patient may be unusually sensitive to stroboscopic stimulation and may respond with either generalized myoclonus (photomyoclonus) or a generalized seizure (photoconvulsion). Other patients show generalized EEG abnormalities compatible with mild encephalopathy.

Treatment of withdrawal seizures usually does not require anticonvulsants. The seizures are brief and do not recur. The long-term administration of anticonvulsants in patients with generalized withdrawal seizures is not reasonable because of poor patient compliance, both while sober and especially while drinking. In addition, sudden withdrawal of anticonvulsants may predispose to or cause seizures, and when combined with alcohol abstinence may increase the risk of seizures.

A fourth manifestation of the withdrawal syndrome is *delirium tremens*. This term is reserved for the rare, serious state of profound confusion, vivid hallucinations, tremors, insomnia, and signs of increased autonomic nervous system activity with fever, tachycardia, dilated pupils, and profuse sweating. Of 266 consecutive admissions of alcoholic patients to Boston City Hospital, only 5% had delirium tremens. Mortality rates are from 5% to 10%, and higher in the presence of concomitant illness. Intercurrent infection or injury worsens the prognosis, and hyperthermia and peripheral vascular collapse are the usual causes of death. The course is most often benign, lasting several days, and the patient rarely remembers the period of delirium.

The mechanism of the withdrawal syndrome is unknown. Nutritional deficiency does not appear to play a primary pathogenetic role. A number of ethanol-induced changes in neuronal activity have been postulated to contribute to withdrawal seizures. Recent attention has been focused upon changes in the function of voltage-dependent calcium channels, which admit calcium into neurons in response to membrane depolarization. Experimental evidence suggests that enhancement of calcium flux may contribute to the pathogenesis of withdrawal syndromes. Calcium channel antagonists are being studied for their efficacy as treatment modalities.

The management of alcohol withdrawal syndrome should include the following:

- Careful search for infection, either CNS (*e.g.*, meningitis) or otherwise (*e.g.*, pneumonia), and space-occupying intracranial lesion (*e.g.*, subdural hematoma). A brain-imaging study followed by lumbar puncture (if not contraindicated) and EEG are often required.
- Maintenance of fluid intake, electrolyte and acid-base balances, and metabolic functions. The major medical complications include water and electrolyte imbalance, vascular collapse, pneumonia, cirrhosis, gastritis, and hyperthermia. A ketotic acidosis may occur in the alcoholic during times of malnutrition, with normal or low blood glucose and normal or elevated lactate. Large volumes of fluid can be lost because of sweating. Careful and continuous monitoring of intravascular fluid status with appropriate replacement must be continued for several days.
- Thiamine and multivitamin administration. Thiamine in a dose of 50 mg to 200 mg, half intravenously (IV) and half intramuscularly (IM) should be given, and thiamine may be added to the intravenous solutions. When the patient is eating, 100 mg orally of thiamine may be given daily.
- Prevention of hypoglycemia. Blood glucose must be checked frequently because hypoglycemia is a complication of alcoholic binges, especially in patients with impaired liver function.
- Control of agitation. The agitated, hallucinating patient can be dangerous to himself as well as to hospital personnel. A well-lighted room and the presence of a responsible family member help to maintain the patient's contact with reality. Sedatives may be necessary to control agitation: chlordiazepoxide in doses of 25 mg to 100 mg orally or IM every 3 to 4 hours as needed; or diazepam 5 mg to 10 mg IV every 5 to 15 minutes until patient is calm, then 5 mg to 10 mg orally or IV every 1 to 4 hours as needed (a total dose of 200 mg may be required in the first few hours, and 1200 mg over 3 to 4 days). It is important to see if the patient is awake before administering sedatives, and sedative orders should not be written on a continuous basis. A cumulative dose effect can be seen with delayed metabolism of such drugs, resulting in excessive sedation if used injudiciously. Paraldehyde and clonidine have also been used successfully.

NUTRITIONAL DISEASES

Several of the neurologic complications of alcohol on the nervous system are thought to be caused by nutritional deficiency that occurs secondary to chronic alcoholism. These diseases include Wernicke's encephalopathy, Korsakoff's psychosis, polyneuropathy, alcohol amblyopia, and pellagra. In the alcoholic, thiamine deficiency results from inadequate dietary intake, reduced gastrointestinal absorption, decreased hepatic storage, and impaired use of the vitamin. Thiamine deficiency can also complicate hyperemesis, starvation, gastric plication, renal dialysis, cancer, and the acquired immunodeficiency syndrome.

WERNICKE–KORSAKOFF DISEASE

Wernicke's disease is a neurologic syndrome characterized clinically by the triad of eye movement disorders, ataxic gait, and mental status changes. The ocular disturbances consist of nystagmus, paralysis of the lateral recti, or paralysis of conjugate gaze. Nystagmus, which may be either vertical or horizontal, is the most frequent abnormality. When cranial nerve VI paralysis occurs, it is usually bilateral, although not symmetrical. The ataxia involves both stance and gait, and may be so severe in the acute stage that the patient cannot stand. The gait is broad-based and ataxic; heel-to-shin testing is severely compromised. Three mental symptoms predominate. First, the most common sign is that of a quiet, confusional state. The patient is apathetic, inattentive, and indifferent to his surroundings. Spontaneous speech is minimal, and communication is difficult. Second, the symptoms of delirium tremens or its variants may be present (*i.e.*, disorders of perception). Third, there may be a selective abnormality of memory, termed *Korsakoff's psychosis* (see later text).

The typical pathologic changes seen in Wernicke's encephalopathy include discoloration of structures surrounding the third ventricle, aqueduct, and fourth ventricle; in occasional acute cases, petechial hemorrhages; and in chronic cases, atrophy of the mamillary bodies. The latter has been demonstrated by magnetic resonance imaging (MR).

Korsakoff's psychosis is characterized by a disabling memory disorder. There is impaired ability to recall events and other information that has been well established prior to the onset of the illness, and a dramatically impaired ability to acquire new information. Remote memory tends to be better preserved than recent memory. Cognitive impairment, for example, of mathematical skills and abstract thinking, may also be present. The patient may show little spontaneity and initiative. Confabulation, although frequently described as the hallmark symptom of Korsakoff's psychosis, is not essential for the diagnosis.

The biochemical basis of Wernicke–Korsakoff disease appears to be thiamine deficiency. Due to the role of thiamine in the metabolism of glucose by the cerebrum, impaired glucose utilization most likely plays a major role in the pathogenesis. The ophthalmoplegia, nystagmus, and ataxia can be reversed by the administration of thiamine alone. The ocular signs are the most sensitive to thiamine. An index of thiamine deficiency can be estimated by the blood ketolase activity. Transketolase is one of the enzymes in the hexose monophosphate shunt and requires thiamine-dependent cocarboxylase as a cofactor. Treatment with thiamine should be started immediately, with 50 mg IV and 50 mg IM.

Although the confusional state appears to clear with thiamine treatment, memory deficit and confabulation are much less responsive. These symptoms recover slowly if at all. Recent studies implicate the excitatory neurotransmitter glutamic acid, generated as a result of impaired glucose metabolism, as a potential producer of the pathologic lesions of Wernicke's encephalopathy. This raises the prospect that antagonists to the N-methyl-D-aspartate receptor might improve the generally poor outcome of this condition.

It should be mentioned that Wernicke's syndrome can be precipitated by giving alcoholic patients intravenous solutions containing glucose without any concomitant vitamin supplementation. The carbohydrate load may diminish marginal thiamine stores and induce the syndrome. As a rule, alcoholic patients seen in the emergency room or office should be given thiamine supplementation in an attempt to prevent Wernicke–Korsakoff disease.

NEUROPATHY

A common effect of chronic alcoholism is peripheral neuropathy. The extent and severity are extremely variable. Some patients are asymptomatic, although sensory and motor deficits and hyporeflexia may be found on examination. Many patients complain of weakness, paresthesias, and pain. Other patients may be so severely affected they cannot walk. Symptoms usually evolve insidiously, initially distally with proximal progression. The legs are affected exclusively or more severely, and prior to the arms. Motor and sensory symptoms may occur concomitantly. Paresthesias may be described as burning or dull, and constant. Examination discloses various degrees of loss of motor, sensory, and muscle-stretch responses. A distal, symmetrical polyneuropathy is the rule, but alcoholics are also predisposed to pressure-induced mononeuropathies. Histologically, the polyneuropathy is indistinguishable from many neuropathies of other causes.

Evidence for the nutritional cause includes the frequent association with Wernicke's encephalopathy and beriberi, the failure of excessive alcohol ingestion to produce neuropathy in patients receiving nutritional supplementation, and the predominantly demyelinating neuropathy seen in most patients. The precise nutritional deficiency has not been defined, and treatment should be instituted with daily B vitamins. Physical therapy may be helpful, but recovery from alcoholic polyneuropathy is often slow and incomplete.

ALCOHOL AMBLYOPIA

This condition is characterized by dim or blurred vision, the finding of a reduction of visual acuity, and the presence of a characteristic centrocecal scotoma, all indicative of optic neuropathy. The latter finding helps to differentiate alcohol amblyopia from other causes of optic nerve or chiasmal disease. These changes develop over several weeks and are always bilateral and generally symmetrical. The condition is also seen in the nutritionally deprived not using alcohol (*e.g.*, prisoners of war), and a genetic predisposition (*i.e.*, inborn error of metabolism) is suspected. Deficiencies of B vitamins riboflavin, thiamine, and B_{12}, and deficient cyanide detoxification have been implicated. Although pathologic changes have not been well documented, reported changes include degeneration of the optic nerves and, less frequently, degeneration of the chiasm and optic tract. Treatment consists of a good diet and the administration of B vitamins. Improvement usually occurs with this regimen and is inversely related to the severity of impairment. Recovery may be incomplete.

PELLAGRA

Pellagra produces an encephalopathy characterized by fatigue, insomnia, and irritability, and occasionally by a confusional psychosis. Alcoholic pellagra, like pellagra of other causes, is known to be caused by a deficiency of nicotinic acid. Since the enrichment of bread with niacin, this condition has become rare.

The hallmark pathologic finding is degeneration of the large cells of the motor cortex, but other CNS areas, such as the spinal cord, may show changes. Treatment consists of a nutritious diet and the administration of niacin.

ALCOHOLIC DISEASES OF UNKNOWN PATHOGENESIS

This is a diverse group of neurologic and muscle disorders of unknown etiology associated with chronic alcoholism. To date, evidence of a nutritional cause is lacking.

ALCOHOLIC CEREBELLAR DEGENERATION

Alcoholic cerebellar degeneration is a common and highly characteristic syndrome. This disorder occurs more frequently in men. Clinically patients demonstrate a wide-based gait, truncal instability of varying degrees, and ataxia of the legs with relatively preserved upper extremity coordination. Less frequently, other neurologic signs such as nystagmus and dysarthria are found. Most often the syndrome evolves over weeks to months, but it may evolve over years or begin abruptly. The ataxia cannot be distinguished from that of Wernicke's encephalopathy although it is usually more chronic and severe, and not accompanied by the behavioral signs of the latter.

The pathologic changes are as distinctive as the stereotyped clinical syndrome. Marked and restricted degeneration of all neurocellular elements, particularly the Purkinje cells, occurs in the midline cerebellar structures, especially the anterior and superior vermis. Cerebellar cortical atrophy can be seen on computed tomography (CT) or MR scanning, but half of alcoholic patients with this finding are not ataxic. Because of its similarity to the cerebellar changes seen in Wernicke's encephalopathy, some believe that thiamine deficiency plays a role in the pathogenesis. Electrolyte disturbance and direct toxic effect have also been postulated. Improved nutrition and vitamin supplementation are recommended but have proved to be of little benefit.

MARCHIAFAVA-BIGNAMI DISEASE

This rare complication of chronic alcoholism, first described in Italian men addicted to red wine, may also occur in the nonalcoholic. The clinical features vary but resemble those of frontal lobe disease with a gradual and progressive dementia, confusion, seizures, and apathy. Bilateral frontal lobe signs such as grasp and suck reflexes may occur, in addition to rigidity and tremor. The characteristic autopsy findings are demyelination of the corpus callosum and adjacent white matter, and can be demonstrated on CT and MR scans. The etiology is unknown, and there is no specific treatment. It is a rare condition and much less likely to account for altered mental status in the alcoholic than conditions such as hepatic encephalopathy, cerebral cortical atrophy, Wernicke–Korsakoff disease, and a space-occupying intracranial lesion.

CENTRAL PONTINE MYELINOLYSIS

This is a rare disorder of the cerebral white matter affecting chronic alcoholics, in addition to non-alcoholics with liver disease, malnutrition, anorexia, burns, cancer, Addison's disease, or severe electrolyte disturbance. Clinical signs include spastic bulbar paralysis and paraplegia or quadriplegia. It is seen more commonly in the undernourished alcoholic who has suffered weight loss, nausea, vomiting, and electrolyte disturbances, particularly hyponatremia.

The most common gross pathologic lesion is pallor in a triangular area at the base of the pons. Nearly all myelin sheaths are destroyed, with initial sparing of axons. The pathogenesis is most likely related to rapid changes in the levels of water in the brain. It has been observed as a sequela of rapid correction of both acute and chronic hyponatremia. The occurrence of central pontine myelinolysis in patients with no or mild electrolyte disturbance indicates that frequently associated disorders, such as alcoholism and chronic liver disease, probably contribute to its production in a yet to be explained manner. MR is superior to CT in detecting the characteristic demyelinative lesion but may be unremarkable early in the course. There is no specific treatment, although corticosteroids have been effective in reducing the severity of experimentally produced lesions in rats. Considerable controversy exists regarding prevention. Most clinicians agree that correction of symptomatic hyponatremia to a serum sodium concentration of not greater than 120 mmol to 130 mmol/liter is advisable, and that correction should not be at a rate greater than 2 mmol/liter per hour, and 25 mmol/liter in 48 hours.

CEREBRAL CORTICAL ATROPHY AND DEMENTIA

Postmortem neuropathologic examination in alcoholic patients frequently discloses diffuse cortical atrophy and ventricular enlargement. These changes can be detected antemortem by CT and MR scanning. The clinical correlate of these changes is imprecise. Although many such patients are demented, some show little functional, cognitive, or neurologic impairment. However, neuropsychological testing of nonintoxicated alcoholic patients often reveals impairment. Although the cognitive deficits are usually mild, severe dysfunction ranges from selective amnesia (anterograde and retrograde) to dementia. The pathogenesis is unknown, but experimental evidence has demonstrated abnormalities of dendrites in the hippocampus.

ALCOHOLIC MYOPATHY

Alcohol is able to cause dysfunction of both cardiac and skeletal muscle, the latter being under-recognized. Abnormal muscle biopsies are found in 46% of ambulatory alcoholics and 60% of those hospitalized. Because malnutrition is not required for the development of myopathy, a direct toxic effect upon skeletal muscle is likely. Several types of myopathic syndromes affecting skeletal muscle exist and can be divided into acute and chronic myopathies. In the acute group, the first involves painless proximal weakness that develops during or shortly after heavy drinking and is associated with hypokalemia. The more dramatic myopathy involves sudden, severe pain, tenderness, and diffuse edema of the muscles. Renal damage and hyperkalemia usually are found. Myonecrosis is indicated by high serum muscle enzymes (creatine phosphokinase, aldolase) and myoglobin in the urine. Recovery usually occurs, but renal damage may be permanent. Another myopathic syndrome is characterized by muscle cramps without marked weakness and may be rather asymmetrical. Muscle enzyme levels are elevated; fibrillations and myopathic changes are demonstrated on electromyography and muscle necrosis (especially Type I fibers) upon biopsy.

The chronic form of myopathy associated with alcohol is rather uniform. It presents as a slowly progressive and painless weakness, with atrophy of the hip and shoulder girdles as the hallmark. A coexisting polyneuropathy is common, but biopsy reveals preferential atrophy of Type II fibers. If the patient stops drinking and consumes a normal diet, this condition also improves.

DISORDERS SECONDARY TO CIRRHOSIS OR PORTAL SYSTEMIC SHUNTS

HEPATIC ENCEPHALOPATHY AND COMA

Hepatic coma, or acute hepatic encephalopathy, is an episodic disorder of consciousness associated with severe liver disease (i.e., cirrhosis). Initial mental confusion precedes progressive drowsiness and coma. The confusional state is characteristically associated with asterixis, or liver flap. This sign may be observed in a variety of metabolic encephalopathies and, although common in hepatic encephalopathy, is not diagnostic.

The EEG is a sensitive indicator of impending coma and becomes abnormal early in encephalopathy. Initially seen are paroxysms of bilaterally synchronous slow waves that later become continuous. High-voltage, asynchronous slow waves, that is, triphasic waves, signifying a metabolic disturbance, may appear early or late.

There are several hypotheses to explain the pathogenesis of hepatic encephalopathy. A disturbance of nitrogen metabolism with an increase in ammonium has led to the *ammonia hypothesis* and is supported by the documented effectiveness of therapies aimed at preventing hyperammonemia. The hallmark neuropathologic change in patients with hepatic encephalopathy is a diffuse increase in the number and size of protoplasmic astrocytes in the cerebral cortex, lenticular nuclei, thalamus, substantia nigra and dentate, and pontine nuclei (nerve cells appear to be unaffected). This is also a finding in hyperammonemia of other causes. More recent work suggests that inhibition of the CNS through the *"GABA-ergic" system* may contribute to the neurologic manifestations in hepatic encephalopathy. GABA, the principal inhibitory neurotransmitter in the brain, and one of its receptors can be modified by benzodiazepines, potentiating GABA's inhibitory effect. In experimental studies in animals and humans, benzodiazepine receptor antagonists have caused marked improvement in hepatic encephalopathy. In addition, levodopa has been observed to result in transient clearing of consciousness in patients with hepatic encephalopathy.

The current treatment aims to reduce the intestinal production of ammonia. Gastrointestinal bleeding, if present, must be arrested as quickly as possible. Gastric aspiration is indicated for an upper gastrointestinal source, and cleansing enemas may be of additional value. Administration of all narcotic, sedative, or tranquilizer medications should be stopped. The diet must be altered to a low protein content with adequate caloric supplementation. Multivitamins should be administered, oral neomycin (4 g to 6 g/day in divided doses) given to eliminate urease-producing organisms from the bowel, and oral lactulose to acidify the colonic contents and facilitate ammonia transport to the stool. Surgical excision of the colon carries a high mortality but is associated with improved dietary protein tolerance and improvement in hyperammonemia and neurologic symptoms. Infectious diseases, especially of the CNS (signs of which may be masked by the metabolic encephalopathy), must be ruled out. Electrolyte imbalance, especially hypokalemia and alkalosis, must be avoided.

ACQUIRED HEPATOCEREBRAL DEGENERATION

This has been described as a chronic form of hepatic encephalopathy. It may occur following several episodes of acute encephalopathy or in the absence of a history of the acute form. Clinical features include tremor, asterixis, choreic movement, myoclonus, dysarthria, ataxia of gait, or impairment of intellectual function. The condition may evolve over months to years, causing increasing debility. Signs of corticospinal tract disease and a diffuse, slow wave abnormality on EEG are seen. Hepatic function is markedly abnormal (elevated serum ammonium is usually present), and jaundice, ascites, and esophageal varices are common. Portacaval shunting is uniformly present. Although the symptoms may resemble Wilson's disease, the lack of family history, Kayser–Fleischer rings, or disordered copper metabolism facilitates differentiation. As in acute hepatic encephalopathy, a diffuse increase in the size and number of protoplasmic astrocytes is observed. In addition, there is diffuse necrosis of the cortex, subjacent white matter, striatum, and cerebellar white matter. Nerve cells may appear swollen with chromatolysis (Oplaski cells). Similar cells are seen in Wilson's disease. Treatment measures are similar to those outlined for acute hepatic encephalopathy but are much less effective.

QUESTIONS AND DISCUSSION

1. A 52-year-old alcoholic is admitted to the hospital because of severe weakness. He also complains of sensory loss, especially in a stocking distribution in both lower extremities. The patient is too weak to stand and has difficulty sitting erect due to weakness of his axial musculature and neck. Examination reveals severe proximal and mild to moderate distal weakness of all extremities; severely impaired light touch, position, and vibratory sensations in the distal lower extremities; and absent knee and ankle jerks bilaterally. What is your diagnosis?

Examination reveals evidence of a sensorimotor polyneuropathy (hyporeflexia, distal sensory and motor deficits) but does not explain the severe proximal and axial weakness. This clinical picture suggests an alcoholic myopathy superimposed upon a more chronic symmetrical polyneuropathy.

Confirmatory studies might include serum potassium, renal function tests and urine for myoglobin, muscle enzymes, thyroid function tests, electromyography with nerve conduction studies, and muscle and nerve biopsy. Management would include abstinence from alcohol, nutritional and vitamin supplementation, and physical therapy.

2. A 46-year-old chronic alcoholic is reported to have suffered a grand mal seizure 12 hours after his last drink. The onset of the seizure was unwitnessed, and various abrasions and contusions, some appearing recent and some older, are noted about the head. Upon arrival in the emergency room, the patient is alert but confused. The paramedic team instituted an intravenous solution containing 5% glucose. What diagnostic and therapeutic measures would you institute?

The timing (peak incidence at 12 to 24 hours) and type (grand mal) favor a diagnosis of withdrawal seizure. However, the seizure may have had a partial (*i.e.*, focal) onset that was not appreciated by observers, with secondary generalization. Furthermore, the signs of recent head injury should initiate a search for a space-occupying brain lesion (*e.g.*, subdural hematoma). A CT or MR of the head is mandatory. A search for infection and metabolic disturbance is also indicated, and an EEG may be helpful. Thiamine deficiency should be assumed in this setting, and thiamine should be given parenterally as per routine (especially after the administration of intravenous glucose, which might precipitate Wernicke's disease). After determining the seizure type, a decision can be made regarding the requirement for long-term anticonvulsant therapy.

3. You are asked to see a 57-year-old alcoholic who has been transferred from another hospital with a tentative diagnosis of brain-stem stroke. He was admitted because of malnutrition, weight loss, and vomiting, and was treated for an electrolyte disturbance. He was found earlier this morning with a severe neurologic deficit. Upon examination, he appears cachectic, alert, and able to comprehend but is unable to give a history due to severe dysarthria. Examination reveals weakness of facial and tongue

movements and severe weakness of, and increased deep tendon reflexes in, all extremities. He grimaces to deep pain in all extremities. A CT of the head without contrast shows only mild cerebral atrophy. What additional studies might you recommend, and are there any other diagnostic possibilities?

Another reasonable consideration to explain this clinical picture is central pontine myelinolysis. The history of recent vomiting, finding of undernourishment, and history of possible hyponatremia with correction would be strongly suggestive. Treatment would be supportive, and any further hyponatremia corrected slowly. An MR done at some point during the hospital course might show the characteristic lesion of the pons.

SUGGESTED READING

Adams RD, Foley JM: The neurological disorder associated with liver disease. Res Publ Assoc Res Nerv Ment Dis 32:198, 1953

Adams RD, Victor M, Mancall EL: Central pontine myelinolysis. Arch Neurol Psychiatry 81:154, 1959

Bansky G, Meier PJ, Riederer E et al: Effects of the benzodiazepine antagonist flumazenil in hepatic encephalopathy in humans. Gastroenterology 97:744, 1989

Charness ME, Simon RP, Greenberg DA: Ethanol and the nervous system. N Engl J Med 321:442, 1989

Reuler JB, Girard DE, Cooney TG: Wernicke's encephalopathy. N Engl J Med 312:1035, 1985

Victor M: The alcohol withdrawal syndrome. In Seixas F, Eggleston S (eds): Alcoholism and the central nervous system. Ann NY Acad Med 215: 210, 1973

Victor M, Adams RD: The effect of alcohol upon the nervous system. Res Publ Assoc Res Nerv Ment Dis 32:526, 1953

Victor M, Adams RD, Collins GH: The Wernicke–Korsakoff Syndrome and Related Neurologic Disorders Due to Alcoholism and Malnutrition. Philadelphia, FA Davis, 1989

Peripheral Neuropathy

Morris A. Fisher

CLINICAL FEATURES AND SCIENTIFIC BACKGROUND

The peripheral nervous system (PNS) encompasses those parts of the nervous system that lie outside the confines of the brain, brain stem, and spinal cord. As such, it consists of those portions of the primary sensory neurons, lower motor neurons, and autonomic neurons that are outside the central nervous system (CNS). By definition, therefore, the PNS includes the cranial nerves, the spinal nerves with their roots and rami, the peripheral nerves, and those aspects of the autonomic nervous system that are outside the CNS.

The concept of the PNS is artificial because all parts of the PNS are connected with CNS structures and are therefore subject to pathologic processes that affect the CNS. Nevertheless, there are disease processes that seem to involve preferentially or primarily the PNS, and it is therefore useful to consider this system as a nosologic entity.

All parts of the PNS are associated with Schwann cells or the comparative ganglionic cells, the satellite cells. This anatomic commonality may account for some of the pathologic aspects of the PNS. More significantly, the normal function of all parts of the PNS are dependent on the normal functioning of the nerve cell bodies from which the motor and sensory axons originate. Since the foot is supplied by nerve fibers whose cell bodies lie at the level of the upper lumbar vertebrae, the physiologic mechanisms involved in maintaining normal nerve function are considerable. There is a constant transport system from the nerve cell bodies to their most distal axonal projections, and this system is necessary for maintaining normal nerve (and muscle) function. There is also transport so that the cell bodies are influenced by distal events. This system provides the conduit by which agents such as herpes virus may reach the nerve cell body. Given the complexity and length of the structures involved, it is not surprising that the normal functioning of the PNS is frequently disturbed.

ANATOMY

Except for the cranial nerves, peripheral nerves separate at the level of the roots. The dorsal roots contain afferent ("sensory") fibers that are located either pre- or postganglionic to the dorsal root ganglion on their way to the spinal cord. The ventral roots consist of efferent ("motor") fibers that originate from the lower motor neurons. The resultant mixed ("motor" and "sensory") nerves are the structures for providing information to and from the CNS throughout the body. In the thoracic and upper lumbar region, these nerves are joined by sympathetic fibers after these fibers have synapsed in the ganglionic chain adjacent to the vertebral column. The parasympathetic outflow originates either in the cranial region (cranial nerves III, VII, IX, and X) or in the sacral region passing distally as the pelvic splanchnic nerves (Fig. 12-1).

Individual muscles and areas of skin are supplied not only by particular nerves but also by fibers that originate in particular roots. This feature of the PNS is important clinically, as will be discussed further on. The PNS distribution in the limbs is superficially complex because of the routing that occurs

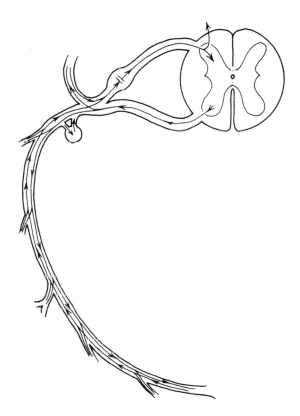

FIG. 12-1. Drawing of peripheral nerve originating from (1) ventral root with cells of origin in the anterior horn of the spinal cord and (2) dorsal root with a dorsal root ganglion. The postganglionic dorsal root fibers pass to the dorsal horn or more superiorly in the spinal cord. The posterior primary ramus extends dorsally, whereas the anterior primary ramus is the main extension of the peripheral nerve. Sympathetic fibers join the peripheral nerve by way of the sympathetic ganglion.

in the brachial and lumbosacral plexi involving the upper and lower limbs, respectively.

Individual nerves are composed of bundles of individual nerve fibers called *fascicles*, which, in turn, are surrounded by connective tissue. All of the motor fibers and many of the sensory fibers are surrounded by myelin. Myelin is formed by foldings of Schwann cell membranes. These supporting cells are ubiquitous throughout the PNS. In myelinated fibers, the junction of sheaths from two adjacent Schwann cells occurs at what are referred to as *nodes of Ranvier*. Most sensory fibers and all autonomic fibers are either poorly myelinated or nonmyelinated. It is important to emphasize, however, that all nerve fibers—even those that are unmyelinated—are ensheathed by Schwann cells.

Nerves are supplied by nutrient arteries which arise from adjacent blood vessels. The arterial supply is richly collateralized both to and within the nerves themselves. The result is a system remarkably resistant to large vessel ischemia.

INDICATIONS OF NEUROPATHIC INJURY

The symptoms and signs of neuropathic injury can be anticipated from the preceding discussion. If nerves to muscles are disrupted, weakness may be present, and atrophy of muscle fibers can occur. Cramping with fatigue is a common symptom. Reflexes may be decreased or lacking if the afferent or efferent nerves that subserve the reflex are disturbed.

A wide range of sensory disturbances are found. With complete loss of innervation, there may be total loss of feeling—anesthesia. This rarely happens because of the considerable overlap of sensory nerve supply. More commonly, alterations in sensation are found. A decrease in sensory perception is referred to as *hypoesthesia*, an increase in this perception is known as *hyperesthesia*, unusual feelings such as "pins and needles" are called *paresthesias*, and unpleasant sensations such as burning are called *dysesthesias*. A decrease in perception of position and vibration is attributed to dysfunction in the larger fibers, whereas diminished pin and temperature sensation is thought to indicate abnormalities in the smaller fibers.

Autonomic dysfunction may result in vasomotor disturbances as well as in alterations in sweating. Trophic changes of the skin and nails can be found resulting from repeated injury and inadequate repair. The skin may become smooth and glossy, hair may decrease (or occasionally increase), and the nails may become thickened.

ANATOMIC DISTRIBUTION

Motor and sensory changes caused by PNS disease occur in the distribution of the roots, the plexi, or the peripheral nerves themselves. Charts are readily available that show these distributions. Although superficially complex, with even limited practice the information becomes readily usable. None of the motor or sensory charts are absolute. The information has been obtained indirectly based on root or nerve injury. Given the potential variability, particularly in sensory distribution, it is not surprising that there may be variations from patient to patient. It is hopeless to attempt to fit each patient into a circumscribed view of normal. General patterns of root and nerve distribution are reliable, and it is important to rely on these patterns (Fig. 12-2).

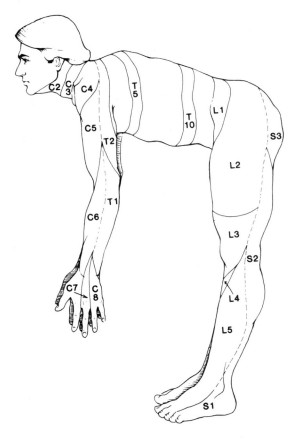

FIG. 12-2. Sequential nature of the cutaneous root distribution as shown with the individual in the quadruped position.

The muscles of the shoulder girdle are innervated mainly by the C5 root, those of the arm by C5 and C6 (triceps brachii C7), those of the forearm by C7 and C8, and those of the hand by C8 and T1. In the lower extremity, the thigh muscles are supplied by the L2, L3, and L4 roots. Those muscles of the anterior leg are innervated mainly by L5, those of the posterior leg by S1, and the small muscles of the foot by S1 and S2.

The root sensory distribution can be visualized with the individual in the anatomic position. In general, C1–C4 innervate the back of the head, the neck, and the shoulder region; C5 innervates the lateral aspect of the arm; C6 innervates the lateral portion of the forearm extending into the hand involving the thumb and index finger; C7 innervates the midportion of the hand and ring finger; and C8 innervates the more medial portion of the hand including the little finger. The posterior aspect of the upper extremity is then supplied by T1 and T2 and the torso is innervated sequentially by T2–L1, with T5 at about the level of the nipples and T10 at the umbilicus. The anterior thigh is supplied by L1, L2, and L3; the anterior leg and foot are supplied predominantly by L4 and L5; the posterior aspect of the lower extremity is supplied by S1 and S2; and the region of the anus is supplied by S3, S4, and S5.

The three main terminal nerves of the brachial plexus in the upper extremity are the radial, ulnar, and median nerves. The radial nerve innervates the extensor muscles as well as providing much of the cutaneous supply to the extensor surface of the arm, forearm, and hand. The median nerve is predominant in supplying the forearm flexors as well as the muscles of the thenar eminence controlling thumb movement. The remaining intrinsic hand muscles are innervated by the ulnar nerve. The median and ulnar nerves supply the cutaneous sensibility to the hand, with the ulnar territory encompassing the little finger, half of the ring finger, and adjacent palmar surface, whereas the median nerve provides the remaining cutaneous innervation (Fig. 12-3).

In the lower extremity, the femoral nerve supplies the knee extensors in the thigh as well as the cutaneous branches for the anterior thigh and medial aspect of the leg and foot (by way of the saphenous nerve). The posterior thigh muscles controlling knee flexion, as well as all the muscles of the leg and foot, are innervated by the sciatic nerve. The anterior tibial (peroneal) branch of the sciatic nerve supplies the anterior compartment of the leg,

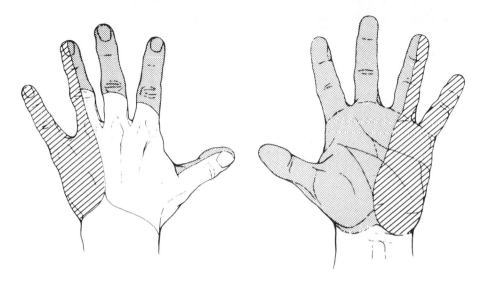

FIG. 12-3. Cutaneous innervation of the hand by the radial (*clear section*), median (*stippled section*), and ulnar (*diagonal lines*) nerves.

that is, those muscles that affect dorsiflexion of the ankle and toes as well as foot eversion, whereas the posterior tibial portion of the sciatic nerve innervates those muscles affecting plantar flexion. The cutaneous distribution is comparable. The anterior leg and dorsum of the foot are supplied by branches of the anterior tibial nerve, whereas the posterior aspect of the leg and plantar aspect of the foot are innervated by branches of the posterior tibial nerve. The medial plantar aspect of the foot and toes is supplied by the medial plantar nerve, whereas their more lateral aspect is supplied by the lateral plantar nerve terminal equivalents of the upper extremity median and ulnar nerves, respectively.

Table 12-1 indicates selected muscle movements with their innervation, and Table 12-2 shows a schema of the cutaneous innervation of the limbs. Neither these tables nor the preceding discussion are meant to be a complete presentation of peripheral nerve distribution. Rather, it is hoped the information will provide a framework to allow clinical use of the material. Referral to more detailed charts can then be made in an active and meaningful manner.

PATTERNS OF ABNORMALITY

Derangements of motor, sensory, and autonomic function may be present with lesions at the level of the roots, plexi, or peripheral nerves. Sensory loss, for example, involving the lateral aspect of the leg combined with weakness of dorsiflexion of the toes would be consistent with a lesion of the L5 root; motor and sensory changes in the distribution of both the axillary and radial nerves would be compatible with injury to the posterior cord of the brachial plexus; and weakness as well as atrophy of intrinsic hand muscles combined with sensory loss involving the median aspect of the palmar surface of the hand, the little finger, and adjacent half of the middle finger would indicate an ulnar nerve lesion.

There are four major categories of PNS disease, based on the anatomic distribution of the abnormality.

The most common type is the *symmetric polyneuropathy*, in which the distal extremities are primarily affected with decreased sensation and often abnormal uncomfortable sensations (dysesthesia). The signs and symptoms of neuropathy usually start in the feet, and clinical findings are present at the level of the knees often before they are found in the hands (glove and stocking neuropathy). Diabetic polyneuropathy is a common example, although uremia and drug or toxic exposure are associated with the same pattern. One possible basis for this distribution of neurologic findings is related to the

TABLE 12-1. Selected Muscle Movements and Their Innervation

JOINT	MOVEMENT	MUSCLES*	PERIPHERAL NERVES*	SPINAL SEGMENTS*
Upper Extremity				
Shoulder	Abduction	Deltoid	Axillary	C5
	Lateral (external) rotation	Infraspinatus	Suprascapular	C5
Elbow	Flexion	Brachialis	Musculocutaneous	C5, C6
		Biceps brachii		
	Extension	Triceps brachii	Radial	C7, C8
Radial-ulnar	Supination	Biceps brachii	Musculocutaneous	C6
		Supinator	Radial	
	Pronation	Pronator teres	Median	C7
Wrist	Dorsal flexion (extension)	Extensor carpi radialis longus and brevis	Radial	C7
	Palmar flexion	Flexor carpi radialis	Median	C7
		Flexor carpi ulnaris	Ulnar	
(Thumb)	Palmar adduction	Interossei	Ulnar	T1
	Palmar abduction	Abductor pollicis brevis	Median	C8
	Extension	Extensor pollicis longus et brevis	Radial	C7, C8
	Opposition	Opponens pollicis	Median	T1
(Finger) excluding thumb	Adduction	Palmar interossei	Ulnar	T1
	Abduction	Dorsal interossei	Ulnar	T1
	Extension (metacarpophalangeal joints)	Extensor digitorum	Radial	C7, C8
		Extensor indicis		
		Extensor digitis minimi		
Lower Extremity				
Hip	Flexion	Iliopsoas	Femoral	L2
	Extension	Gluteus maximus	Inferior gluteal	S1, S2
	Adduction	Adductor magnus	Obturator	L2, L3
		Adductor brevis		
		Adductor longus		
	Abduction	Gluteus medius	Superior gluteal	L4, L5
Knee	Extension	Quadriceps Femoris	Femoral	L3, L4
	Flexion	Biceps femoris	Sciatic	S1
		Semitendinosus		
		Semitendinosus		
Ankle	Dorsiflexion	Tibialis anterior	Peroneal	L4
	Plantar flexion	Gastrocnemius	Posterior tibial	S1, S2
		Soleus		
	Inversion	Tibialis posterior	Posterior tibial	L4, L5
		Tibialis anterior	Peroneal	L4
	Eversion	Peroneus longus et brevis	Peroneal	L5
(Large toe)	Extension	Extensor hallucis longus	Peroneal	L5

*Only main controlling muscle, nerve, and roots listed.
Joint action listed because (1) it can be easily tested and (2) muscle, nerve, and root control is relatively simple. Parentheses indicate action at more than one joint.
Note: Terminal divisions of the brachial plexus can be tested at the thumb. Hip action controlled by muscles innervated by L2–S2 roots.

TABLE 12-2. Schematic Cutaneous Innervation of the Limbs

EXTREMITY*	LATERAL	ANTERIOR	MEDIAL	POSTERIOR
Upper				
Arm	C5 Axillary Radial		Medial cutaneous nerve of arm T2	
Forearm	C6 Musculocutaneous		Medial cutaneous nerve of forearm T1	
Hand and fingers†	Thumb Index C6 C6		Middle Ring Little C7 C8 C8	
Lower				
Thigh	Lateral femoral cutaneous	Femoral L2,L3	Obturator	Posterior cutaneous nerve of the thigh S2
Leg	Peroneal L5		Saphenous L4	Sural S1, S2
Foot		Peroneal L5		Plantar nerves S1

*Portions of the posterior midline areas of the arm and forearm are supplied by branches of the radial nerve.
†For cutaneous distribution, see Figures 12-2 and 12-3.

need to transport material along the entire length of the nerves. Even if the primary pathology then involves the nerve cell body, the manifestations of the disorder would be at the distal parts of the nerve.

The second type of neuropathy is *mononeuropathy*, in which a single nerve is damaged (wrist drop—radial nerve; foot drop—peroneal nerve). Compressive lesions are a frequent cause. *Mononeuropathy multiplex*, in which multiple single peripheral nerves are damaged, is particularly common in diabetes and polyarteritis nodosa. *Plexopathies* result from injury to the nerves in brachial, lumbar, or sacral plexi. Idiopathic brachial neuritis, traumatic injury to the brachial plexus, and retroperitoneal or apical lung tumors are common causes. More proximal injury produces root dysfunction. Motor or sensory loss is then in a dermatomal rather than peripheral nerve distribution. Disk and vertebral bone disease are among the conditions associated with these *radiculopathies*.

PATHOLOGY

The pathologic processes affecting nerves involve primarily myelin or axons, or both. In demyelinating processes, myelin is lost from individual nerve fibers. Characteristically, this occurs in a segmental fashion. There may be marked slowing and even block of conduction. The former is most pronounced in the inherited demyelinating neuropathies, whereas the latter is common in acquired, probably immunologically mediated, processes. Secondary axonal changes occur, but the axons are generally well preserved. As a result, clinical recovery in the acquired neuropathies can be both rapid and complete if remyelination occurs.

Primary axonal degeneration is associated with a large number of exogenous toxins and metabolic derangements. These processes may affect the nerve cell bodies as well as the axons and may be manifest as a dying back of the distal portion of the axon. Secondary demyelination occurs in those fibers with axonal damage. The disrupted myelin may be in the form of a ball or ovoids, but segmental demyelination may also be present. Recovery occurs by regeneration of axons, which often must then reinnervate denervated structures; as a result, recovery may be slow and incomplete.

With physical injury to nerves, the injury may be limited to paranodal demyelination with associated conduction block and rapid recovery (neuropraxia). If axons are interrupted (axonotmesis), total degeneration (Wallerian) of the axons and myelin occurs distal to the site of injury. Since the Schwann cell basal lamina and endoneurial tissue remain intact, axonal regeneration commences promptly after injury. If both the axon and surrounding connective tissue are disrupted (neurotmesis), Wallerian degeneration is inevitable and axon regeneration is limited by distorted connective tissue. Neuromas and aberrant regeneration may occur.

The potential pathologic processes that affect the PNS are similar to those that affect other systems. Metabolic or toxic derangements (*e.g.*, vitamin deficiencies, uremia, alcoholism, heavy metals, industrial solvents, and certain medications) frequently result in nerve dysfunction. Vascular abnormalities affecting nerves usually involve the medium and small arteries, and these abnormalities may be found in rheumatoid arthritis, polyarteritis nodosa, and temporal arteritis. The polyneuropathy of diabetes mellitus may be metabolic in origin, whereas the mononeuropathies seen in this disease probably have a vascular etiology. Idiopathic polyneuritis (Landry–Guillain–Barré syndrome) is representative of an inflammatory process. This probably has an immunologic basis, as do the neuropathies seen in paraproteinemias and macroglobulinemia. Leprosy is a common infectious process affecting nerves. A genetic basis for PNS dysfunction such as peroneal muscular atrophy (Charcot–Marie–Tooth disease) is also not uncommon. Schwannomas and neurofibromas are representative tumors. Trauma is a frequent cause of nerve injury.

DIAGNOSIS

As in other areas of neurology, the physical examination remains a powerful tool for the evaluation of disorders of the PNS. The examination need not be subtle, but it must be accurate. Motor and sensory distributions of a polyneuropathy, mononeuropathy, or radiculopathy can often be appreciated.

The action of individual muscles should be tested and rated as normal strength or mildly, moderately, or markedly decreased. One cannot test all muscles. Concentration must be in those areas that aid in the analysis of the particular problem. Frequently, an evaluation of total muscle strength acting at a joint is sufficient, for example, wrist flexion rather than the individual action of the flexor carpi radialis and ulnaris.

An accurate sensory examination need not be tedious. Again, concentration on areas relevant to the diagnostic question is important. A circumscribed area of sensory deficit often can be best outlined by the patient. This area can then be analyzed in more detail for light touch and pain sensations using a finger and a safety pin, respectively. (Separate pins should be used for each patient so as not to spread hepatitis.) A distal to proximal area of sensory change can be outlined in a similar fashion. Position sense can be tested by moving relevant joints. Slight movements of distal joints should be appreciated accurately. A 128-cycles per second (cps) tuning fork with the base placed on bony prominences is used for testing vibration. The examination should start from the most distal area of potential abnormality. One need then test more proximal locations only if the patient does not perceive the duration of the vibration at the more distal site. A finger of the examiner touching the same bony region as the tuning fork can aid in evaluating the patient's sensitivity.

The most valuable ancillary study for analysis of PNS disorders is electromyography (EMG). This is best viewed as an extension of the neurologic examination. The data are only consistently meaningful if the study is approached in this framework. This is important because EMG, although totally harmless, does entail some discomfort. As a result, reliable information obtained in an efficient fashion is crucial, and this, in turn, must depend on the experience and skill of the electromyographer.

EMG consists of two basic parts. The first part is an evaluation of the conduction in nerves. The second part involves analysis of the electrical activity in muscles—the EMG *per se*. The data can define the location of a lesion as well as aid in understanding the pathophysiology.

Conduction in motor fibers is determined by stimulating electrically and recording the resultant evoked motor response. Muscle fiber contraction is associated with electrical activity caused by the movement of charged ions across membranes, and this electrical activity can be recorded. Latency refers to the time from the stimulus to the onset of the electrical activity. The latency will be shorter if the stimulus is closer to the muscle than if it is more distant. The time difference between a distal and more proximal latency divided by the distance between the two stimulating points enables a conduction velocity to be determined, that is, distance/time = conduction velocity (CV). When recording from muscle, a CV can be determined only if stimulation is performed at at least two points. The unknown time for transmission in slow-conducting terminal nerve fibers as well as across the junction between the nerve and the muscle is then "subtracted out" (Fig. 12-4).

Electrical responses from afferent (sensory) fibers may also be recorded. Since the amplitudes of these evoked afferent responses are several orders of magnitude less than the evoked motor responses,

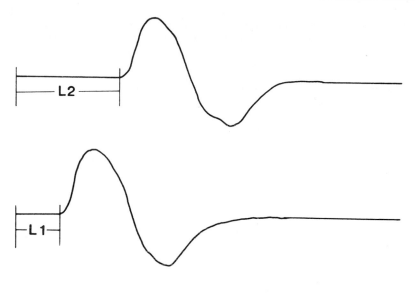

$$cv = d/L2-L1$$

FIG. 12-4. Evoked motor responses with the shorter latency L1 resulting from stimulation closer to the recording site in comparison with the latency L2 resulting from stimulation of the nerve at a more proximal site. The conduction velocity (CV) in the nerve is determined by dividing the distance (d) between the stimulating sites by the latency differences.

the sensory potentials are more difficult to record. At the same time, a meaningful CV can be obtained from a single latency because a CV may be calculated from the time taken to traverse a particular distance, since there is no unknown time across the region of the neuromuscular junction.

The amplitude of evoked motor or sensory responses is a less accurate indicator of normality than is the latency. Amplitude may be affected by the site of the recording as well as by the amount of tissue between the electrical generator in the muscle or nerve and the recording electrodes. Nevertheless, the amplitudes of the evoked efferent or afferent responses reflect the amount of electrical generating tissue. Decreased amplitude responses, focal nerve injury, and side-to-side comparisons of response amplitudes can be particularly helpful.

The different fibers in a particular nerve conduct impulses at different rates. There is a linear relation between fiber size and conduction velocity, with the largest fibers conducting at the fastest velocities. If activity in the largest fibers is lost, then conduction will be slowed. The degree of slowing that may be present with axon loss alone, however, is considerably less than that which may be found with demyelination.

In addition to slowed conduction and decreased amplitude, nerve injury can produce altered configuration and dispersion of evoked responses. These changes in evoked responses can define the location of focal nerve dysfunction. Temporal dispersion is characteristic of demyelinating injury, as is conduction block. In the latter, the size of the response is meaningfully decreased or even absent during stimulation proximal to the block. The result may be a striking picture in which nerve function is lost but conduction studies distal to the region of focal demyelination are entirely normal since those portions of the nerve distal to the block may be entirely normal.

Studies are available (*i.e.,* H reflexes and F responses) which monitor conduction in nerve fibers to and from the spinal cord. These studies are important since proximal nerve injury may be present even in the absence of injury to the more distal nerves which are usually evaluated electro-diagnostically.

The electrical activity generated by muscles can be recorded from the muscle surface but is best appreciated by a needle electrode in the muscle itself. The resultant electrical activity can then be monitored, amplified, and displayed.

At rest, there is no electrical activity. Some activity is usually seen as a needle is moved through muscle ("insertional activity"), but these responses stop when needle movement stops. As a muscle contracts, there is increasing activity. This consists of the firing of motor units. A motor unit is composed of a lower motor neuron in the anterior horn of the spinal cord, its motor axon, and the muscle fibers innervated by that axon. Increasing force of contraction results primarily from the recruitment of more units, although an increased rate of firing also contributes to the increase in muscle tension. This increased muscle activity with increasing force of muscle contraction is readily appreciated during routine EMG. More electrical activity is seen; the amount of visible baseline without motor unit activity decreases; and the audio amplification of the muscle activity becomes increasingly prominent (Fig. 12-5).

Each motor unit is composed of muscle fibers scattered widely throughout a particular muscle. The number of muscle fibers in a motor unit varies with the fineness of control required. For example, there may be only six muscle fibers per motor unit in the eye muscles, but up to several thousand in some of the large postural muscles. The simultaneous contraction of all the muscle fibers in a motor unit results in the usual integrated smooth, triphasic electrical response (Fig. 12-6). Motor unit size varies not only between muscles but also within muscles. The larger motor units have more muscle fibers, and therefore, with discharge will generate more electrical activity than smaller units. The larger units, therefore, will generally be of larger amplitude. During normal reflex or voluntary recruitment, motor units are activated sequentially according to size, with the smaller units discharging first. As a muscle contracts, not only are more units activated but they are also larger. In comparison to

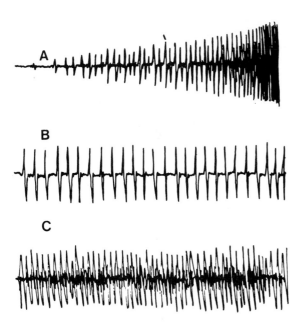

FIG. 12-5. Drawings of motor unit recruitment patterns. (A) Normal pattern with increasing number and size of motor units with increasing force of muscle contraction. (B) Repetitive firing of a single large motor unit characteristic of neuropathies. (C) A "rich" pattern of many small motor units even at low levels of muscle tension seen in myopathies. Amplitude calibrations in the ratio of 1:5:0.5 for A:B:C.

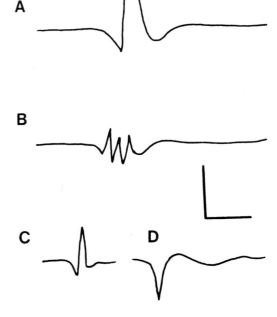

FIG. 12-6. Tracings of (A) normal triphasic motor unit potential, (B) polyphasic potential, (C) fibrillation, and (D) positive sharp wave. Calibrations vertical (microvolts)—A and B, 500; C and D 50; horizontal milliseconds A and B, 5; C and D, 2.

direct tension measurements, amplitude of a particular motor unit is a poor indicator of motor unit size because of (1) the potential variation of muscle fiber organization within a particular motor unit and (2) the relation of the recording needle to those muscle fibers. Motor unit duration, however, provides a reliable estimate of relative motor unit size, with the larger motor units having the larger motor unit durations.

When there is a disruption of the normal connection between nerve and muscle (*i.e.*, denervation), abnormalities appear at rest 1 to 3 weeks after injury that can be detected by EMG. Individual muscle fibers may discharge at rest, and this type of electrical activity is referred to as *fibrillations* or *positive sharp waves*. This activity is not visible clinically. Other types of abnormal spontaneous activity may be present, such as runs of complex potentials (complex repetitive discharges). Particularly in disorders of the motor neuron itself, irregular contractions of entire motor units may appear; these contractions are called *fasciculations*. They are visible clinically and can be present in normal individuals, especially with fatigue.

EMG activity from single muscle fibers can be recorded by using special electrodes. This technique is particularly useful for defining abnormalities of the neuromuscular junction, which may be seen in rapidly progressive neuropathic injury or with reinnervation. This technique has also been used to define the physiologic characteristics of abnormal discharges as well as of normal and abnormal motor units.

In neuropathies, there is a loss of functioning axons. Fewer motor units than normal may be found on voluntary activation of a muscle. At its most extreme, only a single motor unit may be seen to discharge within the recording field of the electrode, even with maximum muscle contraction. In association with these changes, the motor units may be larger than normal. The muscle fibers that have been denervated may be reinnervated by the remaining viable axons of remaining motor units. As a result, these motor units may be larger than normal and also more complex in configuration. Small, complex (polyphasic)-appearing motor unit potentials, however, may also be found. Although these latter potentials are considered more characteristic of myopathies caused by a loss of functioning muscle fibers within motor units, they are seen in neuropathic injury during reinnervation. As motor axons grow into muscle that has lost its innervation, new motor units are formed, and these new units will initially be small and possibly polyphasic because they include a relatively limited number of muscle fibers. A reduced number of motor units, especially if they are large and associated with electrophysiologic evidence of denervation, would be characteristic of a neuropathic process.

These may be the only electrophysiologic findings in those neurogenic processes caused by loss of motoneurons such as amyotrophic lateral sclerosis (ALS). More commonly in neuropathies, slowing of conduction is present and provides evidence of nerve dysfunction. Prominent slowing with no or relatively little denervation would be consistent with a demyelinating process. Borderline to mildly slowed conductions associated with clear and relatively diffuse axonal injury would indicate predominant axonal injury. Low-amplitude evoked responses are most characteristic of axonal dysfunction because of loss of functioning nerve or muscle tissue.

EMG studies can provide information not only about the severity and duration of a neuropathic process but also about the prognosis of nerve injury. The patient's symptoms may not correlate with the degree of nerve involvement. Dysesthesias may occur with relatively minor, partial nerve injury, whereas severe, diffuse nerve abnormalities may be accompanied by few complaints. Normal conduction and lack of denervation several weeks after the onset of nerve dysfunction would indicate a good prognosis because this pattern would indicate functional, but not necessarily structural, abnormalities of the nerve. This is a common clinical situation, for example, in Bell's palsy caused by disruption of facial nerve function.

Nerve biopsies can be performed, especially of the sural nerve. At times the information may be pathognomonic, such as in infiltrative neuropathies (*e.g.*, amyloidosis and metachromatic leukodystrophy). "Teased" fiber preparations allow an examination of individual fibers, and thereby more accurate analysis of the pathology of nerve injury.

SPECIFIC PERIPHERAL NEUROPATHIES

The prime consideration in treating peripheral neuropathies is usually defining the underlying cause. The neuropathies associated with hypothyroidism, carcinoma, and vitamin deficiencies, for example, improve with treatment of these conditions. Uremic neuropathies can resolve after transplantation, and nerve dysfunction related to

TABLE 12-3. Disorders of the Peripheral Nervous System

SYSTEMIC DISEASES	VITAMIN DEFICIENCY	EXOGENOUS TOXINS
Diabetes mellitus	Thiamine	Chloramphenicol
Hypothyroidism	Pyridoxine	Cis-platinum
Renal failure	Niacin	Dapsone
Intestinal malabsorption	Riboflavin	Diphenylhydantoin
Acute intermittent porphyria	Folic acid	Disulfiram
Amyloidosis	Vitamin B_{12}	Ethionamide
Acromegaly		Glutethimide
Leprosy		Gold
Diphtheria		Hydralazine
Lyme disease		Isoniazid
Mycoplasma		Metronidazole
Rheumatoid arthritis		Nitrofurantoin
Systemic lupus erythematosus		Nitrous oxide
Polyarteritis nodosa		Perhexiline maleate
Wegener's granulomatosis		Pyridoxine
Carcinoma		Thalidomide
Waldenströms macroglobulinemia		Vincristine
Multiple myeloma		*Heavy metals*:
Cryoglobulinemia		Arsenic
Benign monoclonal gammopathy		Lead
Paraproteinemia		Thallium
		Industrial agents:
		Solvents:
		n-Hexane
		Methyl-n-butyl-ketone
		2,5 Hexanedione
		Carbon disulfide
		Trichlorethylene
		Acrylamide
		Dimethylaminopropionitrile
		Dichlorophenoxyacetic acid
		TOCP
		Organophosphorus compounds

drugs (vincristine, heavy metals [lead], and industrial solvents [N-hexane, acrylamide]), can all improve by removing the offending agent. A representative list of systemic disorders and toxic causes associated with peripheral neuropathy is presented in Table 12-3. Disulfiram, dapsone, and vincristine can all cause peripheral neuropathies and yet are used to treat conditions in which peripheral neuropathy is a common presentation—alcoholism, leprosy, and carcinoma. Three specific neuropathies are discussed in the following sections—inflammatory polyradicular neuropathy of the Guillain–Barré syndrome, idiopathic facial nerve paresis (Bell's palsy), and diabetic neuropathy.

ACUTE INFLAMMATORY POLYRADICULONEUROPATHY— THE GUILLAIN–BARRÉ SYNDROME

Of remitting polyneuropathies, acute inflammatory polyradiculoneuropathy (AIPN), also known as Guillain–Barré syndrome, is the most common, estimated to occur at a rate 1.5/100,000 persons. AIPN occurs most commonly in young adulthood and early middle age, preceded in almost half of patients by an antecedent infectious illness that usually clears before neurologic dysfunction begins. The hallmarks of the syndrome are progressive, often severe, ascending weakness, complete tendon areflexia, high spinal fluid protein, possible cranial nerve and respiratory compromise, and substantial or complete spontaneous recovery. Weakness develops over hours to days but should not progress longer than 4 weeks. The severe motor compromise, short duration of progression, and elevated cerebrospinal fluid (CSF) protein with few (<10 mononuclear cells/mm^3) are features that distinguish this syndrome from others. Sensory loss may be mild but should be looked for carefully since abnormalities of sensation help differentiate this syndrome from other conditions that may appear similar, including hypokalemia, botulism, and poliomyelitis. Pathologically, there is widespread inflammatory segmental demyelination most prominent proximally and presumably immunologically mediated. Prominent axonal injury and marked decrease in evoked motor response amplitudes argue for a slow recovery.

Although there are characteristic clinical features, the variability of clinical presentation in actual practice should be emphasized. These include ataxia, ophthalmoplegia, and hyporeflexia (Miller Fisher syndrome) and facial diplegia with cardiac arrhythmias. The CSF protein may not be initially elevated, and repeated lumbar punctures may be necessary to demonstrate an increased protein with the associated characteristic dissociation between protein and cells. EMG studies may reveal prominent slowing of nerve conduction, but evidence of conduction block associated with segmental demyelination and proximal conduction abnormalities may be the only findings. As indicated, an estimate of the degree of axonal injury on EMG examination has prognostic implications.

AIPN is considered idiopathic in origin. Syndromes similar to AIPN, however, may be found in conditions such as acute intermittent porphyria, Hodgkin's disease, and less commonly with other neoplasms, hepatitis, infectious mononucleosis, Lyme disease, and recently acquired HIV infection. Certain toxic neuropathies such as with thallium may be similar.

Although recovery may be slow, the characteristic history of AIPN is one of almost complete improvement. As such, the most important treatment is symptomatic, particularly respiratory support and monitoring autonomic dysfunction. Steroids have

been previously advocated, but have not been beneficial and they are possibly detrimental. Plasmapheresis can hasten recovery and appears particularly indicated for those severely involved with respiratory compromise and if used within 7 days of onset.

A syndrome similar to AIPN may sometimes occur in a chronic (CIP) or a chronic relapsing (CIRP) form. These forms are probably variants of the same condition. In comparison to AIPN, the onset is often more gradual; antecedent infections are less common; and sensory symptoms and signs are more frequent. As in AIPN, the basic pathologic process is an inflammatory segmental demyelination, but there is also a loss of myelinated fibers. Onion bulbs are found due to repeated episodes of demyelination with remyelination. The CSF again shows high protein and relatively few cells at some stage in the illness, but may be normal at the time of a particular examination. EMG studies characteristically show slowed conduction. Nerve biopsy may be helpful for the diagnosis. The differential between the chronic inflammatory neuropathies and inherited demyelinative neuropathies may sometimes be difficult and may only be resolved by examining family members. In contrast to AIPN, steroids are thought helpful in CIP and CIRP. Immunosuppressive agents have also been used, and plasmapheresis has produced a temporary improvement. Treatment with high-dose intravenous immunoglobulin has recently been reported effective in CIP and possibly AIPN.

IDIOPATHIC FACIAL PARALYSIS (BELL'S PALSY)

Unilateral weakness of the facial muscles occurs when cranial nerve VII (the facial nerve) is damaged. Disease at the pontine nucleus of the nerve causes the same distribution of facial paresis but is uncommon when compared with the more peripherally placed lesions. Tumors, abscesses, vascular disease, or trauma can all cause this distribution of complete unilateral facial paresis, although these causes are rare. *Bell's palsy* is the term used to describe facial paralysis of undetermined origin that occurs acutely and has a usual natural history of good recovery. The popularized statement that Bell's palsy occurs in the United States every 13 minutes (20 persons 100,000/yr) emphasizes the frequency of this affliction. Because the facial nerve travels through the internal auditory meatus and later gives off branches for the stapedius muscle and for taste sensation on the tongue, patients with

Bell's palsy may complain of ipsilateral hyperacusis and decreased taste sensibility in addition to weak facial muscles.

The cause of Bell's palsy remains obscure, but modern microsurgical techniques have permitted *in situ* examination of the nerve during paralysis. Marked edema with the nerve under tension is consistently seen during the acute phase. However, the cause of the edema and its relation, either causal or reactive, to the paralysis are unknown. However, pressure on the cranial nerve VII can compromise its vascular supply and precipitate or aggravate weakness. An ischemic basis for neurologic dysfunction may underlie Bell's palsy. This could occur from direct vascular dysfunction and thrombosis of the vasonervora, the tiny vessels supplying the nerve itself. Alternatively, a primary inflammatory process, viral or immunologic, may induce edema with secondary vascular compromise. The result of both processes is anoxia to the nerve with resultant vasodilatation, transudation of fluid, and further pressure effects in the confined pathway of cranial nerve VII.

The clinical picture of Bell's palsy is a peripheral facial weakness occurring rapidly, occasionally attended by aching pain around the jaw or behind the ear. The specific constellation of signs and symptoms depends on the anatomic area of involvement. Although cranial nerve VII is predominantly a motor nerve to the muscles of the face, there are sensory components. As the facial nerve leaves the pons and enters the internal auditory meatus along with the acoustic nerve, it carries fibers for lacrimation, salivation, and taste. The nerve then descends through the petrous bone, at which point the fibers to the lacrimal glands branch off. The taste fibers depart in the chorditympani and cross the middle ear. Only motor fibers to the face emerge from the stylomastoid foramen. If the patient suffers with unilateral facial weakness that involves the forehead and lower face, cranial nerve VII has been damaged at or distal to the styloid mastoid foramen. If the same facial weakness is seen in association with decreased taste perception on the anterior part of the tongue on the ipsilateral side of the facial weakness, cranial nerve VII has been damaged more proximally before the chordi-tympani branches off. If cranial nerve VII is damaged in the internal auditory meatus, facial weakness, altered taste perception, and hyperacusis (related to paralysis of the stapedius muscle) will be encountered.

Recovery usually begins within a week, and 75% of patients fully recover over a period of several weeks. Some permanent motor deficit occasionally remains. In some patients, synkinetic or aberrant motor movements develop secondary to faulty and misguided reinnervation.

Steroids have been advocated on the premise that they reduce swelling within the facial canal and thereby diminish vascular compression so that proper oxygenation occurs. This theoretically would interrupt the pathologic cycle. Adour and colleagues studied the effect of oral prednisone on 194 patients with Bell's palsy compared with 110 untreated patients. The steroid dose was 40 mg for 4 days, tapering within 8 days. They reported that the treated group recovered more fully and had fewer complications, although side effects related to drug treatment occurred in 4% of the patients. Furthermore, the two groups were not entirely comparable because severely affected patients accounted for 42% of the original control group and only 30% of the steroid group. Furthermore, the investigators were so convinced that prednisone was superior to no treatment that they abandoned a double-blind format midway into the study. Complete facial recovery was seen in 89% of steroid-treated patients and in 64% of nontreated patients. Some investigators have suggested that the positive steroid effect is maximal if the treatment is started within the first few days of facial weakness, whereas others have felt steroids benefit patients at all points of their illness.

However, not all investigators feel that steroids are selectively effective in Bell's palsy. In a small group of patients treated with vitamins, full recovery occurred in 65% of patients compared with 60% in the steroid group. In a large prospective and randomized study, 88% of steroid-treated and 80% of nontreated control patients recovered full strength. The incidence of residual autonomic synkinesis from probable regenerating neural fibers was less prominent in the steroid-treated group.

The overall excellent prognosis of Bell's palsy with or without steroid treatment is confirmed in all studies. Approximately 15% to 30% of Bell's palsy patients show some residual weakness, but severe weakness is usually seen in only 2% to 4%. The pharmacologic basis of steroid activity focuses on general anti-inflammatory or vasoactive properties with no presumed activity on neuronal function *per se*.

NEUROPATHY ASSOCIATED WITH DIABETES MELLITUS

Diabetes mellitus is common and is commonly associated with nerve dysfunction. The incidence of neuropathic abnormalities in diabetes has been estimated to range from about 5% to 95%. The wide discrepancy relates to differing criteria and techniques used to diagnose PNS injury in these patients. A balanced view would probably indicate a prevalence of 50% to 60% of some form of neuropathy in diabetic patients. The prevalence increases with the duration of the disease, but diabetic nerve dysfunction may be the initial sign of diabetes. Given the various presentations and probable pathogenesis, it is best to think in terms of diabetic neuropathies rather than a single entity.

Polyneuropathies, mononeuropathies, plexopathies, radiculopathies, and autonomic neuropathies are all found individually or in combination in diabetes, and diabetes can therefore be associated with abnormalities at any level of the PNS. Asymptomatic diabetics may show decreased nerve conductions that can normalize with improved control of blood sugar. A distal sensory or sensorimotor polyneuropathy is the commonest type of diabetic neuropathy. A "stocking-glove" sensory loss is characteristic. A loss of position, vibration, and light touch as well as decreased reflexes are prominent features of the "large fiber" pattern. Relatively pronounced loss of pain and temperature sensation in association with pain indicate predominant "small fiber" injury. The pain may have a dull, aching quality in the limbs and also a distal, burning discomfort most prominent at night. Rarely, there is a pattern of sensory ataxia, pain, and arthropathy (diabetic "pseudotabes"). The "small fiber" and "pseudotabetic" patterns may be associated with autonomic dysfunction including an involvement of the gastrointestinal, cardiovascular, and genitourinary systems. Autonomic dysfunction can also occur without other evidence for a neuropathy. Postural hypotension, diarrhea, impotence, urinary retention, and increased sweating are examples of symptoms that may be caused by a diabetic autonomic neuropathy. The painful, asymmetrical, proximal weakness of the legs found in diabetes (diabetic amyotrophy) is probably due to the involvement of the lumbar plexus. Clinical patterns of a polyradiculopathy may occur, particularly in association with a history of weight loss. Isolated peripheral nerve lesions are common. These mononeuropathies can affect almost every major peripheral nerve as well as the cranial nerves, particularly the extraocular muscles. The onset of symptoms is characteristically abrupt and frequently painful. Diabetes may present as peroneal palsies.

The pathogenesis of diabetic neuropathies is varied. Metabolic derangements are commonly considered the basis for the polyneuropathies. Accumulation of sorbitol or depletion of myoinositol in nerves are current theories. There is experimental evidence, however, that edema secondary to structural changes in endoneural blood vessels may be the primary cause. The abrupt onset of painful, focal lesions in the diabetic mononeuropathies is similar to that of other vascular neuropathies and has led to the concept that these neuropathies are due to occlusion of the small, nutrient blood vessels supplying nerves. This finding has not, however, been confirmed pathologically.

The natural history of diabetic mononeuropathies, amyotrophies, and polyradiculopathies is one of improvement, even if occasionally slow. The course of diabetic polyneuropathies varies; some diabetic neuropathies will improve, many will plateau, and some will steadily progress. A severe disability is the exception; however, the pseudotabetic variety is generally progressive and more disabling. Pain, particularly the distal burning dysesthesias, can be a major problem in the polyneuropathies. The manifestations of the autonomic neuropathy may be subclinical but are not infrequently incapacitating. The prognosis for the autonomic neuropathy is among the worst of the diabetic neuropathies.

Good metabolic control is probably helpful for both preventing and ameliorating diabetic neuropathies, and good control of blood sugar should therefore be a goal in these patients. Other therapies are symptomatic. An eye patch is helpful in patients with the self-limited diabetic ophthalmoplegia, as may bracing in those with peroneal palsy. Diphenylhydantoin, carbamazepine, and tricyclic antidepressants have been helpful in the painful sensory neuropathies, and analgesics are reasonable in the acute pain associated with mononeuropathies. Trophic ulcers of the feet may require changes in shoe size, debridement, and antibiotics. Standard medical regimens should be tried for autonomic dysfunction. These regimens include codeine phosphate and diphenoxylate for diarrhea, support stockings and fluorocortisone for postural hypotension, and regular voidings assisted by suprapubic pressure in those with bladder atony. Nighttime lights can assist walking in those patients with sensory loss by preserving visual cues.

FUTURE PERSPECTIVES

The potential for an increased understanding of peripheral neuropathies is exciting. Newer techniques of histopathologic evaluation, including electron microscopy, teased fiber preparations, and morphometric analysis of nerves, have already added meaningfully to our understanding of both normal and abnormal nerves. Similarly, more sophisticated forms of electrophysiologic analysis should allow for a better evaluation of nerve dysfunction. These techniques include recording from single muscle fibers (single fiber EMG); computer analysis of motor unit firing, which can relate the amount of electrical activity generated by a muscle to the force; and increasing routine use of a wider range of electrophysiologic responses. These responses allow for evaluation of conduction in the more proximal portions of nerves and possibly for analyzing the effect of peripheral nerve dysfunction on motorneuron firing. The recording of cortical responses evoked by peripheral nerve stimulation (somatosensory evoked responses) not only allows for a more detailed evaluation of certain peripheral nerve injuries but also provides a possible technique for evaluation at the interface between peripheral and CNS dysfunction.

Immunologic studies are becoming increasingly important for understanding the pathogenesis of nerve disorders as well as providing guides to therapy. Patients with a clinical picture similar to ALS but with conduction block on electrophysiologic examination and elevated titers to ganglioside GM_1 have been treated successfully with immunosuppressive agents. Finally, basic research in the physiology, biochemistry, immunobiology, and axonal transport of nerves provides a dynamism that makes an interest in peripheral nerves continually rewarding.

QUESTIONS and DISCUSSION

1. A 64-year-old patient with a 10-year history of insulin-dependent diabetes mellitus complains of burning dysesthesias in the feet. Examination reveals a mild decrease in strength at the toes and ankles, absent Achilles' reflexes, and decreased pin, touch, and vibration to the knees as well as a decreased position sense in the toes. Electrodiagnostic studies indicate prolonged motor conduction velocities, no sensory potentials, and evidence of denervation distally in the lower extremities. Sensory conductions in the upper extremities are slowed.

   Four weeks later, the same patient develops weakness in the left leg associated with some pain in the region of the left knee. An examination 3 weeks after onset reveals relatively more prominent decreased pin and touch sensation in the lateral aspect of the left leg and dorsum of the left foot, as well as lack of dorsiflexion and eversion of the left ankle. EMG examination shows no evoked motor response stimulating at the fibula head and denervation in the left tibialis anterior, peronei, and extensor digitorum brevis muscles.

   Is the history in the first or second part of the first question indicative of a polyneuropathy, mononeuropathy, or radiculopathy?

   Are both of these histories compatible with a diabetic etiology?

The description in the first part of the first question would be characteristic of a polyneuropathy. The clinical and electrodiagnostic examinations reveal a diffuse sensorimotor neuropathic process most prominent distally.

The history and findings in the second part, by contrast, would indicate a mononeuropathy of the left peroneal (anterior tibial) nerve. Clinically, there is sensory loss, motor weakness, and EMG abnormalities in the distribution of that nerve.

Diabetes mellitus can produce both a polyneuropathy and a mononeuropathy, not infrequently in the same patient. The polyneuropathy is probably secondary to the metabolic derangements of the illness, whereas the mononeuropathy may be vascular in origin.

A significant diabetic polyneuropathy is probably an argument for careful diabetic control. Diabetic mononeuropathies usually resolve with time because of the partial nature of the nerve injury secondary to the ischemic insult. A short leg brace to aid in dorsiflexion of the left ankle could be important for this patient during the recovery period.

2. A 50-year-old woman has a 6-month history of pain in the right wrist. A diagnosis of hypothyroidism has recently been made. This pain awakens the patient at night, usually within several hours of falling asleep. She has noticed clumsiness in the use of that hand and complains of paresthesias radiating into the thumb and index fingers. Recently, she has noted some discomfort in the left wrist. An examination reveals paresthesias and pain on tapping the wrists bilaterally (positive Tinel's signs), weakness of the right abductor pollicis brevis muscle, and numbness involving the right thumb, index finger, and middle finger as well

as the adjacent one-half of the ring finger. There is also numbness involving the lateral half of the palmar surface of the right hand.

This history most likely represents mononeuropathy of which nerve? Where is the lesion located? Is the process probably unilateral or bilateral? EMG examination reveals a prolongation of the median distal motor latencies and a lack or slowing of median sensory potentials, more prominent on the right. Are these findings consistent with your diagnosis?

The case presentation would be compatible with a diagnosis of a carpal tunnel syndrome (CTS). This syndrome is a mononeuropathy caused by "entrapment" of the median nerve as it passes through the carpal tunnel at the wrist. A positive Tinel's sign is a common clinical finding in an area of partial nerve injury, and a progression of this sign distally can be used to follow regeneration after a nerve has been severed. Characteristic electrodiagnostic findings in the CTS are those that indicate median nerve dysfunction at the level of the wrist, that is, prolonged motor conduction stimulating the nerve at the wrist and recording from median innervated thenar hand muscles as well as prolonged conduction when stimulating the digital nerves of median innervated fingers and recording at the wrist. The history would suggest a bilateral process—an assumption confirmed by the electrodiagnostic studies. Bilateral involvement in the CTS is present in approximately 25% of the cases. This syndrome is frequently part of several systemic illnesses including hypothyroidism. A CTS may be the presenting complaint in a patient with abnormal thyroid function.

Initial treatment would consist of therapy for the hypothyroidism as well as splinting the wrists to limit movement. If these measures failed, the transverse carpal ligaments should probably be surgically sectioned. Steroid injections can produce symptomatic relief, but the long-term effectiveness and the possible harm of this therapy have been debated.

3. A 55-year-old patient on vincristine therapy has developed progressive weakness over several weeks, resulting in an inability to walk. An examination reveals a mild "stocking-glove" sensory loss to pin with preserved position sense, absent reflexes in the legs, and moderate to marked weakness in the legs and mild to moderate weakness in the arms, most marked distally. Electrodiagnostic studies reveal borderline, slow motor conduction velocities with considerable evidence of denervation, again most prominent distally.

Does this polyneuropathy involve primarily axons or myelin, and what is the appropriate treatment?

The history and clinical findings would be typical for a polyneuropathy secondary to vincristine therapy. The prominent denervation indicates disruption of the normal connections between nerve and muscle. Combined with the borderline slowing of conduction velocities, the primary disease is of axons rather than of myelin, that is, an axonal type of neuropathy. The treatment, of course, is to stop the vincristine.

4. A 35-year-old man has a 6-month history of weakness in the hands that now involves the legs. An examination reveals atrophy and fasciculations in the intrinsic muscles of the hands, weakness that is distally more prominent in the upper than in the lower extremities, hyperactive reflexes, and extensor plantar responses bilaterally. Sensory testing is unremarkable. Electrodiagnostic examination reveals normal motor and sensory conduction studies in the presence of denervation and decreased activation of motor units in all four extremities. Many of the motor units are both large and polyphasic. A cervical myelogram has been unremarkable.

This would be characteristic of a neuropathic process at what level of the motor unit? What is the most likely diagnosis? Would a sural nerve biopsy be helpful for the evaluation of this neuropathy?

The history and findings would be consistent with a diagnosis of ALS. The extensor plantar responses and hyperactive reflexes would indicate some involvement of the long motor system tracts in the CNS, but the atrophy and fasciculations would be consistent with involvement of the lower motor neurons. This is confirmed by the electrodiagnostic studies, which indicate a chronic motor neuropathic process not readily explained by a process primarily affecting peripheral nerves, plexi, or roots. The normal conduction velocities indicate preservation of at least some of the fast-conducting (i.e., largest) motor axons. Since the pathologic process involves strictly efferent (i.e., motor) fibers, a sural nerve biopsy would not be helpful. The sural is a sensory nerve and therefore contains only afferent fibers.

The important point is that nerve dysfunction may involve either motor or sensory fibers only. In ALS, the primary pathology is at the lower motor neuron level in the anterior horns of the spinal cord. It may be argued this is not an illness of the PNS. Conversely, since ALS involves the cell bodies of efferent fibers with resultant abnormalities in nerve and muscle, the illness might be considered a prototypical neuropathy.

SUGGESTED READING

Adour K, Wingerd M, Bell D et al: Prednisone treatment for idiopathic facial paralysis. N Engl J Med 287:1268, 1972

Asbury AK, Gilliatt RW (eds): Peripheral Nerve Disorders. Boston, Butterworths, 1984

Asbury AK, Bolis L, Gibbs CJ Jr.: Workshop on autoimmune neuropathies: Guillain–Barré syndrome. Neurology 40:381, 1990

Dyck PJ, Thomas PK, Lambert EH et al (eds): Peripheral Neuropathy, Vols 1 and 2. Philadelphia, WB Saunders, 1984

Kelly JJ Jr: Peripheral neuropathies associated with monoclonal proteins: A clinical review. Muscle Nerve 8:138, 1985

Kimura J: Electrodiagnosis in Diseases of Nerve and Muscle. Philadelphia, FA Davis, 1983

Pestronk A: Motor neuropathies, motor neuron disorders, and antiglycolipid antibodies. Muscle Nerve 14:927, 1991

Ropper AH: The Guillain–Barré syndrome. N Engl J Med 326:1130, 1992

Schaumberg HH, Spencer PS, Thomas PK: Disorders of Peripheral Nerves. Philadelphia, FA Davis, 1983

Stalberg E, Trontelj JE: Single Fiber Electromyography. Old Woking, England, Miravalle Press, 1979

Sumner AJ (ed): The Physiology of Peripheral Nerve Disease. Philadelphia, WB Saunders, 1980

Tuck RR, Schmelzer JD, Low Pa: Endoneurial blood flow and oxygen tension in the sciatic nerves of rats with experimental diabetic neuropathy. Brain 107:935, 1984

Waxman SG (ed): Physiology and Pathobiology of Axons. New York, Raven Press, 1978

Vertigo and Dizziness

Judd M. Jensen

" All of Gaul can be divided into three parts. "
Julius Caesar

———————————— • ————————————

Of all the reasons patients seek medical attention, few engender more frustration on the part of physicians than the simple statement "Doctor, I'm dizzy." The purpose of this chapter is to discuss an approach to the problem of vertigo and dizziness that should lead to a correct diagnosis in most patients. Second, the various diagnostic entities are reviewed with emphasis on their clinical presentations, appropriate work-up, and possible therapies.

LET THE PATIENT TELL HIS STORY

In assessing patients with the various "dizzy" syndromes, it is particularly important for physicians to keep their questions open-ended during history taking. Direct questions like "Does the room spin?" or "Do you feel like you're going to pass out?" are often answered in the affirmative by most patients, thus reducing the diagnostic value of the reply. The best approach is to force the patient to describe his symptom complex by simply asking "What do you mean by dizzy?" Most patients are able to provide enough description so that classification of their symptom complex into one of three dizziness

"types" described in the following can be made. Further questioning usually allows the physician to narrow the diagnostic possibilities within each category and often make an accurate diagnosis based on the history alone.

DEFINITIONS

VERTIGO: TYPE 1 DIZZINESS

Patients who have vertigo describe a false sensation of movement. Most commonly, they report that their environment is spinning around them or that they are spinning in a stationary environment. However, the sensation of feeling impelled forward, backward, or to either side is also vertiginous. Others describe "tilting" of their environment or a "back-and-forth" feeling. These patients have a disorder of their vestibular system. They seek medical attention either with an acute episode of vertigo, usually associated with nausea, vomiting, and ataxia, or with a history of recurrent attacks of vertigo.

PRESYNCOPE: TYPE 2 DIZZINESS

Patients who have presyncope describe their dizziness as "light-headedness" or "feeling like I'm going to pass out." This sensation is usually associated with generalized weakness, visual blurring or black-

171

William J. Weiner and Christopher G. Goetz, eds. *Neurology for the Non-Neurologist,* Third Edition. Copyright © 1994, 1989 by J. B. Lippincott Company. Copyright © 1981 by Harper and Row Publishers, Inc.

ing out, diaphoresis, shortness of breath, or palpitations. The patient usually looks pale to an observer. It should be noted that occasionally patients with presyncope will report vertigo during their episodes, presumably due to inadequate perfusion in the brain-stem vestibular nuclei. This can lead to diagnostic confusion with the primary vestibular syndromes, although the remainder of the clinical picture usually distinguishes the two types of dizziness. Type 2 dizziness is typically episodic and is caused by a transient reduction in global cerebral perfusion. Therefore, it is a primary cardiovascular problem rather than a neurologic one.

DYSEQUILIBRIUM: TYPE 3 DIZZINESS

Dysequilibrium is a more complex syndrome than the previous two types and is occasionally misdiagnosed in the elderly as "vertebrobasilar insufficiency." These patients experience their dizziness primarily when standing and walking. They feel better when they are seated or supine. Their dizziness tends to be constant when they are walking, although its severity can vary with environmental stresses. Crowds and difficult walkways (*e.g.*, ramps, escalators, and stairs) exacerbate their symptoms. Patients describe their problem as "bad balance," "poor equilibrium," "swaying," or "just dizzy." The causes of this syndrome are numerous. Disease is present at one or more points in the complex system required for bipedal balance and ambulation.

VERTIGO SYNDROMES: TYPE 1 DIZZINESS

ANATOMY, PHYSIOLOGY, AND PATHOPHYSIOLOGY

Vertigo is a symptom of disease in the vestibular system. This system is usually divided into "peripheral" and "central" components. The peripheral vestibular apparatus includes the labyrinth, which is located in the petrous portion of the temporal bone, and the vestibular portion of the eighth cranial nerve, which connects the labyrinth to the brain stem and is located in the internal auditory canal and cerebellopontine angle. The labyrinth is divided into three semicircular canals that sense head rotation and the otoliths (utricle and saccule) that sense head position relative to the pull of gravity. The central vestibular apparatus consists of the vestibular nuclei at the pontomedullary junction in the brain stem, which receive impulses from the eighth cranial nerve and have rich connections with the nuclei controlling eye movements and the cerebellum. Normally, the paired labyrinths supply balanced tonic impulses to the central nervous system (CNS) regarding the position of the head and its movements. Vertigo occurs when a pathologic process acutely disrupts the input from one labyrinth. The remaining unbalanced contralateral input produces the false sensation of movement. With time, the CNS will adjust to unilateral input. Vertigo is thus typically acute and episodic. A pathologic process that slowly disrupts the input from one labyrinth either will be asymptomatic or will produce a dysequilibrium syndrome—Type 3 dizziness.

NEIGHBORHOOD SIGNS

The physician must determine whether a patient's vertigo is of central or peripheral origin. The presence of one or more "neighborhood" signs and symptoms may be helpful in making this distinction. The most important neighborhood symptoms in peripheral vestibular lesions are hearing loss and tinnitus. These occur in diseases affecting the cochlea, the middle ear, and the acoustic portion of the eighth cranial nerve. Processes that disrupt the vestibular portion of the eighth nerve in the cerebellopontine angle or the internal auditory canal usually also affect the acoustic portion. Likewise, labyrinthine processes may also affect the cochlea or middle ear. "Central" processes affecting the brain stem and cerebellum almost never cause hearing loss or tinnitus; thus, the presence of these symptoms almost excludes central disease.

Eighth cranial nerve and cerebellopontine angle mass lesions (*i.e.*, acoustic neuroma) often present with progressive hearing loss and/or tinnitus and can have associated facial weakness, facial sensory loss, and/or a depressed corneal reflex. However, it is distinctly unusual for such lesions to produce either an acute vertigo syndrome or recurrent attacks of vertigo. When acoustic neuroma and other mass lesions of the eighth nerve and cerebellopontine angle produce dizziness, it is more commonly a Type 3 dysequilibrium syndrome related to slow destruction of the vestibular portion of the eighth cranial nerve or pressure on the brain-stem vestibular nuclei.

The vertigo seen in central vestibular syndromes is frequently accompanied by one or more neighborhood symptoms and signs. Importantly, it is often the presence of such additional findings that clearly defines the vertigo as central in origin. The list of possible neighborhood signs and symptoms includes diplopia, cortical blindness, homonymous hemianopsia, dysarthria, dysphagia, bilateral extremity weakness or sensory symptoms, and unilateral or bilateral facial weakness or numbness.

Ataxia in the form of unilateral upper or lower extremity incoordination, finger-to-nose dysmetria, heel-to-shin dysmetria, inability to stand with the feet together or to walk without a wide base is present to a variable degree in most patients during their attacks of vertigo whether the vertigo is peripheral or central in origin. Ataxia is a sign of cerebellar dysfunction and is seen in vertigo syndromes because of the rich vestibulocerebellar connections. These signs of ataxia should resolve as the vertigo resolves, and their persistence in the absence of vertigo should raise the question of a structural lesion in the brain stem or cerebellum.

NYSTAGMUS

Nystagmus is present in most vertigo syndromes. The character of the patient's nystagmus may be helpful in distinguishing peripheral and central causes of vertigo. Nystagmus of peripheral origin is *unidirectional*; that is, the fast component of the nystagmus always beats in the same direction no matter which direction the patient is looking. For example, with a left peripheral vestibular lesion the fast component of the nystagmus will be to the right on left lateral gaze, right lateral gaze, or vertical gaze. Nystagmus of peripheral origin is *mixed*; that is, it typically has both a horizontal and a rotatory component. Finally, peripheral nystagmus is *suppressed by fixation*. Most physicians check for nystagmus by having the patient fix his gaze on the examiner's index finger and then moving the finger from side to side and up and down. This technique suppresses nystagmus of peripheral origin. The physician can check for nystagmus while the patient is not fixing his gaze. The simplest method is to observe the patient's eye movements as he gazes from side to side in the room without fixing his central vision on any object. Alternatively, the patient's eye movements can be observed with a flashlight when the lights are off in the room or when the patient's eyes are closed (the corneal movement can be seen under the eyelid).

Nystagmus of central origin is typically *multidirectional* (*i.e.*, the fast component of the nystagmus changes with the direction of gaze). *Pure horizontal, pure vertical,* or *pure rotatory* nystagmus is almost always central. Unfortunately for diagnostic purposes, nystagmus of central origin can mimic peripheral nystagmus by being unidirectional or of a mixed form. Peripheral lesions, however, almost never produce multidirectional or pure forms of nystagmus. Perhaps the best means to distinguish central from peripheral nystagmus is by the response to fixation. Central nystagmus is *never suppressed* and is frequently enhanced by fixation.

In general, the nystagmus of central vestibular disorders is more prominent and more persistent than the nystagmus of peripheral vestibular origin. It is also often said as a corollary that peripheral vertigo is paradoxically more intense than central vertigo, but this is not as consistent a finding as the difference in intensity of the nystagmus.

ELECTRONYSTAGMOGRAPHY

Electronystagmography (ENG) can be a useful test in evaluating patients with disorders of the vestibular system. The technique takes advantage of the rich connections between the vestibular and oculomotor nuclei. This examination requires skill and experience to perform and interpret. Unfortunately, the results do not always provide the clinician with definitive answers. At best, ENG can determine the presence of vestibular dysfunction, establish the unilateral or bilateral nature of the dysfunction, and distinguish central from peripheral vestibular dysfunction.

CAUSES OF RECURRENT EPISODES OF VERTIGO

BENIGN PAROXYSMAL POSITIONAL VERTIGO

Benign paroxysmal positional vertigo (BPPV) is the most common cause of recurrent vertigo. The history is characteristic: The patient reports that a few seconds after assumption of a certain head position (usually supine in bed) he experiences the sudden onset of vertigo, which lasts 15 to 60 seconds and then resolves. The patient may also note that if he puts his head into the same position a second or third time (within a brief interval), the vertigo will be less intense each time. The key historical features are the characteristic head position (there can be more than one), the brief latency to onset of vertigo, and the fatigability of the vertigo with repeated trials.

The patient's symptom complex can frequently be reproduced in the office with the Hallpike maneuver. This maneuver begins with the patient sitting on the examination table. He is then put in a supine position with the head hanging over the edge of the examining table and extended 30°. If vertigo does not begin within 30 seconds, the patient is returned to the sitting position; the head is turned to the right, and the patient is again made supine with the head extended. The maneuver can be tried with the head turned to the left if this position also does not produce vertigo. Usually one of these three positions produces a brief episode of vertigo and nystagmus after a short latency period. However, a failure to produce vertigo with the Hallpike maneuver does not rule out BPPV and a positive test is not specific for BPPV.

This syndrome is most commonly "idiopathic" but is also commonly seen after an episode of head trauma. Any patient who develops positional vertigo after head trauma needs an ear, nose, and throat (ENT) evaluation to rule out a perilymph fistula (see later text). The natural history of the idiopathic syndrome is typically a waxing and waning course over months to years. Most cases improve or resolve with time. A rare case may be so debilitating for the patient that section of the posterior ampullary nerve is required. Post-traumatic BPPV almost always resolves within 6 months. Both the idiopathic and post-traumatic BPPV syndromes can be improved with the use of a specific physical therapy regimen. Meclizine is not useful.

This entity is not associated with hearing loss, tinnitus, or other vestibular system neighborhood signs. The presence of any of these should prompt a search for an alternate diagnosis. Structural lesions of the cerebellopontine angle and posterior fossa can rarely mimic BPPV. All patients with BPPV should have either an audiogram or brain-stem auditory evoked responses (BAERs) as a screening test. No further work-up is required if either examination is normal. If the screening test is abnormal, however, then an imaging study of the posterior fossa is necessary. Magnetic resonance imaging (MR) is the optimum technique for this evaluation. Computed tomography (CT) is the best alternative if MR is unavailable.

POSITIONING VERTIGO

Most vestibular disorders of peripheral or central origin can produce *positioning vertigo*, and this may be a source of confusion when evaluating a patient who notes that his vertigo can be produced or exacerbated by a change in head position. This symptom lacks the specificity of head position (usually any change in head position will produce positioning vertigo), the latency to onset of vertigo, and the fatigability with repeated trials seen in BPPV. Positioning vertigo is not a specific syndrome like BPPV but rather a symptom of the underlying vestibular disorder.

MÉNIÈRE'S DISEASE

This syndrome is characterized by repeated attacks of vertigo and tinnitus that continue for hours to days and are superimposed on progressive hearing loss. Patients may have nausea, vomiting, and ataxia during their acute attacks, which may be separated by weeks, months, or years. These patients do not have vestibular system neighborhood symptoms and signs, except for the tinnitus and hearing loss. This disorder is thought to be caused by intermittent swelling of the semicircular ducts in the labyrinth. The etiology is unknown. Low-frequency hearing is lost first. All patients should have bilateral audiometry and an imaging study of the posterior fossa (MR or CT).

Acute attacks are treated with bed rest, intravenous fluids, antihistamines, and phenothiazines. There are reports of efficacy in reducing the frequency of attacks and slowing the hearing loss with the use of thiazide diuretics or propranolol. The value of these medications, however, has not been conclusively proved. Approximately 80% of patients will experience spontaneous remission within 5 years. Some patients will have frequent, disabling attacks of vertigo, and surgical ablation can be considered in these patients. A labyrinthectomy is performed if hearing is already lost. If hearing is preserved, vestibular nerve section is the optimal therapy.

Many patients with Ménière's disease will have positioning vertigo during their acute episodes and for a variable time (days to weeks) after the episode has resolved. In addition, some patients develop a chronic dysequilibrium syndrome between their attacks of vertigo. This is a conversion of Type 1 to Type 3 dizziness. This conversion can occur with many of the Type 1 syndromes; its pathophysiology and therapy are discussed later.

MIGRAINE

The vestibular nuclei in the brain stem receive their blood supply from branches of the basilar artery; therefore, it is not surprising that migrainous vasospasm of the basilar artery can produce vertigo. Other neurologic symptoms such as scintillating scotoma, homonymous hemianopsia, cortical blindness, diplopia, dysarthria, ataxia, paresthesias, and quadriparesis may also be seen with vertigo in this syndrome. Hearing loss and tinnitus, however, are not associated with basilar artery migraine.

These patients are usually young, and the history is typically dominated by the severe headache that follows the vertigo. In some patients, however, the headache may not be prominent, whereas in others the headache may not always follow the vasospastic component of the syndrome. This latter phenomenon is called a *migraine equivalent* and should be considered in a patient with isolated attacks of vertigo who also has a history of vertigo followed by headache. The treatment of basilar artery migraine is similar to the treatment of other migraine syndromes and is not discussed here.

PERILYMPH FISTULA

This syndrome is characterized by episodes of vertigo precipitated by a change in head position, coughing, sneezing, straining, swallowing, loud noises, or air travel. There may or may not be associated tinnitus and hearing loss. These symptoms occur because of a small tear in either the oval or the round window. Many, though not all, patients have a history of head trauma. The diagnosis is made by pneumatic otoscopy, a procedure that typically reproduces the patient's symptom complex. Most patients will heal spontaneously, but surgical correction is possible for those patients who have persistent symptoms.

TEMPORAL LOBE EPILEPSY

Vertigo can rarely be experienced as part of a temporal lobe seizure. These patients typically have other clinical manifestations including alteration of consciousness, automatisms, and postictal disorientation, so distinguishing this syndrome from the other recurrent vertigo syndromes is usually straightforward. An electroencephalogram (EEG) is not part of the routine work-up of patients with vertigo.

CAUSES OF A SINGLE, ACUTE EPISODE OF VERTIGO

ACUTE PERIPHERAL VESTIBULOPATHY

The pathophysiology of this syndrome is poorly understood and has resulted in a confusing nomenclature. The terms *acute labyrinthitis, vestibular neuronitis*, and *acute vestibulopathy* have all been applied to a similar clinical syndrome. It is characterized by the acute or subacute onset of severe vertigo, nausea, vomiting, and ataxia. The patient usually remains incapacitated for hours to days and then slowly returns to normal over several more days. Positioning vertigo is common during the acute stage and may remain for a time after the continuous vertigo has resolved: Likewise, a Type 3 dizziness or dysequilibrium syndrome may occur after the true vertigo resolves. In some patients, this may remain a troublesome problem for several weeks. Some patients will experience recurrent attacks of acute vestibulopathy.

This common clinical syndrome occurs in people of all ages. Although theories of a viral or "postviral" origin abound, there is no consensus regarding the etiology or pathophysiology. The disease process affects the "peripheral" vestibular system, and therefore the nystagmus seen has characteristics typical of "peripheral" lesions. Hearing loss and tinnitus are not typical but are seen in some patients. Some authors believe that the presence of these symptoms distinguishes labyrinthitis from vestibular neuronitis (the auditory symptoms being present only in the former). However, many patients presenting with an episode of vertigo, hearing loss, and tinnitus will have Meniere's disease. Other vestibular system neighborhood signs are not seen in acute vestibulopathy.

Acute vestibulopathy can sometimes be difficult to distinguish from a posterior circulation vascular event. Therefore, older patients (greater than 60 years) with a history of vascular disease and patients with risk factors for vascular disease (e.g., diabetes mellitus and hypertension) should have a posterior fossa imaging study performed when they present with an acute vertigo syndrome. This procedure is necessary to exclude a small brain-stem or cerebellar hemorrhage or infarction. All other patients need only an audiogram or BAERs for a screening work-up. Posterior fossa imaging is necessary only if the screening test is abnormal.

Therapy consists of bed rest, intravenous fluids, phenothiazines, and antihistamines for the acute vertigo. The treatment for those patients who develop Type 3 dizziness is discussed later.

VERTEBROBASILAR VASCULAR DISEASE

Most of these patients have a history of cerebrovascular disease (CVD) or, at least, risk factors for CVD. The clinical syndrome is characterized by the sudden onset of vertigo, which is usually not as severe as that seen in acute vestibulopathy and other peripheral vestibular disorders. There may or may not be associated nausea, vomiting, and ataxia. If a headache or stiff neck is present, the diagnosis of a cerebellar hemorrhage should be considered and a CT scan should be obtained immediately. Hearing loss and tinnitus are not seen in this syndrome; however, one or more other vestibular system neighborhood signs are usually present. The nystagmus has the characteristics of a central vestibular disorder. Many neurology texts make the point that the diagnosis of vertebrobasilar ischemia should never be made when the patient's sole complaint is vertigo and that other brain-stem symptoms or signs must be present. The advent of MR has made it clear that there are patients with brain-stem or cerebellar ischemic events or even small hemorrhages whose only symptom is vertigo. Therefore, as noted earlier, all patients at risk for CVD should have a posterior fossa imaging study as part of their evaluation. MR is the optimum study; if it is unavailable, CT with thin cuts of the posterior fossa should be able to exclude a small hemorrhage.

The presence of a cerebellar hemorrhage requires intensive care unit monitoring and possible surgical decompression. Vertigo can be seen as part of a progressive basilar artery thrombosis, and systemic anticoagulation with heparin may be indicated in these patients. Otherwise, all patients need a complete cardiac examination and an electrocardiogram (ECG). If either suggests a cardiac lesion that could be a source of emboli, then an echocardiogram or Holter monitoring may be necessary. Patients should be treated with antiplatelet agents unless a cardiac embolic source is found. In the latter case, warfarin therapy should be considered depending on the clinical setting. Transcranial Doppler evaluation may be helpful in evaluating patients with posterior circulation ischemia, as this technique can detect stenosis of the vertebral or basilar arteries. Anticoagulation can be considered when significant stenosis is identified. Carotid duplex examination is generally not indicated in the work-up of patients with vertebrobasilar ischemia. Similarly, carotid endarterectomy is not indicated to improve vertebrobasilar ischemia. While an acute dysequilibrium syndrome (without vertigo) can be caused by a brain-stem or cerebellar stroke, chronic Type 3 dizziness and dysequilibrium are not symptoms of vertebrobasilar insufficiency.

MULTIPLE SCLEROSIS

Vertigo is a common symptom in multiple sclerosis and can be the presenting symptom or a recurrent symptom. The vertigo is often not as severe as that seen in peripheral vestibular disorders, and the patient may or may not have nausea, vomiting, and ataxia. Hearing loss is rare but does occur. Most patients have or have had other neurologic symptoms corresponding to other areas of demyelination in the CNS. The diagnosis of multiple sclerosis, however, should be considered in a young person with an acute attack or recurrent attacks of vertigo, particularly if the nystagmus suggests a central vestibular disorder. In cases where the nystagmus is indeterminate, ENG may be useful in distinguishing a central from a peripheral lesion. A specific work-up for multiple sclerosis includes MR of the brain, evoked potentials, and a lumbar puncture to evaluate cerebrospinal fluid for oligoclonal bands and an elevated IgG/albumin ratio. Therapy consists of adrenocorticotropic hormone (ACTH) or corticosteroids for the inflammatory demyelination and phenothiazines and antihistamines for the vertigo.

HEAD TRAUMA

Most patients who complain of "dizziness" after an episode of head trauma will not have true vertigo but rather the Type 3 dizziness typical of a "post-concussive syndrome." Type 1 symptoms, however, can result from head trauma. Two diagnostic possibilities have already been discussed under BPPV and perilymph fistula. A basilar skull fracture can also lacerate the vestibular portion of the eighth cranial nerve and cause vertigo. Most of these patients have other significant injuries, including a hearing loss and facial nerve palsy. Any patient who complains of constant vertigo after an episode of significant head trauma needs skull x-rays, a head CT scan with bone windows, and an ENT evaluation.

PRESYNCOPE: TYPE 2 DIZZINESS

Presyncope is a cardiovascular problem, not a neurologic one. The patient's symptom of "light-headedness" and feeling of faintness are caused by a *globally* diminished cerebral blood flow. If the reduction in cerebral blood supply exceeds the brain's minimum requirements, loss of consciousness or syncope results. Although these patients may have "neurologic" symptoms such as visual blurring or "blacking out," facial or extremity paresthesias, generalized weakness, and even vertigo, they also typically have autonomic symptoms like diaphoresis, palpitations, and nausea.

Most patients with Type 2 dizziness have their symptom complex reproduced by hyperventilation, even if hyperventilation syndrome is not the suspected diagnosis. This procedure produces a global reduction in cerebral blood flow by reducing arterial PCO_2 and thus causing arterial vasoconstriction. Thus, reproduction of the patient's symptom complex by this maneuver confirms the presence of a Type 2 syndrome. For the procedure to be helpful diagnostically, it must be performed in a rigorous manner with good patient effort. A handkerchief or tissue should be placed 12 to 15 inches away from the patient's face, and he should be instructed to breathe rapidly and deeply for 3 minutes, moving the handkerchief or tissue with each breath.

A few other points about Type 2 dizziness are worth making. Presyncope is *not* a type of transient ischemic attack (TIA). That syndrome is due to a *focal* area of ischemia in the brain, not a *global* reduction in blood flow. Consequently, CT scan, carotid duplex, and cerebral angiography are not indicated in the evaluation of Type 2 dizziness. Likewise, presyncope is not a type of seizure, and an EEG is not a useful part of the work-up.

CAUSES OF PRESYNCOPE

HYPERVENTILATION SYNDROME

Hyperventilation syndrome, a common cause of Type 2 dizziness, occurs in two forms. The first is found in the acute, high-grade hyperventilator who develops the complete syndrome of light-headedness, visual blurring, and perioral and digital paresthesias. The episodes usually occur when the patient is anxious or excited, and the patient is usually aware of feeling "short of breath." Most of these patients are young women, and their symptoms can usually be easily reproduced in the office with hyperventilation. The second form, found in the chronic, low-grade hyperventilator, typically occurs in anxious, pressured, hard-driving individuals who start overbreathing when they are in stressful situations. These people are usually unaware that they are hyperventilating and do not feel short of breath. Visual blurring and paresthesias are not usually present. Their symptoms can also be reproduced in the office with hyperventilation, but it is frequently difficult to convince these patients that overbreathing is the cause of their problem. Both forms of hyperventilation syndrome are often part of an underlying anxiety disorder. Reassurance regarding the benign nature of their symptoms is the most important treatment. Instruction to blow into a plastic or paper bag during the acute attacks is often helpful. Anxiolytic agents may be useful in selected patients.

ORTHOSTATIC HYPOTENSION

Orthostatic hypotension is also a common cause of Type 2 dizziness, particularly in the elderly. The symptoms almost always occur when the patient is standing and are frequently maximal just after the patient rises from the sitting or supine position. Gravity decreases venous return to the heart, resulting in a decline in left heart filling. The autonomic nervous system is normally able to adjust peripheral resistance, cardiac rate, and contractibility so that cardiac output and blood pressure are maintained. However, if the patient is hypovolemic from fluid loss or diuretic therapy, is pharmacologically vasodilated, or has his compensatory autonomic responses blunted by medication or disease, cardiac output and blood pressure may fall sufficiently to produce Type 2 symptoms. In these patients, a significant orthostatic drop in blood pressure can usually be demonstrated in the office and the procedure will frequently reproduce the patient's complaint. The blood pressure should always be checked with the patient going *directly* from the supine to the standing position. It should be noted that asymptomatic but demonstrable orthostatic blood pressure changes are common in the elderly. If the patient's history does not suggest orthostatic hypotension and the orthostatic maneuver does not reproduce his symptoms, then the observed fall in blood pressure may not be the cause of his dizziness.

The most common causes of orthostatic hypotension are diuretic and other antihypertensive medications. Other causes of this syndrome include autonomic neuropathy, primary orthostatic hypotension, Shy–Drager syndrome, and internal bleeding.

Symptomatic orthostatic hypotension from antihypertensive medications should be dealt with by adjusting the patient's regimen. The "neurologic" causes of chronic orthostatic hypotension are treated in a similar manner. Elastic stockings are the best initial treatment. If these do not provide complete relief, then sodium chloride tablets can be added cautiously if they are not contraindicated by hypertension, congestive heart failure, hepatic cirrhosis, or renal failure. The mineralocorticoid fludrocortisone acetate can be used in refractory cases. The initial dose is 0.05 mg (one-half tablet) three times a week. The blood pressure and serum electrolytes must be monitored closely.

VASODEPRESSOR OR VASOVAGAL PRESYNCOPE

This patient's history is usually diagnostic. The episode of dizziness occurs either in a hot, crowded room or in the setting of sudden pain or strong emotion. The patient is always standing and may have premonitory symptoms of yawning, diaphoresis, and pallor. The reductions in blood pressure and cerebral blood flow are caused by a sudden, reflex dilation of the resistance arterioles. It usually occurs in young, otherwise healthy patients but can occur in the elderly. Hot, crowded rooms favor vasodilation and could produce symptomatic hypotension in an elderly person with otherwise compensated mild orthostatic hypotension. The only treatments for this syndrome are reassurance and avoidance of the precipitating circumstances.

CARDIAC PRESYNCOPE

Cardiac presyncope is usually caused by an arrhythmia that produces a sudden drop in cardiac output and thus a fall in cerebral perfusion. Common offending arrhythmias include sick sinus syndrome, paroxysmal supraventricular tachycardia, atrial fibrillation–flutter, complete heart block, and ventricular tachycardia. This diagnosis should be *strongly* considered in any patient whose Type 2 dizziness occurs while he is sitting or supine. A work-up includes an ECG and Holter monitoring, although it is often difficult to diagnose the arrhythmia without repeated and prolonged monitoring.

Exercise-related Type 2 dizziness may be caused by aortic stenosis or idiopathic hypertrophic subaortic stenosis (IHSS). An echocardiogram is useful in the diagnosis of these conditions. Finally, paroxysmal episodes of light-headedness and dizziness can be a manifestation of coronary ischemia. These episodes are sometimes called *angina equivalents*, as the patients may not experience chest pain. This diagnosis should be considered in any patient with unexplained episodes of Type 2 dizziness and the appropriate risk factors.

CAROTID SINUS HYPERSENSITIVITY

Carotid sinus hypersensitivity is primarily a disorder of the elderly in which the carotid sinus in the neck becomes abnormally sensitive to pressure and produces episodes of bradycardia and decreased cardiac output. Classically, this syndrome was described in men who wore tight collars; however, that history will not be present in most patients with this disease. It should be suspected in middle-aged or elderly patients with unexplained bouts of presyncope or syncope. The diagnosis is made by light carotid massage under strictly controlled conditions (*i.e.*, the presence of a crash cart and personnel skilled in cardiopulmonary resuscitation [CPR]). The treatment is placement of a permanent pacemaker.

MICTURATION PRESYNCOPE

Micturation presyncope is the usual cause of a "dizzy spell" when the patient gets up at night to urinate. It is due to the sudden peripheral vasodilation that may occur at the end of urination, resulting in a drop in systemic blood pressure and cerebral perfusion. The reflex vasodilation is more likely to occur with a full bladder; thus, patients should be instructed to empty their bladders completely before retiring for the night. The presence of a mild, usually asymptomatic orthostatic blood pressure drop will predispose patients to this problem.

HYPOGLYCEMIA

Although this metabolic derangement does not cause reduced cerebral blood flow, its symptoms are similar to those of presyncope and thus this diagnosis should be considered in evaluating patients with Type 2 dizziness.

Most patients with symptomatic hypoglycemia are insulin-dependent diabetics who either did not consume an adequate caloric load for their insulin dose or took an excessive dose of insulin. Oral hypoglycemic agents are occasionally unpredictable in their action and can produce symptomatic hypoglycemia. Early diabetics who are not yet on therapy can have "reactive" hypoglycemia from surges of insulin. This occurs typically 2 to 5 hours after eating and is more often manifested by diaphoresis and palpitations than light-headedness and other "neurologic" symptoms. The diagnosis is made by documenting serum hypoglycemia while the patient is symptomatic. In general, a serum glucose of less than 50 mg/dl is necessary to produce central nervous system (CNS) symptoms. Insulin-secreting tumors can produce the same symptoms.

DYSEQUILIBRIUM: TYPE 3 DIZZINESS

Disequilibrium is a common problem in the elderly but can be seen in younger patients after a Type 1 episode or after mild head trauma. The symptom complex tends to be present primarily during ambulation and is usually improved in the sitting or supine position. These patients complain of feeling unbalanced and insecure when walking. They often tend to hold onto walls and furniture when they walk. They may complain that their heads feel "fuzzy," "thick," or "out of sorts."

There are several etiologies of Type 3 dizziness, and many patients have more than one contributing cause. Before these causes are discussed, a review of the physiology of human balance mechanisms may be helpful in understanding this syndrome.

NORMAL MECHANISMS OF EQUILIBRIUM

Gravity and environmental stimuli are constant challenges to bipedal locomotion. Several things must occur to ensure proper maintenance of an upright posture and smooth ambulation. First, the CNS must get adequate sensory input regarding the body's position in space, particularly relative to the ground; second, the CNS must be able to correctly process the sensory input; and third, an appropriate motor response must be mounted to meet the environmental challenge. Deficits in one or more of these steps result in imbalance or dysequilibrium.

Four sensory inputs determine the position of the body in space. The most important of these inputs is vision. Distortion or loss of visual input is a serious blow to the maintenance of equilibrium. Anyone who has attempted to walk around wearing glasses with the wrong refraction can appreciate how distortion of visual input can cause "dizziness." The vestibular system is the second most important sensory input for balance. It provides information regarding movement and the relationship of the head to the ground. Acute, unilateral disturbances in the vestibular system produce vertigo, but slowly progressive bilateral or healing vestibular lesions produce a dysequilibrium syndrome. Position sense in the joints and muscles of the lower extremities is the third input necessary for normal equilibrium. The fourth sensory modality necessary for balance is hearing; this sense gives the brain information about the environment, which it can compare with the other sensory modalities. The simple exercise of walking down the street or through a crowded mall with one's ears filled with cotton will demonstrate how diminished hearing can cause "dizziness."

PROCESSES THAT DISTURB EQUILIBRIUM

A broad range of diseases can interfere with sensory input, central integration, or motor response and therefore produce dysequilibrium. Some patients with Type 3 dizziness have disease at only one level in this physiologic loop. Many patients, however, have disease at multiple levels or with multiple facets of the same level (i.e., multiple sensory deficits). This broad spectrum of possibilities offers a diagnostic challenge to clinicians.

ABNORMALITIES OF SENSORY INPUT

Any disease process that disturbs normal vision can produce Type 3 dizziness. Diseases that distort vision tend to cause more problems than those that produce visual loss alone; however, both can cause dysequilibrium. Degenerative disease of the vestibular system, slowly growing neoplasms (acoustic neuroma), toxins (aminoglycoside antibiotics), and residual dysfunction after an acute vestibular disorder can all cause Type 3 dizziness. Peripheral neuropathies, as in diabetes mellitus or chronic alcoholism, can produce enough sensory loss in the lower extremities to prevent adequate sensory input for balance. Spinal cord disease, like spondylitic cervical myelopathy, can also produce significant lower extremity sensory loss. Finally, hearing loss can contribute to Type 3 dizziness.

ABNORMALITIES OF CENTRAL INTEGRATION

Any process that produces a global impairment in CNS function can cause dysequilibrium. Dizziness is a common complaint in patients who have dementia. Although many of these patients have multiple etiologic factors in their Type 3 syndrome (i.e., sensory deficits and poor motor response), poor central integration of their sensory input is often a contributing factor. Likewise, patients with metabolic encephalopathy of any etiology may have a disruption of central integrative processes and dysequilibrium. Medications, particularly those with sedative side effects, may impair central integration. Many sedative medications also have toxic effects on the vestibular system.

ABNORMALITIES OF MOTOR RESPONSE

There are three major elements in human motor function: the pyramidal system, the extrapyramidal system, and the cerebellum. Disturbance in any one of these elements can produce an improper or inadequate motor response and thus Type 3 dizziness. Parkinson's disease, a degenerative disorder of the extrapyramidal system, produces bradykinesia, rigidity, a flexed posture, and loss of postural reflexes. Dizziness is a common complaint in this syndrome, because patients are unable to mount a smooth motor response to their environmental challenges and they feel imbalanced. Cerebellar disease of any type (*e.g.*, alcohol-related, degenerative, or neoplastic) produces gait ataxia and dysequilibrium. Frontal lobe dysfunction from degenerative disease, hydrocephalus, or neoplasm results in a gait disorder that prevents a normal motor response. Spondylitic cervical myelopathy may produce spasticity in the lower extremities (in addition to the sensory loss described earlier) that interferes with smooth motor function.

DIAGNOSTIC EVALUATION OF TYPE 3 DIZZINESS

An evaluation of patients with Type 3 dizziness should focus on finding reversible or treatable etiologies of this syndrome. All patients should have their medication regimen reviewed. Drugs that are vestibulotoxic or cause clouding of consciousness should be stopped or reduced in dosage. A metabolic screen should be obtained in all patients to evaluate for hepatic and renal insufficiency, electrolyte imbalance, and thyroid dysfunction.

All patients should be asked about visual problems and, if present, a complete ophthalmologic evaluation should be obtained. Likewise, patients should be questioned about hearing loss or tinnitus. If either of these symptoms is present, audiometry or BAERs should be performed. If a *unilateral* abnormality is demonstrated, an imaging study of the posterior fossa should be done. Bilateral abnormalities should prompt an ENT evaluation. Inquiry should also be made about a history of Type 1 symptoms (vertigo). All such patients should have an audiogram or BAERs.

Patients should be questioned about sensory loss and paresthesias in the feet. Patients with Type 3 dizziness due to lower extremity sensory loss frequently have exacerbation of their symptoms when they walk into a dark room or close their eyes while they are shampooing in the shower. This etiology of Type 3 dizziness can be screened for in all patients with the Romberg maneuver. This test requires that the patient stand with his feet together and then close his eyes. If the procedure *reproduces* or worsens his dizziness, then sensory loss is suggested as an important etiologic factor. If the patient's lower extremity deep tendon reflexes are hypoactive or absent, a peripheral neuropathy is the most likely

cause of the sensory loss and an appropriate work-up should be ordered. If reflexes are hyperactive, then spinal cord disease is likely and appropriate radiologic studies should be obtained.

A formal neurologic consultation should be considered in most patients with Type 3 dizziness, as a careful, detailed neurologic examination is very helpful in the evaluation. Subtle signs of parkinsonism, ataxia, spasticity, and frontal lobe gait dysfunction may only be appreciated by someone experienced in neurologic disorders. Early parkinsonism may be manifested only by masked facies and a shuffling gait—tremor need not be present. Mild ataxia can be tested for by asking the patient to stand with his feet together (eyes open). If this maneuver reproduces a feeling of dysequilibrium, then ataxia is suggested and posterior fossa imaging may be necessary. Spasticity is manifested by stiff leg movements when walking and hyperactive deep tendon reflexes. Such findings may require MR of the spinal cord or myelography. Frontal lobe gait disorders are manifested by difficulty in initiating gait from a standing position and difficulty in lifting the feet off the floor. Such findings also require radiologic imaging of the brain.

Patients with Type 3 dizziness who have no identifiable cause should undergo ENG, as cerebellopontine angle tumors (particularly acoustic neuroma) can present with a dysequilibrium syndrome. Most of these patients present with unilateral hearing loss or tinnitus and will have subtle signs of facial sensory loss, a depressed corneal reflex, or mild facial palsy. However, slow destruction of the vestibular portion of the eight cranial nerve can produce Type 3 dizziness, and not all patients are aware of their hearing loss. ENG will pick up subtle evidence of vestibular dysfunction and will also diagnose bilateral vestibular damage or degeneration that can present as a dysequilibrium syndrome. All patients with a *unilaterally* abnormal ENG require posterior fossa imaging.

THERAPY FOR TYPE 3 DIZZINESS

Many patients with this syndrome are treated with antihistamines such as meclizine. This medication, which has significant potential sedative side effects in the elderly, is usually not helpful and may make the patient's symptoms worse. Other vestibulotoxic or sedative medications should be stopped or reduced in dosage. Metabolic derangements should be corrected to the extent possible. Some visual problems (*i.e.*, cataracts) are remedial, and improvement in hearing may be possible in some patients with a hearing aid.

If a peripheral neuropathy is discovered, its cause should be elucidated and therapy, where possible, instituted. Spondylitic cervical myelopathy may improve with decompressive laminectomy. Parkinson's disease can be treated with dopaminergic agents, and frontal lobe dysfunction secondary to hydrocephalus may be ameliorated with a shunt process.

Despite the aforementioned therapeutic possibilities, a significant number of patients will have no definitive therapy for their Type 3 dizziness. Many of these patients can benefit from the following treatment modalities.

The use of a light cane may be beneficial for some people. Patients with motor dysfunction can use it to steady themselves and stabilize their gait. Patients with sensory loss (*e.g.*, visual, auditory, or lower extremity) can drag the cane along the ground to provide themselves with extra sensory stimulation. A soft cervical collar (usually best worn with the clasp in front) can decrease aberrant or asymmetrical input from diseased vestibular apparatuses and thus reduce the sensation of dysequilibrium.

Patients who are experiencing Type 3 dizziness while recovering from a Type 1 episode and other patients with degenerative or toxic vestibular disorder may benefit from vestibular exercises. These maneuvers are designed to "retrain" the diseased vestibular system with repeated stimulation.

The patient should attempt to find a straight walkway, 20 to 30 feet long, in the home. The patient begins the exercise by walking. The feet should be spread wide apart, and the arms should be outstretched laterally and parallel to the floor. The patient should walk up and down the walkway, narrowing the distance between the feet with each pass until the balls of the feet touch with each step. The procedure is then repeated with the arms held tightly at the side. It is then performed a third time with the arms outstretched in front of the patient, parallel to the floor. When this procedure is completed the whole exercise is repeated with the eyes *closed*. The entire procedure should take 20 to 30 minutes and should be performed twice a day.

Finally, some patients may benefit from low doses of a central stimulant such as ephedrine or methylphenidate. These medications must be used cautiously in elderly patients, particularly those with hypertension and cardiac disease.

QUESTIONS AND DISCUSSION

1. J.D. is a 42-year-old white man who experienced the sudden onset of vertigo, nausea, vomiting, and ataxia 3 weeks ago. The vertigo, nausea, and vomiting resolved in 48 hours, but the patient still complains bitterly of "dizziness" and states that he can't go back to work because "I walk like a drunk." When questioned, he admits that his dizziness is present only when he is standing or walking and seems to resolve when he is sitting or supine. He denies hearing loss and tinnitus. There is no associated visual blurring, diaphoresis, or pallor. His neurologic examination is normal except that he tends to veer to the right when walking. How would this patient's current symptoms of dizziness be categorized?

    A. Type 1—vertigo
    B. Type 2—presyncope
    C. Type 3—dysequilibrium
    D. Malingering
    E. Not classifiable

The correct answer is (C). This patient's syndrome began as a Type 1 disorder; however, as the vertigo resolved, it converted to a Type 3 dysequilibrium syndrome. This is a common sequela to acute vestibulopathy and is due to a residual mismatch between the input from the paired vestibular systems. The symptoms usually resolve over several weeks, and recovery is usually hastened with the use of vestibular exercises.

2. S.T. is a 28-year-old white woman who complains of a 2-week history of "everything spinning around." The episodes are precipitated by any type of head movement in the horizontal or vertical plane. The vertigo begins immediately with repeated head movements. The patient denies hearing loss and tinnitus but does recall a 2-week episode of "numbness" below her waist about 3 months ago. When she is asked to follow the examiner's finger with her eyes, coarse, horizontal nystagmus is noted on lateral gaze bilaterally and vertical nystagmus is present on upgaze. Her neurologic examination is otherwise remarkable only for questionable bilateral Babinski signs. The most likely diagnosis is:

A. Depression
B. BPPV
C. Meniere's disease
D. Multiple sclerosis
E. Perilymph fistula

The correct answer is (D). This patient's symptoms are typical of positioning vertigo, a nonspecific symptom that can be seen in any vestibular disorder. The multidirectional pure horizontal and pure vertical nystagmus that is not suppressed by fixation is essentially diagnostic of a central vestibular disorder. The history of transient neurologic symptoms in the lower extremities would make multiple sclerosis a strong diagnostic consideration. The position-related vertigo of BPPV is usually produced by a single head position; there is a latency of 10 to 60 seconds to the onset of vertigo; and the vertigo tends to fatigue with repeated trials. Ménière's disease can be associated with positioning vertigo, but there is also a history of hearing loss and tinnitus. Finally, in both BPPV and Ménière's disease the nystagmus would have characteristics of peripheral vestibular disease (*i.e.,* unidirectional, mixed, and suppressed by fixation).

3. H.L. is a 69-year-old black man who complains of "dizzy spells." The patient describes 10 to 12 episodes in the last 6 weeks of sudden visual "blackouts" and feeling "like I'm going to pass out." His wife notes that he breaks out in a cold sweat during the attacks and looks "glassy-eyed." The episodes last 30 to 60 seconds and the patient feels "fine" afterward. There is no history of vertigo, hearing loss, tinnitus, or other focal neurologic symptoms. The spells are not related to body position or exercise and have occurred in many different situations, including watching TV and eating in a restaurant. The patient's neurologic examination is normal, and 3 minutes of hyperventilation reproduces his symptom complex. This patient's dizziness should be categorized as:

A. Type 1—vertigo
B. Type 2—presyncope
C. Type 3—dysequilibrium
D. Vertebrobasilar insufficiency
E. Hypoglycemia

The correct answer is (B). The patient's symptoms are typical of those caused by globally diminished cerebral perfusion. Vertebrobasilar insufficiency causes focal areas of ischemia and focal neurologic

symptoms. The episodes are too brief and too discrete for hypoglycemia attacks.

What is the most likely etiology of this patient's Type 2 dizziness?

A. Hyperventilation syndrome
B. Vasovagal attacks
C. Orthostatic hypotension
D. Cardiac arrhythmia
E. Aortic stenosis

The correct answer is (D). Hyperventilation should reproduce the symptom complex in all Type 2 patients, because by lowering arterial PCO_2 it causes cerebral vasoconstriction and globally diminished cerebral blood flow. The diagnosis of hyperventilation syndrome must be made by other criteria (*i.e.,* the situations of stress or anxiety in which it typically occurs). Vasovagal or vasodepressor attacks are also situational (*e.g.,* hot, crowded room or sudden emotion) and always occur when the patient is upright. Likewise, orthostatic hypotension occurs only when the patient is on his feet. Aortic stenosis produces exercise-related presyncope. Most patients with Type 2 symptoms that occur when sitting or supine will have a cardiac arrhythmia.

Which of the following conditions can produce Type 3 (dysequilibrium) dizziness?

A. Chronic renal failure
B. Diabetes mellitus
C. Aminoglycoside antibiotic toxicity
D. Spondylitic cervical myelopathy
E. Parkinson's disease

The answer is that all of the aforementioned conditions can produce Type 3 dizziness. Chronic renal failure is associated with a peripheral neuropathy that diminishes sensory input from the lower extremities and thus presents normal balance. In addition, the metabolic encephalopathy of uremia may inhibit proper central integration of the sensory modalities required for balance and thus exacerbate the feeling of dysequilibrium. Diabetes mellitus is also associated with a peripheral neuropathy; however, this disease is also frequently complicated by retinopathy, which decreases input from the most important sensory modality for balance. Aminoglycoside antibiotics can damage the vestibular portion of the eighth cranial nerve and produce a dysequilibrium syndrome. Cervical spinal cord compression can decrease sensory input from the lower extremities and cause spasticity, which impedes the proper motor response for balance and ambulation. Parkinson's disease also prevents a smooth motor response to environmental stresses and therefore Type 3 dizziness.

SUGGESTED READING

Baloh RW: The Essentials of Neurotology. Philadelphia, FA Davis, 1984

Baloh RW, Honrubia V: Clinical neurophysiology of the vestibular system. Philadelphia, FA Davis, 1984

Baloh RW, Honrubia V, Jacobson K: Benign positional vertigo: Clinical and oculographic features in 240 cases. Neurology 37:371, 1987

Brandt T: Vertigo and dizziness. In Asbury AK, McKhann GM, McDonald WI (eds): Diseases of the Nervous System: Clinical Neurobiology, pp 561–576. Philadelphia, WB Saunders, 1986

Brandt T, Daroff RB: The multisensory physiological and pathological vertigo syndromes. Ann Neurol 7:195, 1980

Brandt T, Daroff RB: Physical therapy for benign paroxysmal position vertigo. Arch Otolaryngol 106:484, 1980

Drachman DA, Hart CW: An approach to the dizzy patient. Neurology 22:323, 1972

Harner SG: Clinical findings in patients with acoustic neurinoma. Mayo Clin Proc 58:721, 1983

Jonas S, Klein I, Dimant J: Importance of Holter monitoring in patients with periodic cerebral symptoms. Ann Neurol 1:470, 1977

Lipsitz LA: Syncope in the elderly. Ann Intern Med 99:92, 1983

Nelson RL: Hypoglycemia: Fact or fiction? Mayo Clin Proc 60:844, 1985

Troost TB: Dizziness and vertigo in vertebrobasilar disease. Stroke 11:301–314, 1980

Zee DS: Vertigo. In Johnson RT (ed:) Current Therapy in Neurologic Disease, pp 8–13. St. Louis, CV Mosby, 1985

Behavioral Neurology

Christopher G. Goetz
Robert S. Wilson

Bizarre or altered behavioral patterns are traditionally felt to relate to psychiatric disorders or generalized delirium from drugs, toxins, or metabolic imbalances. However, some specific neurologic conditions present with remarkably consistent behavioral abnormalities. These conditions have equally consistent anatomic substrates and, when identified by an astute diagnostician, they suggest specific causes and treatments. In this chapter, five conditions are discussed, each with a prominent behavioral and seemingly psychiatric presentation, but with a pathologic basis related to a specific neurologic dysfunction. These conditions are temporal lobe epilepsy, fluent aphasia, Wernicke's encephalopathy, transient global amnesia, and herpes encephalitis.

These strange disorders are not rare, and their complexity often relates not to management problems but instead to accurate identification. The topic is thus particularly pertinent to the non-neurologist, who is most likely to be the first person to interview and evaluate these patients.

ANATOMIC BASIS— PAPEZ CIRCUIT

It is well recognized that the ability to recall and engender memories is intimately linked to the emotional makeup of such memories. Furthermore, several clinical conditions demonstrate combined and prominent memory-emotional alterations, suggesting that the anatomic basis of these two functions may be linked. In 1937, the neuroanatomist Papez published a treatise describing an anatomic circuit that linked those nuclei and paths that appear important to many aspects of emotional–behavioral integration. This circuit has been named the *Papez circuit* and is probably the most important circuit for clinicians dealing with behavioral abnormalities to know. Familiarity with this circuit allows one to think systematically about the anatomic foundations of behavioral neurology.

The circuit is schematically diagrammed in Figure 14-1 (*A*), with anatomic nuclei and paths identified in the sagittal brain section of Figure 14-1 (*B*). As indicated, the pathway is circular, providing continual reintegration of information. The two focal cortical areas most prominently involved are the cingulate cortex and the hippocampus of the temporal lobe. Diffuse cortical impulses travel into the hippocampus, an area felt to be particularly important to memory and emotional expression. This information travels forward in the fornix path to the mamillary bodies of the hypothalamus and continues to the anterior lobe of the thalamus, and further to the midline cingulate cortex, which finally projects diffusely to cortical regions.

Familiarity with this circuit is useful, since disease anywhere along the pathway will be expected to

William J. Weiner and Christopher G. Goetz, eds. *Neurology for the Non-Neurologist*, Third Edition. Copyright © 1994, 1989 by J. B. Lippincott Company. Copyright © 1981 by Harper and Row Publishers, Inc.

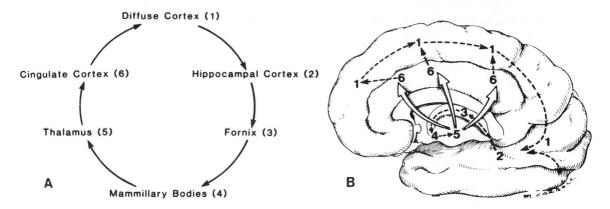

FIG. 14-1. Papez circuit (*A*) Schematic diagram of brain regions connected by the Papez circuit. (*B*) Anatomic diagram of brain regions numbered in *A* with arrows indicating the direction of general informational flow.

demonstrate aberrant emotional behavior, although not necessarily the same pattern. This knowledge allows the clinician to focus immediately on a finite number of nuclei and connecting paths to explain abnormal behavioral symptoms if they have a focal anatomic basis. Clearly, "diffuse cortical input" is important to remember because toxic and metabolic encephalopathy often present with agitated behavior or a change in personality. The other areas, however, are focal, and identification of disease at these levels can lead to rapid intervention. Reference will be made back to the circuit throughout this chapter.

TEMPORAL LOBE EPILEPSY

Also referred to as psychomotor epilepsy and partial complex seizure, psychomotor or psychosensory variety, temporal lobe epilepsy (TLE) may manifest itself with intermittent spells of bizarre behavior, including babbling nonsense and frank visual and auditory hallucinations, all related to organic disease of the central nervous system (CNS). Differentiation of this disorder from psychotic disorders like schizophrenia can be difficult and yet essential because their treatments are drastically different. Certain specific characteristics are helpful in establishing abnormal behavioral patterns as probable epilepsy, and they are the focus of this discussion.

TLE represents an abnormal electrical discharge that begins in one temporal lobe and usually crosses rapidly to involve both sides of the brain. Four helpful identifying characteristics of TLE include:

1. Distinct temporal pattern of the spells
2. Presence of an aura
3. Presence of peculiar motor behaviors called *automatisms*
4. Specific type of loss of consciousness

Not all are necessarily seen in every TLE patient, but the presence of even one suggests this diagnosis.

The distinctive temporal pattern of TLE refers to repeated, but intermittent, and paroxysmal changes in behavior, not necessarily linked to any emotional provocation. The behavioral changes are brief, lasting seconds to minutes. Often, before any visible behavioral change can be appreciated by an observer, the patient experiences a stereotypic and fixed sensation, known as an *epileptic aura*. The aura represents the beginning of the seizure and can help in localizing the focus, or source, of the seizure activity. The aura may be olfactory, in which the patient suddenly smells a strange, often pungent odor, or it may be a gustatory sensation, or a strange abdominal "butterflies" feeling, also called *epigastric rising*. Emotional changes of sudden unfamiliarity with one's environment, "jamais vu," or sudden intense familiarity with the surroundings, "déjà vu," are seen, and there may be intense and vivid auditory or visual hallucinations. The aura and area of the temporal lobe cortex that are felt to relate to the seizure focus are listed in Table 14-1. The presence of this stereotypic aura and sudden unprovoked change in behavior help to quickly identify a TLE patient. The aura is sensed by the patient and is not identified by the clinician, except by interview. The patient may not necessarily link the strange aura to his spells, so that information must be specifically solicited.

The presence of automatisms is also useful in the diagnosis of TLE. These activities appear as the seizure spreads in the amygdala region of the temporal lobe. The movements may range from rather primitive movements (lip smacking, eye blinking, or chewing motions) or may be highly complex (dressing and undressing, piling objects on top of one another). Again, these are stereotypic and rather fixed from one spell to another so that a detailed record of two or more episodes helps to establish the pattern of behavior.

The peculiar loss of consciousness in TLE is also helpful. After the aura, which of course the examiner cannot see unless it involves automatisms, there is a sudden loss of contact with the environment. Unlike in other generalized seizures, these patients only rarely fall to the floor, shake all over, urinate, and bite their tongue. Instead, they lose consciousness but maintain body tone and may walk around, but "in a daze, out of contact" with the environment. When the spell is over, the patient is usually amnestic for the seizure except that he may recall the beginning of the seizure and hence recount, if specifically asked, the details of the aura. Immediately after the spell, the patient is usually confused and sleepy. If restrained during this period, he may strike out randomly at people who may try to assist. However, these patients are generally not violent in a specifically goal-directed manner either during or after their seizures. As strange as their behaviors may be, focused violence, like tracking a person with a gun or retrieving a kitchen knife

out of a drawer and stabbing a victim, is far outside the repertoire of TLE.

Two specific examples will help to delineate the methods used in diagnosing TLE.

Case 1 A quiet 34-year-old right-handed woman is admitted for observation after she suffered head trauma on a city bus. She was the cause of an unprovoked fist fight on the bus and reports, "They said I did it but I don't remember a thing."

The question is whether this patient suffers from (1) head trauma with retrograde amnesia, (2) social deviant behavior, claiming ignorance to avoid responsibility, or (3) amnesia and bizarre behavior related to TLE. To differentiate TLE from the other two disorders, the interview focuses on the characteristics of TLE.

In discussing this event with the patient, it is found that this is only one of many violent episodes in this woman's life. Each episode is similar in that she cannot understand why she gets into fights, being a quiet, shy person, and she says that the events are never precipitated by an argument. She says she has no warning and that "that's all I remember." However, when specifically asked about smells, taste, sounds, and visions, she states that she usually starts thinking of a peculiar tune that always recurs in her head before a fight and makes her nervous for those last few seconds. Importantly, this major clue is only gleaned from specific questioning.

When the victim of the fight, who is in the next hospital room, is interviewed, he comments that he and the patient were sitting quietly in the bus when suddenly the patient started fidgeting in her purse, picking at items, and smacking her lips loudly. She then started walking around the bus babbling noises and picking at her clothes. The bus was crowded and the patient bumped into several passengers. A minute later, she seemed to start swinging randomly at people. The man was hit in the head, fell over, and hit his face on the bus seat. As they were both taken to the hospital, this man no-

TABLE 14-1. Temporal Lobe Foci and Related Auras

FOCUS	AURA
Uncus	Smell, taste
Cingulate cortex	Change in emotional perception—déjà vu, jamais vu, euphoria, sense of sudden doom
Insula	Epigastric rising sensation
Amygdala	Pupillary dilatation, photophobia, automatisms
Association temporal cortex	Auditory, visual hallucinations

ticed that the belligerent woman seemed now considerably confused and sleepy.

The characteristic aura, the paroxysmal quality of the repeated episodes by history, and the automatisms of lip smacking and clothes picking with amnesia all suggest TLE. An electroencephalogram (EEG) demonstrated epilepsy, and anticonvulsant medications have virtually abolished the episodes.

Case 2 A 16-year-old boy on the psychiatric unit with a diagnosis of schizophrenia and hallucinatory behavior is evaluated by the neurologist because of a single generalized seizure. On being interviewed, this patient says: "It's just like before, but this time much worse." Several times each week this patient sees "the man," a blurry but discernible bearded man who silently beckons him forward verbally. As this happens, everything in the patient's environment becomes suddenly more distinct, clearer, and more colorful, with a clear sense of familiarity and warmth. Then a strange feeling of dread and a "fog" come over the patient, in that the patient then appears to lose touch for approximately 5 minutes. He has no recollection of this period of losing touch, but the family says that he walks around in the house mumbling strange noises that are sometimes prayers, and at the same time bows his head back and forth in a seemingly ritualistic manner. After this, he lies down and sleeps for approximately 2 hours. The same stereotypic pattern occurred immediately before the generalized seizure.

This patient again shows the stereotypic aura, which is hallucinatory this time, along with the sense of emotional familiarly with the environment. Stereotypic repetition of episodes and the automatisms with amnesia and sleepiness afterward strongly suggest TLE. In regard to this latter episode in which there was a generalized motor seizure with bilateral shaking, this pattern can be seen with TLE

when the seizure activity spreads throughout both sides of the brain. An EEG study with nasopharyngeal recordings demonstrated abnormal epileptiform activity, and on medication the patient has shown remarkable improvement. This case demonstrates the important interface between psychiatric symptoms and clear focal neurologic disease.

Table 14-2 serves as a summary and outlines additional guidelines for differentiating TLE episodes from psychotic bizarre behaviors of schizophrenia. These patterns are clinically useful, although no absolute rules hold true.

ANATOMY AND CLINICAL FINDINGS

The anatomic lesions of TLE naturally relate to the temporal lobe and, depending on the area damaged, will give rise to different auras (see Table 14-1). As can be seen, some of these nuclei are primary portions of the Papez circuit, and the others have direct input into the circuit.

In examining a patient with TLE, static findings may include a homonymous hemianopia or a homonymous quadrant anopia, especially in the superior fields (Fig. 14-2). Because these fibers pass through the temporal lobe *en route* to the occipital cortex, the superior quadrant anopia should be specifically sought.

Much has been written about psychopathology in TLE patients. Although the seizures and bizarre behavior are intermittent, interictal or between-seizure abnormalities are often attributed to TLE. Problems such as sedation, inattention, and depressed mood may be seen as dose-related side effects of antiepileptic medications. If toxicity can be ruled out, the most common psychiatric problem in epilepsy is depression. Although not specific to TLE, research suggests rates of depression as high as 75% in some clinical samples. Paradoxically, depression may appear after seizure control is accom-

TABLE 14-2. Clinical Distinctions Between TLE Behavior and Schizophrenia

	TLE	SCHIZOPHRENIA
Environmental precipitants	Rare	Frequent
Duration of attack	0.5–5 min	May be days
Aura	Usual	Lacking
Injury to others	Rare and undirected	Unpredictable—may be directed or undirected
Disturbance of consciousness	Present	Lacking or only mind clouding
Symptoms and signs after attack	Sleepy, confused	Lacking

TLE = temporal lobe epilepsy.

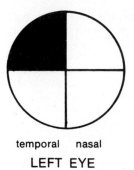
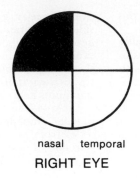

| temporal   nasal | nasal   temporal |
| **LEFT EYE** | **RIGHT EYE** |

FIG. 14-2. Visual field defect associated with right temporal lobe disease, termed *left superior quandrantanopsia.*

plished, suggesting that seizures, like electroconvulsive therapy (ECT), may serve to elevate mood, possibly through opioid mechanisms. Aggressive behavior is often attributed to TLE. There is, however, no good evidence of a disproportionate level of aggressive or violent behavior in TLE or epilepsy. Aggressive behavior may be seen following a seizure, but it is typically nondirected and random, occurring when the patient is aroused or restrained. The hypothesis that TLE is characterized by a distinct personality profile has not been supported by recent research. On the other hand, psychiatric signs and symptoms in general are more commonly seen in TLE than in other forms of epilepsy, particularly in patients with severe, uncontrolled TLE.

ETIOLOGY

TLE is often seen in patients with a history of birth trauma. Brain tumors, both primary and metastatic, may also involve the temporal lobe and present early with characteristic TLE. Subacute onset of TLE with fever should suggest encephalitis, specifically resulting from herpes simplex, which has a predilection for the temporal lobes. EEG findings are discussed in Chapter 7. Drugs useful in the control of TLE are listed in Table 14-3, along with usual doses, plasma levels, and common side effects.

FLUENT APHASIAS

Aphasia is a specific language deficit that occurs without weakness of the articulatory muscles and is due to cortical brain disease. The two basic types of aphasia are subfluent and fluent. The former group is not difficult to diagnose and would not be confused with psychiatric disease, since in most

TABLE 14-3. Drugs Used in the Control of TLE, Doses, Therapeutic Plasma Levels, and Common or Important Side Effects

DRUG	DAILY ADULT DOSE (mg/kg)	PLASMA LEVEL (μg/ml)	TOXICITY
Primidone*	10–25	7–15 primidone 20–40 phenobarbital	Lymphadenopathy, nausea, vomiting, sedation, ataxia
Carbamazepine*	7–15 (in two doses)	4–10	Agranulocytosis, nausea, vomiting, sedation, ataxia
Valproic acid*	15–30 (divided doses)	50–100	Nausea, vomiting, sedation, elevated liver enzymes, ataxia
Phenytoin	4–7	10–20	Lymphadenopathy, nausea, vomiting, sedation, vitamin K and folate deficiency, ataxia
Phenobarbitol	1–5	15–40	Sedation, hyperactivity in children, vitamin K deficiency, ataxia

*Indicates drug preferentially recommended for TLE as opposed to other forms of seizures.

cases an obvious right hemiparesis accompanies the change in speech pattern. The fluent aphasias, however, are not associated with motor problems, so that these patients present with behavioral alterations in the form of strange speech. The adage taught to young neurologists that in evaluating an acute behavioral change, one must always rule out fluent aphasia is applicable to all clinicians.

Aphasic problems occur with focal dominant hemisphere disorders. For most people, the left hemisphere is dominant for speech, although in a small percentage of left-handed persons the right hemisphere may be dominant. Subfluent aphasias relate to frontal lobe disease, and fluent aphasias relate usually to dominant temporal or temporoparietal damage. Since the temporal lobe is involved in the Papez circuit, behavioral alterations in fluent aphasias are expected and characteristic.

In contrast to the frustration and depressed affect common in subfluent aphasia, fluent aphasics are often seemingly unaware of their deficit and unconcerned. Patients may not realize that their speech is incomprehensible to others. In extreme cases, these patients may blame their inability to communicate on others to the point of frank paranoia. Impulsivity is also observed. The combination of such behaviors can result in serious management problems.

The evaluation of aphasia is usually rapid and requires no unusual implements. Table 14-4 outlines the manner of examination, which has three focal points. First, by listening to the patient's spontaneous speech, one decides whether the speech is subfluent, slow, and sparse or fluent, rapid, and free flowing. This evaluation makes no judgment on content of speech but instead on rhythm and ease of word production. Second, the examiner asks the patient to follow a verbal command—"Show me a spoon," "Raise your left hand," and so forth and tests his ability to comprehend. This integration of auditory information helps to distinguish various aphasias and localizes the disease. The command must be verbal, and the investigator must discipline himself not to use nonverbal communication during this task. Third, the patient is asked to repeat a sentence—first a reasonable phrase, such as "Today is Tuesday; tomorrow I will phone Bill," and then a nonsense phrase such as "No ifs, ands, or buts." These three simple maneuvers can be performed by confused or intoxicated patients and by patients with short attention spans. However, they are not performed by aphasics. Furthermore, the pattern of disability in the three tasks isolates the specific areas of dominant cortical dysfunction.

The patient who is usually diagnosed as confused, agitated, and often schizophrenic is the patient with a Wernicke's aphasia (not to be confused with Wernicke's encephalopathy, which is discussed in the next section).

The following case history will help to typify this syndrome and emphasizes the common confusion between this condition and the word salad of schizophrenia.

Case 3 A 65-year-old hypertensive right-handed woman was well until 3 hours before an evaluation in the emergency room. Her family lived with her and reported that after lunch the patient took a 40-minute nap; upon awaking she "began speaking nonsense—crazy talk." Her past medical and psychiatric history was negative, and no similar events had ever occurred.

The patient is alert and talkative, but her speech has no discernible sense. Phrases such as "oh, me, why not, should we, what now, amen Moses" are spoken rapidly and spontaneously. She can follow no verbal commands nor will she repeat simple phrases. The family feels she may be poisoned or has gone crazy.

TABLE 14-4. Major Types of Aphasia with Guides to Their Rapid Identification

NAMES	FLUENCY	FOLLOW COMMANDS	REPEAT	FOCAL DAMAGE	ASSOCIATIVE PROBLEMS
Broca's	Subfluent	Yes	No	Dominant frontal lobe	Right hemiparesis
Wernicke's	Fluent	No	No	Dominant temporal lobe	Visual field abnormalities, no weakness
Conductive	Fluent	Yes	Yes for short phrases; cannot repeat "no ifs, ands, or buts"	Dominant connecting fibers between Broca's and Wernicke's area	Visual field abnormalities or mild weakness, decreased sensation on right side of body and face

The highlights of this case are the patient's age, the acute onset, the characteristic speech pattern, and the easily retrieved results of an accurate aphasia testing screen. Importantly, in a patient who is 65 years old without prior psychiatric history, the new onset of schizophrenia, regardless of how bizarre the behavior or speech may be, would be exceptional.

ETIOLOGY

Wernicke's fluent aphasia is usually seen with dominant temporal lobe disease in the form of cerebrovascular accidents or sometimes tumors. The rapid onset in an elderly individual suggests the former, whereas a more indolent course can be seen with tumors. When this speech pattern is encountered, the clinician should immediately focus attention on the dominant temporal lobe. Associated findings often include the superior quadrant anopia (Fig. 14-2), and temporal lobe seizures may be an associated phenomenon.

The other fluent aphasia, the conduction aphasia, does not appear as a seemingly psychiatric illness; thus it will not be discussed in detail. These patients speak fluently and usually make sense, except that they mix up words or make new words (paraphasic errors). Although they can repeat simple sentences, they have trouble with nonsense phrases like "no ifs, ands, or buts." The disease here localizes to the arcuate fasciculus of the parietal lobe connecting the temporal and frontal speech areas. Strokes and tumors are again the likely causes, although sometimes Wernicke's aphasia, as it resolves, tends to become a conduction aphasia. Anomic aphasia, in which the patient is fluent and behaviorally appropriate, but has trouble finding the proper word, is seen as other forms of aphasia resolve.

WERNICKE–KORSAKOFF'S SYNDROME

Wernicke–Korsakoff's syndrome, also known as Wernicke's encephalopathy–Korsakoff's psychosis, represents a neurologic emergency. The important triad of Wernicke's encephalopathy is behavioral alterations, extraocular movement abnormalities, and ataxia. These symptoms occur to a greater or lesser extent with a selective memory impairment, and when this memory impairment is marked the syndrome is then called Korsakoff's psychosis. The

two diseases are the same, but are referred to with different terms depending on the degree of memory deficit. The pathogenesis of this syndrome relates to vitamin deficiency in the form of vitamin B_1, or thiamine. Patients at high risk for this syndrome are, first, alcoholics who obtain calories through the alcohol but do not receive essential vitamins. Patients with prolonged emesis or with gastric bowel resection can also suffer with thiamine deficiency. Occasionally, voluntary starvation in the form of political protest, psychotic disturbances, or unsupervised treatment of obesity can also induce this syndrome. Finally, and important to surgical patients, hyperalimentation can be associated with Wernicke's encephalopathy when water-soluble B vitamins are not included in the formula.

The behavioral picture of Wernicke's encephalopathy–Korsakoff's psychosis ranges among three different presentations. The patient with acute Wernicke's encephalopathy shows global confusion and his demeanor is usually quiet and apathetic. He is alert and responsive, but inattentative, and he appears fatigued. Occasionally, a patient may be more agitated, especially if that patient is undergoing delirium tremens associated with alcohol withdrawal. The usual presentation, however, is one of an affable but dull affect.

In the partially treated patient or in the early stages of chronic disease, the affect becomes more bright, and the patient becomes more loquacious. The memory deficits become more apparent as the patient is less globally confused. He is nonhesitant in his speech, and it is at this point that the famed confabulatory aspects of Korsakoff's psychosis may be seen. Confabulation is not an essential component of Korsakoff's psychosis; the characteristic trait of this condition is the preferential loss of recent memory.

The patient with chronic Wernicke–Korsakoff's syndrome is typically alert and oriented but displays characteristic deficiencies in recent and remote memory. The recent memory deficit is usually profound and consists of an inability to make an enduring record of daily experiences. The remote memory deficit is temporally graded such that more remote events are relatively more accessible to recall. Thus, a patient asked to name presidents since World War II may recall Truman and Eisenhower but not their successors. Confabulation is not typically seen in chronic patients. Behaviorally, such patients are usually apathetic and indifferent, with occasional outbursts of irritability.

In diagnosing this syndrome, the neurologic signs of extraocular muscle palsy or nystagmus and ataxia are important features to recognize. In many ways, the patient with acute Wernicke's encephalopathy looks like a drunkard, in that he has trouble walking; he may have nystagmus from the alcohol itself; and he has an altered affect. Because of the similarity, it is a common adage that a patient seen in the emergency room who is drunk should be given an injection of thiamine (1) to treat possible Wernicke's encephalopathy and (2) to prevent a future episode of the condition. The chronic patient is difficult to manage because, although the extraocular movements improve quickly with thiamine therapy and the ataxia improves to a moderate extent, the memory problems are least abated by thiamine therapy. There has been new interest in the treatment of memory deficits with presumed cholinergic precusors like lecithin or choline chloride, but these agents have not been tested extensively. The dose of thiamine given is usually 50 mg intravenously (IV) and 50 mg intramuscularly (IM) or 100 mg muscularly. B vitamins should be continued orally until the patient resumes a normal diet.

ANATOMIC BASIS

The unifying basis for this disorder involves the Papez circuit where there is capillary proliferation at the level of the mamillary bodies. In some cases in which the mamillary bodies are spared, the anterior lobe of the thalamus is involved. Additional pathologic findings may involve cerebellar and diffuse cortical degeneration. Although the clinical picture of Korsakoff's psychosis should immediately suggest vitamin deficiency and disease that at least includes the mamillary bodies, it can be seen in diseases that involve other aspects of the Papez circuit. The same syndrome has been reported in patients who recover from a viral encephalitis with prominent hippocampus involvement. Such clinical overlap again emphasizes the importance of the Papez circuit in localizing diseases that involve both memory and affective disorders.

TRANSIENT GLOBAL AMNESIA

The syndrome of transient global amnesia occurs in middle-aged or elderly patients who usually have diabetes or hypertension, or who are at high risk for cerebrovascular disease. Physical or emotional stress often precedes the amnestic episode.

When the spell begins, the patient will be unable to learn new information from that time forward until the end of the spell. His memory for events that day and the preceding day are almost always poor. Memory for prior events will be better, although hazy memory losses will still be detectable sometimes even for events that took place years before the amnestic spell. The syndrome is transient and clears completely within 24 hours, except for a permanent amnesia for the episode itself. Significantly, the patient's affect is often bland during the episode, although family members are distressed.

These patients are often brought to medical attention when the family notes that they repeatedly ask the same questions and seem unable to remember the answer and sometimes deny that an answer has been given. At the same time, these patients may perform complex tasks during an episode without difficulty, as long as these tasks were learned prior to the event.

These patients are not globally confused. In testing orientation, however, they may report the wrong answer because they cannot integrate changes in place and time. When asked to do arithmetic calculations or use logical processing, they respond appropriately.

Memory testing during an attack demonstrates a marked inability to establish new memories despite preserved attention, language, and higher cognitive functioning. If the physician leaves the room of a patient with this disorder, he will have to reintroduce himself when he returns. Recent memory function is deficient in such patients regardless of which sensory system is employed in the memory tasks, so that visual, tactile, and auditory memories are disturbed. The retrograde amnesia is such that the activities of the previous days may be only dimly recollected during the episode. The retrograde amnesia is occasionally more extensive, affecting memories formed years before the episode. Confabulation is notably lacking in these patients. Upon recovery, there is no recollection of the episode itself, and there is typically a permanent retrograde amnesia for events occurring in the hour or so prior to the episode.

This syndrome with its peculiar constellation of memory and behavioral features can be highly confusing unless it is recognized.

The anatomic basis for transient global amnesia is felt to relate to poor vascular profusion to the posterior and undersurfaces of the temporal lobes by the vertebral basilar vessels. In this sense, it is a transient ischemic attack in almost all instances, although the prognosis for these patients has been said to be better than for those patients with other forms of transient ischemic attacks. Associated vertebral basilar symptoms, such as vertigo, nausea, and mild ataxia, may accompany this syndrome, but they clear quickly. Because this syndrome is so often a single episode without recurrence, it is important to identify it as such.

On the other hand, the additional features of impaired cognition (orientation, language, judgment), other focal neurologic signs or symptoms observed during or following the episode, or epileptic features or visual symptoms like flashing lights or a homonymous hemianopsia should prompt consideration of alternate diagnosis and further evaluation.

In patients whose amnesic episodes are brief (*e.g.*, less than one hour) and/or recurrent, temporal lobe epilepsy should be considered, and treatment with anticonvulsant medications can be successful. In patients with focal neurologic signs or symptoms during or subsequent to the amnesic episode, tumors and cerebrovascular disease should be considered, and the prognosis may be more guarded. If the amnesia includes additional disorientation and/or inattention, drug ingestion, especially with anticholinergic or sedative drugs, may be the cause.

Transient global amnesia is most often confused with psychogenic amnestic states. Hysterical amnesia may occur abruptly but is frequently associated with a specific precipitating event with retention of memory for other events within the time interval. One does not see the profound yet selective deficit in recent memory, nor the temporally graded retrograde amnesia.

In the more severe hysterical amnesia, such as in fugue states, there is the characteristic disassociative behavior with an additional loss of personal identity, a feature not seen in transient global amnesia. In contrast to the transient global amnesia patient, the hysterical patient will often acknowledge that the memory is poor, but will have an inappropriate affect, "*la belle indifférence.*"

Because the episodes tend not to recur, no pathologic studies have been performed on patients with typical transient global amnesia. The anatomic basis of this syndrome, however, is felt to relate to temporal lobe disease of the area involved in the Papez circuit. The combination of memory problems and bland affect helps to direct the clinician to focus on the Papez circuitry in the differential diagnosis.

The unifying points of this chapter have been that abnormal behavior can be a manifestation of focal neurologic disease, and the lesions responsible for such behaviors are mainly predictably located somewhere in or near the Papez circuit. Using the Papez circuit as the foundation, one has two major diagnostic advantages. First, one can analyze behavior with a systematic rigorous discipline provided by neuroanatomy. Second, because this is an anatomic circuit, one has the plasticity to integrate diseases that may be of different etiologies, affect different nuclei in the brain, and yet present with similar clinical presentations.

HERPES SIMPLEX ENCEPHALITIS

Herpes encephalitis affects primarily the temporal lobes and leads to necrosis and hemorrhagic destruction of brain tissue. The mortality rate in herpes simplex encephalitis has been reduced, but the prevalence of neurologic deficits among survivors remains high. These deficits are almost exclusively in the behavioral realm. Temporal lobe seizures already described are a common presenting feature of this disease. The most common sequela is an amnesia that can be isolated with sparing of other cognitive functions. The amnesia consists of an inability to form enduring memories. In more severe cases, the deficit in recent memory is accompanied by alterations in language, perception, and intelligence such that global dementia is seen. This linguistic disorder typically resembles a fluent aphasia with poor comprehension and paraphasic or nonsensical speech. Profound perceptual problems may also be seen; patients may be unable to recognize family members or friends (prosopagnosia) or common objects (visual agnosia). The most striking sequelae of herpes simplex encephalitis, however, are the often bizarre behavioral and emotional changes which, in the extreme, resemble those reported by Kluver and Bucy in primates after bilateral removal of the temporal lobes. In humans, the syndrome is sometimes referred to as a *limbic dementia* and consists, in addition to the visual agnosia, of emotional placidity, distractability, and alterations in sexual behavior. Thus, patients are often apathetic with flat affect and may show childlike compliance. In humans, the hypermetamorphosis consists of manual and oral exploration of the environment with placement of objects in the mouth. Episodes of bulimia may be seen along with ingestion of inappropriate material. The sexual changes consist primarily of inappropriate comments and overtures. The Kluver–Bucy syndrome is not diagnostically specific; the symptom complex may also be seen with head trauma, Alzheimer's disease, and Pick's disease. The behavioral alterations in herpes simplex encephalitis are typically less extreme than the full Kluver–Bucy syndrome and they consist of episodically inappropriate behavior, personality changes, delusions, and hyposexuality. Such behavioral sequelae are frequently viewed as psychogenic by the family and may be resistant to traditional forms of psychiatric treatment.

QUESTIONS AND DISCUSSION

1. Patients at high risk for developing Wernicke's encephalopathy include:

   A. Patients with posthepatitis cirrhosis
   B. Hospitalized patients receiving intravenous hyperalimentation
   C. Alcoholics
   D. Health food advocates who consume large quantities of B vitamins

The correct answers are (B) and (C). Wernicke's encephalopathy relates to thiamine deficiency. Patients who do not receive vitamins in hyperalimentation will eventually become depleted, as will patients whose dietary caloric intake involves only alcohol. Cirrhosis *per se* is not associated with water-soluble vitamin problems, and patients ingesting megavitamins may develop many other problems, but certainly not Wernicke's encephalopathy.

2. A patient says he has a seizure disorder. He is under arrest for having destroyed his friend's apartment and beaten up his girlfriend. He says, "I didn't mean to. I don't remember a thing." This behavior could represent TLE or could alternatively be antisocial behavior by a patient trying to plead ignorance. Along with an EEG, what facts will help you decide that the patient's behavior is probably related to a seizure?

   A. After an argument, the patient raced after his girlfriend, caught her in the parking lot, and beat her up.
   B. He was observed to exhibit picking movements of his hands and lip smacking before any belligerent behavior began.
   C. The fighting and destructive behavior oc-

curred when the girlfriend tried to restrain the patient from rising out of his chair.
   D. The patient says this happened three times before: "I know when I'm going into a spell because I hear a strange buzz in my ears. That's all I remember, everything else is a complete blank."

The correct answers are (B), (C), and (D). Automatisms like those described in (B) are common in TLE; the aura of primative auditory sensation is helpful, since the primary auditory cortex is in the temporal lobe. The destructive combative behavior should be *nondirected*—the patient will not chase after someone, but instead will be *combative* only if restrained or somehow confined. Running after his girlfriend in the midst of an argument and searching for her in a dark parking lot is a highly directed violent activity.

3. Transient global amnesia is felt to relate to vascular insufficiency in the distribution of which cerebral vessel or vessels?

   A. Frontal lobe anterior cerebral arteries
   B. Parietal lobe middle cerebral arteries
   C. Hippocampal posterior cerebral arteries
   D. Carotid arteries

The correct answer is (C). The vertebrobasilar system provides the vascular supply to the hippocampus, specifically by the posterior cerebral artery.

4. Other conditions besides transient global amnesia that are part of the differential diagnosis of amnestic syndromes include:

   A. Anticholinergic drug effect
   B. Psychomotor epilepsy
   C. Head trauma
   D. Migraine headaches

All are true, and it is important to consider clinically the differential diagnosis of amnestic syndromes.

5. Match the anatomic area of disease most consistently related to each clinical condition.

   A. Bilateral hippocampal regions
   B. Temporal lobe
   C. Mamillary bodies
   D. Dominant temporoparietal lobe

   1. Psychomotor epilepsy
   2. Transient global amnesia
   3. Wernicke's encephalopathy
   4. Fluent aphasia

The correct answers are (A) and (2); (B) and (1); (C) and (3); and (D) and (4).

6. During or after herpes encephalitis which of the following occur?

    A. Temporal lobe seizures
    B. Aphasia
    C. Amnesia
    D. Childlike affect and hypersexual behavior

The answers are (A), (B), (C), and (D).

During the encephalitis, and as a residual, seizures may occur and they may be difficult to control. Because the spells may not have generalized shaking, tongue biting, and incontinence associated with them, they may not be appreciated as epileptic aphasia. Especially fluent forms can occur, since the dominant temporal lobe may be diseased, and when both temporal lobes are affected, amnesia and Kluver–Bucy syndrome may occur.

SUGGESTED READING

Benson, DF: Aphasia, alexia, and agraphia. New York, Churchill Livingstone, 1979

Bogen JE: Wernicke's region—where is it? Ann NY Acad Sci 280:834, 1976

Engel J, Caldecott–Hazard S, Bandler R: Neurobiology of behavior: Anatomic and physiological implications related to epilepsy. Epilepsia (Suppl 2)27:53, 1986

Flor–Henry P: Lateralized temporal-limbic dysfunction and psychopathology. Ann NY Acad Sci 280:777, 1976

Geschwind N: Aphasia. N Engl J Med 284:654, 1971

Greenwood R, Bhalla A, Gordon A et al: Behaviour disturbance during recovery from herpes simplex encephalitis. J Neurol Neurosurg Psychiatry 46:809, 1983

Hanibert G: Emotional disturbance and temporal lobe injury. Compr Psychiatry 19:441, 1978

Hodges JR, Warlow CP: The aetiology of transient global amnesia: A case-control study of 114 cases with prospective follow-up. Brain 113:639, 1990

Luria AR, Hutton JT: Modern assessment of the basic forms of aphasia. Brain Lang 4:190, 1977

Papez JW: A proposed mechanism of emotion. Arch Neurol Psychiatry 38:725, 1937

Pincus JH, Tucker GJ: Behavioral Neurology. New York, Oxford University Press, 1974

Pritchard PB, Lombroso CT, McIntyre M: Psychological complications of temporal lobe epilepsy. Neurology 30:227, 1980

Victor M, Adams RD, Collins GH: Wernicke–Korsakoff's syndrome—a clinical and pathological study of 245 patients. Contemp Neurol Sci 1:1, 1971

Alzheimer's Disease and Other Dementias

David A. Bennett
Jacob H. Fox

Loss of cognitive function associated with age was recognized in antiquity. The concept of acquired dementia occurring prior to old age, however, developed more slowly. By the middle of the 19th century, neurosyphilis was recognized as a major cause of dementia in young and middle-aged persons; reports subsequently appeared describing cases of dementia associated only with cerebral atrophy. In the early 20th century, Alzheimer presented the clinical history and detailed postmortem findings of a 51-year-old woman with progressive dementia. For the next 60 years, the term *Alzheimer's disease* referred to an uncommon progressive dementia in young or middle-aged persons. The much more common dementia of older persons was attributed to the effects of cerebral atherosclerosis ("hardening of the arteries") or the inevitable manifestations of aging. In the past 25 years, however, it has become apparent that most of these elderly persons have Alzheimer's disease.

Many persons with dementia are cared for by their primary care physician; only a small proportion are managed in specialized dementia centers. Unfortunately, because physicians often do not look for or recognize dementia, many others are not recognized as having the condition. A recent survey found that many physicians do not take advantage of formal, published diagnostic criteria for dementia, and many do not perform structured mental status tests. Dementia often develops over

many years. For much of this time, the patient is not totally disabled and is more functional in a familiar and stable environment. Further, many families are determined to care for demented relatives. Therefore, despite the lack of effective therapy for cognitive dysfunction at this time, increased awareness of dementia enables physicians to more readily detect potentially treatable dementing conditions and to modify the effects of the less treatable conditions on the patient and family.

DEMENTIA

Dementia refers to acquired intellectual deterioration in an adult. Evaluating a person for dementia involves determining whether there has been a loss of cognitive function relative to a previous level of performance. Typically, evidence is obtained through the clinical history from a knowledgeable surrogate and is documented by mental status testing. In some situations, when the clinical history is not adequate, test results from a single evaluation can be contrasted with the estimated premorbid level of ability. In cases of progressive dementia, formal neuropsychological performance testing on two or more occasions over a period of 6 to 12 months may be necessary to document decline.

Criteria for dementia have been developed by the National Institute of Neurological and Communi-

195

cative Disorders and Stroke (NINCDS) and the Alzheimer's Disease and Related Disorders Association (ADRDA). The NINCDS–ADRDA criteria require unmistakable deterioration in at least two cognitive domains relative to the patient's previous level of function. This is determined by a history of intellectual decline and must be documented by formal mental status testing. The NINCDS–ADRDA criteria for dementia do not require that the loss of cognitive function be severe enough to interfere with impaired social and occupational functioning, as dictated by some other criteria.

The terms *benign senescent forgetfulness* and *age-associated memory impairment* have been proposed to refer to some persons with evidence of cognitive impairment who do not meet present clinical criteria for dementia. Some of these persons will, upon follow-up evaluation, develop dementia. At present, there is no way to make this prediction. When effective drug therapy for dementia becomes available, this issue will assume greater importance.

ALZHEIMER'S DISEASE

EPIDEMIOLOGY

Prevalence estimates suggest that Alzheimer's disease affects about 10% of persons over the age of 65, making it one of the most common chronic diseases of older persons. The occurrence of Alzheimer's disease is strongly related to age. Therefore, the rapid growth of the oldest population age groups is expected to have a profound effect on the public health problem posed by this disease.

Other than age, there are no well-documented risk factors for Alzheimer's disease. Persons with lower educational attainment may be at greater risk of Alzheimer's disease, as they are for developing many other common chronic diseases. It is usually assumed that low education is a marker for other variables important in the causation of disease. Head trauma, cigarette smoking, and aluminum exposure have also been evaluated.

CLINICAL FEATURES

The clinical evaluation of persons for Alzheimer's disease has four objectives: (1) to determine if the person has dementia; (2) if dementia is present, to determine whether its presentation and course are consistent with Alzheimer's disease; (3) to assess evidence for any alternate diagnoses, especially if the presentation and course are atypical for Alzheimer's disease; and (4) to evaluate evidence of other, coexisting, diseases that may contribute to the dementia, especially conditions that might respond to treatment. The clinical history should focus on the temporal relationship between the loss of different cognitive functions and the development of behavioral disturbances and impairment of physical function.

The most common initial symptom of Alzheimer's diseases is difficulty with memory. The family will report that the patient has left important tasks undone, such as bills unpaid and appointments not kept. The onset of this disease may be almost imperceptible but will typically progress to become a more serious problem in a few years' time. The family members will no longer feel comfortable leaving messages with the patient, and they will have to remind him about the same things innumerable times. After the memory disorder becomes apparent, the family will notice other disorders of cognition. Difficulty in balancing a checkbook is a common early complaint. Difficulty in carrying out normal occupational duties may also be seen if the patient is still employed. Confusion in following directions can also be a common earlier symptom, and if the patient is driving a car, he may get lost (an event that frequently precipitates the first evaluation by a physician). Frightening lapses of memory, such as leaving on a gas stove, may also occur.

As the disease progresses, difficulty in communication becomes more apparent. The patient may have difficulty in remembering simple words or names and may be unable to participate in normal conversation. Reading and writing will also be impaired, as will simple activities of daily living, such as bathing and dressing. The patient may not recognize family members, which causes the family great distress and dismay. The family will become afraid to leave the patient alone, and the patient will require constant attention.

Agitation, hallucination, delusions, and even violent outbursts may be seen at any time during the course of the illness. Previous personality traits may be exaggerated or may be obscured completely by new behavior patterns. Changes in sleep–wake patterns may also disrupt normal living patterns. These types of symptoms are particularly difficult for the family and place a great burden on the caregiver.

A general physical decline is not seen until the latest stages of the illness. Incontinence may be seen at any time and may initially reflect the patient's inability to find the bathroom. As the illness progresses, there seems to be a true loss of bladder control and ultimately even bowel function. The loss of the ability to walk is also said to be an occurrence seen at the late stages of the illness. This, however, may be due to excessive restraining and tranquilization in an institutional setting rather than to the natural history of the illness. Many patients with even the most profound dementia seem to maintain the ability to walk until some type of medical or orthopedic disaster occurs. An inability or unwillingness to eat and also seizures may occur in the later stages of Alzheimer's disease.

Atypical presentations can be seen in Alzheimer's disease. Patients with progressive aphasia, apraxia, and lengthy periods of isolated memory disorders may ultimately have Alzheimer's disease. The clinical diagnosis is less certain in these patients, and a neurologic consultation is appropriate.

The typical history in Alzheimer's disease is a gradually progressive dementia over several years. The average patient with Alzheimer's disease lives approximately 8 years from the onset of symptoms, although the variation may be from a few years to 20 years. There may be plateau periods during which a deterioration is not obvious; however, a lengthy plateau would be unusual in Alzheimer's disease. There is no clear evidence that the age of onset determines the natural history. Younger patients generally tend to have more speech disorders as the illness progresses, but longevity does not seem to vary significantly with the age of onset. Obviously, the older the patient, the more prone he is to other medical problems that might cause an early death. One question that is asked frequently by the family is whether the physician can predict the course of the illness. No proven methods are yet available to make predictions. Alzheimer's disease is associated with increased risk of death, especially among those patients in institutions. In the community, persons with Alzheimer's disease who have mild or moderate cognitive impairment have survival comparable to that of persons without the disease. By contrast, those with more severe cognitive impairment or cachexia have a much greater risk of dying.

DIAGNOSIS

Formal, standardized assessment of cognition is required to make a diagnosis of dementia and Alzheimer's disease. A wide range of measures are available for this purpose. Several brief measures (*e.g.*,

the Mini–Mental Status Examination and the Blessed Orientation, Memory Concentration Test) are suitable for use at the bedside or in the physician's office. Although they may help distinguish persons with dementia from persons without dementia, they are less effective in distinguishing Alzheimer's disease from other dementias.

In the office or hospital, routine mental status testing should include checking the patient's orientation by asking for his full name, the day of the week, the day of the month, the month and the year, where he is, and also his age and date of birth. Show the patient four or five objects and then ask him to name them twice (*e.g.*, a coin, safety pin, keys, and a comb). Tell the patient that you will ask him to recall the objects in a few minutes. Then check the patient's knowledge of common events by asking him for the names of well-known public figures (*e.g.*, the president, governor, or mayor). Ask the patient to repeat some numbers (the typical patient can remember six numbers forward and three or four backward). Then ask him to do some simple calculations (*e.g.*, multiplication, addition, and "serial sevens"). Ask the patient to repeat a simple phrase; to follow a two-step direction (*e.g.*, "point to the ceiling, then point to the floor"); and to do something with his right hand and then his left hand (*e.g.*, "make a fist with your left hand," followed by "salute with your right hand"). Ask the patient to write his name; to write a brief phrase to dictation (*e.g.*, "Today is Monday"); and then to draw something (usually a clock). Also ask the patient to read a simple phrase. Finally, ask him to recall the four or five objects that you showed him previously.

This mental status test can be administered in a few minutes and gives the clinician much of the required information. In order to make a diagnosis of dementia, a deficit should exist in more than one area of cognition. Patients with early Alzheimer's disease may have profound memory problems with only mild deficits in other aspects of cognition. As the disease progresses, language and other aspects of cognitive dysfunction typically become more obvious.

PHYSICAL EXAMINATION

The most important function of the neurologic examination in evaluating persons with dementia is in diagnosing conditions other than Alzheimer's disease. The general physical examination is usually normal in Alzheimer's disease. The neurologic examination (excluding the mental status testing) is also usually normal. Minor parkinsonian features (rigidity and bradykinesia), myoclonic jerks, frontal lobe signs (grasp reflex, snout and glabellar signs), and similar abnormalities on examination may occasionally be seen, especially later in the course of the illness. Any other significant abnormality of the neurologic examination should alert the physician to the possibility of a diagnosis other than Alzheimer's disease.

GENETICS

Evidence suggests that there is a genetic component to Alzheimer's disease. In some families, several members may be affected in a pattern consistent with an autosomal dominant mechanism of inheritance, and there are reports that Alzheimer's disease is linked, in some families, to the 21st chromosome. First-degree relatives of patients with Alzheimer's disease may also be at an increased risk for development of the disease. Second, although the concordance rate for monozygotic twins is less than 100%, it is higher than for dizygotic twins. Finally, nearly all persons with Down's syndrome develop the pathology of Alzheimer's disease, an observation that has focused attention on the role of the 21st chromosome in Alzheimer's disease (see sections on pathology and etiology).

LABORATORY INVESTIGATION

There is no reliable antemortem diagnostic test for Alzheimer's disease. The purpose of laboratory testing is to identify other conditions that might cause or exacerbate dementia. These tests routinely include a brain scan and blood tests (see Table 15-1).

The purpose of morphologic imaging with magnetic resonance imaging (MR) or computed tomography (CT) is to look for evidence of another disease process that can cause or contribute to cognitive impairment, including stroke, tumor, or hydrocephalus. MR is superior to CT because it is subject to less artifact, it provides greater contrast

TABLE 15-1. Laboratory Aids in the Differential Diagnosis of Dementia

ROUTINE TESTS	CONDITIONS
Vitamin B_{12}	B_{12} deficiency
T4 or TSH	Hypothyroidism
RPR, FTA, MHA-TP	Syphilis
Brain scan (CT or MR)	Vascular disease (MR more sensitive but less specific), mass lesions, hydrocephalus, demyelinating diseases and leukodystrophies (MR superior)

OTHER TESTS	CONDITIONS
Lumbar puncture	Chronic meningitis, syphilis, inflammatory disease(s)
Electroencephalography	Creutzfeld–Jacob disease, epilepsy
Single photon emission computed tomography	Pick's disease and frontal lobe dementias
Drug screen/levels	Delirium due to drug toxicity
Heavy metal screen	Lead, mercury, arsenic, copper poisoning
Sedimentation rate autoimmune profile	Inflammatory disease(s)
Angiography	Inflammatory disease(s)
Cerebral biopsy	Inflammatory disease(s)
Chemistry profile	Chronic metabolic disturbances, endocrinopathies
Complete blood count	Chronic infections, anemia
Human immunodeficiency virus	HIV encephalopathy
Ceruloplasmin	Wilson's disease
Long-chain fatty acids	Adrenoleukodystrophy
Arylsulfatase A	Metachromatic leukodystrophy
Chest x-ray	Cardiopulmonary disease, lung tumors
Electrocardiogram	Cardiopulmonary disease

between gray and white matter, and coronal images which provide excellent views of the mesial temporal lobes can easily be obtained. With agitated patients, however, CT is often preferred because the image can be obtained more quickly. There is also strong research interest in using morphologic imaging as a direct diagnostic tool for Alzheimer's disease. At the present, these are not at the stage of being suitable for wide clinical use.

Single photon emission computed tomography (SPECT) imaging reflects cerebral blood flow and is used as an index of local cerebral metabolic rate. Although SPECT and positron emission tomography (PET) are useful research tools, these procedures are not currently at a stage at which they are clinically useful tests for the presence of Alzheimer's disease.

DIFFERENTIAL DIAGNOSIS

The differential diagnosis of dementia should emphasize potentially treatable disorders that may cause, or exacerbate, dementia. Although reversible disorders are uncommon, their importance justifies a thorough evaluation of each patient.

TOXIC/METABOLIC CONDITIONS

Many toxic/metabolic conditions produce a delirium, and rarely dementia. Delirium differs from dementia by the onset and duration of cognitive impairment, and level of consciousness. The onset of cognitive impairment in delirium is typically hours or days, and it lasts days to weeks; in addition, patients are either hyper- or hypoalert.

Drug toxicity is a common reversible cause of delirium in the elderly. Older persons may be more susceptible than younger persons to drug side effects on cognition. This is due to many factors, including altered drug kinetics and use of multiple medications in older persons with several illnesses or complaints ("polypharmacy"). Clinicians should also be alert to the possibility of drug side effects further impairing cognition in persons with pre-existing cognitive impairment. A typical presentation is the rapid worsening of dementia following the administration of a new drug (or following the reinstitution of a previous medication that the patient has not taken for some time), with or without altered level of consciousness. Psychotropics such as neuroleptics and sedative–hypnotics, and cardiovascular medications, especially antihypertensives, are common offending agents.

METABOLIC AND HEMATOLOGIC DISORDERS

Hypothyroidism has been recognized for many years as being associated with an organic brain syndrome. Although clinical manifestations of myxedema are usually seen, a patient may occasionally present with dementia without other manifestations of hypothyroidism. Similar cases are seen with disorders of calcium metabolism, especially hypercalcemia, and also with an electrolyte imbalance.

Chronic liver and renal disease are frequently associated with an organic brain syndrome. However, it is unusual for these diseases to be present without prominent manifestations of the primary illnesses. Repeated episodes of hypoglycemia can cause dementia, although in this case, the history is usually clearly episodic rather than gradual.

Pernicious anemia can cause an organic brain syndrome even without hematologic or other neurologic findings. Whether this is also true for folate deficiency is unclear. Various types of neurologic dysfunction have been reported with folate deficiency, including organic brain syndromes. There are some cases in the literature of organic brain syndromes without any other findings that did reverse with folic acid treatment. This deficiency syndrome, however, is not as clearly described as that of B_{12}.

Korsakoff's syndrome, due to thiamine deficiency, presents with an anterograde amnesia in which the patient is unable to learn new information. Classically, it develops in the wake of an acute Wernicke's encephalopathy with confusion, ophthalmoplegia, and ataxia. However, many patients with Korsakoff's syndrome do not present with a Wernicke's encephalopathy. Although alcoholism is the most frequent setting for this syndrome in developed countries, it may also be associated with other conditions leading to nutritional deficiency, including starvation, malnutrition, protracted vomiting, and gastric resection. It can also be precipitated by administration of carbohydrates to patients with marginal thiamine stores.

VASCULAR DEMENTIA

Vascular dementia includes all dementia syndromes resulting from ischemic, anoxic, or hypoxic brain damage. It is, therefore, a markedly heterogeneous group of conditions. The concept of multi-infarct dementia (MID) suggests that vascular dementia is due to the combined effect of multiple, discrete cerebral infarctions. However, currently, the classification of the vascular dementia syndromes is unsettled, and MID is now considered one of many vascular dementia syndromes.

A history of multiple strokes, an abnormal physical examination with focal neurologic findings, and the presence of vascular risk factors in a person with dementia are suggestive of vascular disease but do not prove that the dementia is related to cerebrovascular disease. Both Alzheimer's disease and stroke are common among older persons. They often occur in the same individual by chance alone. Therefore, it is important that an attempt be made to temporally relate the onset, or worsening, of cognitive impairment to a stroke. There is no typical neuropsychological profile of persons with vascular dementia, as the behavioral manifestations are dependent on the vascular territory involved, and this may differ widely among patients. However, persons with vascular dementia rarely present with the insidious onset of memory loss characteristic of early Alzheimer's disease.

Recently, white matter lesions on MR or CT have attracted considerable attention. Although white matter lesions are commonly found in elderly persons, their etiology and significance remain controversial. Many demented persons with white matter lesions on MR or CT have Alzheimer's disease at autopsy. Therefore, although the presence of vascular dementia should be supported by evidence of vascular disease on CT or MR, the presence of these lesions does not necessarily indicate that the dementia is of vascular origin.

Careful control of vascular risk factors such as hypertension and cigarette smoking may alter the natural history of this illness. The value of drugs such as aspirin in preventing the progression of MID is still unknown.

Vasculitides can also cause cognitive dysfunction and psychiatric symptoms, often associated with focal motor signs and seizures. An elevated Westergren erythrocyte sedimentation rate often suggests that further evaluation for a specific immunologic disease is warranted. Further evaluation may require electroencephalography, cerebrospinal fluid studies, and/or angiography. In some cases, meningeal and cerebral artery biopsy are necessary for definitive diagnosis.

SYMPTOMATIC HYDROCEPHALIC DEMENTIA

No other syndrome causing dementia has generated such intense interest (and frustration) among neurologists as normal pressure hydrocephalus. The syndrome consists of gait disturbance, dementia, and incontinence. The onset usually occurs over several months, although the disease may present more acutely. As opposed to Alzheimer's disease, the dementia is mild compared with the gait disturbances, although some cases have been associated with prominent dementia without major gait abnormalities.

Brain scans typically demonstrate hydrocephalus with enlargement of ventricles out of proportion to sulci. Several studies have attempted to determine predictors of improvement following ventricular shunting. Useful clinical indices include motor signs preceding cognitive dysfunction, short duration of dementia prior to surgery, and the presence of a known cause, such as traumatic or spontaneous subarachnoid hemorrhage, meningitis, or partial obstruction.

Some patients with gait problems or dementia will improve with CSF shunting procedures; however, the insertion of a shunt is not a benign procedure, especially in geriatric patients. Those patients with dementia and prominent gait problems and those patients with a previous history of meningitis, subarachnoid hemorrhage, or serious head trauma should be considered as candidates for the normal pressure hydrocephalus syndrome. When the patient is younger, the gait problem greater, and the onset of dementia more recent, the approach to treatment should be more vigorous.

DEPRESSION

Loss of interest in hobbies and community activities, apathy, weight loss, and sleep disorders may be interpreted by the family as depression, although they actually may result only from dementia. In some cases, depression coexists with dementia. It is useful to ask the caregiver about symptoms suggesting dysphoric mood such as crying, complaining, or even suicidal ideation. Depression may contribute to impairment of activities of daily living, and rarely to the cognitive deficits. If impairment in activities of daily living exceeds what is expected for the severity of cognitive dysfunction, the possibility of a coexisting depression should be considered. Pseudodementia, a syndrome of depression with impaired cognition in which treatment of the depression relieves the cognitive deficit, has been described but is probably rare.

INFECTIONS

Cognitive impairment is the most common neurologic manifestation of acquired immunodeficiency syndrome (AIDS) and may precede the development of other signs of infection with the human immunodeficiency virus (HIV). Patients with the AIDS dementia complex present with forgetfulness and poor attention, typically over several months. The memory impairment is typically less striking than that seen in Alzheimer's disease. Other signs of AIDS should be sought, and, if found, a high index of suspicion for other infections should be maintained.

Chronic meningitis, especially cryptoccal meningitis, can present as dementia, although there are almost always other associated signs and symptoms. The same can be said for neurosyphilis. Brain abscesses, like brain tumors, can present solely with dementia, although focal findings are usually also present. Creutzfeldt–Jakob disease has been shown to be caused by a slow virus. Its onset is subacute rather than chronic, and there are other neurologic abnormalities such as myoclonic jerks, extrapyramidal findings, and visual disturbances, as well as the organic brain syndrome. Its significance far outweighs its frequency in that similar causes are being suggested for some of the other illnesses.

MASS LESIONS

Brain tumors are frequently associated with organic brain syndromes. Classically, there are also major focal findings and signs of increased intracranial pressure. However, it is well recognized that brain tumors, especially in the "silent" areas of the brain, may present exclusively as a change of personality and intellectual decline. Subtle focal findings can usually be demonstrated on the neurologic examination, but they are occasionally lacking. Similar comments may be applied to subdural hematomas, especially in the geriatric age group.

PARKINSON'S DISEASE

Dementia is common among persons with Parkinson's disease. It is unclear at this time to what extent this reflects the coincidental occurrence of two diseases of the elderly. Clearly, however, many persons with Parkinson's disease with dementia do not have concomitant Alzheimer's disease. The dementia of Parkinson's disease has been referred to as "subcortical" dementia, characterized by forgetfulness, slowing of thought processes, apathy or depression, and an inability to manipulate acquired knowledge. The term, however, is controversial and should be considered a syndrome or symptom complex. Whether it serves as a useful construct remains a matter of debate.

PICK'S DISEASE

Pick's disease is a degenerative dementia of unknown etiology. Clinically similar cases, often called *lobar dementia* or *dementia of the frontal lobe type*, may have the same pathogenesis. Classically, personality changes precede intellectual decline. When cognitive changes begin, language may be affected before memory. MR or CT scans may reveal predominantly frontal and temporal lobe atrophy.

PATHOLOGY

The general pathologic features of Alzheimer's disease have been described. Grossly, there is atrophy and dilatation of the ventricles. Microscopically, there are large numbers of neuritic plaques and neurofibrillary tangles. Both of these lesions can be seen in the brains of older persons without dementia; however, they are found in greater numbers in the neocortex, hippocampus, and amygdala in persons with Alzheimer's disease. The current pathologic criteria for Alzheimer's disease, in fact, are based on the demonstration of a sufficient number of neuritic plaques and neurofibrillary tangles on microscopic examination. It is not clear at this time, however, whether there is a qualitative difference between these pathologic indices in persons with dementia *vs* persons without dementia.

Plaques are composed of a central extracellular proteinaceous amyloid core, surrounded by dystrophic axon terminals. Some evidence suggests that amyloid is neurotoxic and that its deposition is the initial event in plaque formation. By contrast, others propose that it accumulates after the neurites degenerate. Of interest is the fact that the amyloid comes from a larger precursor protein coded on the 21st chromosome, and a point mutation in this gene has been reported in some families with Alzheimer's disease.

The major constituents of neurofibrillary tangles are paired helical filaments. Evidence suggests that these tangles may be composed of abnormally phosphorylated proteins. The mechanism of this process is currently under intense investigation.

Cerebrovascular amyloid (amyloid angiopathy) is also a common finding in persons with Alzheimer's disease, as are granulovacuolar degeneration and Hirano bodies.

ETIOLOGY AND PATHOGENESIS

The only well-documented risk factor for Alzheimer's disease is age. Despite extensive investigations over the past several years, including intoxications with metals (*e.g.*, aluminum and mercury), viral infections, and disordered immune function, the etiology of Alzheimer's disease remains an enigma. As already mentioned, there appears to be a genetic component to Alzheimer's disease, and most efforts are now aimed at elucidating the mechanism of plaque and tangle formation. The fact that the clinical manifestations and rate of progression vary considerably among individuals within families or twin pairs suggests that, as with most chronic diseases, environmental factors may interact with genetic susceptibility to produce Alzheimer's disease.

TREATMENT

Currently, there is no effective pharmacotherapy for the cognitive dysfunction in Alzheimer's disease. However, there are many areas in which intervention can improve quality of life for both the patient and the caregiver. Successful intervention requires that the physician work effectively with providers of many other medical and nonmedical services. In general, four areas should be discussed with the family: (1) community resources, (2) advocacy, (3) behavior management, and (4) experimental therapies and procedures.

COMMUNITY RESOURCES

Most major cities now have a local chapter of the ADRDA (now called the Alzheimer Association). The address and phone number of the local chapter can be obtained from the national headquarters at 70 East Lake Street, Chicago, IL, 60601, 312-853-3060 or 800-572-6037. The association provides information regarding local support services for both the patient and the caregiver from other persons facing similar problems. Community services include adult day-care programs, inpatient and outpatient respite care programs, nursing home special care units, and hospice services.

Most patients with Alzheimer's disease in the mild to moderate stage can be cared for at home, assuming a caregiver is available and willing to assume this responsibility. This decision can only be made by the family. It is not appropriate for the physician (or others not involved in daily care) to insist on home care when the family finds this objectionable. Many patients do well in the day-care setting, and this greatly alleviates the burden on the caregiver. Family support groups, usually sponsored by the Alzheimer Association, are also helpful. The caregiver's mental and physical health

must be maintained. This ultimately benefits the patient since a sane, healthy caregiver can manage a patient with Alzheimer's disease longer and better than one who is overwrought and exhausted. The caregiver must have rest, and other family members should be urged to take turns in caring for the patient. Nursing home placement, however, is ultimately chosen by most families at the later stages of the illness. The family should be advised to seek out a nursing home where activities and exercise are stressed and where tranquilizers and restraints are minimized.

Lastly, it must be stressed that Alzheimer's disease places a tremendous social, economic, physical, and psychological burden on the family. The psychological stress on the family is frequently not dealt with adequately. Stress is placed on the family in general, and particularly on the caregiver. Informal counseling through family self-help groups and formal psychological counseling may be necessary. The physician should be available and supportive throughout the course of the illness.

When the patient's death is drawing near, an open discussion of the family's desire for intervention should be initiated. A family occasionally feels that aggressive intervention is mandatory to the very end. Most families, however, are against resuscitation and life-support equipment. Patients with Alzheimer's disease may end up intubated and on respirators because the physician has never discussed the question of resuscitation with the family. The physician's role is obviously to be supportive and informative. Most families have a clear feeling of what the patient would have wanted and they need only be asked in advance.

ADVOCACY

Because patients with Alzheimer's disease may eventually lose all decision-making capabilities, it is important that, at the time of the initial diagnosis, the physician alert the patient and family of the need to make decisions regarding living wills and trusts, power of attorney, and guardianship. The determination of power of attorney or guardianship is fundamental to making economic or ethical decisions regarding the care of the patient. Many patients with mild cognitive impairment are legally competent to execute a valid power of attorney, placing in the hands of another person decisions regarding his health and estate. Guardianship must be imposed upon a patient who has become incompetent to render informed consent. Advice in legal matters by a competent and sympathetic attorney is often of great value.

Dementia appears to be a risk factor for unsafe motor vehicle operation. Although most demented persons stop driving on their own, or after encouragement from family members, many others continue to drive after disease onset. This can be a particular problem in this age-group, in which many of the women do not drive.

BEHAVIORAL MANAGEMENT

The course of Alzheimer's disease is often punctuated by neuropsychiatric disturbances. Among these, depression, alterations of sleep–wake cycles, and aggressiveness may respond to pharmacologic intervention. Few controlled studies exist from which to guide the dose and duration of pharmacotherapy. In persons with dementia and depression, studies of imipramine, L-deprenyl, and methylphenidate have demonstrated marginal efficacy. In persons with disturbances of sleep, a low-dose, sedating neuroleptic may be preferable to hypnotics for the nondepressed Alzheimer's disease patient with a significant sleep disorder. Persons with coexistent depression should be treated with an antidepressant.

Physical aggression may have the most severe consequences for the family, eventually leading to institutionalization of the patient. Numerous studies have addressed the pharmacologic management of behavioral disturbances among patients with Alzheimer's disease. The majority of studies, focusing on neuroleptics such as thioridazine, haloperidol, and loxapine, have shown small benefits. Thioridazine, starting at 10 mg in the evening, can be tried. It can be gradually (e.g., each week) increased. The more potent neuroleptics should be reserved for the acutely and uncontrollably agitated patient. It is important to be aware of side effects such as increased confusion and extrapyramidal signs.

EXPERIMENTAL TREATMENT

Several neurotransmitter systems that appear to be affected in Alzheimer's disease and play a role in the cognitive dysfunction provide the basis of neurotransmitter replacement therapy. Dysfunction of the cholinergic system in Alzheimer's disease and evidence that this system is involved in human cognition spawned numerous clinical trials of cholinergic agents. Investigations following five basic strategies (precursor loading, increasing release, decreasing degradation, activating receptors,

or stimulating the intracellular second messengers) have met with limited success. Several other neurotransmitter systems and peptidergic systems are also affected in Alzheimer's disease. Agents affecting these systems, however, have also met disappointing results. Ergoloid mesylate (Hydergine) is the only drug currently approved by the Food and Drug Administration for use in dementia. However, despite numerous therapeutic trials, its efficacy has never been firmly established.

QUESTIONS AND DISCUSSION

1. A 75-year-old man with a 2-year history of gradually declining cognitive function presents with an acute worsening of his mental status, hallucinations, and a decreased level of consciousness. What may be going on?

   A. Alzheimer's disease
   B. Chronic tubercular meningitis
   C. Alzheimer's disease with a new superimposed infection
   D. Alzheimer's disease and a change in the patient's living environment

The answers are (C) and (D). The 2-year history of declining cognitive function resembles Alzheimer's disease, but the acute deterioration suggests more of a "toxic encephalopathy" in the context of preexisting Alzheimer's disease. Major diagnostic considerations would include the recent use of drugs that may impair cognition, some type of febrile illness, or a metabolic disturbance. The work-up would usually consist of drug screen and systemic blood work. Occasionally, a new focal process can also cause this, such as a cerebral infarct or hemorrhage in one of the "silent" areas of the brain. If a careful examination reveals no focal abnormalities, and the diagnosis remains dubious, a CT scan or MR scan should be done. A patient who has recently moved to a new environment may also decompensate suddenly since he no longer has the social cues and references that aided him previously.

2. What is the current status of treatment for Alzheimer's disease?

   A. Lecithin is advocated for reversing memory loss and preventing strokes.
   B. Agitation can be treated, but physicians must be careful to avoid oversedation.

C. Aspirin is effective in dilating cerebral blood vessels.

The answer is (B). Unfortunately, no direct treatment for Alzheimer's disease is currently available. Attempts at the replacement of acetylcholine and other neurotransmitters have been unsuccessful, although therapeutic trials are continuing.

Complications of Alzheimer's disease can be treated. Agitated behavior is the most common complication, and the major tranquilizers can be useful in this context. The physician should be careful to use no more than the exact amount of medication required, because patients with Alzheimer's disease are particularly sensitive to the side effects of these medications.

3. What is the clinical difference between Alzheimer's disease and multi-infarct dementia?

A. CT scanning will detect differences.
B. Multi-infarct dementia is more rapidly progressive and is associated with depression.
C. Multi-infarct dementia is usually accompanied by other focal signs in addition to the mental decline.
D. The two terms are synonymous.

The answer is (C). There is no absolute way of differentiating these two clinical syndromes. The history in Alzheimer's disease is generally that of a gradual progressive dementia with a normal general neurologic examination and an imaging procedure that shows atrophy. The medical history is also usually negative. The more characteristic picture of multi-infarct dementia is that of a stepwise deterioration in neurologic function with a background of risk factors for cerebrovascular disease, particularly hypertension. Minor focal abnormalities might be found in the neurologic examination, although not always, and imaging procedures, particularly MR scanning, may show signs of numerous small infarcts. A significant number of patients, particularly elderly ones, have elements of both syndromes and, therefore, complete differentiation is sometimes impossible.

SELECTED REFERENCES

Bennett DA, Evans DA: Alzheimer's disease. DM 34:1, 1992

Bennett DA, Gilley DW, Wilson RS et al: Clinical correlates of high signal lesions on magnetic resonance imaging in Alzheimer's disease. J Neurol 239:186, 1992

Breitner JCS, Murphy EA, Folstein MF et al: Twin studies of Alzheimer's disease: An approach to etiology and prevention. Neurobiol Aging 11: 641, 1990

Cummings JL, Benson DF: Dementia: A Clinical Approach, 2nd ed. Boston, Butterworth–Heinemann, 1992

Evans DA, Scherr PA, Cook NR et al: Estimated prevalence of Alzheimer's disease in the United States. Milbank Mem Fund Q 68:267, 1990

Folstein MR, Folstein SE, McHugh PR: "Mini-mental state": A practical method for granting the cognitive state of patients for the clinician. J Psychiatr Res 12:189, 1975

Gilley DW, Wilson RS, Bennett DA et al: Cessation of driving and unsafe motor vehicle operation by dementia patients. Arch Intern Med 151:941, 1991

Jarvik LF, Berg L, Bartus R et al: Clinical drug trials in Alzheimer's disease: What are some of the issues? Alzheimer Dis Assoc Disord 4:193, 1990

Katzman R, Jackson JE: Alzheimer's disease: Basic and clinical advances. J Am Geriatr Soc 39:516, 1991

Mayeux R: Therapeutic strategies in Alzheimer's disease. Neurology 40:175, 1990

Schneider LS, Pollock VE, Lyness SA: A meta-analysis of controlled trials of neuroleptic treatment in dementia. J Am Geriatr Soc 38:553, 1990

Neurotoxic Effects of Drugs Prescribed by Non-Neurologists

Christopher G. Goetz
Cynthia L. Comella

Neurotoxicology is a growing field of clinical interest, and physicians are increasingly required to evaluate and treat patients with numerous complications of toxic exposure. The usual compounds discussed in a chapter on neurotoxicology would include metals (*e.g.*, lead, mercury, and arsenic), industrial toxins (*e.g.*, organic solvents, gases, pesticides, and other environmental toxins), and biologic toxins (*e.g.*, bacterial exotoxins, animal poisons, venoms, and botanical poisons). Syndromes associated with these toxins, however, are not frequently encountered by the non-neurologist. On the other hand, many drugs that are commonly prescribed by treating physicians may precipitate neurotoxic signs or exacerbate underlying neurologic disease. The neurologic complications of drugs commonly prescribed for the medical management of ambulatory adults are discussed in this chapter.

ANTIBIOTICS

PENICILLINS

Penicillin and related agents rarely cause nervous system toxic effects, although seizures and myoclonic jerks have been reported with high intravenous (IV) doses. Such effects appear more commonly in elderly patients with compromised renal function. Meningitic inflammation may enhance neurotoxic effects by promoting the penetration of these drugs into the central nervous system (CNS) and decreasing their egress. Polyneuritis with paresthesias, paralysis, and loss of tendon reflexes has also been reported.

AMINOGLYCOSIDES

The toxicity of all aminoglycoside antibiotics, *neomycin, kanamycin, streptomycin, gentamycin, tobramycin,* and *amikacin,* are similar. The two major adverse effects are (1) damage of the eighth cranial nerve and hearing apparatus, and (2) a potentiation of neuromuscular blockade. Cochlear and vestibular damage is the result of direct toxicity of these drugs. Auditory toxicity is more common with the use of amikacin and kanamycin, whereas vestibular toxicity predominates following gentamycin and streptomycin therapy. Tobramycin is associated equally with vestibular and auditory damage. The incidence of clinical ototoxicity due to these drugs ranges from 5% to 25% depending on whether audiometry is used to detect hearing deficits. Aminoglycoside hearing loss is usually irreversible and may even progress following the discontinuation of drug therapy.

A potentially fatal neurotoxic effect of all aminoglycosides is a neuromuscular blockade. The aminoglycosides act similarly to curare and block the

William J. Weiner and Christopher G. Goetz, eds. *Neurology for the Non-Neurologist*, Third Edition. Copyright © 1994, 1989 by J. B. Lippincott Company. Copyright © 1981 by Harper and Row Publishers, Inc.

neuromuscular junction. Aminoglycosides also possibly potentiate ether and other anesthetics during surgery. Sudden or prolonged respiratory paralysis due to aminoglycosides may be reversed by the administration of calcium or neostigmine.

ANTIFUNGAL AGENTS

The *polymyxins* are related closely to the aminoglycosides in structure and neurotoxicity. The incidence of neurotoxic reaction has been estimated at 7%, and syndromes other than neuromuscular blockade include paresthesias, peripheral neuropathy, dizziness, and seizures. Respiratory paralysis, however, is the most serious neurotoxic reaction. An underlying renal dysfunction predisposes to the neuromuscular blockade induced by this drug group. Signs of neuromuscular blockade include diplopia, dysphagia, and weakness.

Amphotericin B is widely used against systemic fungal infection. When the drug is used intrathecally, seizures, pain along the lumbar nerves, mononeuropathies (including foot drop), and chemical meningitis have occurred.

ANTITUBERCULOUS DRUGS

Isoniazid (INH) has been associated with neurotoxic effects felt to be related to drug binding of pyridoxine and resultant excessive vitamin excretion. A prominent polyneuropathy is associated with chronic INH administration, and symptoms include paresthesias, diminished pain, touch, and temperature discrimination, and eventual weakness. Seizures, emotional irritability, euphoria, depression, headache, and psychosis may rarely occur. The neurotoxic reactions due to INH are dose-related and are more common in "slow inactivators." In these patients, neurotoxic reactions can be prevented or diminished by the administration of pyridoxine at a dose of 50 mg daily. Patients who intentionally or inadvertently overdose acutely with INH may develop severe ataxia, generalized seizures, and coma. Supportive measures, anticonvulsants, and pyridoxine should be administered to these patients.

Rifamycin is frequently administered with INH. Neurologic side effects are uncommon but may include headache, dizziness, inability to concentrate, and confusion. Less commonly, signs of peripheral neuropathy may develop. *Ethambutol* precipitates a reversible optic neuritis, as well as a more generalized peripheral neuropathy. A metallic taste in the oral cavity is frequently associated with ethambutol therapy and may be due to an impairment of receptor activity.

ANTIVIRAL DRUGS

The treatment of selected viral infections in non–HIV-positive individuals has become possible over the past few years. The neurologic complications of HIV and the drugs used to treat it will be discussed elsewhere.

Acyclovir can be administered either intravenously or orally. Acyclovir is used orally for the treatment of localized or ophthalmic varicella zoster, treatment of minor herpes simplex virus, and reducing the severity of varicella. Neurologic side effects are rarely associated with oral acyclovir. However, seizures, encephalopathy, hallucinations, and coma have been described, as has tremor.

Amantadine has been used to prevent influenza A infections. This agent, in addition to its antiviral action, also appears to have anticholinergic and dopaminergic effects, which has lead to its use in mild Parkinson's disease. The neurologic side effects associated with amantadine include sedation, confusion, myoclonus, hallucinations, delirium, and seizures. As amantadine is excreted through the kidney, the presence of renal impairment may reduce its clearance, causing it to accumulate in the body and resulting in amantadine toxicity.

OTHER COMMONLY PRESCRIBED ANTIBIOTICS

Sulfonamide, pyrimethamine, and *trimethoprim* are used mainly in the treatment of urinary tract infections (UTIs). They are generally considered safe drugs and are not associated with marked neurotoxicity. They may, however, cause headache, fatigue, tinnitus, and acute psychosis. Some signs may mimic meningitis. On the second or third day of therapy, patients may complain of difficulty in concentrating and impaired judgment. *Nitrofurantoin* is also used commonly in the treatment of UTIs. A polyneuropathy is the major toxic syndrome with this drug. Similar to the Guillain–Barré syndrome, this neuropathy is usually subacute and begins in the distal extremities, often with sensory complaints of paresthesias and numbness. The neuropathy ascends and involves the motor system with progressive weakness and areflexia. The discontinuation of the drug is essential, and not all patients will recover. The prognosis appears to relate most significantly to the extent of the neuropathy at the time of drug withdrawal.

Chloramphenicol has been associated with toxic encephalopathy and symptoms of confusion and delirium when high doses were used. Underlying neoplastic disease and liver and renal dysfunction may predispose to excessive drug accumulation and toxic encephalopathy. A reversible optic neuritis has been associated with prolonged therapy with high doses (>2 g/kg). The optic neuropathy is sudden in onset and is associated with decreased visual acuity and ocular pain. Ototoxicity has been associated with chloramphenicol installation into the middle ear, although patients had multiple drug therapy in most cases. Finally, a peripheral neuropathy may occur, and this complication often accompanies the optic neuropathy. The neuropathy is predominantly sensory, so that patients complain of numbness and paresthesias. In patients who are receiving phenytoin or phenobarbital, chloramphenicol will inhibit the metabolism of these drugs so that there will be a marked elevation in anticonvulsant blood levels in these patients. This effect occurs quickly, and therefore immediate adjustment of the anticonvulsant dose must be effected to avoid toxicity. The practical management of seizure patients who require chloramphenicol must include the careful monitoring of the blood level of the anticonvulsants.

Tetracycline can be associated with pseudotumor cerebri or increased intracranial pressure. The syndrome is characterized by headache, papilledema, elevated spinal fluid pressure and, in babies, bulging fontanels. Significant vestibular toxicity has also been associated with a tetracycline derivative, minocycline.

Erythromycin is probably the least toxic of the commonly used antibiotics from a neurologic perspective. An uncommon side effect is temporary hearing loss. Erythromycin interacts with carbamazepine, thus the anticonvulsant levels increase rapidly when erythromycin is introduced.

CARDIAC DRUGS

GLYCOSIDES

Digitalis and related agents are the mainstay of treatment for congestive heart failure. Neurologic complications of digitalis therapy have been recognized for almost 200 years and are characterized by nausea, vomiting, visual disturbances, seizures, and syncope. Adverse effects on the CNS reportedly occur in 40% to 50% of patients with clinical digitalis toxicity and may occur before, simultaneously with, or after the signs of cardiac toxicity develop.

The most frequent and often the first sign of clinical intoxication is nausea, which appears to be due to central mechanisms rather than gastrointestinal irritation. The incidence of digitalis-related visual disturbances has been estimated at 40%, and although these symptoms may occur as an isolated symptom, they may usually occur concomitantly with other toxic signs. Blurred vision, reversible scotomas, diplopia and defects of color vision, and total amaurosis represent the spectrum of optic side effects.

Seizures are most commonly seen in pediatric patients. The incidence of digitalis-related seizures is difficult to estimate since other seizure etiologies (*i.e.*, arrhythmia) are so high in cardiac patients. Transient mental aberrations felt to be caused by intermittent cerebral hypoperfusion resemble transient global amnesia. Syncope, probably due to conduction delay or hyperactivity of baroreceptors, has also occurred in digitalis toxicity. Other neurotoxic reactions include facial neuralgia, paresthesias, headache, weakness, and fatigue. Cerebral symptoms consisting of confusion, delirium, mania, and hallucinosis have been reported in as many as 15% of patients with digitalis toxicity. Although the mechanism for the symptoms is unknown, it is felt that they are not the result of altered cardiac function.

ANTIARRHYTHMICS

Quinidine is mainly used in treating auricular fibrillation. Nervous system manifestations are usually not significant, but with overdosage or in susceptible individuals the following may occur: headache, nausea, vomiting, blurring of vision, ringing of the ears, flushing, palpitations, and even convulsions. A precipitous drop in blood pressure related to vagal influences can cause syncope, vertigo, and respiratory arrest (on rare occasions).

Lidocaine-induced CNS toxicity occurs commonly and may relate to its rapid absorption across the blood–brain barrier. The syndrome appears to relate to a diffuse excitement of neuronal systems with an early prodrome of altered behavior. Garrulousness and loss of inhibitions may be the prominent feature, as may agitation or psychosis. Circumoral numbness, diplopia, and tinnitus may also occur, with progressive muscle twitches and tremors. Generalized myoclonic seizures and finally CNS and respiratory depression are seen with higher doses. In both the cardiac and surgical patients, hypoxia and acidosis develop rapidly if the lidocaine syndrome is not reversed. Treatment focuses on adequate oxygenation and support, because the half-life of bolus lidocaine given acutely is 6 to 8 minutes. Since repeated injections, however, change the kinetics of lidocaine and prolong its half-life to approximately 90 minutes, more long-lasting effects can be seen.

Procainamide may cause lightheadedness and even syncope due to the hypotensive action. Additionally, a lupus erythematosus syndrome can develop in patients on procainamide and 80% of patients receiving the drug for 6 months have antinuclear antibodies; these antibodies clear with the withdrawal of the agent. During lupus-like syndrome, encephalopathy with confusion and agitation can develop. Procainamide also has a curare-like effect at the neuromuscular junction and hence can precipitate myasthenia gravis or exacerbate it.

Tocainide hydrochloride is a new antiarrhythmic agent that is structurally and pharmacologically similar to lidocaine, except that it is well absorbed when given orally. Tocainide has been proven effective in managing various ventricular arrhythmias; however, because it crosses the blood-brain barrier, it frequently causes several neurologic side effects, which include lightheadedness, dizziness, tremor, twitching, paresthesias, sweating, hot flashes, blurred vision, diplopia, and mood changes. Peak plasma concentrations of tocainide occur within 1 to 2 hours of ingestion; the plasma half-life is 12 to 15 hours in patients with unimpaired renal and hepatic systems. CNS side effects appear to be linearly related to the dose.

Bretylium is a parenteral antiarrhythmic drug used in the prophylaxis and treatment of ventricular fibrillation and life-threatening ventricular arrhythmias that do not respond to first-line agents such as lidocaine. The antiarrhythmic mechanisms of bretylium in humans are not clearly defined, but in animals it increases the ventricular fibrillatory threshold and also the action potential duration and effective refractory period. It induces a state of chemical sympathectomy.

The most significant side effect of this drug is severe supine and orthostatic hypotension. Patients report dizziness, light-headedness, vertigo, and faintness. Bretylium may also rarely cause flushing, hyperthermia, confusion, paranoid psychosis, mood changes, anxiety, lethargy, and nasal stuffiness.

Amiodarone is an orally effective antiarrhythmic drug that, like bretylium, slows repolarization in various myocardial fibers and raises the threshold for ventricular fibrillation. Early reports of adverse effects include corneal microdeposits, thyroid dysfunction, and cutaneous photosensitivity. Recently, however, toxic neurologic side effects have been described and, in a series of 54 patients studied, these side effects were the most common reason for either altering or discontinuing amiodarone therapy.

A reversible syndrome of tremor, ataxia, and peripheral neuropathy without nystagmus, dizziness, encephalopathy, or long-tract signs developed in 54% of these patients. Tremor occurred earliest and most frequently (29%). The 6- to 10-Hz flexion-extension movements in the fingers, wrists, and elbows were indistinguishable from essential tremor. Thirty-seven percent of the patients reported ataxia associated with falls, staggering, and difficulty in dressing the lower limbs. The ability to walk was seriously impaired in 18% of the patients. None of these patients had pre-existing gait problems and none had sensory or long-tract abnormalities on examination. Peripheral neuropathy associated with this drug was first reported in 1974 and continues to account for a significant portion of the neurologic toxicity reported today. The neuropathy is sensorimotor in type and generally causes numbness and tingling of all four extremities. Proximal weakness occasionally accompanies the paresthesias. Sural nerve biopsies have been examined and have revealed demyelination with mild axonal loss in some cases. Lamellated inclusions of lysosomal origin were found in all cell types in the nerves and are a characteristic finding of this neuropathy.

DIURETICS

Diuretics are divided into three principal groups: thiazide, loop, and potassium-sparing. Diuretics most frequently cause extracardiac side effects as a direct result of the electrolytes lost or retained in the renal system. Each group can, however, cause adverse effects that are indirectly linked to electrolyte and water balance.

The *thiazide* diuretics have been reported to cause syncope, acute muscle cramps and pain, hyporeflexia, weakness, flaccid paralysis, and epileptiform movements. The deterioration of mental function, including the development of coma, can be precipitated with thiazide administration in patients being treated for cirrhosis. Thiazides given concomitantly with triamterene and amantadine can increase the likelihood of neurotoxicity from the amantadine.

If loop diuretics, particularly *furosemide*, are given quickly and in high doses, they can cause deafness and paresthesias. If they are given to a patient who is also receiving lithium chronically, loop diuretics can alter the renal clearance of lithium and increase the risk of lithium toxicity and fluid electrolyte abnormalities. Loop diuretics can also potentially increase the success with which succinylcholine blocks the neuromuscular junction in anesthetized patients.

Potassium-sparing diuretics, including spironolactone and triamterene, have been reported to cause confusion, drowsiness, muscle weakness, paresthesias, dizziness (although this may be a result of cardiac rhythm changes), and headache.

SYMPATHOLYTICS

Methyldopa can cause sedation, which is usually transient in nature, but may persist in as many as 5% of patients. Mood alterations including depression are not uncommon, although most patients who develop behavioral changes usually have a prior history of affective illness. The depressive state is reversible on withdrawal of the drug. Parkinsonism, resulting from dopamine antagonism, has been reported several times; however, considering the widespread use of this agent, this is probably rare. Other minor neurologic complaints associated with methyldopa include confusion, dizziness, headaches, and syncope.

Clonidine is an alpha$_2$-noradrenergic agonist, and some people have suggested that this drug induces an overall decrease in norepinephrine release, possibly through a presynaptic mechanism. Sedation is the most common adverse neurologic effect of clonidine. Other less common neurotoxic reactions include depression, nightmares, and reversible dementia syndrome.

Reserpine was historically a popular drug in the treatment of hypertension, but disabling neuropsychiatric side effects have limited its current use. Drug-induced parkinsonism can occur and is felt to relate directly to the depletion of central dopaminergic stores by reserpine. This effect may occur in patients with no prior neurologic deficits or can be seen as a marked and sudden exacerbation of already present, but mild, Parkinson's disease. Psychiatric depression with early morning awakening, melancholy, loss of appetite, and diminished self-confidence are also seen with reserpine therapy and may also relate to central neurotransmitter depletion. This effect is more common with higher dosage and in patients with a history of prior affec-

tive disturbance. Drug withdrawal does not always result in immediate reversal, and early symptoms of depression should alert the physician to discontinue therapy.

Propranolol is one of the multiple beta-adrenergic receptor blockers currently in clinical usage in the United States. Propranolol is used mainly in the medical management of angina pectoris, hypertension, and certain cardiac arrhythmias. Propranolol seems to promote hypotension by reducing cardiac output and by reducing renin synthesis, possibly by CNS effects not yet elucidated.

Neuropsychiatric symptoms occur frequently during treatment with propranolol. Lassitude or insomnia and depression are the most common reactions, although vivid nightmares, hypnagogic hallucinations, and psychotic behavior have been reported with high-dose (more than 500 mg/day) propranolol therapy. The nighttime behavioral problems can often be avoided by eliminating doses after 8 PM. More recently, psychotic symptoms and confusion have been seen even with low-dose therapy and especially in two classes of high-risk patients—those with prior histories of major psychiatric illness and those with hyperthyroidism. This toxic psychosis clears promptly after the withdrawal of the drug. The pharmacology of propranolol-induced psychosis is unclear, although pre- and postsynaptic noradrenergic inhibition has been implicated (as has serotonergic antagonism). Orthostatic light-headedness, mild unsteadiness of gait, and dizziness may also be seen and may relate to the hypotensive effect of the drug. Paresthesias and slurred vision also occur. Sexual impotency, which is reversible with the withdrawal of the drug, can be particularly troublesome, and the physician must often ask the patient specifically about the problem in order to learn of it. This side effect can often be overlooked or misinterpreted by the patient, family, and physician in a rehabilitation setting after a myocardial infarction or after cardiovascular surgery. Propranolol has also been reported to unmask signs of hypoglycemia in predisposed individuals. Finally, propranolol has been reported to exacerbate or precipitate myasthenia gravis in susceptible individuals because of its curare-like depolarization blockade of nicotinic receptors. A long-acting propranolol preparation is now available and may be associated with fewer neurologic side effects. In order to avert side effects of nonselective beta blockage, selective beta$_1$ antagonists have been developed. Neurologically, however, these drugs have the same types of side effects as seen with propranolol and its derivatives.

Prazosin competitively blocks the vascular post-synaptic alpha-adrenergic receptors and is the first of a class of similar antagonists derived from quinazoline. The selective affinity of prazosin for alpha-receptors allows it to block the contractile response of vascular smooth muscle to norepinephrine, consequently lowering mean arterial pressure and peripheral resistance. Like other antihypertensives that cause vasodilatation, prazosin causes hypotension; dizziness and faintness have been reported in up to 50% of patients receiving this drug. These are most pronounced after the first dose(s) or in patients who have had a hiatus from the drug and are reinstituting treatment. Hypotension can be minimized if the initial dose is small and is given at bedtime. Other CNS side effects include headache, dry mouth, nasal stuffiness, lassitude, hallucinations, depression, paresthesias, nervousness, and priapism.

VASODILATORS

Hydralazine is the only direct-acting vasodilator generally available for the treatment of chronic hypertension. The neurologic side effects of hydralazine are few and uncommon in clinical practice. Peripheral neuropathy characterized by diffuse numbness and tingling is the only consistent neurotoxic reaction and is felt to be due to a direct toxic effect of the drug.

Verapamil, nifedipine, and *diltiazem* are calcium-entry blocking agents that decrease coronary vascular resistance and increase coronary blood flow. Each of these drugs selectively inhibits the transport of slow channel calcium ions in cardiac tissue. These slow channel ions link myocardial excitation to contraction and help control energy storage and use. Verapamil is used primarily to treat or prevent supraventricular tachyarrhythmias; nifedipine and diltiazem are used primarily to treat angina. These agents all have antihypertensive properties.

The extracardiac side effect profile is similar for all three drugs. The most prominent symptoms of toxicity are associated with excessive vasodilatation; patients complain of dizziness, light-headedness, flushing, headache, and increased fatigue. Adverse neurologic effects may also include confusion, tremor, paresthesias, insomnia, sedation, equilibrium changes, blurred vision, weakness, and nervousness. The calcium-entry blocking agents should generally be used cautiously with beta-adrenergic blocking agents because the risk of severe hypotensive side effects is compound. In addition, both verapamil and nifedipine can increase serum digoxin levels, thus compounding the potential risk of digitalis toxicity. Flecainide has been associated with tremor and dystonia. Mexiletine has been associated with an action tremor that increases in incidence as blood levels increase.

ANGIOTENSIVE CONVERTING ENZYME INHIBITORS

Captopril has been used in the United States to treat moderate to severe hypertension, based on its effect on the renin-angiotensin-aldosterone (RAA) axis. This cascading hormonal axis simultaneously maintains systemic arterial pressure and sodium balance by detecting and correcting even small changes in renal perfusion. Alongside the increased understanding of the RAA axis has come the discovery of drugs that specifically and selectively inhibit the RAA cascade.

Few neurologic side effects have been reported; however, in a large multinational study, 5% of the participating patients reported symptoms of hypotension, including dizziness, light-headedness, and vertigo. These symptoms were generally transient and mild and most frequently occurred in patients who were sodium or water depleted. Dysgeusia occurred in between 2% and 4% of patients participating in this small trial. The incidence of taste change or loss increased in patients with impaired renal function.

GASTROINTESTINAL AGENTS

Common gastrointestinal problems include the hypermotility disorders with vomiting and/or diarrhea; hypomotility disorders, with constipation; or excessive acid secretion leading to "heartburn" or ulcerations. A wide variety of drugs are commonly recommended for these disorders. Fortunately, neurologic complications from these frequently prescribed agents are infrequent.

LAXATIVES

There are only a few neurologic complications associated with the drugs used to treat constipation. *Docusate sodium* (Colace) is a stool softener that occasionally causes nausea or a bitter taste. The long-term use of nonprescription laxatives may cause neurologic complications arising secondary to depletion of electrolytes. Profound muscle weakness may occur from the potassium depletion following chronic laxative intake. The irritant purgatives, such as cascara, may damage the myenteric plexus of the colon, leading to a reduction of intestinal motility and a worsening of constipation.

ANTIEMETICS

Of the antiemetic drugs, several commonly prescribed agents act as dopamine receptor blockers in similar fashion to the neuroleptic drugs described below. *Metoclopramide* (Reglan), *prochlorperazine* (Compazine), and *promethazine* (Phenergan) are three widely used antiemetics with neuroleptic properties. Sedation may occur as an early complaint with the introduction of these agents. In addition, acute dystonia, with distressing involuntary spasms of head, neck, eyes, facial, and trunk muscles may occur, particularly in children treated with prochlorperazine. If not recognized by the clinician, these acute, sometimes bizarre symptoms may be inaccurately thought to have a psychogenic etiology. The treatment of the acute dystonia from the dopamine receptor blocking antiemetics is the administration of anticholinergic agents.

In addition to acute dystonia, these dopamine receptor antagonist, antiemetic agents may cause a parkinsonian syndrome, clinically indistinguishable from idiopathic Parkinson's disease. Those of more advanced age appear to be more susceptible to this neurologic complication and may even be treated with antidopaminergic agents if the symptoms are not recognized as being associated with the medication. Akathisia may also occur as a side effect of these medications. If these agents are used on a long-term basis, as in the treatment of chronic esophageal reflux, the potentially irreversible symptoms of tardive dyskinesia may even occur.

A different type of agent with predominantly anticholinergic effect, *scopolamine* is prescribed for the treatment of motion-induced nausea and vomiting. Recently, scopolamine has become available in a long-acting, transdermal patch preparation. The neurologic side effects of scopolamine are those associated with blockade of muscarinic receptors. The most frequent is xerostomia. The reduction in saliva production, if severe, can lead to mucosal ulcerations and dental problems. Other peripheral effects of scopolamine include blurred near vision resulting from alterations in accommodation, reduced sweating, and urinary retention from effects on bladder muscles. A potentially irreversible effect of the anticholinergic agents is the exacerbation of closed-angle glaucoma with the potential for causing blindness.

The CNS side effects of these drugs include sedation and confusion. Losses in recent and immediate memory can occur at high doses. Finally with toxicity, delirium and hallucinations have been described.

ANTIDIARRHEALS

Drugs used to symptomatically alleviate diarrhea frequently contain morphine or morphine derivatives. These compounds act to reduce the propulsive contractions of the small bowel and colon. The neurologic adverse effects from these agents include sedation, respiratory depression, and coma, typically with pupillary constriction.

Anticholinergic agents have also been used to treat symptoms of diarrhea. *Diphenoxylate-atropine* (Lomotil) is a widely prescribed antidiarrheal agent. Overdoses of this agent most frequently cause a predominantly opioid intoxication.

Some antidiarrheal compounds, for example, Donnatal, are combinations of morphine derivatives and from one to three different anticholinergic agents. Donnatal contains phenobarbital, hyoscyamine, atropine, and scopolamine. Although each component is present only in small amounts, patients taking several tablets a day or elderly persons may experience significant side effects.

Bismuth compounds, as found in the nonprescription *bismuth subsalicylate* (Pepto-Bismol), have been recommended for the treatment of "traveler's diarrhea." The neurologic sequelae of these agents are rare. There have been reports of an acute reversible psychotic reaction following excessive use of these compounds as a result of acute bismuth toxicity. More commonly, tinnitus is noted with large doses, arising from the salicylate component in this compound.

ANTIACIDITY AGENTS

The magnesium and aluminum antacids, if taken in large quantities or with renal impairment, may cause neurologic symptoms secondary to alteration in electrolytes. Sucralfate is an aluminum compound that coats the gastric mucosa. Although little of this agent is absorbed directly, sucralfate may reduce the absorption of phenytoin and, in those taking this anticonvulsant, may result in a drop in phenytoin levels below the therapeutic range.

The H_2-receptor antagonists inhibit acid secretion from the parietal cells. Currently, four H_2-

receptor antagonists are approved for use in the United states. *Cimetidine* (Tagamet) is the first to be developed. Other more recently developed H_2-receptor antagonists include *ranitidine* (Zantac), *nizatidine* (Axid), and *famotidine* (Pepcid). The neurologic complications of these medications include lethargy, confusion, depression, hallucinations, and headache. Individuals developing unexplained encephalopathic symptoms who are treated with these drugs may improve with the discontinuation of these agents. Additionally, the effect of cimetidine and, to a lesser degree, the other H_2 blockers on the cytochrome P-450 enzymes in the liver may alter the pharmacokinetic profile of other drugs undergoing hepatic degradation, including warfarin and phenytoin.

RESPIRATORY AGENTS

ADRENERGIC DRUGS

Of the three types of adrenergic receptors (alpha, $beta_1$, $beta_2$), it is the $beta_2$ receptor that mediates bronchodilation. The first sympathomimetics available for the treatment of asthma were not $beta_2$ selective (*metaproterenol, isoproterenol, epinephrine, ephedrine*); therefore, in addition to dilating bronchiolus, they also produced significant cardiac and CNS effects. The introduction of $beta_2$-selective agents (albuterol, terbutaline) resulted in a reduction in the number of adverse effects. These agents are most efficiently administered by inhalation, resulting in benefit with minimal side effects. When these agents are administered parenterally, there may be nausea, vomiting, headache, and a variable-amplitude postural and action tremor associated with these agents.

XANTHINE BRONCHODILATORS

The xanthine compounds include *aminophylline* and *theophylline*. These agents are now prescribed only for those patients suffering with chronic rather than intermittent symptoms of bronchoconstriction. Theophylline is metabolized primarily in the liver, and drugs that affect hepatic enzymes, including tobacco, may alter the metabolism of theophylline. Liver disease, heart failure, and pulmonary disease tend to slow the metabolism of theophylline, sometimes resulting in toxicity even at low dosages. The therapeutic serum concentration of theophylline is 10 μg to 20 μg/ml. The side

effects from theophylline tend to be dose-related. However, even in the therapeutic range, neurologic side effects may occur. These include nausea, nervousness, insomnia, and headache. Although usually associated with toxic levels of theophylline, seizures may also occur in the high therapeutic range, particularly in the elderly, with a history of previous brain injury. This latter group is likely to develop prolonged seizures with a poor outcome. The mechanism of theophylline-induced seizures is not clearly understood. In otherwise healthy asthmatics, the seizures are typically short-lived with a good outcome. A recently described neurologic side effect observed in children is the occurrence of acquired stuttering, which resolves with the discontinuation of this drug.

PSYCHIATRIC DRUGS

NEUROLEPTICS

Phenothiazine drugs and *haloperidol* are antipsychotic agents with the common property of dopaminergic receptor blockade. As a class, they are associated with various important neurologic complications, which include sedative effects, autonomic dysfunction, acute dystonic reactions, akathisia, parkinsonism, and the late complication of tardive dyskinesia. The sedation and encephalopathy associated with these drugs may relate primarily to their anticholinergic properties. Although these drugs can reduce agitation in young patients, the anticholinergic effects may lead to confusion in elderly patients and may induce paradoxical agitation rather than sedation. These drugs may lower the seizure threshold and have been associated occasionally with exacerbation of pre-existing epilepsy. The management of acute encephalopathy caused by neuroleptics involves the general maintenance of life systems. Physostigmine 1 mg to 2 mg IV may reverse anticholinergic toxicity.

A curious neurotoxic sign associated with neuroleptic management is neuroleptic malignant syndrome, which includes extrapyramidal signs and severe hyperthermia. Laboratory findings usually include transient elevations of serum aldolase or creatine kinase. The treatment of neuroleptic malignancy syndrome involves, first, the patient's removal from heat sources. The neuroleptic should be stopped and the patient should be placed in a cool environment. Ice packs about the body and ice water stomach lavage may be instituted. When the rectal temperature drops to 38°C, these dramatic efforts at cooling can be stopped, since patients have been reported to experience seizures when temperatures drop too rapidly. Dantrolene, an agent that acts at the muscle, can be used to decrease rigidity and lower body temperature. Doses range from 1 mg to 10 mg/kg IV in four divided doses. Levodopa can also be used, and bromocriptine has been tried with success.

Neuroleptics may also induce dystonias early in the course of neuroleptic treatment or after a new dosage increase in chronically treated patients. The manifestations are diverse and may include oculogyric crises, painful postures of the head and neck, and forced tongue protrusion. Acute management involves IV or IM injection of an anticholinergic agent. This treatment will ameliorate the dystonia within minutes, but since the anticholinergic effect is short-lived, oral anticholinergic agents should be prescribed for the next 24 to 48 hours.

Drug-induced parkinsonism occurs usually after weeks of therapy and will respond to low doses of anticholinergic drugs. Since most parkinsonian signs are self-limited, the need for anticholinergic drugs should be re-evaluated every 2 months.

Tardive dyskinesia is an abnormal involuntary movement disorder that occurs after chronic exposure to neuroleptics. The movements are usually stereotypic or choreic and involve predominantly the linguofaciobuccal muscles. In patients on neuroleptics who develop this syndrome, an attempt to remove the neuroleptics should be made if the patient's psychiatric condition permits. If the movements do not resolve after neuroleptics, reserpine may be used, usually between 1 and 2 mg/day. Side effects of reserpine, however, include hypotension and drug-induced depression as well as parkinsonism.

ANXIOLYTICS

Benzodiazepines are commonly prescribed anxiolytic agents. The therapeutic index of these agents is 10 to 30 times that of the barbiturates and, hence, their absolute toxicity is less. However, since these agents are so widely used, adverse reactions are frequently reported. The predominant toxic symptom is drowsiness or paradoxical excitation. Withdrawal seizures have also been reported. Dry mouth, tachycardia, dilated pupils, and depressed bowel sounds may occur early after the introduction of benzodiazepines because of possible anticholinergic effects. Withdrawal symptoms include excessive apprehension, anorexia, nausea, postural tremulousness, insomnia, and confusion. Withdrawal symptoms are best handled in the hospital, and barbiturates are usually substituted.

Meprobamate is widely used to treat anxiety, and the major toxicity of this drug relates to sedation and ataxia. Sedation is enhanced when meprobamate is consumed along with other drugs, including tricyclic antidepressants, monoamine oxidase inhibitors, and possibly ethanol.

ANTIDEPRESSANT AGENTS

Tricyclic antidepressants induce an acute encephalopathy that is characterized by agitation, confusion, mydriasis, and sometimes convulsions. Tremor and myoclonus may be prominent motor features of this syndrome. Medical complications of these drugs include complex cardiac arrhythmias and heart block. Generalized support measures should be instituted for the patient who takes an overdose of tricyclic antidepressants. *Physostigmine*, a centrally active cholinesterase inhibitor, given 1 to 2 mg IV will often awaken a patient from coma. This finding suggests that much of the toxic mental alteration relates directly to central anticholinergic toxicity.

Tricyclic antidepressants may also precipitate a more chronic neurotoxic syndrome in which tremor and sedation or insomnia are the prominent features. The tremor is usually postural or intentional and resembles that seen with amphetamine intoxication or use of lithium. Currently, most tricyclic antidepressants can be monitored with plasma levels, so that intoxication can be detected at early stages.

Newer generation antidepressants have been developed in order to be more selective on the nor adrenergic or serotonergic systems. Many of these agents (*e.g., trimipramine, amoxapine,* or *maprotiline*), however, still have significant anticholinergic side effects that would include blurred vision, urinary retention, and confusion. Trazodone can cause priapism.

Monoamine oxidase (MAO) inhibitors are drugs that have been used for decades in the treatment of depression. The characteristic of acute monoamine oxidase inhibitor intoxication is hyperpyrexia, with fevers as high as 108°F. Coma, tachycardia, tachypnea, dilated pupils, and profuse sweating occur. Rapid recovery after hemodialysis suggests that this means of therapy is effective. A second cataclysmic syndrome is the hypertensive crisis associated with combined use of MAO inhibitors with tyramine products or other centrally active agents. Cheese, chicken livers, chocolate, wine, and some forms of herring have been associated with this syndrome in patients ingesting MAO inhibitors. Much less dramatic and also more common are mild side effects, such as mild dizziness, a generalized weakness, dysarthria, and confusion that can occur in patients receiving therapeutic doses of these agents.

Lithium carbonate is well established as an effective agent in the treatment of manic-depressive illness. Neurotoxic effects are not rare, and the most common and annoying effect is a fine postural intention tremor, which may be seen even in therapeutic doses. A reduction of the dosage will usually either eliminate the tremor or significantly reduce its intensity. The beta-adrenergic blocker propranolol may prove beneficial. Toxic confusional states may also occur with lithium and, if this develops, lithium blood levels should be checked. Ataxia, seizures, and coma can occur in high doses (serum levels exceeding 2.0 mEq/l). There is no specific antidote for severe lithium intoxication. After severe intoxication, residual symptoms including ataxia, nystagmus, choreoathetoid movements, and hyperactive deep tendon reflexes have been reported.

HYPNOSEDATIVE AND OTHER AGENTS

Barbiturates are usually used to manage seizure disorders but are still used to calm patients and facilitate sleep. Drowsiness is a common complaint associated with their use, and ataxia (often without nystagmus) can develop when the plasma level rises above 50 μg/ml. In higher doses, severe ataxia, nausea, vomiting, and nystagmus predominate. A second encephalopathic syndrome occurs in children on phenobarbital and is highly distinctive. Instead of somnolence, these children develop remarkable agitation and hyperactivity. This can give the picture of attentional deficit disorder (ADD), or childhood hyperactivity. Patients with chronic toxic exposure to barbiturates show ataxic gait, slurred speech, and periods of intermittent agitation. Tremors and confusion, as well as diplopia and nystagmus, are characteristic.

Ethchlorvynol has a rapid onset and a short duration of action. The common side effects associated with its use are a strange mint-like aftertaste, dizziness, nausea, vomiting, and facial paresthesias. Idiosyncratic reactions characterized by marked excitation and histrionic behavior have also occurred. Chronic abuse of this drug results in both tolerance and physical dependence. Withdrawal symptoms resemble those seen with delirium tremens and may be especially severe in elderly patients.

Methaqualone may induce transient and persistent paresthesias and other signs of peripheral neuropathy. Paradoxical restlessness and anxiety instead of sedation and sleep are also reported with this drug. As with many of the drugs already mentioned, methaqualone with alcohol may have addictive sedating effects. Other drug interactions include enhanced effect of MAO inhibitors and tricyclic antidepressants. Delirium and marked myoclonus may also occur in patients who acutely overdose with these drugs.

Disulfiram is used in the rehabilitation of alcoholics, since high levels of acetaldehyde accumulate when alcohol is ingested with the drug. Chronic disulfiram therapy is associated with two distinct neurotoxic syndromes, an encephalopathy and a neuropathy. The encephalopathy is usually acute or subacute in onset, characterized by delirium and paranoid and psychotic behavior, and is often confused with the diagnosis of schizophrenic reaction. The behavioral response to neuroleptics or other psychotrophic drugs is generally not marked, a finding that should suggest a toxic cause; withdrawal of disulfiram and mild sedation with supportive care (but without neuroleptic therapy) are recommended in the treatment of disulfiram encephalopathy.

Disulfiram is also associated with a rare, axonal distal sensory/motor polyneuropathy. The recovery after drug withdrawal both clinically and pathologically suggests a dying back or distal axonopathy rather than new degeneration secondary to the loss of nerve cells. It is not known whether disulfiram is the responsible agent or whether a toxic metabolite induces the neuropathy. Disulfiram is possibly metabolized to carbon disulfide, a compound capable of causing an axonal neuropathy in humans and animals.

ANTI-INFLAMMATORY AGENTS

SALICYLATE COMPOUNDS

Because of their ready availability in most households, *salicylates* represent a common source of intoxication, accounting for the largest yearly number of serious childhood poisonings. In acute intoxication, the prominent neurologic and respiratory signs may immediately suggest the correct diagnosis and direct prompt and appropriate intervention. The neurologic manifestations of salicylate toxicity include a rapid and dramatic alteration in consciousness and global function with convulsions and coma. Confusion and restlessness are seen early, leading within a few hours to excitability, tremor, incoherent speech, and often delirium or hallucinosis. This phase has been referred to as a "salicylate jag" to indicate its similarity to alcoholic inebriation, although euphoria and elation are conspicuously absent with salicylates. After this phase, a gradual depression in the level of consciousness occurs with a rapid lapse into coma. Seizures are especially common in children and are usually generalized. The pathophysiology of the convulsions appears to relate to combined effects of metabolic and respiratory disturbances. In infants, salicylate intoxication induces a marked hypoglycemia, and seizure activity is especially hazardous in this young age-group. Diplopia, dizziness, and decreased visual acuity can also be seen with salicylate intoxication. Involvement of the audiovestibular (eighth cranial) nerve can lead to tinnitus, vertigo, and complete deafness. This complication is more common with chronic salicylate intoxication and is seen especially in elderly patients treated for arthritic or headache conditions where aspirin or salicylate compounds are ingested daily. The treatment of salicylate toxicity involves minimizing drug absorption, hastening drug elimination, correcting acid–base disturbance, and treating existing neurologic or medical complications. Induced emesis in the awake patient is the most effective means of emptying the stomach. Enhanced elimination is affected by alkalinization of the urine or by peritoneal or hemodialysis. Careful fluid and electrolyte management is tantamount and depends on the age of the patient and the stage of intoxication. The complications of hypoglycemia in infants must be anticipated and thereby prevented. Seizures are usually treated with phenytoin and phenobarbital.

There is a poor correlation between the serum salicylate levels and the clinical severity of intoxication. Despite apparently adequate treatment and progressive lowering of toxic plasma salicylate levels, sudden and unexplained deaths are not rare.

STEROIDS

Steroids induce three neurotoxic syndromes: increased intracranial pressure (pseudomotor cerebri), toxic encephalopathy, and myopathy. Infants are more likely than adults to develop steroid-related, increased intracranial pressure, hydrocephalus, and papilledema. This syndrome may occur while patients are receiving steroids or after withdrawal. The pathophysiology of this syndrome is unknown, although it may relate to water intoxication. When it occurs, patients have been treated for weeks or months with steroid compounds.

In contrast, steroid-induced toxic encephalopathy may occur within days of steroid introduction. The behavior is varied and fluctuant, ranging over 24 hours from momentary euphoria to depression to fully developed psychosis. Depersonalization and motor retardation may make these patients difficult to manage during the intoxicated phase. Paranoia with visual and auditory hallucination and markedly delusional thinking may predominate. Although this syndrome typically occurs early in the course of steroid therapy, cases exist where mental decline developed after more than 3 months of treatment. Doses of medication do not clearly correlate with symptoms, although the encephalopathy is generally more frequent in high-dose treatment groups. Patients with a prior history of psychiatric care or depression may be at higher risk for encephalopathy than other patients. Suicides have occurred, making this encephalopathy a significant source of potential morbidity. Treatment focuses on withdrawal of the steroid and medical and psychiatric support. Steroids can sometimes be reintroduced later without the reappearance of the problem.

Steroid myopathy, characterized by proximal weakness and atrophy, appears unrelated to the actual duration of drug treatment, and type II fibers appear to be selectively affected. Patients complain of progressive weakness that focuses primarily on the proximal muscles (shoulders and thighs).

Because the steroid compounds alter coagulation factors, secondary hypercoaguable states can occur, resulting in cerebrovascular disease. Rapid withdrawal of steroids induces the behavioral manifestations seen clinically in Addison's disease. These manifestations are secondary phenomena and are not related directly to drug neurotoxicity.

NONSTEROIDALS

The nonsteroidal anti-inflammatory agents account for approximately 4% of the prescription market. There are a variety of types currently available, and ibuprophen is even available in low doses as a nonprescription drug. Despite widespread use, these agents infrequently cause significant neurologic adverse effects. The most common neurologic side effect is headache. Other rare but serious central disturbances include confusion, hallucinations, and overt psychosis. Although not well evaluated in controlled studies, some have suggested that there may be subtle cognitive and memory changes associated with these agents, particularly in the more elderly patient. Another infrequent yet important side effect described is the occurrence of aseptic meningitis. Initially reported in 1978, there have been subsequent case reports in which *ibuprofen* was the most commonly associated drug, although *sulindac, naproxen,* and *tolmetin* have also been implicated. From these case reports, it appears that young women with connective tissue disorders are the most likely to develop this side effect. The clinical picture is that of aseptic meningitis, with fever, chills, and meningismus. The cerebrospinal fluid has an elevated protein, a pleocytosis of granulocytes, and a normal or reduced glucose. The underlying mechanism for this syndrome is felt to be a hypersensitivity reaction to the drugs. Although an infectious source for meningitis must be sought, no communicable agent has been isolated. The meningeal syndrome resolves with the discontinuation of the nonsteroidal only to recur, sometimes more rapidly and severely, if treatment is reinitiated.

Indomethacin has proved to be a potent anti-inflammatory drug but appears less efficacious than salicylates in the treatment of arthritis and rheumatoid variants. Its mode of action is still uncertain, but it may act by way of inhibition of prostaglandin synthesis. CNS toxicity is one of the most frequent dose-limiting factors, precluding the use of indomethacin in 30% to 50% of patients. Neurotoxic effects consist of headaches, depression, agitation, and, rarely, hallucinations. Ataxia, clumsiness, and impaired postural reflexes may also occur, although slow increases in dosage may prevent their development.

Phenylbutazone, used in the treatment of ankylosing spondylitis, is not associated with marked neurotoxic effects. An alteration in the sensation of taste is the most frequently reported neurologic side effect. Phenylbutazone alters the metabolism of phenytoin and, in seizure patients, may be associated with anticonvulsant toxicity or increased seizure activity.

Naproxen has been associated with adverse neurologic reactions in approximately 8% of patients. These effects include headache, drowsiness, vertigo, inability to concentrate, and depression. Because of its protein-binding affinity, naproxen can be associated with phenytoin toxicity in seizure patients. By displacing phenytoin from proteins, naproxen causes higher levels of unbound phenytoin to circulate, so that toxic signs develop even though the total serum phenytoin level remains in the therapeutic range.

Sulindac is another recently marketed nonsteroidal anti-inflammatory agent recommended for use in various types of arthritis. Its mode of action may be the inhibition of prostaglandin synthesis by one of its metabolites, a sulfide. The neurotoxicity of sulindac has been estimated between 1% and 10%, with headache and dizziness being most common. Vertigo, tinnitus, and decreased hearing occur in less than 1% of reported patients. Paresthesias, peripheral neuropathy, and transient blurring of vision are rare, but more clinical experience is needed to confirm the true incidence of these reactions.

HORMONES

Oral contraceptives have become widely prescribed, and related neurotoxic syndromes have emerged with disturbing frequency. The most alarming side effect is cerebrovascular disease. The risk of cerebrovascular accidents on oral contraceptives is increased in young women, and stroke syndromes in young women who are on birth control pills are three to eight times more frequent than in those who are not taking oral contraceptives. The symptoms of transient ischemic attacks and stroke syndromes may be varied. In hemispheric strokes, dominant hemispheric lesions provoke aphasias and right hemiparesis. Left hemiparesis with hemisensory loss in the face and body follow a right middle cerebral artery occlusion. Brain-stem cerebrovascular accidents presenting with "crossed-syndrome" (*e.g.*, decreased sensation on the right face with decreased sensation on the left body or decreased strength of the right face with decreased strength of the left body) follow vertebrobasilar disease of the brain-stem circulation. The treatment for such strokes involves the removal of the oral contraceptives and the general rehabilitation efforts used in other forms of cerebrovascular disease. Angiographic findings more typical of embolic disease are usually seen with oral contraceptive–induced strokes, although thrombotic disease also occurs. High estrogen–containing oral contraceptives are associated with more cerebrovascular disease than are other contraceptive products.

Chorea is another serious problem related to oral contraceptives. The involuntary movements appear days or weeks after starting birth control pills and may be more frequent in patients with prior history of Sydenham's (rheumatic) chorea. The chorea usually starts abruptly and may involve only one side of the body (hemichorea). Theoretically, the early childhood chorea of rheumatic fever relates to striatal vasculopathy, and estrogens during adult life may precipitate a chemical alteration that unveils the long quiescent lesion. A similar phenomenon occurs occasionally during pregnancy when a woman develops severe involuntary movements that terminate when the pregnancy ends (chorea gravidarum). Birth control chorea may disappear within 48 hours after medication is stopped, although the abatement may take longer.

Neuro-ophthalmologic signs also occur with patients who are taking oral contraceptives. Pseudotumor cerebri may occur in patients who are often not the typically obese women with pseudotumor cerebri in other settings. Vascular headaches (migraines) may also appear for the first time or suddenly change in pattern when oral contraceptives are started. Common migraine (without an aura) may become classic migraine, with patients beginning their headache syndrome with symptoms or signs of focal cerebral dysfunction. In cases where migraines appear for the first time, increase in frequency, or become focal, a cessation of oral contraceptives is suggested.

Various other neurologic disorders are occasionally associated with the use of oral contraceptives. Seizures may change in pattern of frequency. Carpal tunnel syndrome of median nerve neuropathy or other pressure neuropathies may occur related to the increased fluid retention associated with oral contraceptives. Drug-induced and reversible myasthenia gravis has also rarely been reported.

VITAMINS AND ADDITIVES

Vitamins are vital trace substances, and neurologic syndromes are generally associated with deficiency syndromes. However, since health enthusiasm has reached passionate proportions for many individuals, especially Americans, clinicians are encountering neurotoxic syndromes associated with these seemingly safe agents. Of the fat-soluble vitamins, vitamin A is directly associated with neurotoxicity, and vitamin D can alter bone and renal metabolism, causing secondary neurologic dysfunction. Of the water-soluble vitamins, only pyridoxine (B₆) is established to provoke neurologic complications.

Vitamin A, clearly required for normal growth, vision, reproduction, and maintenance of epithelium, in high doses accumulates and can induce the syndrome of increased intracranial pressure (pseudotumor cerebri). Foods high in vitamin A include broccoli, cabbage, and liver, although dietary hypervitaminosis A is most unusual. Medically, vitamin A is used in the treatment of acne vulgaris and other dermatologic illnesses. Whereas the generally recommended daily allowance is 5,000 IU, individual capsules can contain five times that value, with subjects often ingesting 100,000 IU daily. At these doses, intoxication will develop over several months; at 200,000 IU daily, intoxication may develop within weeks. Recent publicity about vitamin A's cancer preventive properties may increase the number of people who self-expose themselves to this product.

Early signs of increased intracranial pressure include headaches, blurred vision, transient obscuration of vision, and sixth cranial nerve paresis. On funduscopic examination, gradual papilledema develops without further signs of focal neurologic deficit. No neurologic clue exists to establish the etiology, but the skin changes, organomegaly, and history of vitamin ingestion will establish the diagnosis. Since vitamin zealots are often "antimedication," these patients must be specifically questioned about vitamins.

Vitamin D when given in massive amounts mobilizes bone calcium and phosphorus. When there is bone demineralization and degeneration, nerve root and spinal cord compression can occur. Alterations in the calcium balance can produce generalized weakness, muscle aches, cramps, and mild metabolic encephalopathy. Meningeal symptoms and trigeminal neuralgia are two additional reported findings without clear pathogenesis. The latter may relate to bony foraminal alterations. When renal impairment occurs, progressive secondary encephalopathy, not directly related to the vitamin, develops and coma may result.

Pyridoxine, or *vitamin B₆*, has recently been implicated in a highly selective toxic syndrome provoking a sensory ataxia and dorsal root gangliar dysfunction. Widely used, especially by women to treat premenstrual tension and edema, pyridoxine induces this neurotoxic syndrome in occasional patients consuming chronic daily doses of 2 g or more. Gradually, the patient notes difficulty walking, with lightning-like dysesthesias in the back. Numbness of the extremities occurs and importantly, facial dysesthesias, so uncommon with most toxic neuropathies other than trichloroethane, quickly develop. Areflexia, stocking-glove sensory loss, and profound sensory ataxia with preserved strength are typical. On electromyography, marked slowing of the sensory nerve conduction is seen with normal motor conduction.

Tryptophan is an amino acid that has become popular for management of insomnia and behavioral changes related to the menstrual cycle (premenstrual syndrome). Myalgia and eosinophilia have been reported in numerous patients, as well as a progressive neuropathy affecting primarily the lower extremities with aching weakness. In some instances, patients are so disabled that they are wheelchair-bound and need ventilatory assistance. Cessation of exposure to tryptophan and plasma exchange have been associated with clinical improvement in some cases.

QUESTIONS AND DISCUSSION

1. Match the cardiac drug with a prominent side effect.

    A. Propranolol
    B. Digitalis
    C. Alpha methyldopa
    D. Lidocaine

    1. Visual disturbance in as many as 40% of patients
    2. Depression and impotency
    3. Garrulous, uninhibited behavior
    4. Parkinsonism
    5. Peripheral neuropathy in 25%

The correct answers are (A) and (2); (B) and (1); (C) and (4); and (D) and (3). Propranolol and other beta-antagonists can cause depression and impotency that can be obscured in the rehabilitative setting after a myocardial infarction or surgery. Digitalis has prominent visual side effects, and patients often complain of halos around everything. Alpha methyldopa can cause or aggravate parkinsonism, and lidocaine is often associated with a bizarre and alarming change in behavior.

2. Factors that contribute to the acid-base abnormality of salicylate intoxication include the following:

    A. Salicylates initially depress medullary breathing activation.
    B. Salicylates are acids that displace bicarbonate and can also lead to ketosis.

    C. Myoglobinuria usually precipitates renal shutdown and metabolic acidosis.
    D. All of the above.

The answer is (B). Salicylates initially activate the medullary breathing center and cause respiratory alkalosis. Later, at high doses, the medullary breathing center can be inhibited. In addition, salicylates induce and enhance the chemosensitive response and are acids as described in (B). The net response is a metabolic acidosis with either a respiratory acidosis or alkalosis. Myoglobinuria is not a feature of salicylate intoxication.

3. True statements regarding birth control pills and neurologic disability include:

    A. Peripheral neuropathy of the axonal type can mimic multiple sclerosis.
    B. Cerebrovascular accidents usually relate to cardiac valvular vegetations.
    C. Chorea often resolves within days or weeks of drug cessation and is rarely a permanent sequela of oral contraceptive ingestion.
    D. Papilledema when it occurs is due to the steroid-induced hypervitaminosis A.

The answer is (C). Birth control pills are not associated with a peripheral neuropathy, but instead their toxicity relates predominantly to a CNS function. Cerebrovascular accidents are an alarming complication of these drugs in young women and may be of embolic or thrombotic origin. They do not relate specifically to valvular vegetations. Chorea often occurs within days of the first ingestion of birth control pills and may promptly stop after drug cessation. Only in rare instances (usually a hemiballistic syndrome) will the chorea be long-standing after drug cessation. In such cases, a static cerebrovascular accident is hypothesized to underlie the chorea as opposed to the transient chorea, which probably relates to a hormonally induced functional alteration in dopaminergic sensitivity at the striatum. Papilledema, when it occurs in patients on birth control pills, may have multiple etiologies, including venous thrombosis and pseudotumor cerebri. It does not appear to relate to hypervitaminosis A.

4. Five neurologic complications of neuroleptic therapy are listed below. Indicate whether they are usually:

A. Acute, occurring minutes or hours or, at most, days after starting the drug
B. Subacute, occurring days, weeks, or a few months after starting the drug
C. Chronic, occurring after several months or years of drug treatment

1. Dystonia
2. Parkinsonism
3. Chorea
4. Tremor
5. Oculogyric crises

The answers are (A) and (1) or (5); (B) and (2) or (4); (C) and (3). The acute neurologic side effects related to neuroleptic drugs are dystonia and akathisia. The contorted posture of dystonia is frightening to see or experience. An oculogyric crisis, with the eyes thrown back and the neck usually hyperextended, is only one example of a dystonic complication of neuroleptics. Recently, a late-onset dystonia has been described as within the realm of tardive dyskinesia, but this is probably uncommon. Tardive dyskinesia should be mainly considered a choreic or stereotypic disorder and is the major chronic side effect of neuroleptic drugs. The subacute problem associated with neuroleptic medication is parkinsonism, which may include any of the following: tremor, bradykinesia, rigidity, or postural reflex compromise.

5. True statements regarding the use of anti-emetic drugs include:

A. Metoclopramide is particularly useful in Parkinson disease patients with nausea secondary to their dopaminergic medication.
B. Children receiving prochlorperazine for gastrointestinal distress are least likely to have neurologic complications.
C. In a patient using a scopolamine patch who reports acute right eye pain, an emergency visit to an ophthalmologist and removal of the patch should be recommended.
D. Scopolamine may cause drug-induced parkinsonism by a similar mechanism as the neuroleptics.

The correct answer is (C). Scopolamine is an anticholinergic agent that may exacerbate narrow-angle glaucoma, with painful symptoms in the eyes. If not recognized and treated emergently, this may result in blindness. Both metoclopramide and prochlorperazine are dopamine receptor blockers, similar to the neuroleptics. Hence both agents may cause drug-induced parkinsonism or worsen pre-existing Parkinson's disease. Children treated with these drugs are at more risk for developing acute

dystonic reactions. In contrast, scopolamine, being an anticholinergic agent, does not cause drug-induced parkinsonism.

6. In patients receiving theophylline, which of the following is true?

A. Seizures occur only if serum levels are in the toxic range.
B. Theophylline is a useful agent in an elderly patient with congestive heart failure and a previous stroke with a history of intermittent asthma.
C. A child receiving IV infusions of theophylline is at increased risk for developing acute dystonic reactions.
D. The pharmacokinetics of drugs metabolized in the liver may affect the metabolism and serum levels of theophylline.

The answer is (D). Theophylline is metabolized by the hepatic enzymes. Other drugs metabolized in the liver may alter theophylline metabolism, affecting the serum levels. The seizures associated with theophylline may occur in the therapeutic range. In particular, patients with previous brain injury are at increased risk. Congestive heart failure may increase theophylline levels even when the drug is administered at recommended doses. Theophylline is a xanthine compound without dopamine receptor activity and is not known to cause acute dystonic reactions.

SUGGESTED READING

Dahls FH, Ma KK, Bird TD: Theophylline-associated seizures with "therapeutic" or low toxic serum concentrations: Risk factors for serious outcome in adults. Neurology 41:1309, 1991

Giménez-Roldàn S, Mateo D: Cinnarizine-induced parkinsonism. Clin Neuropharmacol 14:156, 1991

Goetz CG: Neurotoxins in Clinical Practice. New York, SP Medical and Scientific Books, 1985

Heiman-Patterson TD, Bird SJ, Parry GJ et al: Peripheral neuropathy associated with eosinophilia–myalgia syndrome. Ann Neurol 28:522, 1991

Hoppmann RA, Peden JG, Ober SK: Central nervous system side effects of nonsteroidal anti-inflammatory drugs. Arch Intern Med 151:1309, 1991

Lipsy RJ, Fennerty B, Fagan TC: Clinical review of the histamine-2 receptor antagonists. Arch Intern Med 150:745, 1990

Miller LG, Jankovic J: Persistent dystonia possibly induced by flecainide. Mov Disord 7:62, 1992

Silverstein A (ed): Neurological Complications of Therapy: Selected Topics. Mt. Kisco, NY, Futura, Publishing Co., 1982

Spencer PS, Schaumburg HH (eds): Experimental and Clinical Neurotoxicology. Baltimore, Williams & Wilkins, 1980

Vinken PJ, Bruyn GW, Cohen MM et al (eds): Handbook of Clinical Neurology, Vols 36 and 37: Intoxications of the Nervous System. Amsterdam, North Holland Publishing Company, 1979

Sequelae of Minor Closed Head Injuries

Charles M. D'Angelo

The National Center for Health Statistics, a branch of the United State Department of Health, Education, and Welfare, records almost 8 million head injuries yearly. Of these, 1.5 million are classified as major head injuries, including severe cerebral concussion, cerebral contusion, and intracranial hemorrhage. Fortunately, over 6 million cases are classified as minor head injuries. Many excellent textbooks deal with the diagnosis and treatment of the severe head injury patient. This chapter deals with the patient who has a minor head injury; typically, the patient sustains a head injury, is evaluated in an emergency facility, and is sent home soon after the injury or after 24 to 48 hours observation. This chapter is a discussion of dire possibilities; a discussion of suspicions that should arise when confronted by a patient who complains of a headache or mild neurologic deficit after a head injury.

SCALP INJURIES

The scalp has five layers: skin, subcutaneous tissue, galea aponeurotica, loose areolar tissue, and periosteum. Superficial contusions, abrasions, or lacerations of the scalp seldom pose a problem for the patient. A delayed wound infection occasionally necessitates a consultation with the family doctor. Local wound care results in good healing, because the scalp is well vascularized.

Three conditions can be a problem: subgaleal hematoma, subgaleal infection, and subperiosteal hematoma. The galea aponeurotica has abundant blood vessels. Injuries that lacerate the galea can be associated with excessive bleeding. An improper closure of the wound, which does not tightly approximate the galea, can result in arterial bleeding into the loose areolar layer, a *subgaleal hematoma*. The hemorrhage can extend throughout the loose areolar space, confined by the superior eyelids, zygomatic arch, and superior nuchal line. The patients return a few hours to a few days after skin closure with a "pumpkin head." The loose areolar layer is contaminated occasionally by bacteria during injury or wound closure. The resultant *subgaleal infection* is associated with fever, headache, and marked scalp tenderness. A "pumpkin head" condition will sometimes develop.

Injuries that tear the periosteum cause subperiosteal bleeding. This bleeding further separates the periosteum from the underlying calvarium, a *subperiosteal hematoma*. The mass of a subperiosteal hematoma can be large and disfiguring. The mass slowly recedes without treatment. Since the soft center is surrounded by a ring of firm periosteum, a subperiosteal hematoma can be misdiagnosed as a depressed skull fracture. A tangential view skull roentgenogram differentiates the two possibilities. The elevated periosteum incites new bone formation. The resultant bony lump can cause undue anxiety but resolves without treatment.

221

William J. Weiner and Christopher G. Goetz, eds. *Neurology for the Non-Neurologist*, Third Edition. Copyright © 1994, 1989 by J. B. Lippincott Company. Copyright © 1981 by Harper and Row Publishers, Inc.

SKULL FRACTURES

Skull fractures, like fractures elsewhere in the body, are classified as simple, compound, or comminuted. A skull fracture in and of itself has little clinical significance. A skull fracture indicates that the intracranial contents have been subjected to significant rotational force and could be damaged. A skull fracture alerts the physician to possible "impending" intracranial complications. The site and course of a fracture are important. A linear fracture traversing the middle meningeal groove or a major venous sinus can cause an epidural hematoma or subdural hematoma, respectively. Linear fractures approaching the foramen magnum are associated with posterior fossa subdural hematomas: such fractures are termed *complicated fractures*.

Skull fractures with a break in the scalp are called *compound fractures*. Fractures that enter the various skull sinuses (*e.g.*, mastoid sinus, sphenoid sinus, or frontal sinus) also communicate with the external environment and are compound fractures. Such fractures may herald the development of pneumocephalus, cerebrospinal fluid (CSF) fistula, or meningitis. A sinus air–fluid level or the presence of intracranial air seen on a skull roentgenogram indicates a compound skull fracture.

Fractures of the skull base, *basilar fractures*, are seldom seen on routine roentgenograms. The most common sites of basilar fractures are the cribiform plate and petrous bone. Cribiform plate fractures should be suspected in patients with periorbital eccymoses (raccoon sign), anosmia, or CSF rhinorrhea. Petrous bone fractures are often accompanied by mastoid ecchymosis (Battle's sign), hemotympanum, CSF otorrhea, and CN VII dysfunction. Basilar skull fractures can traverse neural foramina with injury to cranial nerves. The suspicion of a basilar skull fracture should alert the treating physician to the possibility of impending CSF fistula and meningitis.

At the time of impact, a fracture edge may lacerate the dural and subarachnoid membranes, trapping the membranes in the fracture line. CSF flows into the trapped membranes and cannot exit. The expanding, trapped CSF forms a cyst, known as a *leptomeningeal cyst*, that erodes or expands the fracture line. Such cysts are not uncommon in children and cause the so-called *growing* or *spreading fracture*.

CEREBROSPINAL FLUID FISTULA

All CSF fistulae have a defect in the dura-arachnoid membranes, which allows CSF to escape from the subarachnoid space. CSF fistulae commonly present clinically as CSF rhinorrhea or otorrhea. Traumatic CSF fistulae occur in 2% to 3% of patients with head injuries. There is little correlation between the severity of the head injury and the development of a CSF fistula. Almost 50% of patients who had a traumatic CSF fistula had no loss of consciousness or only a brief loss of consciousness at the time of injury.

A CSF fistula may be immediate or delayed. Immediate CSF rhinorrhea ceases spontaneously within 1 week in 85% of patients; immediate otorrhea ceases within 1 week in nearly all cases. Delayed CSF rhinorrhea usually occurs within 3 months of the head injury.

The most common cause of CSF rhinorrhea is a basilar fracture involving the cribiform plate of the frontal fossa. Basilar fractures entering the frontal, ethmoid, or sphenoid sinuses may also cause CSF rhinorrhea. Otorrhea is caused by fractures of the petrous bone involving the mastoid air cells. It is interesting that a petrous bone fracture can cause CSF rhinorrhea. In such cases, the tympanic membrane is intact and the communication with the nasal cavity is by way of the eustachian tube.

A CSF fistula should be suspected in any patient who develops signs or symptoms of meningitis after a head injury. A headache that increases in intensity in the erect position is a suspicious symptom. Occasionally, a patient describes an intracranial "swooshing" sensation (pneumocephalus) with inhalation. The appearance of clear, water-like fluid draining from the nose is highly suspicious. The fluid often "pours out" in the head-dependent position. CSF may often be seen behind the eardrum.

The diagnosis can be confirmed if collected nasal fluid, uncontaminated by blood, contains greater than 30 mg glucose per 100 ml. CSF glucose may be less than 30 mg/100 ml if meningitis is present. Dextrostix testing is unreliable because the tape often turns positive due to sugar in normal nasal mucus. The diagnosis of a CSF fistula can be suspected if a routine skull roentgenogram reveals pneumocephalus. A definitive diagnosis may require the extra-arachnoid detection of radioimmunosorbent assay (RISA) or ^{99m}Tc serum albumin injected into the lumbar subarachnoid space. Detection of radioactivity in the nasal cavity or auditory canal confirms the diagnosis of CSF fistula but does not always indicate the site of the leak. Often a contrast-enhanced computed tomography (CT) scan will reveal a collection of contrast material, "puddling," at the site of the fistula.

POST-TRAUMATIC MENINGITIS AND ABSCESS

Head trauma as the leading cause of meningitis in adults highlights the clinical importance of CSF fistulae. Meningitis occurs in 3% to 50% of patients who have traumatic dural fistulae. The infection rate tends to be high if the CSF leak persists for 7 days or longer. In 85% of the patients with meningitis, the etiologic organism was *Pneumococcus*. Unlike pneumococcal meningitis in the general population, the mortality rate in patients with CSF fistulae is less than 10%. Meningitis due to CSF fistulae should be treated aggressively with antibiotics determined by CSF sensitivity studies.

The question of whether or not prophylactic antibiotics should be used in patients with CSF fistulae is controversial. Some centers in which prophylactic antibiotics were employed reported the development of meningitis due to highly resistant strains of organisms. Many centers, therefore, do not use routine prophylactic antibiotics. We, however, obtain a nasal and pharyngeal culture on all patients with a CSF fistula. If signs of meningitis occur, we institute antibiotic therapy based on the "predomi nate growth" in the cultures until CSF sensitivity studies are complete.

Because of the proximity of the undersurface of the frontal lobes of the brain to the cribiform plate, a frontal lobe abscess can develop in a patient with a CSF fistula. Symptoms may be nonspecific, such as a headache and mild obtundation. Spinal fluid may be normal. The diagnosis is confirmed by using brain scan techniques.

INTRACRANIAL EXTRA-AXIAL LESIONS

EPIDURAL HEMATOMA

Epidural hematoma, a mass of clotted blood between the inner skull table and the dura, is the best known neurosurgical emergency, yet the diagnosis is often delayed, resulting in mortality rates exceed-ing 90% in some series. The classic description of an acute epidural hematoma progresses as follows: a blow to the head causing a linear fracture crossing the middle meningeal groove of the temporal bone; brief loss of consciousness; a regaining of consciousness ("lucid interval"); arterial bleeding with an expanding epidural mass; increasing intracranial pressure with obtundation; tentorial herniation with contralateral hemiparesis and ipsilateral pupillary dilatation; decerebrate rigidity; respiratory irregularity; and death. This classic presentation occurs in less than 10% of cases of epidural hematomas.

In many cases, there is no loss of consciousness or the patient never regains consciousness. Up to 60% of epidural hematomas form in patients with minimal underlying brain damage and no loss of consciousness, or a brief period of being "dazed." Furthermore, although most epidural hematomas are associated with fractures crossing the middle meningeal groove, the middle meningeal vein, not the artery, is often lacerated. The evaluation of cerebral compression is, therefore, slower, extending over several hours or days, or occasionally weeks. Likewise, about 30% of epidural hematomas do not occur in the temporal area but are located in the frontal or occipital areas or posterior fossa. An epidural hematoma should be suspected in any patient sustaining a skull fracture.

SUBDURAL HEMATOMA

Bleeding into the subdural space commonly occurs by two mechanisms: (1) During a rotational injury of the brain, the frontal or temporal poles are severely contused or lacerated; bleeding from the contused brain extends into the subdural space; and (2) during a rotational injury of the brain, veins bridging the subdural space from the cerebral cortex to the dura are torn, with venous bleeding directly into the subdural space. The second mechanism is more common in patients with cerebral atrophy (*i.e.*, the elderly and alcoholics).

Subdural hematomas are classified arbitrarily according to the time interval between the head injury and the development of clinical manifestations. Acute subdural hematomas occur within 4 days of trauma; subacute subdural hematomas occur between 4 and 14 days; and chronic subdural hematomas occur after 14 days.

Unlike the acute subdural hematoma, the *chronic subdural hematoma* initially forms in the absence of underlying brain injury. Indeed, the initial injury is often trivial or forgotten altogether. The venous hemorrhage is encapsulated by a membrane. The atrophic brain allows the development of a large mass that shifts the cerebral structures initially without a significant increase in intracranial pressure. Patients present with a headache and obtundation. The depressed level of alertness or awareness overshadows the neurologic deficit.

SUBARACHNOID HEMORRHAGE

Trauma is the most common cause of subarachnoid hemorrhage, and subarachnoid bleeding is the most common hemorrhage following trauma. Abrasions, contusions, and lacerations of the cortical surface produce bleeding into the subarachnoid space. The blood can cause meningeal irritation with headache, nuchal rigidity, and photophobia in an otherwise normal patient.

Blood in the subarachnoid space can incite fibrosis within the basal CSF cisterns, impeding normal CSF flow. Patients may develop hydrocephalus several days to several weeks after a head injury. The clinical picture is similar to so-called normal pressure hydrocephalus with the development of mental deterioration, urinary incontinence, and gait dysfunction. Ventriculomegaly is seen on CT or magnetic resonance imaging (MR) scans of the brain.

INTRACRANIAL INTRA-AXIAL LESIONS

At the moment of impact, the skull and the intracranial contents are suddenly accelerated or decelerated. The intracranial structures are subjected to severe rotational stresses during acceleration or deceleration. During rotation, cortical surfaces may be damaged by bony protuberances of the cranial vault; or white matter–gray matter junctions may shear from one another. Such shearing rotational injuries include concussion, contusion, and intercerebral hemorrhage.

CONCUSSION

Cerebral concussion denotes the loss of consciousness without significant anatomic damage to the brain. This brief loss of awareness may be due to rotational stress that temporarily blunts neural activity in the reticular activating system (RAS) of the brain stem. The membrane potential may change due to a breakdown of "tight junctions." The severity of the concussion is quantified by the duration of amnesia. The duration of amnesia is the length of amnesia following impact (retrograde amnesia) plus the length of amnesia prior to impact (anterograde amnesia). The duration of unconsciousness is usually overestimated by observers. Therefore, it is helpful to record the time interval between "the first thing and the last thing remembered" after and before the accident. A cerebral concussion itself is of little clinical significance; its importance is in the fact that it may be the first warning of more severe neurologic injuries. Patients who sustain a cerebral concussion should consequently be observed for a progressive neurologic deficit. This observation may be done by hospital personnel or reliable family members.

CONTUSION

Cerebral contusions occur usually on the undersurface or the poles of the frontal lobes, or the poles of the temporal lobes. The frontotemporal poles are the common sites damaged by bony prominences during rotation. Subpial hemorrhage and edema formation occur at the site of the contusion. The swelling may not be significant or maximal for 2 to 4 days after impact. The patient is awake and alert after the initial concussion. Increasing intracranial pressure, decreased level of consciousness, and focal neurologic deficit may develop later as the contusion mass increases in bulk.

HEMATOMA OR HEMORRHAGE

If the cerebral contusion is severe, the cerebral tissue can be disrupted with intracerebral bleeding. The site of bleeding, like cerebral contusion, is most common in the frontotemporal region. The development of a neurologic dysfunction may be delayed because the hemorrhage is delayed. The initial hemorrhage may be small, and signs develop only when surrounding edema increases the mass effect.

CRANIAL NERVE INJURIES

A dysfunction of any cranial nerve may be seen following closed head injury. A cranial nerve can be sheared, stretched, contused, or lacerated as it transverses bony protuberances or through bony canals. Cranial nerves may be involved directly in fractures of the skull base. The olfactory nerve (CN I) is most often injured.

OLFACTORY NERVE (CN I)

The loss of smell (anosmia) or the perversion of smell (parosmia) occurs in 5% of patients who sustain a head injury. Anosmia is reported in 40% of patients exhibiting CSF rhinorrhea after a head injury. The olfactory filaments can be sheared from the olfactory bulb during the rotation of the brain, or the filaments can be injured by fractures through the cribiform plate. Because CN I is often not evaluated in an emergency situation, the dysfunction may not be detected until weeks after the head injury when the patient complains of changes in the sense of taste or smell. Many patients regain the sense of smell within 2 years but are annoyed by parosmia during the recovery period. This condition cannot be treated effectively.

FACIAL NERVE (CN VII)

An injury to the facial nerve is next in frequency; however, it is only one-third as common as an injury to CN I. Because of the proximity of the facial and vestibuloacoustic (CN VIII) nerve as it courses through the petrous bone, either one or both of these nerves can be injured by transverse fractures of the petrous bone. Fractures near the internal auditory meatus usually involve CN VII and CN VIII with ipsilateral peripheral facial weakness (*i.e.*, the forehead musculature is involved as well as the face), ageusia in the anterior two-thirds of the tongue, and ipsilateral deafness. Fortunately, such injuries are less common than trauma to the facial nerve further along its course, which results in ipsilateral facial paresis or paralysis. The onset of facial weakness 4 to 5 days after an injury, especially in patients with hemotympanum, suggests a swelling of the nerve in the facial canal. Such patients should be started on a course of corticosteroids and should be evaluated for possible facial nerve decompression. Computerized visual field testing aids in discovering small scotomata.

TRIGEMINAL NERVE (CN V)

The Gasserian ganglion of the trigeminal nerve is occasionally traumatized when fractures of the petrous bone involve Meckel's cave. A complete dysfunction of the ganglion is rare. A spotty decrease in facial sensation usually occurs. Corneal sensation may be decreased, resulting in corneal laceration or conjunctival inflammation.

OPTIC NERVE (CN II)

The optic nerve is rarely injured by basilar skull fractures. A delayed discovery of scotomata is noted occasionally during a visual field examination. Such scotomata are probably due to a contusion of the optic nerve in the optic foramen.

OCULOMOTOR NERVE (CN III) AND ABDUCEUS NERVE (CN VI)

A dysfunction of CN III and CN VI are usually caused by an increased intracranial pressure with uncal herniation. Consequently, pupil inequality and diplopia are noted more often in acute head injury. A residual dysfunction such as ptosis, pupillary dilation, and paresis of outward gaze may be noted by an examining physician on a future occasion.

CAROTID CAVERNOUS FISTULA

Sixty percent of carotid cavernous fistulae, or pulsating exophthalmus, result from a head injury. A traumatic tear in the intracavernous portion of the carotid artery, or one of its small branches, forms an arteriovenous communication in the cavernous sinus. The unrestricted flow of arterial blood into the cavernous sinus increases venous pressure within the cavernous sinus as well as in the superior and inferior orbital veins that drain the orbit. Almost all clinical signs and symptoms are due to the increased pressure within the cavernous sinus and orbital venous system. The force required to produce a tear in the intracavernous arterial structures is not known, but it is generally assumed to be severe enough to cause a basilar skull fracture. The signs and symptoms of the fistula occur usually ipsilateral to the site of the fistula. Bilateral findings can occur in patients with severe bilateral basilar skull fracture, with large patent intercavernous veins, and in patients with elastic-collagen disorders, such as the Ehlers–Danlos syndrome.

The most common clinical features are pain, intracranial bruit, pulsating exophthalmus, chemosis, ophthalmoplegia, and diminished visual acuity. A *headache*, usually described as a steady or pulsating "fullness," occurs in the ipsilateral supraorbital region: It is increased in the head-dependent position. The *intracranial bruit* is ipsilateral and incessant, and it is the patient's most annoying symptom. The machinery-like bruit can also be heard by the physician using a stethoscope, which is pressed lightly over the orbit. The bruit is diminished by compression of the ipsilateral carotid artery in the neck. *Exophthalmus* usually averages 8 mm but may reach 24 mm, with consequent restriction of globe movements. Decreased orbital venous drainage results in increased interstitial fluid of the conjuctiva, or *chemosis*. Severe chemosis causes eyelid eversion with further inflammation of the conjunctiva. *Diplopia* is most often due to compression of the abduceus nerve (CN VI) in the cavernous sinus. The diplopia is most marked with lateral gaze. Paresis of the oculomotor nerve (CN III) or trochlear nerve (CN IV) also occurs, but it is only half as common as an abduceus dysfunction. Venous stasis within the orbit causes retinal ischemia and *decreased visual acuity* or blindness.

The diagnosis of carotid cavernous fistula should be suspected in any patient presenting with signs of a basilar skull fracture, such as CSF rhinorrhea and periorbital or mastoid ecchymoses. The diagnosis is confirmed by cerebral angiography.

POST-TRAUMATIC EPILEPSY

The incidence of chronic seizures following non-penetrating, closed head injuries is approximately 5%. The causal relationship between the occurrence of a head injury and the development of chronic seizures is controversial. Multiple factors determine the likelihood of developing chronic seizures following a closed head injury. The factors include the patient's age, focal brain injury, diffuse brain injury, the site of brain injury, and the time of the first seizure.

AGE

The development of a chronic seizure disorder is influenced by the age of the patient at the time of injury. Children under 5 years of age, and particularly under 1 year of age, frequently have a seizure immediately following a head injury; however, few children develop a chronic seizure disorder. Patients who are 16 years of age or older and who have an early post-traumatic seizure are more likely to have chronic seizures than their counterparts who are under 16 years of age.

FOCAL BRAIN INJURY

Focal cortical lacerations, such as those that occur with depressed skull fractures, may be associated with chronic seizures in 60% of patients. Likewise, 40% of patients with deeper cerebral lesions, as seen with intracerebral hematomas, develop chronic seizures. The likelihood of developing a chronic seizure disorder appears to be related to the severity of the focal cerebral lesion.

DIFFUSE BRAIN INJURY

The degree and duration of cerebral hypoxia influence the onset of chronic seizures. The more severe the ischemic brain damage, the greater the likelihood of developing seizures. In this regard, the presence of post-traumatic amnesia that lasts for more than 24 hours increases the likelihood of developing a chronic seizure disorder.

SITE OF BRAIN INJURY

Chronic seizures more commonly follow injuries near the central sulcus of the brain than injuries to frontal or occipital poles.

TIME OF FIRST SEIZURE

Seizures that occur within 24 hours of a head injury probably have no prognostic implications for further seizures. Chronic seizures have been reported in only 3% of patients who had a seizure during the first week following a head injury but in 25% of patients who had a seizure during the first week.

The development of chronic seizures following a head injury is problematical. For example, in one series of 265 patients, 8% "developed" their first seizure 10 years or more after their head injury. Furthermore, 50% of patients who develop post-traumatic seizures will cease seizing spontaneously with the use of anticonvulsant therapy.

POST-TRAUMATIC SYNDROME

The post-traumatic or postconcussion syndrome often receives little attention. The problem is not life threatening, yet it can disable a patient for weeks to months. Symptoms include headache, dizziness or giddiness, memory loss, poor concentration, nervousness, disturbed sleep, and decreased libido.

The etiology is still unknown; however, a loss of neuron membrane "tight junctions" may play a role in these vague "psychogenic complaints." The result of the neurologic examination is usually normal. The symptoms last for 2 to 6 weeks in most cases but can be present for 1 to 2 years. The occurrence of the syndrome is more likely in patients who sustain a mild head trauma (*i.e.*, a short duration of amnesia following cerebral concussion). It is more common in women, in people of average intelligence, and in assembly line workers. The diagnosis is made by the multiplicity of symptoms and the exclusion of a significant structural lesion. CT and MR scanning can exclude mass lesions. Labyrinthine testing of auditory evoked potentials helps evaluate the complaint of dizziness. The treatment consists of reassurance, rest, and analgesics.

Although the patient usually has many bothersome complaints that interfere with his usual work routine, it is important that he return to work as soon as possible. If a patient with the post-traumatic syndrome is initially disabled because of his headache or inability to concentrate, it is difficult to discontinue his disability 2 months later when he may still complain of his original symptoms. The physician should indicate to the patient's employer, if necessary, that the patient's symptoms may persist for a long time. Every effort should be made to have him return to work, even at a reduced work load if necessary. The granting of disability can be the greatest problem area for the treating physician.

NECK INJURIES

Following a head injury, an examination of the neck is often cursory or omitted. Injuries of the cervical vertebrae and carotid arteries can consequently be overlooked. The cervical spine is flexed, extended, and rotated in almost all head injuries. Roentgenograms of the cervical spine including views from the odontoid process to the C7–T1 interspace should be obtained in patients sustaining a significant head injury and in patients complaining of neck, upper extremity, or suboccipital pain.

Bruises on the neck should alert the examining physician to the possibility of carotid artery injury. Intimal tears of the carotid artery result in clot formation and possible cerebrovascular accident (CVA). Auscultation for carotid artery bruits should be part of the post-traumatic examination.

PITUITARY INJURY

At the time of impact, small hemorrhages may occur in the pituitary stalk or anterior lobe of the pituitary gland. Disorders of water retention and menstrual cycle are not uncommon after head injuries. Damage to the pituitary stalk can decrease the release of antidiuretic hormone (ADH) resulting in increased thirst, polyurea, dehydration, and hypernatremia (diabetes insipidus). Injuries to the hypothalamic-pituitary axis may cause an unphysiologic increase in ADH production with water retention and hyponatremia (inappropriate ADH syndrome). Cerebral edema may occur.

Menstrual irregularity may occur for 2 to 3 months following a head injury. The cause is probably damage to the anterior lobe of the pituitary gland.

QUESTIONS AND DISCUSSION

1. A 23-year-old man sustains a severe closed head injury during a motorcycle accident. He regains almost all neurologic function and is discharged from the hospital 5½ weeks after injury. Ten weeks after injury, his parents took him to their physician and stated that he was "getting worse." Specifically, he is incontinent of urine, intermittently confused, and "clumsy." The most likely diagnosis is:

   A. Meningitis
   B. Hydrocephalus
   C. Brain-stem CVA
   D. Cervical myelopathy
   E. Subdural hematoma

The answer is (B). Subarachnoid hemorrhage is common during any head injury. The subarachnoid blood may obstruct normal CSF channels, causing ventricular dilation. The enlarged ventricles compress white matter tracts and cause changes in mentation, gait, and urination.

2. A 37-year-old woman was discharged from the hospital 5 days after admission for a "cerebral concussion" incurred in an automobile accident. The discharge summary reads: "cerebral concussion—no neuro deficit." Two weeks after discharge, she complains to her physician that she cannot smell. Her examination is normal except for periorbital ecchymosis. Which diagnosis is possible?

A. CSF fistula
B. Basilar skull fracture
C. Brain abscess
D. All of the above
E. None of the above

The answer is (D). Anosmia indicates a possible fracture of the cribriform plate. Such basilar fractures can communicate with the "outside world," resulting in a CSF fistula and secondary infection.

3. Intracranial air seen on "routine" post-trauma skull roentgenograms may indicate:

A. CSF fistula
B. Depressed skull fracture
C. Epidural hematoma
D. Subdural hematoma
E. Intracerebral hematoma

The answer is (A). Pneumocephalus is an indicator of a rent in the cranial vault. CSF may exit; bacteria may enter.

4. A 72-year-old man is sent home from an outpatient emergency facility after being seen following a fall in his garage. He has no neurologic deficit. He is seen again 9 days later because "he sleeps all the time." The neurologic examination is normal. The most likely diagnosis is:

A. Subclinical meningitis
B. Hyponatremia secondary to pituitary injury
C. Impending CVA
D. Subdural hematoma
E. Post-traumatic seizures

The answer is (D). Subdural hematomas are more common in patients with cerebral atrophy, such as the elderly and chronic alcoholics.

5. The post-traumatic syndrome occurs most frequently following:

A. Acute subdural hematoma
B. Craniotomy for cerebral aneurysm
C. Closed head injury with severe temporal lobe contusion
D. Minor closed head injury
E. Traumatic CSF fistula and meningitis

The answer is (D). The post-traumatic syndrome occurs more frequently following a minor head injury. Indeed, among individuals sustaining a minor head injury, post-traumatic headache is more common in patients who were dazed than in those experiencing 30 minutes of amnesia.

SUGGESTED READING

Annegers JF et al: Seizures after head trauma: A population study. Neurology 30:683, 1980

Brown FD, Mullan S, Duda EE: Delayed traumatic intracerebral hematomas. J Neurosurg 48:1019, 1978

Feeney DM, Walker AE: A prediction of post-traumatic epilepsy: A mathematical approach. Arch Neurol 36:8, 1979

Fleischer AS, Patton JM, Tindall GT: Cerebral aneurysms of traumatic origin. Surg Neurol 4:233, 1975

Friedman WA: Head injuries. Ciba Clin Symp 35:1, 1983

Grossman RG, Gildenberg PL: Head Injury: Basic and Clinical Aspects. New York, Raven Press, 1982

Gurdjian ES, Webster JE: Head Injuries. Boston, Little, Brown, 1958

Guthkelch AN: Benign post-traumatic encephalopathy in young people and its relation to migraine. Neurosurgery 1:101, 1977

Hall S, Bornstein RA: The relationship between intelligence and memory following minor or mild closed-head injury: Greater impairment in memory than intelligence. J Neurosurg 75:378, 1991

Healy CB: Hearing loss and vertigo secondary to head injury. N Engl J Med 306:1029, 1982

Jeret JS, Mandell MA, Anziska B, et al: Clinical predictors of abnormality disclosed by computed tomography after mild head trauma. Neurosurgery 32:9, 1993

Kihlberg JK: Head injury in automobile accidents. In Caveness WF, Walker AE: Head Injury, pp 27–36. Conference Proceedings. Philadelphia, JB Lippincott, 1966

Leech PJ, Paterson A: Conservative and operative management for cerebrospinal fluid leakage after closed head injury. Lancet 1:1013, 1973

Lende RA, Erickson TC: Growing skull fractures of childhood. J Neurosurg 18:479, 1961

Lobato RD, Rivas JJ, Gomez PA, et al: Head-injured patients who talk and deteriorate into coma. J Neurosurg 75:256, 1991

Markwalder TM: Chronic subdural hematomas: A review. J Neurosurg 54:637, 1981

Masters SJ: Evaluation of head trauma: Efficacy of skull films. Am J Neuroradiol 1:329, 1980

Schechter PJ, Henkin RI: Abnormalities of taste and smell after head trauma. J Neurol Psychiatry 37:802, 1974

Walker AE, Caveness W, Critchley M: The Late Effects of Head Injury. Springfield, IL, Charles C. Thomas, 1969

Wilkins RH, Rengachary SS: Trauma. In Wilkins RH, Rengachary SS (eds): *Neurosurgery*, pp 1531–1688. New York, McGraw-Hill, 1985

Wrightson P, Gronwall D: Time off work and symptoms after minor head injury. Injury 12:445, 1981

Youmans JR: Neurological Surgery, Vol 4, Chaps. 56–71. Philadelphia, WB Saunders, 1982

Neuromuscular Diseases

Hans E. Neville
Steven P. Ringel

Neuromuscular diseases primarily involve the anterior horn motor neuron, the peripheral nerve (see Chap. 12), the neuromuscular junction, or the muscle. Weakness is a common symptom, but compared with disorders of the central nervous system (CNS), it may be accompanied by striking muscular atrophy and diminished muscle tone. Patients may also present with muscle pain, stiffness, cramps, twitching, limb deformities, or myoglobinuria.

This chapter discusses the clinical presentations of neuromuscular diseases and their diagnostic evaluation. Following the classification of disorders (Table 18-1), individual diseases will be described in detail and principles of management covered.

Since the original publication of this book there have been significant developments in the genetics of neuromuscular disorders. Accordingly, we have added the latest information on chromosome localization, gene determination (when known), and data on DNA diagnostic testing available to the clinician for genetic counseling (Table 18-2).

CLINICAL PRESENTATIONS

WEAKNESS

The mode of onset, location, and progression of weakness are important diagnostic features. The rapid onset of weakness is characteristic of most diseases of the neuromuscular junction, the Guillain–Barré syndrome, and acute electrolyte disturbances. Remissions and relapses suggest myasthenia gravis, periodic paralysis, or potassium depletion. Insidious and slowly progressive weakness occurs in many diseases. Three patterns of weakness frequently encountered are proximal, distal, and cranial. Each pattern is associated with typical symptoms that are mentioned frequently by the patient and with signs that are easily observed even before individual muscles are tested. These features are usually absent in patients with nonorganic complaints, who may have vague symptoms and demonstrate normal strength.

Proximal weakness is characteristic of myopathies and the spinal muscular atrophies. These patients will report difficulty in climbing stairs or arising from low chairs due to weakness of the hip and knee extensors. When standing from a chair, they will lean forward and push with their hands on the armrests. In arising from the floor or a squatting position, they may require one or more supports with the hands on the floor, knees, and thighs (Gowers' maneuver, Fig. 18-1). Their gait has a waddling appearance due to a weakness of hip fixators. Knee extensor weakness may cause the leg to "give out." The knee is kept locked, gradually leading to hyperextension (back-kneeing), which in turn produces an exaggeration of the lumbar lordosis. Shoulder–girdle weakness produces difficulty

William J. Weiner and Christopher G. Goetz, eds. *Neurology for the Non-Neurologist*, Third Edition. Copyright © 1994, 1989 by J. B. Lippincott Company. Copyright © 1981 by Harper and Row Publishers, Inc.

TABLE 18-1. **Classification of Neuromuscular Disorders**

A. Disorders of the anterior horn cell (motor neuron)
1. Spinal muscular atrophies (SMAs)
   Infantile SMA (Werdnig–Hoffmann disease)
   Juvenile SMA (Kugelberg–Welander disease)
2. X-linked spinal and bulbar muscular atrophy (Kennedy's syndrome)
3. Amyotrophic lateral sclerosis (ALS)
4. Poliomyelitis and postpolio syndrome
B. Disorders of peripheral nerve (see Chap. 12)
1. Radiculopathy
2. Plexopathy
3. Mononeuropathy
4. Polyneuropathy
C. Disorders of the neuromuscular junction
1. Myasthenia gravis
2. Eaton–Lambert syndrome
3. Botulism
D. Disorders of muscle
1. Dystrophies
   Duchenne/Becker dystrophy
   Facioscapulohumeral dystrophy
   Limb–girdle dystrophy
   Myotonic dystrophy
2. Myotonic disorders
   Myotonia congenita
   Myotonia dystrophy

3. Inflammatory myopathies
   Polymyositis
   Dermatomyositis
   Inclusion body myositis
   Sarcoidosis
   Polymyalgia rheumatica
4. Metabolic myopathies
   Glycogen storage diseases
      Myophosphorylase deficiency (McArdle's disease)
      Acid maltase deficiency
      Other glycogen storage disorders
   Disorders of lipid metabolism
      Carnitine deficiency
      Carnitine palmityl transferase deficiency
   Mitochondrial myopathies
   Malignant hyperthermia
5. Toxic myopathies
   Alcoholic myopathy
6. Endocrine myopathies
   Thyroid dysfunction
   Parathyroid dysfunction
   Adrenal dysfunction
   Pituitary dysfunction
7. Congenital myopathies
   Central core disease
   Nemaline myopathy
   Myotubular myopathy
8. Periodic paralysis and paramyotonia congenita

in elevating the arms and may be accompanied by scapular winging (Fig. 18-2). With the arms hanging at the sides there is an inward rotation of the shoulders with the backs of the hands facing forward, producing an oblique axillary crease. The high-riding scapulae produce a conspicuous "trapezius hump"; the clavicles slope downward and stand out prominently from the atrophic neck musculature (Fig. 18-3).

Distal weakness, accompanied by sensory loss, is characteristic of neuropathies. Distal weakness with normal sensation is a typical presentation of amyotrophic lateral sclerosis (ALS) (Fig. 18-4) and myotonic dystrophy. These patients find it difficult to manipulate small objects including buttons, and they also have difficulty when eating or using writing utensils. They may complain of "dragging" their legs because of a footdrop, or of frequent tripping on uneven ground. The knees are raised high in walking, while the feet flap limply and the soles are scuffed.

Cranial weakness affects the extraocular, facial, and oropharyngeal muscles and is an important differential feature in diagnosis (Figs. 18-5 and 18-6). Ptosis and ophthalmoparesis occur in disorders of the neuromuscular junction, myotonic dystrophy, and the syndrome of progressive external ophthalmoplegia. Dysphagia and dysphonia may occur in these disorders and also in ALS.

ATROPHY AND HYPERTROPHY

The disuse of a limb will produce a modest degree of muscle atrophy, which is seen after the casting of a fracture or in the hemiplegic limb of a stroke patient. The muscle retains much of its strength in disuse atrophy, and the shrunken-appearing limbs of the elderly may similarly be surprisingly strong.

TABLE 18-2. Neuromuscular Disease Gene Abnormalities

DISORDER	CHROMOSOME (R) RECESSIVE (D) DOMINANT	GENE PRODUCT	ABNORMAL GENE DETECTION BY:	SPECIAL FEATURES
Anterior Horn Cell				
1. Spinal muscular atrophy	5 (R)	1. Unknown	1. Linkage analysis available	
2. Spinal and bulbar muscular atrophy (Kennedy's)	X	2. Androgen receptor	2. PCR; Southern Blot available	2. Gene enlarged (CAG repeats)
3. ALS (familial in 5%)	21 (D)	3. Unknown	3. Linkage analysis in development	
Peripheral Nerve				
1. Charcot–Marie–Tooth disease (TYPE 1)	1,17,X	1. Unknown	1. Fully discussed in another chapter	
Neuromuscular Junction	No known genetic defect	N.A.	N.A.	
Muscle				
1. Duchenne/Becker dystrophy	X	1. Dystrophin	1. PCR; Southern Blot available	1. Prominent gene deletions in 60%–70%
2. Facioscapulohumeral dystrophy	4 (D)	2. Unknown	2. Linkage analysis in development	
3. Limb–girdle dystrophy (recessive)	15 (R)	3. Unknown	3. Linkage analysis in development	
3a. Limb–girdle dystrophy (dominant)	5 (D)	3a. Unknown	3a. Linkage analysis in development	
4. Myotonia congenita	7 (D)	4. Chloride channel defect	4. Linkage analysis in development	

5. Myotonic dystrophy	19	(D)	5. Myotonin (protein kinase)	5. PCR; Southern Blot available	5. Gene enlarged (GCT repeats)
6. Phosphorylase deficiency (McArdle's)	11	(R)	6. Phosphorylase deficiency	6.–10. Diagnosis by assay for enzyme activity and glycogen content; linkage analysis in development	
7. Acid maltase deficiency	17	(R)	7. Acid maltase deficiency		
8. Phosphofructokinase deficiency	1	(R)	8. Phosphofructokinase deficiency		8. Subunits from 2 chromosomes
9. Phosphoglycerate mutase deficiency	7	(R)	9. Phosphoglycerate mutase deficiency		
10. Phosphoglycerate kinase deficiency	X	(R)	10. Phosphoglycerate kinase deficiency		
11. Carnitine palmityl transferase deficiency	1	(R)	11. Carnitine palmityl transferase deficiency	11. Linkage analysis in development	11. Diagnosis by enzyme assay
12. Mitochondrial myopathies	Mitochondrial DNA		12. Defects of one or more electron transport chain proteins	12. PCR; Southern Blot	12. Deletion or point mutation of mitochondrial DNA
13. Myotubular myopathy	X	(R)	13. Unknown	13. Linkage analysis in development	
14. Central core disease	19	(R)	14. Unknown	14. Linkage analysis in development	14. Same gene as malignant hyperthermia
15. Nemaline (rod) myopathy	1	(R)	15. Unknown	15. Linkage analysis in development	
16. Paramyotonia congenita	17	(D)	16.–17. Sodium channel	16.–17. PCR, Southern Blot in development	16.–17. Different defect in same gene
17. Periodic paralysis (hyperkalemic)	17	(D)			

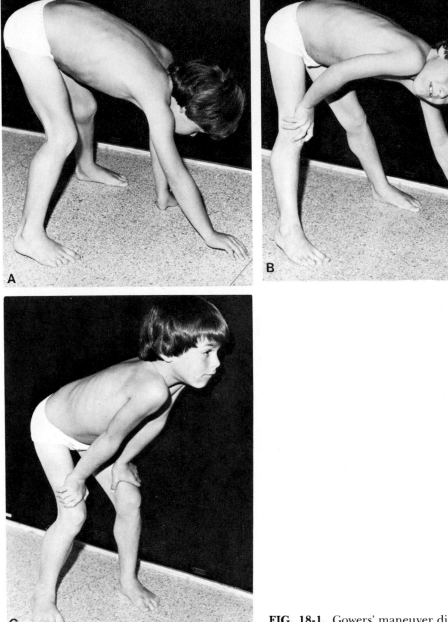

FIG. 18-1. Gowers' maneuver displayed in arising from the floor.

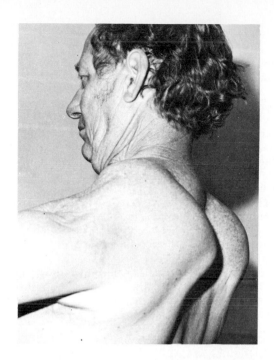

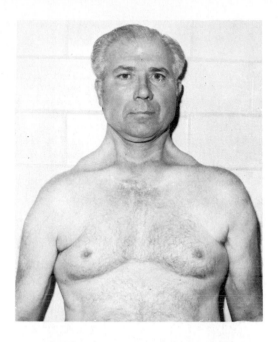

FIG. 18-2. Winging of the scapulae when the arms are elevated.

FIG. 18-3. Shoulder–girdle weakness with "trapezius hump," "step-sign" with prominent down-sloping clavicles, and an oblique anterior axillary crease.

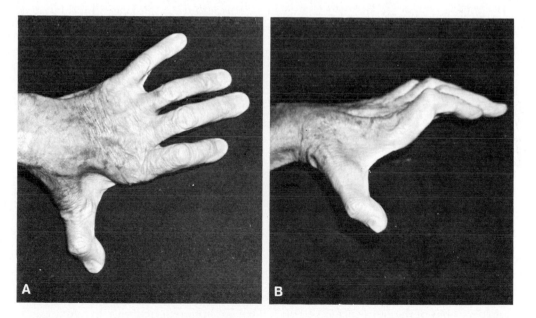

FIG. 18-4. Distal atrophy in motor neuron disease. (*A*) Loss of first dorsal interosseus produces a prominent depression. (*B*) Guttering of the back of the hand.

235

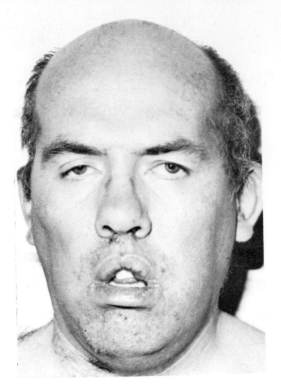

FIG. 18-5. Typical facial appearance in myotonic dystrophy with frontal balding, temporalis and masseter atrophy, ptosis, and protuberant lower lip.

In contrast, patients with neuromuscular disease may have striking muscular atrophy and obvious weakness.

Atrophy of the muscles around the shoulder reveals the underlying bony prominences. The knee or elbow may be greater in circumference than the thigh or arm, respectively. Flattening of the thenar eminence and guttering of the interossei produce a wasted, claw-like deformity of the hand (Fig. 18-4). Several disorders produce characteristic appearances. Examples include "Popeye arms" in facioscapulohumeral dystrophy, "stork legs" in Charcot–Marie–Tooth neuropathy, and the "hatchet-face" appearance in myotonic dystrophy (Figs. 18-5 and 18-6).

Pseudohypertrophy of the gastrocnemius occurs in Duchenne's muscular dystrophy and occasionally in limb–girdle dystrophy and juvenile spinal muscular atrophy (Fig. 18-7). Diffuse hypertro-

phy suggests myotonia congenita, hypothyroidism, or amyloidosis.

PAIN, STIFFNESS, AND CRAMPS

Inflammatory myopathies and other collagen–vascular diseases may produce muscle pain and tenderness, but the absence of these symptoms does not exclude the diagnosis. Rarely, similar discomfort is present with trichinosis, influenza, or an acute denervating disorder. In older patients, pain, aching, and stiffness in the shoulder and hip–girdle muscles should suggest polymyalgia rheumatica. Most patients with limb aching and pain without weakness do not have a neuromuscular disease. The diagnosis of fibrositis or fibromyositis is often evoked particularly in otherwise healthy middle-aged women who have diffuse aches and pains; however, this purported entity has no pathologic foundation.

Stiffness may be a nonspecific symptom, or it may be a symptom of *myotonia*, a phenomenon consisting of a delayed relaxation of the muscle following voluntary contraction or percussion. This produces a difficulty in releasing the grip or initiating movements after a period of rest.

Muscle *cramp*, a prolonged involuntary contraction, is a universal and benign symptom that occurs with increased frequency during unaccustomed exercise, "body building," pregnancy, or electrolyte disturbance. It may also occur in hypothyroidism, partial denervation (especially in ALS), tetany (with hypocalcemia, hypomagnesemia, or alkalosis), and certain metabolic myopathies.

MUSCLE TWITCHING

Fasciculations (the tiny twitches with the terrible reputation) are contractions of muscle fibers in a single motor unit. Fasciculations appearing in a strong muscle are usually benign and are exacerbated by many factors, including fatigue and caffeine. When they occur in a weak muscle they are most frequently associated with ALS, but they also occur after root or peripheral nerve injury. Fasciculations differ from *myokymia*, which consists of brief tetanic contractions of independent small bands of muscle. Myokymia may be benign (upper eyelid twitching) but has been reported with thyrotoxicosis, uremia, tetany, and rare motor unit hyperactivity states. Myokymia occurring in facial muscles suggests multiple sclerosis or a pontine glioma.

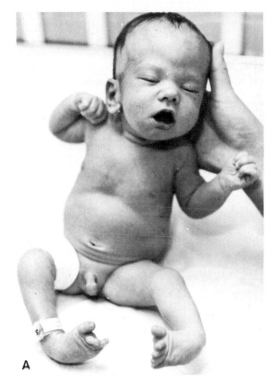
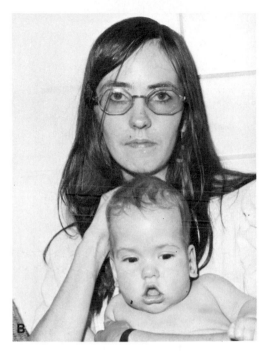

FIG. 18-6. (*A*) Congenital myotonic dystrophy with typical "shark mouth" and club feet. (*B*) Same infant whose evaluation led to the diagnosis of myotonic dystrophy in the mother.

HYPOTONIA

Various unrelated disorders present with infantile hypotonia. The most frequent abnormality in the "floppy baby" is a CNS disease, such as perinatal asphyxia. The hypotonic infant may exhibit normal muscle strength, with the ability to lift its head or limbs against gravity. In the absence of other abnormalities, the prognosis for normal development may be excellent. In infants with obvious weakness, the underlying disorder may be spinal muscle atrophy or a congenital myopathy. Weaknesses of sucking and respiration are serious concomitants, but the prognosis in these disorders varies widely.

DEFORMITIES

Neuromuscular disorders are often associated with skeletal deformities and should be suspected in the patient with unexplained hip dislocation, scoliosis (Fig. 18-8), contracture, or malformation of the feet (*e.g.*, club foot, equinovarus, or pes cavus deformity). Arthrogryposis or multiple congenital limb deformities may occur with various diseases affecting any part of the motor unit (Fig. 18-6).

MYOGLOBINURIA

The syndrome of myoglobinuria consists of weakness and painful swelling of affected muscles in association with headaches, nausea, and vomiting. The urine turns reddish brown within 24 hours and is benzidine- and hemastix-positive. Most episodes are not associated with an underlying neuromuscular disease but are related to unusual circumstances that produce acute muscle necrosis, including trauma, exertion, muscle ischemia, electrical shock, recurrent seizures, or myotoxin agents.

A patient with recurrent myoglobinuria should be evaluated for an underlying neuromuscular dis-

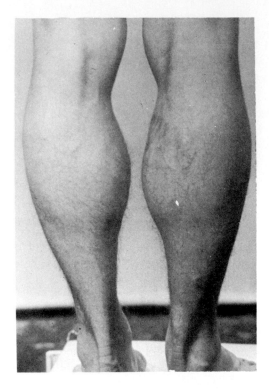

FIG. 18-7. Pseudohypertrophy of the calves.

ease. McArdle's disease, carnitine palmityl transferase deficiency, and acute polymyositis are among the possibilities. The major complication of myoglobinuria is acute renal failure. Affected patients should be hydrated to maintain a high urine output, and serum electrolytes should be closely monitored. Hyperkalemia may require correction.

CLINICAL INVESTIGATION

ENZYME ELEVATION

Muscle necrosis results in elevated levels of "muscle" enzymes including serum creatine phosphokinase (CPK). The highest levels occur in the syndrome of myoglobinuria, Duchenne muscular dystrophy, and polymyositis. Normal or slightly elevated values occur in most of the chronic muscular dystrophies and motor neuron disorders.

ELECTROMYOGRAPHY

Electrophysiologic investigation includes nerve conduction velocity studies, needle electromyography (EMG) examination, and evaluation of neuromuscular transmission. A description of these tests is provided in Chapter 12.

EMG is useful in differentiating *neuropathic* (anterior horn cell and peripheral nerve) from *myopathic* disorders (Fig. 18-9). *Neuropathic* disorders are associated with spontaneous electrical activity of individual muscle fibers, detected as *fibrillation* potentials. Fewer motor units are available for voluntary recruitment, producing a decrease in the electrical interference pattern. Following chronic denervation, surviving motor axons develop collateral sprouts that reinnervate muscle fibers. This results in abnormally large polyphasic motor unit potentials.

In *myopathic* disorders, the random loss of individual muscle fibers results in a decreased size of the motor unit potentials. Many units are recruited

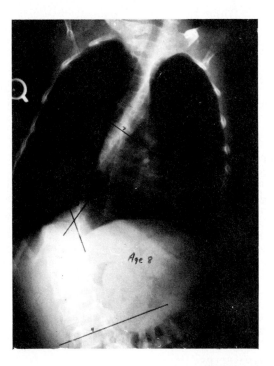

FIG. 18-8. Scoliosis in chronic infantile spinal muscular atrophy. The angle of curvature is measured and followed closely (55° in this patient).

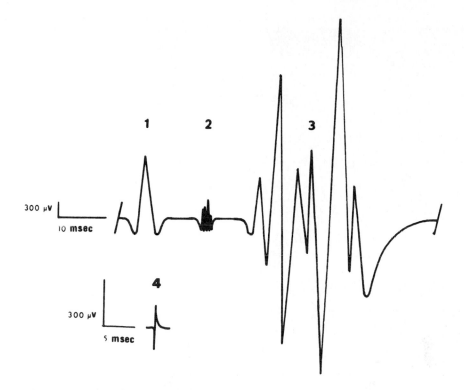

FIG. 18-9. (*1–4*) Single motor unit action potentials recorded by EMG. (*1*) Normal motor unit action potential. (*2*) The *myopathic* potential is brief, small amplitude, and polyphasic. (*3*) The *neuropathic* potential is prolonged, high amplitude, and polyphasic. (*4*) A fibrillation potential is produced by a denervated muscle fiber.

simultaneously during voluntary contraction, producing an increased interference pattern.

In disorders of the *neuromuscular junction*, repetitive stimulation of a peripheral nerve may produce a characteristic change in the amplitude of the muscle twitch. Single-fiber EMG may reveal increased "jitter," a measure of the synchrony of depolarization occurring in muscle fibers nearby.

MUSCLE AND NERVE BIOPSY

Muscle biopsy is performed easily under local anesthesia as an outpatient procedure, allowing histologic, histochemical, ultrastructural, and biochemical studies.

Normal muscle stained for enzyme activity shows a checkerboard distribution of two muscle fiber types (Fig. 18-10*A*); type 1 or slow-twitch oxidative fibers (lightly stained with 9.4 ATP), and type 2 or fast-twitch, glycolytic fibers (darkly stained with 9.4 ATP). With chronic denervation and reinnervation, as in anterior horn cell disorders and neuropathies, fiber-type grouping is seen (Fig. 18-10*B*). In contrast, most myopathies are characterized by the destruction of individual fibers (Fig. 18-10*C* and *D*). Abnormal storage products or an enzyme deficiency can be characterized biochemically. Disorders of the neuromuscular junction are generally associated with a normal muscle biopsy.

The muscle biopsy is useful in the evaluation of patients suspected of having a myopathy, anterior horn cell disease, "paralytic" hypotonia, or a collagen-vascular disorder associated with neuromuscular symptoms. It is particularly valuable in the dystrophies and spinal muscular atrophies, where genetic counseling requires a confident diag-

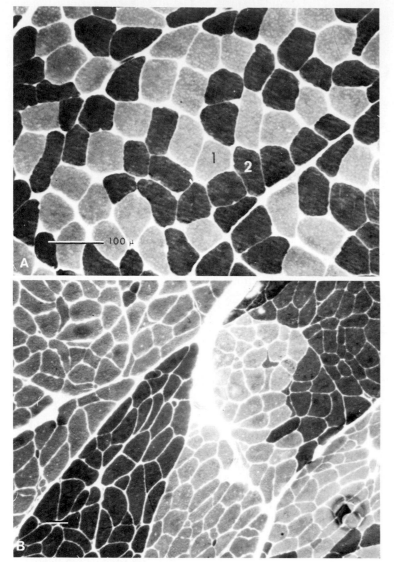

FIG. 18-10. Muscle biopsy. (*A*) Histochemical fiber typing with *p*H 9.4 myofibrillar ATPase shows the checkerboard distribution of type 1 (oxidative) and type 2 (glycolytic) fibers in normal muscle. (*B*) Fiber-type grouping in chronic denervation. (*C*) Histologic stains reveal characteristic features of Duchenne dystrophy, including necrotic and opaque fibers, marked variation in fiber size, and proliferation of connective tissue. (*D*) Mononuclear cell infiltrate around muscle fibers and vessels in polymyositis. Bar = 100 u.

nosis, and in polymyositis, where intensive immunosuppression may be recommended. Muscle histochemistry (particularly fiber typing) is essential whenever a biopsy is performed.

Nerve biopsy is used less frequently because routine histologic sections are rarely of diagnostic use except with vasculitis, amyloidosis, granulomatous disorders, and in the inherited neuropathy HMSN Type 1 (Charcot–Marie–Tooth disease).

GENETICS AND GENETIC TESTING IN NEUROMUSCULAR DISEASE

In the past 10 years molecular biology techniques have produced a torrent of information on the chromosome location of specific genes, gene structure, and segments of DNA so closely "linked" to

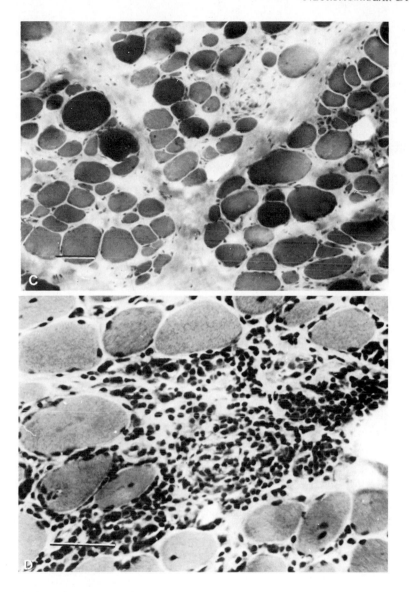

FIG. 8-10 (*continued*)

individual genes that their presence or absence provides important clues about the gene itself. Our aim is to avoid the jargon and complexity of original gene research articles and in this way make the material useful to our audience, the practicing clinician. For those wishing more detailed information, a suitable review of genetics is listed in the references.

Before describing the specific genetic defects known for the various neuromuscular disorders, some basic definitions and concepts will be reviewed here. Disease affecting the motor neuron, the peripheral nerve, and muscle itself may be transmitted in families from generation to generation. Until the seminal work on the structure and function of

DNA by Watson, Crick, and many others in the early 1950s, the molecular events leading to transmission of disease within families remained purely descriptive. Since then progress has been rapid in searching for the chromosome, disease-specific gene sites, the DNA structure of specific genes, their protein product, and the various gene and protein abnormalities associated with specific diseases. Since 1988 the number of neurologic disorders with known gene loci has grown from 61 to 129. And of these 129, there are at least 27 neuromuscular disorders for which the gene locus is known. For many of these disorders where the nucleotide sequence of the specific gene is known, members of an entire family can now be screened to detect affected and unaffected individuals. It is in this latter area that the knowledge of gene location and structure can be put to very practical use. Individuals carrying a defective gene can receive counseling regarding the chances their progeny may inherit the defect, and asymptomatic individuals can be warned of the possible later development of a specific disease. This ability to precisely identify individuals who might develop a disease gives to physicians unique diagnostic and therapeutic opportunities, especially if techniques of gene therapy are eventually successful. To assist the clinician in understanding the sections on genetics sections, some basic definitions and concepts are presented here.

NUCLEAR DNA

This material consists of a "backbone" of alternating sugar and phosphate molecules to which are attached any of four individual bases. These bases (adenine, guanidine, thymidine, and cytosine) are the building blocks of DNA. It is their numbers and sequence that determine the "coding" for individual proteins to be manufactured in the cell cytoplasm. Each chromosome consists of two very long, intertwined DNA strands that are held in close proximity by chemical bonds between bases on each of the strands. This forms the now familiar "double helix" configuration of DNA. Although the bulk of cell DNA is located in the nucleus, a small amount is also found within mitochondria, where its function in coding for mitochondrial proteins is similar to that for nuclear DNA. At various positions along the DNA of a given chromosome within the nucleus, there are specific base sequences that define a particular gene. Information provided by the base sequence is transcribed to build a complementary structure, messenger RNA.

MESSENGER RNA (mRNA)

This material is formed by nuclear processes as a complementary structure to nuclear DNA. Once formed, it is not confined to the nucleus but may pass freely into the cell cytoplasm. Having received a specific message from nuclear DNA, the messenger RNA in concert with ribosomal RNA captures free amino acids and assembles them into a specific protein according to the original DNA code from the cell nucleus.

PROTEIN

The basic building material for structural integrity and metabolic functions in cells. Proteins are continually being manufactured (DNA to mRNA to protein) and destroyed in normal cell processes.

GENE

The specific sequence of bases on a chromosome that codes for the construction of a particular protein. Individual genes are localized to a predictable section of the double helix DNA strand of a given chromosome.

GENE DEFECT

This refers to any abnormality of base sequence in a portion of the DNA strand constituting the gene. The abnormal DNA sequence may transcribe the same error to mRNA, which in turn may manufacture a faulty protein based on the error. The resulting defective protein, in some instances, may cause no particular problem in cell function. In other situations cell function may be seriously compromised to the point of causing cell death.

SOUTHERN BLOT

The long DNA strands constituting the chromosomes may be cut into short fragments of nucleotide sequences by "restriction enzymes," which operate at very specific sites along the DNA. A solution containing the fragments may then be applied to an agarose gel and the gel exposed to an electrical field (electrophoresis) to separate the DNA fragments from one another according to molecular weight. The fragments are then transferred onto a nitrocellulose membrane, where "probes" of DNA complementary to some of the separated DNA fragments can be used to localize a specific DNA sequence. The complementary probe structure will bind to the separated fragment. If the probe has been previously radioactively labeled, the fragment's position on the membrane (and its molecular weight) can be determined. Since the size of fragments resulting from DNA exposure to a given restriction enzyme is known, the size of the fragment identified by a given probe can be determined to be normal, too big, too small, or missing altogether. In this way, smaller than expected genes with missing segments or "deletions" can be identified (Duchenne's dystrophy) or segments that are too large (myotonic dystrophy) can be detected.

DELETIONS AND DUPLICATIONS

A missing sequence of bases within a particular gene DNA is termed a *deletion*. Conversely, an enlargement of base sequences within gene DNA is called a *duplication*. Such sequence anomalies may cause a serious transcription error in the formation of mRNA, which, in turn, will result in the manufacture of a faulty protein or no protein at all.

POINT MUTATION

This is the term designating a gene defect produced by the substitution of one single base for another in the total gene sequence. At critical points this can cause major DNA code errors that result in either defective proteins or total absence of a particular protein.

POLYMERASE CHAIN REACTION

Polymerase chain reaction (PCR) is a technique for increasing the amount of DNA to be studied. Since the amount of DNA material from blood or other tissue is quite small, single-point mutations or small deletions or duplications may escape detection using Southern Blot techniques. By knowing the base pattern on either side of a sequence of interest, the sequence can be manufactured in very large quantities, a process called *amplification*. The amplified sequence can then be detected by Southern Blot methods.

WESTERN BLOT

This technique utilizes an antibody developed against a protein of interest (commonly used to identify dystrophia in muscle). A specimen of tissue containing the protein is solubilized, all proteins separated according to molecular weight by electrophoresis, and the separated proteins transferred to a nitrocellulose membrane. The antibody is then tagged with a suitable marker and applied to the membrane, where it will bind to the protein of interest if that protein is present. The marker locates the protein and allows for quantitation of the amount present and its molecular weight. The method is commonly employed to detect reduced size and amount of dystrophia in Becker dystrophy, or total absence of dystrophia as in Duchenne's dystrophy.

LINKAGE ANALYSIS

It is well recognized that certain specific base sequences on a DNA strand of a given chromosome are passed on to an individual's progeny. Some of these, though carrying no genetic information, are in close geographic proximity to specific genes. Whenever the gene is present on a chromosome, these noncoding nucleotides are also there and are considered "linked" to the gene. This "linkage" of a gene to a nongene sequence is useful in predicting if the gene in question has been passed on to a patient's children. The method is used to detect disease carriers and even for prediction of disease status in unborn fetuses. This indirect method of inferring the absence or presence of the defective gene is useful in cases of DNA point mutations where gene defects may be unknown or too heterogeneous for precise identification.

DISORDERS OF THE ANTERIOR HORN CELL (MOTOR NEURON)

SPINAL MUSCULAR ATROPHIES

Spinal muscular atrophies (SMAs) constitute a group of hereditary disorders characterized by a loss of spinal and cranial motor neurons. Most cases are autosomal recessive.

In acute infantile SMA (Werdnig–Hoffmann disease), symptoms of hypotonia, poor feeding, weak cry, and respiratory distress may be present at birth or may develop after several months. An examination reveals flaccid areflexic extremities, fasciculations of the tongue, pooling of saliva in the posterior pharynx, and paradoxical respiration. Most patients die of respiratory failure by 2 years of age.

A chronic form of infantile SMA presents during the first year of life. Children often learn to sit independently but are rarely able to stand or walk. Sensation and intellect are unaffected. As the disease progresses, skeletal deformities develop, which include contractures at the hips and knees, hip dislocation, and kyphoscoliosis (Fig. 18-8). Many patients survive into adolescence or adulthood, but they ultimately succumb to respiratory insufficiency. Good pulmonary management, including spinal fusion to prevent progressive kyphoscoliosis with its attendant restrictive pulmonary disease, can increase the life expectancy of these patients by many years.

Juvenile SMA (Kugelberg–Welander disease) produces insidious proximal weakness beginning in late childhood or early adolescence, with a clinical appearance similar to limb–girdle dystrophy. The progression is slow, but many patients require a wheelchair by their mid-thirties. The prevention of contractures and scoliosis and good respiratory care are important.

GENETICS

This disorder is inherited as an autosomal recessive trait with the abnormal gene located on chromosome 5. The precise gene location has not yet been determined, and its structure is still unknown. However, linkage analysis can provide useful probabilities as to the likelihood of relatives developing the disorder.

X-LINKED SPINAL AND BULBAR MUSCULAR ATROPHY (KENNEDY'S SYNDROME)

This unusual disorder can be confused with ALS. Patients in their thirties and forties present with swallowing dysfunction, slurred speech, perioral and tongue fasciculations, facial weakness, mild limb weakness, hand tremor, gynecomastia, and impotence. The disorder is very slowly progressive but, unlike ALS, rarely is fatal. Some link to an androgen abnormality had been suspected, but only recently has the precise genetic abnormality been identified.

GENETICS

This strikingly familial disorder results from a gene abnormality on the X chromosome. Thus, only males are affected, there is never male-to-male transmission, and females, though unaffected clinically, are carriers. In this respect the genetics of the disorder are identical to that seen in Duchenne's and Becker's dystrophies. The mutation for the disease occurs within the androgen receptor gene on the X chromosome. Since androgen receptors are present in motor neuron cell membranes, a defect of the receptor somehow is involved in pre-

mature cell death. The specific gene defect is an enlargement of the base coding sequence due to multiple, extra CAG repeats (cytosine-adenine-guanidine). It is termed a *trinucleotide repeat expansion*. An increase of gene size in a genetically determined disorder is unusual, having been described in only two other conditions, the fragile X syndrome and myotonic dystrophy. Testing for this gene defect is available only in some research laboratories at present but may become more widely available for use in identifying asymptomatic males in kindreds where the disease occurs.

AMYOTROPHIC LATERAL SCLEROSIS

Amyotrophic lateral sclerosis (ALS) is characterized by rapidly progressive muscle wasting and weakness resulting from the degeneration of anterior horn (lower) motor neurons, accompanied by varying degrees of spasticity and hyperreflexia due to degeneration of (upper) motor neurons of the pyramidal tract. Most cases occur sporadically, whereas 5% are familial. Asymmetrical weakness and atrophy are common; they produce a foot drop or wasting and claw deformity of the hand (Fig. 18-4). Hyperreflexia in an atrophic fasciculating limb strongly suggests the diagnosis. Within weeks to months, the disease may spread to involve virtually all muscles. A typical advanced case will have an atrophic fasciculating tongue, forced monotonous speech, and relative sparing of facial and eye movements. Many patients succumb to respiratory insufficiency or infection within 2 to 3 years, although 10% survive 10 years or longer, particularly younger patients and those who have a preserved swallowing function.

EMG is the most useful diagnostic procedure. Spinal cord compression is often suspected when cranial weakness is absent; cervical myelography may be indicated in this circumstance. Hyperthyroidism, hyperparathyroidism, chronic lead intoxication, plasma-cell dyscrasia, hexosaminidase A deficiency, or collagen-vascular disease may also be considered in the differential.

The treatment of this rapidly progressive disorder is entirely symptomatic, because the cause remains unknown, and patients often fall victim to advertisements for quick cures. In addition to providing exercise, stretching, respiratory care, adaptive equipment, and bracing, the patient's chronic swallowing dysfunction should be monitored to avoid malnutrition, recurrent aspiration, or choking spells. Specific therapy for this serious complication is included in the section on treatment. Cramps are often bothersome, particularly at night, but they may respond to quinine. Spasticity may be relieved with baclofen or diazepam.

GENETICS

The vast majority of ALS patients have no known genetic predilection for the disease. In the 5% of ALS patients with similarly affected family members often in multiple generations, linkage analysis points to a gene defect on chromosome 21. This work is still under development and not yet available to general physicians.

POLIOMYELITIS AND POSTPOLIO SYNDROME

Acute poliovirus infection in nonimmunized individuals leads to a nonspecific febrile illness, followed by paralytic symptoms in a minority. Although the widespread use of immunization has reduced the frequency of new cases in developed countries, many adult patients still have residual weakness.

Unpredictably, progressive weakness may develop after many years of static deficit. In some cases, this results from unrecognized nerve compression that can easily occur in a weakened extremity. In other patients, the progression of weakness may result from a dysfunction of surviving motor neurons. There is no evidence for viral reactivation.

DISORDERS OF THE PERIPHERAL NERVE

This topic is discussed in Chapter 12.

DISORDERS OF THE NEUROMUSCULAR JUNCTION

MYASTHENIA GRAVIS

Myasthenia gravis (MG) is an autoimmune disorder that is associated with a postjunctional defect of the acetylcholine receptor. It may occur at any age but is most frequent in women in the third decade and men in the fifth decade of life. Fluctuating weakness and fatigue in cranial, limb, or trunk musculature are characteristic. Ocular symptoms, including alternating ptosis, diplopia, and blurred vision, are present initially in more than 50% of patients and eventually in 90%. Facial muscles are often weak, producing a snarling appearance when laughing. Speech becomes increasingly slurred, nasal, or hoarse as the patient continues to talk, and progressive dysphagia with choking and aspiration of food may occur. Neck muscle weakness may be so prominent that the patient uses his hand to prop up his head. Generalized MG frequently involves the respiratory muscles, and sudden respiratory collapse was a serious complication before the advent of modern immunosuppressive therapy.

The clinical course is occasionally fulminating but is characterized more commonly by a gradual progression of symptoms with frequent remissions and relapses. Sudden worsening may occur with an overdose of anticholinesterase medication, superimposed infection, electrolyte disturbance (especially hypokalemia), pregnancy, or emotional stress.

The diagnosis of MG should be considered in any patient who has an unexplained acute weakness, and in patients who demonstrate objective signs of fatigue such as ptosis or diplopia following sustained upward gaze. A possible diagnosis of MG may be strengthened by three tests, any of which may be negative. An intravenous (IV) injection of edrophonium (Tensilon) may briefly correct ptosis, ophthalmoparesis, or limb weakness. Repetitive stimulation of a peripheral nerve may produce a decremental response in the train of muscle twitches. Antibodies to the acetylcholine receptor (AChR) are present in the serum of almost 90% of patients with generalized MG, and they have been shown to produce both a transmission blockade and the destruction of the postsynaptic receptor site of the neuromuscular junction.

The treatment of MG has changed considerably in the last two decades, with increasing recognition of the primary autoimmune disturbance. Anticholinesterase drugs such as pyridostigmine (Mestinon) and neostigmine are still used for symptomatic relief but are no longer the mainstay of treatment. Patients frequently become refractory to these medications during exacerbations of the disease, leading to overdosage and a paradoxical increase in weakness. An overdosage is suggested by signs of cholinergic excess, including abdominal cramping, diarrhea (which may lead to hypokalemia and further weakness), profuse salivation and lacrimation (with increased risk of aspiration), miosis, fasciculations, or cramps. If early signs of ventilatory failure develop, anticholinesterases should be discontinued and intubation should be considered.

Corticosteroids are effective in the treatment of MG. When given initially, a transient exacerbation of weakness may occur in the first 2 weeks with a potential for respiratory failure. Azathioprine is also used, alone or in combination. Intensive immunosuppression is continued for 6 months to 1 year and is then tapered slowly after the patient regains his full strength.

Thymectomy has been recommended for all patients with generalized MG, except the very young and very old. Ten percent of patients harbor a thymoma, but all patients are believed to benefit from surgery. Plasmapheresis and IV immunoglobulin have been advocated for the treatment of acutely weakened patients but must be used with other immunosuppressive therapy since its benefit is transient. Other ancillary measures include the use of ephedrine and potassium and the avoidance of medications known to potentiate neuromuscular blockade, including aminoglycoside antibiotics, propranolol, procainamide, phenytoin, quinine, and curare.

Patients with isolated ocular symptoms (ocular MG) may develop generalized MG, but the risk is low after 2 years. These patients may not require surgery or intensive immunosuppression. MG in childhood differs little from the adult form but is treated conservatively because aggressive treatment may retard growth. Fifteen percent of infants born to affected mothers develop transient myasthenic symptoms such as hypotonia and feeding difficulties, probably due to the transplacental passage of maternal AChR antibodies. These newborns usually respond to anticholinesterase medication and resolve over 6 to 12 weeks. A reversible myasthenic syndrome may develop following chronic use of D-penicillamine.

EATON–LAMBERT SYNDROME

This rare paraneoplastic disorder is characterized by the defective release of acetylcholine from nerve terminals. Unlike MG, cranial muscles are usually spared, patients may have distal paresthesias or dry mouth, and a repetitive stimulation produces an incremental response. The diagnosis mandates a search for malignancy, particularly bronchogenic carcinoma. Symptoms may improve with the removal of the malignancy or by immunosuppression.

BOTULISM

Improperly canned food may contain the toxin of *Clostridium botulinum*, which also impairs the release of acetylcholine. A sudden onset of blurred vision, diplopia, dysphagia, and dysphonia is rapidly followed by a generalized weakness: patients frequently require respiratory support. Recovery is prolonged but may be complete. The diagnosis rests on the isolation of the toxin from stool, gastric contents, or contaminated food, and there is a characteristic electromyographic abnormality.

In infants, honey has been implicated as a source of botulinum spores that germinate in the intestine and produce the toxin, leading to hypotonia and severe constipation.

DISORDERS OF MUSCLE

DYSTROPHIES

DUCHENNE'S AND BECKER'S DYSTROPHY

Duchenne's muscular dystrophy is an X-linked recessive disorder but may be due to a spontaneous mutation in one-third of cases. From the time they first walk, boys who are affected with this disorder have a clumsy waddling gait. An examination reveals a protuberant abdomen resulting from an accentuation of the lumbar lordosis, pseudohypertrophy of the calves (Fig. 18-7), and tight heel cords with a tendency toward toe walking. In arising from the floor, these children adopt a characteristic four-point stance with hands planted first on the ground, then on the knees and thighs as they come to a stand (Fig. 18-1). Mental retardation is common, whereas eye movements, swallowing, and sensation are unaffected. When the child is 9 to 12 years of age, increasing proximal weakness makes independent walking impossible. Once in a wheelchair, these children develop progressive kyphoscoliosis, contractures in all joints, and equinovarus deformity of the feet. In subsequent years, these children become virtually immobile and require complete care. The combination of weak respiratory muscles and kyphoscoliosis drastically reduces pulmonary reserve, and they generally succumb by the late teens or early twenties.

The CPK is markedly elevated (20 to 100 times normal) even before the disease is clinically evident. Muscle biopsy is characteristic, with increased fibrosis, grouped basophilic fibers, large round opaque fibers, and scattered necrosis (Fig. 18-10C).

Although no specific treatment is available, a competent rehabilitative team can improve the quality of life for these patients. The prevention of contractures, particularly the Achilles tendon and iliotibial band, is important early in the disease. A surgical release of contractures along with the use of long leg braces can prolong independent walking for several years. When the patient becomes confined to a wheelchair, the development of kyphoscoliosis can be slowed with proper upright positioning and, in selected cases, spinal fusion. Unfortunately, hip and knee contractures are accelerated by the constant sitting position, so that these children can sleep only on their side and require numerous pads for comfort. Respiratory management and a host of devices that are useful to patients with chronic disability are described in the section on treatment.

GENETICS

These two disorders are the clinical variations of what has been the most thoroughly studied genetically determined primary muscle disease. For many years clinicians and geneticists had known that the disease was transmitted by a gene defect on the X chromosome. Females were known to be asymptomatic carriers, and males would manifest the disease. Duchenne patients were always the most seriously affected, usually dying in their teens or early twenties. Becker patients were considered by many to have a more slowly progressive form of Duchenne's dystrophy. In some patients diagnosed as having facioscapulohumeral or even limb–girdle dystrophy, the latest DNA work has shown them to have, in actuality, Becker's dystrophy.

Investigation of the X chromosome has shown a wide variety of deletions and point mutations that may lead to a total absence of the gene product dystrophia (a cell membrane protein) or the production of a dystrophia that is smaller than expected, present in smaller than expected quantities, or both. In some cases, the nature of the DNA defect may allow for differentiation between the Becker and Duchenne forms of the disease. At present either form of the disease seems related to dystrophia abnormalities, but the situation may be even more complicated with the discovery of several abnormalities in dystrophia-associated glycoproteins as well.

Testing for the presence or absence of dystrophia is technically difficult and, for the moment, should be carried out by a few service laboratories where quality control and high volume assure accuracy. For children suspected of having the disease, a blood specimen should be screened first, since 60% to 70% of cases will demonstrate a deletion or duplication. The abnormality detected in these may even

be specific for either the Duchenne or Becker form of the disease. For the remaining 20% to 30% where no deletion or duplication is found or where the differentiation between Becker and Duchenne is necessary, a small specimen of skeletal muscle obtained by biopsy should be analyzed by Western Blot for determination of dystrophia quantity and quality. If dystrophia is absent, a diagnosis of Duchenne's dystrophy is confirmed; if dystrophia is reduced in quantity, of an abnormal size, or both, a diagnosis of Becker's dystrophy is confirmed. If there is no dystrophia abnormality, another disorder should be considered.

For testing to determine the carrier status of females, it is necessary to obtain blood from the suspected carrier as well as from any affected dystrophic males in the family. Using PCR and Southern Blot techniques, 55% of Duchenne and 70% of Becker patients will demonstrate a DNA deletion or duplication in the dystrophin gene. If the same abnormality is detected in the female subject, she can be considered to be a carrier. If not detected, a linkage analysis of DNA from the various family members' blood can be undertaken to determine the likelihood of her being a carrier. The results of these analyses are best discussed with the carrier suspect and her family by a physician or genetic counselor who is fully acquainted with the techniques and the diseases. Counseling on carrier status is sometimes less than a perfect statistical proposition and requires great care in presentation to a family.

Finally, for the carrier suspect who is already pregnant and wishes to know whether the fetus is affected with Becker's or Duchenne's dystrophy, prenatal diagnosis may be achieved using cells obtained at amniocentesis/chorionic villus biopsy. By PCR techniques described above, any major deletions or duplications may be detected. If none are found and point mutations are suspected, a linkage analysis of the fetal DNA is possible if sufficient numbers of affected and unaffected relatives are available for study.

FACIOSCAPULOHUMERAL DYSTROPHY

This disorder is characterized by a slowly progressive weakness with predominant involvement of the shoulder-girdle muscles and variable amounts of facial and peroneal muscle weakness. Most cases are autosomal dominant. Symptoms begin insidiously in the first two decades of life and progress slowly; the patient's life span may be normal.

The patient may have difficulty whistling, blowing up a balloon, or drinking through a straw. The lips are often pouting (bouché de tapir), and the smile is transverse. During sleep the eyes may remain slightly open. The clavicles are prominent and downsloping (Fig. 18-3). The shoulders droop and are rotated forward, producing an oblique axillary crease. The scapula wing when the patient attempts to elevate the arms (Fig. 18-2) and the trapezius muscles are pushed up prominently. Atrophy of the triceps and biceps contrasts with preserved forearm muscles, producing a "Popeye" appearance. Peroneal muscle weakness with foot drop occurs in some patients, but hip muscles are generally spared and patients retain the ability to walk. Surgical fixation of the scapula to the posterior thoracic wall has occasionally been performed, because many are able to abduct the arm fully when the scapula is forcibly held in place; unfortunately, the scapula may tear loose. General guidelines for treatment are outlined at the end of this chapter.

GENETICS

The gene for this autosomal dominant disease is located on the long arm of chromosome 4. A large cooperative effort, primarily based in Europe, has defined multiple nucleotide sequences closely linked to the gene, but the gene itself is still not specifically localized. Technical difficulties make linkage analysis in affected families so uncertain that the methods are not yet available to clinicians.

LIMB–GIRDLE DYSTROPHY

Limb–girdle dystrophy is associated with a progressive proximal muscle weakness in childhood or adult life, transmitted in a sporadic or autosomal recessive fashion. A wide range of clinical expression has been noted in these patients, suggesting that this is actually a group of related disorders. Facial, tongue, and pharyngeal weaknesses are usually lacking. The shoulder weakness differs from that of facioscapulohumeral dystrophy in that the deltoid is affected and winging is usually less prominent. An anterior axillary fold and neck flexor weakness is usual (Fig. 18-3). Respiratory muscle involvement may occur in some patients. General supportive measures for these patients are outlined at the end of this chapter.

Progressive proximal weakness is a common complaint in the neuromuscular clinic. Many patients with a limb–girdle syndrome are now recognized as having a specific entity such as adult spinal muscular atrophy or polymyositis, which might previously have been classified on clinical grounds as limb–girdle dystrophy.

GENETICS

The search for the gene abnormality in this disorder is difficult since sporadic cases of this rare disorder are not easily analyzed for DNA defects. However, large inbred kindreds of the disease have provided sufficient linkage information to localize the defect to chromosome 15. The extremely rare autosomal dominant form of this disease has been linked to chromosome 5. DNA analysis for this disorder is still in the province of research laboratories and unavailable to clinicians.

MYOTONIC DISORDERS

MYOTONIA CONGENITA

Impaired muscle relaxation is encountered in both autosomal dominant and autosomal recessive varieties of myotonia congenita. Patients complain of difficulty in releasing their hand grip, stiffness of muscles, and difficulty in initiating activity after a prolonged rest. They may report subjective weakness if normal exertion is opposed by myotonia in antagonistic muscles. Muscle hypertrophy is frequent and occasionally produces a Herculean appearance. EMG is useful in establishing the diagnosis, because muscle biopsy is nonspecific. Several medications are helpful in reducing myotonia, including phenytoin, procainamide, quinine, and carbamazepine.

GENETICS

A defect of the chloride channel in skeletal muscle has recently been defined in both the autosomal dominant form (Thompson's disease) and recessive forms of myotonia congenita. The gene abnormality is due to a point mutation within the chloride channel on chromosome 7. At present, linkage analysis may be done on family members in the autosomal dominant form, but the techniques are still not generally available to clinicians.

MYOTONIC DYSTROPHY

A predominantly *distal* weakness, in contrast to most myopathies, is encountered in adults with myotonic dystrophy. Advanced cases have a characteristic facial appearance with ptosis, temporalis and masseter wasting, protuberant lower lip, and thinning of the sternocleidomastoid muscle, producing a typical "hatchet face" appearance (Figs. 18-5 and 18-6). The speech is often dysarthric and nasal, and the patient may complain of dysphagia. As in other autosomal dominant disorders, mild and severe cases may appear in the same family; however, a unique, commonly observed feature is a lack of acknowledgment of symptoms, even in obvious cases (Fig. 18-6B).

Other organ systems are involved in this disorder, leading to cataract formation, impairment of gastrointestinal motility, and endocrine abnormalities. Patients are frequently noted to have low intelligence, no goal orientation, poor work histories, and bizarre personalities. Progressive cardiac conduction abnormalities may lead to sudden death. Serial electrocardiograms (ECGs) are recommended, and a pacemaker should be considered in patients with progressive conduction disturbance. A reduced ventilatory drive may produce symptoms of alveolar hypoventilation including disturbed sleep. General anesthesia should be given cautiously because patients are unduly sensitive to barbiturates and other medications that depress ventilatory drive. The myotonia is generally asymptomatic and does not require treatment. Weakness of the ankles may be improved with polypropylene splints. Proximal weakness is rarely severe enough to prevent walking.

GENETICS

By linkage analysis methods, chromosome 19 has long been known to contain the abnormal gene for this autosomal dominant disease. Only recently has the gene itself been identified, and work continues to characterize the gene product, a protein kinase. The gene defect, surprisingly, consists of an expansion of trinucleotide repeat sequences reminiscent of that described for X-linked spinal and bulbar muscular atrophy. In myotonic dystrophy a noncoding region of the gene is enlarged by multiple GCT repeats (guanine-cytosine-thymidine) numbering from as few as 100 to over 1000. Disease severity roughly correlates with higher numbers of these repeats. It is now thought that the gene region for these repeats is particularly unstable in both male and female gametes during meiosis, resulting in amplification of the repeats. But for unknown reasons such instability is far more serious in the female gamete. Thus, a child of a myotonic mother will usually have a significantly larger abnormal gene (and early, more serious clinical manifestations) than would be expected if the father were the carrier of the defect. The gene instability-amplification during meiosis and correlation of increased gene size with more severe disease may explain the phenomenon of "anticipation" long known to occur in myotonic dystrophy. Testing for this gene defect using Southern Blot techniques is now available to the clinician in many DNA laboratories. The method can be used to screen relatives of affected patients, looking for asymptomatic individuals who might wish to know their status before having children.

INFLAMMATORY MYOPATHIES

An autoimmune disturbance underlies polymyositis (PM) and dermatomyositis (DM), whereas other syndromes may be caused by Coxsackie virus, pyogenic bacteria, trichinosis, sarcoid, or tuberculous granuloma. In polymyalgia rheumatica, an inflammatory process may involve fascia rather than muscle, although patients complain of muscular pain and weakness.

The symptoms and signs of PM and adult-onset DM are identical, with the exception of the characteristic rash of DM. The latter disorder may be a paraneoplastic syndrome in adults. In patients with an associated collagen vascular disease (*i.e.*, systemic lupus erythematosis, rheumatoid arthritis, Sjögren's syndrome), the inflammatory myopathy may be a minor or major manifestation of the disease. Patients with juvenile DM may have a systemic vasculitis with pulmonary fibrosis, myocarditis, gastrointestinal ulcers, cerebral vasculitis, skin ulceration, and calcification.

Although PM may develop at any age, most cases occur in childhood and in the fifth and sixth decades of life. The disease often begins insidiously with systemic features such as fever, arthralgias, myalgias, and Raynaud's phenomenon. Weakness may begin relatively suddenly and may become profound, but more commonly there is a subacute progression of proximal weakness that is not readily distinguishable from other limb–girdle syndromes. Muscle tenderness may be absent. The rash of DM may take several forms, appearing before, after, or in association with the onset of weakness. The upper eyelids often have a lavender or *heliotrope* discoloration, and periorbital edema and flushing of the cheeks occurs in advanced cases. The chest and neck may become reddened and develop telangiectasia. *Gottran's* papules are thickened erythematous patches that occur over the knuckles and other joint extensor surfaces. Skin nodules may break down and exude calcium.

The disease often has a variable course. Some patients have an acute episode with complete recovery, even without treatment. Other patients demonstrate a relapsing, remitting course with incomplete recovery between episodes, or a chronic progressive course that responds poorly to treatment. The serum CPK is elevated in most cases, particularly those with acute onset. A muscle biopsy shows necrosis of muscle fibers, perivascular inflammatory infiltrate, and perifascicular atrophy (Fig. 18-10D).

Corticosteroids are generally prescribed, although some patients may not respond despite the addition of azathioprine or other immunosuppressants. Adult patients who have DM should be screened for an occult malignancy.

Inclusion body myositis is a cause of insidious proximal or distal weakness in adults. Biopsy reveals red-rimmed vacuoles in the muscle fibers, and intranuclear filamentous inclusions. Steroids appear ineffective and the disease progresses slowly.

Polymyalgia rheumatica (PMR) is characterized by muscle pain and stiffness, which is most severe in the morning and has a predilection for the shoulders. It rarely occurs before 55 years of age and is most frequent in women. Other constitutional symptoms may be present, including anorexia, fever, and night sweats. Temporal arteritis (TA), which is manifested by scalp tenderness, temporal headaches, or visual obscuration, is associated with PMR in 20% to 50% of cases and can produce a sudden, permanent blindness. With the exception of the erythrocyte sedimentation rate that is markedly elevated, all tests are usually normal. PMR responds dramatically to low doses of prednisone. High doses are used if TA is suspected or documented by temporal artery biopsy.

METABOLIC MYOPATHIES

GLYCOGEN STORAGE DISEASES

These rare autosomal recessive disorders exhibit the common finding of excess glycogen in skeletal muscle and sometimes other organ systems. Patients with McArdle's disease lack adequate amounts of the enzyme myophosphorylase, which is necessary for the degradation of glycogen into glucose. Painful cramps and myoglobinuria are typical clinical features. The enzyme acid maltase also acts to degrade glycogen into glucose. Symptoms of acid maltase deficiency may vary widely from severe hypotonia, weakness, and early death in infants to the adult form characterized by a slowly progressive limb–girdle syndrome with early respiratory failure.

The other diseases in this group (with deficiency of phosphofructokinase, phosphoglycerate mutase, or phosphoglycerate kinase) are characterized by low or absent levels of enzymes critical to normal cell glycolysis. Clinical symptoms for any of these include exercise intolerance, cramps, and myoglobinuria.

GENETICS

The chromosome loci for these autosomal recessive disorders are known and are summarized in Table 18-2. Testing for the gene defect in affected patients or their relatives is not useful clinically since the diagnosis can be made more readily by muscle biopsy and tissue assay for enzyme deficiencies.

DISORDERS OF LIPID METABOLISM

Carnitine palmityl transferase deficiency also results in exercise-related cramps. The gene locus for this autosomal recessive disorder is now thought to be on chromosome 1, but genetic tests of use to the clinician are not yet available. Carnitine deficiency is associated with a progressive weakness and may produce superimposed attacks of hepatic encephalopathy.

MITOCHONDRIAL MYOPATHIES

Defects in mitochondrial metabolism may underlie various syndromes including progressive external ophthalmoplegia, infantile hypotonia, or adult exercise intolerance. These disorders are often systemic and are accompanied by a failure to thrive, lactic acidosis, or myoclonus epilepsy. They may occur sporadically or through maternal inheritance. Muscle biopsy shows "ragged-red fibers" caused by an accumulation of abnormal mitochondria.

The Kearns–Sayre syndrome is a sporadic disorder that presents in the first two decades of life. It combines muscle weakness with a distinctive triad of progressive external ophthalmoplegia, pigmentary retinal degeneration, and heart block. These patients must be evaluated periodically for a need for a cardiac pacemaker.

GENETICS

As with nuclear DNA, significant deletions or subtle point mutations may occur in mitochondrial DNA. The majority of patients with the Kearns–Sayres syndrome show obvious deletions that lead to major defects in the mitochondrial electron transport chain and striking clinical abnormalities. Several commercial laboratories offer DNA analysis for confirmation of this disorder, although the need for such testing is questionable if the patient's clinical signs are typical and the muscle biopsy shows typical ragged-red fibers.

MALIGNANT HYPERTHERMIA

Patients with malignant hyperthermia are free of symptoms unless exposed to certain anesthetic agents, particularly halothane and succinylcholine. The full syndrome includes an elevation in temperature up to 43°C, muscular rigidity, tachycardia, marked lactic acidosis, myoglobinuria, and refractory cardiac arrhythmias. Untreated cases are uniformly fatal. Anesthesia and the surgical procedure must be terminated immediately, while dantrolene sodium is administered with cooling measures.

The disease is autosomal dominant in many patients, and there may be subtle evidence of an underlying myopathy. There is no reliable confirmatory test, thus patients with a previous episode and their relatives should not receive these agents.

GENETICS

The latest work suggests that a genetic defect closely associated with the gene defect for central core disease on chromosome 19 may be causative for malignant hyperthermia. No DNA testing is available to the clinician at present.

TOXIC MYOPATHIES

A wide variety of medications and toxic compounds can produce either acute muscle necrosis or a slowly progressive chronic myopathy. Alcohol can produce both of these syndromes in the same patient and is the most common myotoxin. The acute myopathy usually follows a binge of drinking and may be accompanied by myoglobinuria. Other drugs and toxins associated with acute myopathy include ipecac, amiodarone, clofibrate, other cholesterol-lowering agents, heroin, aminocaproic acid, chlorthalidone, vincristine (where a sensorimotor neuropathy is usually superimposed), and any substance that produces hypokalemia including diuretics, purgatives, liquorice, carbenoxolone, or amphotericin B.

A chronic proximal myopathy is associated with prolonged corticosteroid therapy, particularly with dexamethasone and fluorinated steroids. A discontinuation leads to a slow recovery. The aforementioned drugs associated with acute myopathy may also produce a chronic myopathy.

ENDOCRINE MYOPATHIES

Hypothyroidism is associated with cramps, mild weakness, and "hung-up" reflexes. Hyperthyroid-ism may produce mild weakness, whereas ophthalmoplegia occurs in Graves' disease.

Hypoparathyroidism may lead to a carpopedal spasm or tetany. Hyperparathyroidism may combine weakness with brisk reflexes, which are reminiscent of ALS.

Acromegaly is associated with a chronic myopathy and the carpal tunnel syndrome. The weakness in Addison's disease and hyperaldosteronism is probably caused by electrolyte disturbances. Cushing's disease may produce the same myopathy as exogenous steroids.

CONGENITAL MYOPATHIES

In distinction to other familial myopathies, a congenital myopathy refers to a group of diseases that are frequently inherited, nonprogressive, or slowly progressive and that display characteristic abnormalities on muscle biopsy. They may present in childhood as a floppy baby with contractures or they may present in adult life. The prognosis varies between the various types, and some infantile cases may improve.

GENETICS

Chromosomes containing gene defects have now been identified for three of the congenital myopathies: 19 for central core disease, chromosome 1 for nemaline rod myopathy, and the X chromosome for one form of myotubular myopathy. DNA testing for these disorders is still not available to clinicians.

PERIODIC PARALYSIS AND PARAMYOTONIA CONGENITA

Patients who suffer from a periodic paralysis experience recurrent episodes of acute weakness separated by periods of normal strength. Carbohydrate loading, strenuous exercise followed by rest, cold exposure, or agents that alter serum or total body potassium may initiate an attack. Most cases are inherited and have been subdivided into hypo-, hyper-, and normokalemic forms depending on the serum potassium level. An identical picture may occur sporadically in association with hyperthyroidism, or with total body potassium depletion associated with diarrhea or diuretics. The diagnosis is aided by provocative tests that alter serum potassium. A muscle biopsy reveals characteristic vacuolar changes. Potassium supplementation and acetazolamide are recommended in the hypokalemic variety. The hyperkalemic variety may respond to acetazolamide, diuretics, or salbutamol. Since respiratory and cranial muscles are rarely affected, the overall prognosis is good.

Paramyotonia congenita is a disorder closely related to the periodic paralyses. Clinical symptoms in this autosomal dominant disorder include cold-induced myotonia and weakness, episodic weakness without potassium abnormality, and production of symptoms with potassium loading.

GENETICS

The structure of the adult human skeletal muscle sodium channel is now known following the successful cloning of the gene for that protein. Point mutations in that gene on chromosome 17 are thought to produce either hyperkalemic periodic paralysis or paramyotonia congenita depending on the substitution of only a single base. DNA tests for these disorders are not yet available outside a few research laboratories but are likely to be developed eventually for use by clinicians.

TREATMENT OF NEUROMUSCULAR DISEASES

The initial reaction of the patient and family to the diagnosis of a neuromuscular disease is often one of despondency and hopelessness. In time, with support and understanding, they may understand that the future is less bleak and that a well-balanced rehabilitative approach will maximize their function, prolong ambulation, deter complications, and create an optimistic environment. The problems that these patients face depend more on the degree of the disability than on the disease that produces it. The treatment of the ambulatory patient is discussed in this section, and an approach to the problems of the weaker wheelchair-bound patient is provided.

All patients are encouraged to maintain a normal range of motion through a program of stretching, while avoiding overexertion. The frozen shoulder is a painful complication particularly in ALS, but is easily avoided. In children, contractures at the hips and ankles may impair walking long before a muscle weakness becomes critical, and this must be prevented. A foot drop may be remedied by a lightweight posterior polypropylene splint that is molded to the shape of the foot and fits into the shoe. An arthrodesis may be necessary for a marked ankle instability. Painful calluses that accompany foot deformities may be treated by a podiatrist. In patients with hip weakness, raising the height of seats with a toilet seat elevator or electric lift chair makes standing without assistance easier. Patients rely heavily on hand supports for getting up from the toilet, getting out of a tub, or going up stairs. Supports must, therefore, be securely anchored. A cane, crutches, or a walker is necessary as the weakness increases. Long leg braces that allow locking of the knee joint may prevent precipitous knee buckling. If a patient becomes temporarily bedridden due to an intercurrent illness, early ambulation is imperative to prevent further atrophy and contracture. In Duchenne dystrophy, the percutaneous release of contractures at the Achilles tendons, iliotibial bands, and hamstrings combined with the use of long leg braces may prolong ambulation for several years.

Weakness of the hands impairs the fine dexterity required for eating, writing, and dressing. Various pieces of adaptive equipment are designed to splint the hand and allow easier grasping. Large-handled utensils, a buttonholer, or a pencil attached to the hand with a Velcro strap may be useful. The patient who has a shoulder weakness can use a long-handled reacher to get objects from cabinets or high shelves.

Visual obstruction due to ptosis may be relieved by lid crutches attached to eyeglasses or by surgery. Head instability due to neck weakness may be improved by wearing a foam collar. Patients who have severe dysarthria can develop alternate means of communication with the help of a speech therapist.

Patients who have dysphagia may benefit from an evaluation including a modified barium swallow and a consultation with a nutritionist and a therapist with experience in swallowing disorders. Occasionally, symptoms are temporarily ameliorated by an inferior constrictor myotomy; however, in advanced cases, the patient may require diversion by esophagostomy or gastrostomy. Salivary secretions that cannot be swallowed may be decreased with amitriptyline or they may be removed with a portable suction unit. Families should be instructed in the Heimlich maneuver.

Palpitations or unexplained syncope due to a heart block can occur with various neuromuscular disorders, particularly myotonic dystrophy and Kearns–Sayre syndrome. These patients may require periodic ECGs or Holter monitoring, and a pacemaker may be indicated. With acute generalized weakness, pulmonary and swallowing function should be monitored in an intensive care unit because respiratory failure or aspiration can develop rapidly, particularly in myasthenia and the Guillain–Barré syndrome.

Respiratory failure is the most serious complication of the nonambulatory patient and is produced by a combination of respiratory muscle weakness, atelectasis, recurrent aspiration, poor cough reflex, and decreased lung volume from progressive kyphoscoliosis. The usual physical signs of pneumonia are often difficult to detect in a patient who has a baseline tachypnea because of small tidal volumes. The patient's family should therefore seek an early medical evaluation if any new respiratory symptoms develop. Daily postural drainage with chest percussion can be performed at home by the family, and immunization should be considered.

Kyphoscoliosis in preadolescent patients (Fig. 18-8) is minimized by a properly fitting wheelchair and polypropylene jackets or braces that restrict lateral movement. Spinal fusion may be suggested if the curve progresses despite conservative therapy. Segmental spinal instrumentation allows early postoperative ambulation and has replaced the use of Harrington rods.

A great deal of mobility and comfort is possible for the patient who is confined to a wheelchair if the wheelchair is properly designed and fitted. Detachable arm rests and swing-away elevating leg rests facilitate transferring and prevent lower extremity contractures and edema that develop if the legs are constantly dependent. Ball-bearing feeders and a lap tray make independent eating possible for the patient who cannot elevate his arms to his mouth, and a thick foam cushion prevents decubiti. A motor-powered wheelchair is useful for patients who lack the upper limb strength or the attendance of another person necessary to propel the chair.

The transfer of an overweight patient in and out of a wheelchair can be difficult even with a hoist, thus reduction diets should be encouraged. A patient with total paralysis will often sleep more comfortably on an air or water mattress that distributes weight evenly, preventing unrelenting pressure and decubiti. A frequent change of position in both the wheelchair and bed as well as padding to support the limbs prevent nerve compression palsies.

Apart from minimizing the physical handicap, the physician must be aware of the patient's social, emotional, and sexual needs. A severely handicapped patient who relies on others for eating, hygiene, and elimination will understandably become depressed over this extreme dependency. Active counseling of the patient and family should be directed toward solutions to the various problems in "personal space" and independence that arise.

The patient in the final stage of a neuromuscular disease will succumb to respiratory failure unless ventilatory support is provided. The thought of prolonging life on a respirator is unacceptable for many patients, but for others considerable satisfaction can still be gained if the environment is supportive. The physician, patient, and family should discuss these options well in advance.

The treatment of patients with chronic neuromuscular weakness requires the services of the primary physician; physical, occupational, and respiratory therapists; an orthotist; a podiatrist; an orthopedist; a nutritionist; a social worker; and a psychiatrist. With proper management, the patient can be educated to compete in a world that is inherently easier for those who are able-bodied.

QUESTIONS AND DISCUSSION

1. A 61-year-old woman is admitted to the hospital with a 4-day history of progressive weakness. Her medical history is unremarkable except for congestive heart failure that is being treated. She had been constipated for several days and she then had diarrhea after taking laxatives. Her examination was remarkable for generalized mild weakness, hypoactive reflexes, and flexor plantar responses. Cognition, cranial nerves, and sensation were normal.

A quadriparesis with intact cognition, a lack of sensory disturbances, and flexor plantar responses are most likely caused by a disorder of the peripheral nervous system.

The differential diagnosis includes the Guillain–Barré syndrome (reflexes are more likely to be absent than diminished), botulism poisoning (lack of cranial nerve dysfunction, especially ocular, is atypical), myasthenia gravis (cranial nerve involvement would also be expected), acute polymyositis, and an electrolyte disturbance.

Useful studies include an electrolyte and serum CPK determination and a sedimentation rate. An EMG–nerve conduction study would be helpful early on, when the physician is looking for decrement with repetitive stimulation (seen in myasthenia and botulism).

This patient's potassium level was 1 mEq/dl due to diuretics and diarrhea, and her strength returned to normal with treatment.

2. A 19-year-old pregnant woman reports that two maternal uncles died of muscular dystrophy at the ages of 15 and 16. She wants to know if her fetus or her 1-year-old daughter may be affected.

Some cases of muscular dystrophy may have actually been spinal muscular atrophy. This is usually an autosomal recessive disorder, and the risk of the woman developing muscular dystrophy would be low.

Death occurring in the teenage years is characteristic of Duchenne dystrophy. This illness in two male siblings would not be due to a spontaneous mutation, and it indicates that their mother was a carrier. Genetic linkage analysis requires blood samples from the affected uncles but is not an option in this case.

Blood samples on mother and daughter as well as fetal cells obtained by amniocentesis can be screened for 70% of patients carrying the abnormal gene. If no deletion is found, linkage analysis can be carried out on all specimens to determine the probabilities of all three having the identical X chromosome. Since there is no linkage information from the two deceased brothers of the pregnant mother, no accurate probability can be given concerning her being a carrier or having passed the abnormal gene on to her fetus. The situation might be clarified if the mother's CPK is significantly elevated, which would argue for her being a carrier. Since CPK levels usually decrease during pregnancy, the finding of normal values would not be helpful. In such a complex situation the assistance of an experienced genetic counselor is advised.

3. A 51-year-old woman is admitted to the hospital because of symptomatic bradycardia. She reports frequent "dizzy spells" for about 1 year, but she has never fainted. She has also had a lifelong stiffness in her hands and a nasal voice, and she trips frequently.

Myotonic dystrophy is suggested by the history of grip myotonia and systemic complaints. Recurrent abdominal pain, gallstones, chronic diarrhea, dyspepsia, and dysphagia are common symptoms. Cardiac conduction disturbances may present with dizziness or may be discovered on a routine ECG. A careful examination for clinical myotonia, as well as for the characteristic facial features, supported the diagnosis in this case. Myotonic dystrophy is a common disorder, although it is frequently overlooked.

An ECG demonstrated a complete heart block, and a pacemaker was implanted during the patient's stay in the hospital. Bilateral foot drop was relieved with polypropylene ankle bracing.

All relatives of this patient should be evaluated clinically for signs and symptoms of this autosomal dominant disorder. Symptomatic relatives can be counseled and followed for the disorder. Asymptomatic individuals can be given information regarding the disease. Should they wish to know their carrier status with certainty, a DNA analysis of blood would provide definite information regarding the presence or absence of trinucleotide repeat sequences. This information would be of use particularly to unaffected individuals planning families.

SUGGESTED READING

Brooke MH: A Clinician's View of Neuromuscular Diseases, 2nd ed. Baltimore, Williams & Wilkins, 1986

Dyck PJ, Thomas PK, Lambert EH et al: Peripheral Neuropathy, Vols 1 and 2. Philadelphia, WB Saunders, 1984

Emery AEH, Rimoin DL: Principles and Practice of Medical Genetics, Vols 1 and 2. New York, Churchill Livingstone, 1990

Engel AG, Banker BQ: Myology, Vols 1 and 2. New York, McGraw-Hill, 1986

Evans RW, Baskin DS, Yatsu FM: Prognosis of Neurological Disorders. New York, Oxford University Press, 1992

Nickel VL, Botte MJ: Orthopedic Rehabilitation. New York, Churchill Livingstone, 1992

Rowland LP (ed). Amyotrophic Lateral Sclerosis and Other Motor Neuron Diseases. Advances in Neurology, Vol 56. New York, Raven Press, 1991

Neurologic Aspects of Cancer

Susan Miguel Snodgrass

Cancer may affect the central nervous system (CNS) in many ways. Primary tumors of the CNS are diagnosed in about 17,000 Americans each year. Though this is only a small fraction of the approximately 1 million new cases of cancer, brain tumors kill more Americans each year than multiple sclerosis and Hodgkin's disease. The emotional implications alone both to the patient and to the family associated with the diagnosis of brain tumor can be insurmountable. The symptoms, ranging from headache at their mildest, to seizures, blindness, paralysis, and cognitive impairment, rob patients of independence and dignity. Their incidence unfortunately is on the rise.

The medical subspecialty of neuro-oncology is not limited to the diagnosis, care, and treatment of the patient with primary tumors of the CNS. It also deals with the neurologic complications of systemic cancer, both metastatic and nonmetastatic, and the complications of its treatment.

Improvements in the treatment of systemic cancer, while increasing survival, have been accompanied by an increase in the incidence of CNS metastasis. While eradicating systemic tumor, micrometastases find a safe haven from most chemotherapeutic agents behind the blood–brain barrier. Brain metastases, affecting about one-quarter of patients, are now seen in patients thought long cured of their systemic disease and not just in the near-terminal. The natural history of other cancers has been changed. CNS metastases are now being diagnosed in tumors thought not to have nervous system spread. In some malignancies, like small cell carcinoma of the lung and acute lymphoblastic leukemia, CNS involvement is so commonplace that brain imaging in the former and lumbar puncture and prophylactic treatment in the latter are a matter of course.

In some cases the nonmetastatic neurologic complications outnumber the metastatic. Encephalopathy is one of these. Although in patients with large tumor burdens this is sometimes attributed to multisystem failure, it is important for the clinician to recognize that this is not always the case. Aside from the diagnosis of CNS metastasis, now made more often antemortem with the help of improved and more readily available neurodiagnostic equipment, the recognition and treatment of electrolyte abnormalities and endocrine dysfunction, which contribute to encephalopathy, can improve the quality of life and improve patient survival.

Advances in the fields of molecular biology have allowed researchers to identify oncogenes that are involved in cell reproduction and when left unmodified can lead to tumor production. Acquired or inherited mutations and deletions in one of the cell's defense mechanisms, the tumor suppressor can allow the cell to be unusually susceptible to the development of certain cancers. This is especially important in neurology, since it has long been recognized that there are associations between brain

William J. Weiner and Christopher G. Goetz, eds. *Neurology for the Non-Neurologist*, Third Edition. Copyright © 1994, 1989 by J. B. Lippincott Company. Copyright © 1981 by Harper and Row Publishers, Inc.

tumors and familial syndromes such as von Recklinghausen's disease.

Recent identification of onconeural antigens (an antigen present in both the nervous system and the tumor) has increased the understanding of certain paraneoplastic syndromes. These are rare but clinically important complications of systemic cancer felt to be antibody-mediated and are discovered before the underlying cancer in 50% of the cases. Their recognition could lead to early diagnosis and treatment for the patient, ultimately leading to a better outcome.

This chapter addresses some of the more common problems in neuro-oncology. The non-neurologist needs to be able to diagnose these conditions in a timely fashion when therapeutic intervention is of the most benefit to the patient.

PRIMARY CENTRAL NERVOUS SYSTEM TUMORS

GLIOMAS

CNS tumors vary greatly between adults and children. Histology is more variable in children, and the location is usually in the posterior fossa. In adults the most common brain tumors are gliomas, including not only the astroglial neoplasms but also oligodendrogliomas and ependymomas (Table 19-1).

Astrocytomas account for 65% to 70% of all gliomas. The term is commonly used to describe low-grade tumors of astroglial origin. These tumors stain positively for glial fibrillary acidic protein (GFAP). Initially gliomas were classified into four histologic grades by Kernohan, using cellularity, pleomorphism, vascularity, and necrosis. More recently a three-tiered system is in vogue that seems to correlate more with survival. In this system the low-grade astrocytoma is hypercellular with varying pleomorphism, lacking the vascular proliferation of anaplastic astrocytoma and the necrosis that is the hallmark of glioblastoma. Average survival is about 1 year with glioblastoma multiforme (GBM) and about double or triple that for anaplastic astrocytoma.

Low-grade astrocytoma encompasses a diverse group of tumors in which both histology and location play key roles. With gross-total resection the objective whenever possible, cerebellar juvenile pilocytic astrocytoma is resected for complete cure, while the inaccessible brain tumor is often irradiated with dismal results. In addition, a substantial

TABLE 19-1. Brain Tumors

	PERCENT OF ALL BRAIN TUMORS
Glioma	40–50
Astrocytoma Grade I	5–10
Astrocytoma Grade II	2–5
Astrocytoma Grades III and IV (GBM)	20–30
Oligodendroglioma	1–4
Ependymoma (all grades)	1–3
Meningioma	12–20
Pituitary tumor	5–15
Neurinomas (primarily VIII)	3–10
Medulloblastoma	3–5

Adapted from Schwartz SI (ed): Principles of Surgery, 5th ed. New York, McGraw-Hill, 1989.

margin for error exists in diagnosis with low-grade tumors resembling stroke, multiple sclerosis, or encephalomalacia and GBMs mistaken for metastases, abscesses, lymphoma, or parasites.

TUMOR BIOLOGY

Recent developments in molecular biologic techniques have allowed researchers to identify growth factors and inhibitors necessary for cell growth and differentiation. Proto-oncogenes have been identified whose products consist of growth factors or their receptors, which unrestrained allow for the development of malignancies. The oncogene c-sis, encoding for part of the platelet-derived growth factor, has been identified in GBM. It is involved in the autocrine system in malignant astrocytomas. C-erbB has been identified in 30% of malignant gliomas and is associated with the transforming growth factor receptor.

The most well-described tumor suppressors are Rb and p53, associated with retinoblastoma and the Li–Fraumeni syndromes, respectively. They are felt to be present ubiquitously and to encode for proteins that go on to bind with virally encoded oncoproteins.

Sophisticated chromosome analysis of GBMs has identified gene abnormalities in chromosomes 10, 13, 17, and 22, with the chromosome 10 abnormality seen only in the most anaplastic tumors. Chromosome 17 abnormalities, however, have been demonstrated to be present in all grades of astrocytomas. It would seem that mutations on chromosome 17, near the p53 gene, may be an early change in the origin of astroglial neoplasms and would help to explain the long-recognized tendency for gliomas to become more malignant with time. It is also of interest that the hereditary neurofibromatosis syndrome Type 1 is associated with chromosome 17 abnormalities and neurofibromatosis syndrome Type 2 is associated with abnormalities of chromosome 22.

PRESENTATION

The presentation of astroglial neoplasms differs with age, location, and histology. Typically an adult presents with headache, seizures, and/or focal neurologic deficit. Increasingly common is the discovery of a brain mass in an otherwise asymptomatic individual. The overall incidence increases with age, and unexplained first seizures in adults should be thoroughly investigated with computed tomography (CT) or magnetic resonance imaging (MR). The presentation is helpful prognostically. Patients with long-standing symptoms and having seizures without focal neurologic deficits or altered mentation seem to do better. Earlier age of onset is also associated with a better prognosis.

Gliomas are usually supratentorial in adults. Low-grade tumors usually appear hypodense by CT and T1-weighted MR and show minimal or no enhancement (Fig. 19-1). GBMs, on the other hand, are often ring-enhancing lesions, sometimes cystic with massive amounts of peritumoral edema. These are generalizations, and the appearance can vary.

TREATMENT

Treatment of patients with glioblastoma depends on the size, location, and clinical setting, and must be individualized. Initial treatment is usually corticosteroids, which reduce cerebral edema and frequently give dramatic symptomatic relief. Anticonvulsants to prevent seizures are usually in order for supratentorial lesions, and care must be taken to follow levels. Drug toxicity should not be mistaken for progression of disease.

Definitive therapy involves surgery whenever possible. Not only does surgery provide symptomatic relief by means of decompression, but it also provides an adequate pathologic specimen. Removal also improves response to adjuvant thera-

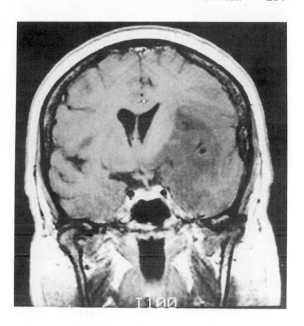

FIG. 19-1. Large, low-grade glioma of the left parietal-temporal lobe.

pies. Along with age under 45, the completeness of removal probably best correlates with improved survival. When removal is not possible, biopsy should be attempted to confirm the diagnosis. Even gross total removal is usually followed by externally delivered radiation therapy. It is given to a wide area, including 1 cm to 2 cm of peritumoral edema in the radiation port. Whole-brain radiation therapy is no longer administered for single, primary lesions given its potential for long-term cognitive dysfunction. Postoperative radiation therapy has been shown to increase median survival from 17 to approximately 36 weeks. With improved techniques a 52-week survival is generally expected.

The role of radiation therapy in low-grade lesions is less clear. Most clinicians still follow surgery with externally delivered radiation therapy. An important exception is the pilocytic astrocytoma, in which median survival already approaches 80% at 10 years. Radiation therapy is probably indicated in those patients undergoing subtotal resection; however, some recent studies failed to show significant differences in median survival, time to malignant transformation, or quality of life when a group of patients with low-grade astrocytomas were treated immediately postoperatively with radiation therapy *vs* a group of patients in whom radiation was withheld until there was progression of disease.

Various strategies have been employed to increase the effectiveness and reduce the toxicities associated with radiation therapy. Hyperfraction, a method of delivering radiation in more frequent, smaller dose per fraction treatments, has been employed. The smaller dose per fraction is felt to be less toxic to the late-responding tissues, the CNS, even when the total dose delivered is higher than with conventional fractionation. There may be slightly improved tumor control, and the delayed toxicities may be lessened. Neither hyperthermia nor radiation sensitizers have been found to be useful in the treatment of gliomas.

CHEMOTHERAPY

The most important restriction in the use of chemotherapy in the treatment of brain tumors is the blood–brain barrier. This unique barrier consisting of endothelial cells and glial foot processes prevents the passage of most oral and intravenously administered hydrophilic drugs. The most commonly used drugs are the lipid-soluble nitroureas. The oral drug lomustine (CCNU) and the injectable carmustine (BCNU) are the most studied. Individual studies using adjunct chemotherapy in addition to surgery and XRT have shown little benefit, though a larger meta-analysis gives a survival advantage to those patients receiving chemotherapy. Long-term survivors were more likely to be found in the chemotherapy arms of these studies.

In vitro testing of other, more hydrophilic compounds have been encouraging. Most notable are the platinum-based drugs such as cisplatin (DDP). Arterial injections of this drug in conjunction with intravenous BCNU is a common therapy in the medical center setting and has shown some promising results in terms of improved survival. Tumors involving multiple vascular territories require intra-arterial injections to each of those territories to be effective, and this limits the usefulness of this technique in many patients. Side effects, including seizures, stroke, and hearing loss, can be devastating and should be considered when counseling patients about available treatment options. The most difficult ethical decisions involve the young, neurologically intact brain tumor patient who has just undergone a gross total resection of a malignant lesion. These patients already have the best survival advantage, and to subject them to yet unproven, potentially hazardous treatment modalities is a decision that needs to be made by well-informed patients in conjunction with qualified physicians in a major medical center setting. Gross total resection followed by externally delivered radiation to 6000 cGy and concomitant intravenous BCNU is still the treatment of choice for many patients. More risky, less well-proven therapies can be utilized at recurrence but always following a re-resection whenever possible. Chemotherapy is not routinely employed as part of the initial treatment of low-grade glioma in adults, though it can be useful at recurrence. Patients should be encouraged to seek care at a center actively involved in national protocols.

BRACHYTHERAPY

Catheters can be surgically implanted into the tumor bed, which later can be loaded with radioactive seeds, usually ^{125}I. These seeds deliver constant low-dose radiation to the tumor bed with limited exposure to surrounding normal tissue. This therapy has been used as "up-front" therapy in conjunction with externally delivered radiation therapy. It has also been employed at the time of recurrence. It has been shown to increase survival in malignant glioma in this setting. Unfortunately, mass effect–producing radionecrosis frequently follows this treatment, necessitating chronic steroid treatment and reoperation in a substantial number of patients. Recurrence distant from the original radiation field, rare in conventionally treated patients, has been increased as well.

IMMUNOTHERAPY

Immunotherapy utilizing either antibodies, immune effector cells, or viruses and cytokines has been shown to have antitumor effects *in vitro*. Radioactively labeled antibodies have been used intravenously, intra-arterially, into the ventricle and into the tumor bed. In a small number of patients, some interesting but short-lived responses have been noted. At the present time antibody therapy seems to be most useful in the treatment of leptomeningeal tumor.

Interferon-alpha and beta have shown limited responses but with significant toxicity. Interleukin-2–activated lymphocytes (LAK cells) have been shown to result in tumor regression in a small number of patients. However, large amounts of peritumoral edema produced by the interleukin necessitated the use of corticosteroids, which are lympholytic. Investigations using lower doses of interleukin-2 are pending. Studies using lymphocytes derived from the tumor bed (tumor-infiltrating lymphocytes, TIF) are also being conducted.

OLIGODENDROGLIOMA

The oligodendrogliomas are a less frequently occurring subclass of glioma. They are derived from oligodendrocytes, the myelin-producing cells of the CNS. Histologically they have a "fried-egg" appearance and stain for myelin basic protein. They tend to present in patients with seizures. They have a tendency to bleed spontaneously and can present with a stroke-like syndrome. Though usually presenting as ill-defined hypodense lesions on CT or T1-weighted MR, they frequently calcify, but rarely enhance.

Oligodendrogliomas are treated by excision. The role of radiation therapy is controversial since oligodendroglioma is by definition a low-grade glioma. It is probably indicated in subtotally resected lesions, and it has shown some survival advantage. Median survival is about 5 years. Chemotherapy has been utilized for recurrent malignant disease. A combination of procarbazine, CCNU, and vincristine (PCV) is now being used in that setting.

MENINGIOMA

Meningiomas represent 12% to 20% of all intracranial neoplasms. They are usually benign lesions originating in the arachnoid layer of the meninges. They are not a malignancy of the brain parenchyma and by definition are "extra-axial." They occur most commonly along the dural folds and cerebral convexities, though they may occur in the spinal cord as well. They may be hyperdense on noncontrasted CT (Fig. 19-2). They are usually isodense to brain parenchyma on both T1- and T2-weighted MR. Enhancement is shown on CT and MR. They are hormonally responsive and occur more frequently in women than men. They are increased in breast cancer patients, and it is important to differentiate a benign meningioma from a metastatic brain lesion. Meningiomas are also increased in von Recklinghausen's disease. There are various histologic subtypes. Papillary and angioblastic varieties are more aggressive.

Clinical presentation is dependent on the size and location of the lesion. Surgical resection is the treatment of choice if treatment is necessary. Recur-

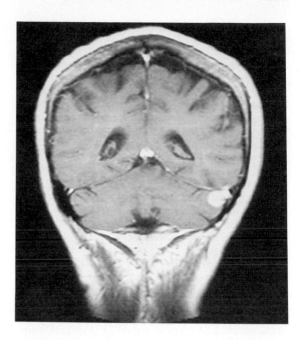

FIG. 19-2. Left-sided tentorial meningioma.

rence has been linked to the degree of resection. Radiation therapy has been used in patients with incomplete resections, especially those having more aggressive histologies. Since meningiomas are usually a relatively benign lesion, frequently found on "routine scans," observation may be an option for certain select patients.

Some meningiomas have been found to be estrogen and/or progesterone receptor positive. Some have D1 dopamine receptors. Hormonal therapy has been used in certain patients with recurrent disease.

PITUITARY TUMORS

The term *pituitary tumor* refers to a diverse group of neoplasms that happen to be located in the sella turcica, the location of the pituitary gland. They can be primary or metastatic. Some pituitary masses are not tumors at all; giant aneurysms and granulomas can also be located in that area. The most commonly occurring tumor is the pituitary adenoma. It is a benign tumor accounting for 5% to 15% of intracranial neoplasms, occurring less frequently than meningiomas.

Pituitary adenoma typically presents with headache, bitemporal visual loss, ocular palsy, and symptoms of hormonal oversecretion or pituitary insufficiency. The most frequent oversecretion syndrome is that produced by the prolactinoma. It is frequently seen in young women presenting with galactorrhea and amenorrhea. The growth hormone–secreting adenoma is the next most common, presenting in children as gigantism and in adults as acromegaly. Overproduction of other pituitary hormones occurs, as do nonsecretory tumors.

The sella turcica is a small, bony midline structure with a dural covering that lies beneath the optic chiasm. It is this relationship, and the chances for permanent visual loss, that often dictate treatment. Small, prolactin-secreting lesions confined to the sella, especially microadenomas, are usually amenable to treatment with dopamine agonists such as bromocriptine. Bromocriptine and a synthetic somatostatin agent called octreotide may be effective in some growth hormone–secreting tumors.

Suprasellar extension, visual loss, medication ineffectiveness, or intolerance may all be indications for surgery. The surgical approach is usually transpenoidal, with minimal morbidity to the patient. Postoperative radiation may be used in certain patients, especially those with large residual or recurrent tumor. Some patients require chronic hormone replacement. All patients deserve a multidisciplinary approach to their care, involving the endocrinologist, ophthalmologist, neurologist, and neurosurgeon.

CHILDHOOD TUMORS

MEDULLOBLASTOMA

Medulloblastomas are malignant tumors of the CNS composed of small cells with scanty cytoplasm and hyperchromatic nuclei. Their cell of origin is not known. They are presumed to arise from the embryologic external granular layer and can be considered to belong to a group of tumors collectively called *primitive neuroectodermal tumors* (PNETs), all of which selectively express a cellular membrane protein called *synaptophysin*. The term *medulloblastoma* refers to those PNETs occurring below the tentorium. They are the most common solid tumor of childhood, second only to leukemia in overall frequency (Table 19-2).

The peak incidence of medulloblastoma is at 5 years. It typically presents as a midline cerebellar

TABLE 19-2. Incidence of Brain Tumors in Children by Histology

TUMOR	PERCENT
Medulloblastoma	25
Cerebral low-grade astrocytoma	23
Cerebellar astrocytoma	13
High-grade astrocytoma	11
Brain-stem glioma	10
Ependymoma	9
Germ cell tumors	2
Other	7

Adapted from Walker RW: unpublished.

mass with symptoms of increased intracranial pressure. Headache, lethargy, nausea, and vomiting are common, as are ataxia and double vision. Increased tumor bulk can fill the fourth ventricle and impede the outflow of cerebrospinal fluid (CSF) and produce hydrocephalus. These symptoms rapidly worsen and are present for a short time before the tumor is diagnosed, 4 months on average. The CT or MR reveals a dense midline posterior fossa lesion (Fig. 19-3). Most patients have hydrocephalus at the time of diagnosis. Other tumors may mimic medul-

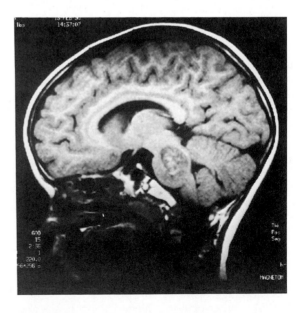

FIG. 19-3. Rare brain-stem primitive neuroectodermal tumor (RNET).

loblastoma, but certain features of the history and scan may help to differentiate them. Cerebellar astrocytomas tend to produce more lateralizing signs. Brain-stem gliomas produce long-tract signs including hemiparesis and spasticity as well as more cranial nerve palsies than the medulloblastoma. Ependymoma, also presenting as a midline lesion, most closely mimics medulloblastoma but produces more cranial nerve palsies. Most of these other tumors are diagnosed after a longer symptomatic period. Intoxications and post–viral encephalomyelitic syndromes may mimic the symptoms and should be considered in the differential in the child with a negative scan. The opsoclonus–myoclonus paraneoplastic syndrome associated with neuroblastoma should also be considered in these children.

Unlike adult brain tumors, medulloblastoma has a predilection for causing micrometastasis to the subarachnoid space. This is referred to as *meningeal seeding*. Distant metastasis can occur as well, especially to the bone and occasionally to the peritoneum. The use of microfilters when a ventriculoperitoneal shunt is required is common practice. Disseminated tumor, present in 20% to 30% of children at the time of diagnosis, is probably the most important predictor of poor outcome. A staging work-up consisting of postoperative scanning of the brain, spinal MR or myelogram, and CSF examination should be done in all patients even if there are no symptoms of metastases. Because of the natural history of this disease, even asymptomatic patients are presumed to have micrometastases and postoperative radiation therapy is given to the cranial-spinal axis in most cases.

Medulloblastoma presenting in very young children is a very difficult disease to treat. These patients are more likely to present with more histologically differentiated, more diffusely metastatic tumors, and to have a worse prognosis. Children under 3 are also more devastated by treatment. The cognitive impairment associated with radiation therapy in this group has led to studies utilizing chemotherapy postoperatively and delaying radiation therapy. Other studies have used chemotherapy in conjunction with reduced-dose radiation therapy. Hypothyroidism is another side effect of radiation therapy in these patients.

The overall 5-year survival for patients with medulloblastoma is about 50%; it is much higher in certain subgroups. This tumor should be considered potentially curable. A classification schema has been developed in an attempt to identify those patients with average vs increased risk for early recurrence. This might allow for treatment modifications, allowing for reduced radiation doses in the patients with average risk and/or identifying those patients who might benefit from adjuvant chemotherapy immediately postoperatively.

EPENDYMOMAS

Ependymomas arise from the ependymal cells lining CSF-filled spaces. This tumor usually presents as a posterior fossa mass arising from the floor of the fourth ventricle in children. It can also present in the hemispheres and spinal cord. In the posterior fossa it produces symptoms of increased intracranial pressure with headache, nausea, vomiting, and occasional cranial nerve palsies. Clinically and radiographically the tumor resembles the medulloblastoma. Surgical resection is the treatment of choice, and the degree of resection is again prognostic for good survival. Eighty-five percent 5-year survival has been reported in patients after complete resection; however, a 45% 5-year survival is the average overall. These tumors, like medulloblastoma, can seed the neuro-axis but do so in a very small percentage of patients. Cranial-spinal postoperative radiation therapy is frequently employed for diffuse ependymomas of the posterior fossa. Local radiation is used for hemispheric and spinal lesions.

Spinal ependymoma accounts for 60% of spinal cord gliomas and may present anywhere along the length of the spinal cord. The tumor has a predilection for the lumbosacral spine. Resection and radiation therapy are utilized. Complete neuroimaging should be employed to ensure that a spinal lesion is not a drop metastasis from the posterior fossa.

Chemotherapy has been used in small children to delay radiation, similarly to medulloblastoma. It may also have a role in the treatment of more malignant lesions and at recurrence.

PRIMARY CNS LYMPHOMA

Primary central nervous system lymphoma (PCNSL) is a rare tumor representing about 1% of intracranial neoplasms. It is a form of non-Hodgkin's lymphoma and is usually of the B-cell variety. It rarely if ever metastasizes systemically. It should not be confused with CNS involvement with systemic lymphoma, which almost always is leptomeningeal and not parenchymal. It is more frequent in patients with inherited, acquired, or iatrogenically induced immunodeficient states. The incidence in transplant patients is greatly increased compared with that in the general population. About 10% of patients with the acquired immunodeficiency syndrome (AIDS) have been shown to be affected in autopsy series.

PCNSL typically presents in the sixth or seventh decade with a slight male predominance. The symptoms are vague, such as headache and personality changes. Neither seizures nor focal neurologic problems are encountered in the average patient. Immunocompromised patients present at an earlier age. PCNSL is hyperdense and brilliantly contrast enhancing on imaging studies. Edema is not a common feature. Multifocal in 50% of the cases, it frequently involves deep midline structures. It resembles toxoplasmosis on scan and often occurs in similar patient populations. It is common practice to treat these lesions empirically with anti-toxoplasmosis medications for 2 weeks and then to follow the patients clinically and radiographically in an attempt to save the patient a biopsy. Steroids should not be used unless the patient is severely compromised neurologically or herniation is imminent. Steroids will reduce the chance of positive cytology if a biopsy is eventually required.

Resection has no place in the treatment of PCNSL. The work-up of these patients should include a brain image, preferably an MRI. A spinal tap can yield positive cytology but more frequently shows nonspecific changes. Slit lamp exam and/or vitreous biopsy may be useful in the 20% of patients presenting with ocular involvement. Bone marrow biopsy may help in some patients, perhaps to differentiate PCNSL from systemic lymphoma or small cell lung cancer. If unable to obtain a diagnosis by these means, a stereotaxic biopsy is in order.

Once the diagnosis is secured, corticosteroids are commonly employed and give great symptomatic relief. They should probably be used with the institution of radiation therapy, which is the mainstay of treatment.

Even with radiation therapy, the prognosis in this disease remains poor. The average life expectancy is about 16 months in the immunocompetent patients and less in immunodeficient ones. Trials involving the use of chemotherapy have shown average survival of 40 months in different series using different chemotherapy regimens. Methotrexate is an effective drug, commonly used intravenously, intrathecally, and intraventricularly in this disease

and has shown great promise. It has been shown to produce measurable levels in the CSF even when given intravenously. Unfortunately, it has significant neurotoxicity, which is increased by prior exposure to radiation therapy.

CNS COMPLICATIONS OF SYSTEMIC CANCER

BRAIN METASTASES

Metastatic tumor to the CNS occurs in about one-quarter of cancer patients, two-thirds of whom are symptomatic. Given 1 million new cases of cancer diagnosed each year in America, the number of patients with symptomatic brain metastases is staggering. It greatly exceeds the number of any single primary tumor type occurring in the adult population. It is one of the feared complications of systemic cancer, as well as one of the most difficult to treat.

The symptoms depend on the size, location, and number of metastases. At times, presenting with headaches, altered mental status (AMS), cranial nerve palsies, paralysis, and seizures, they produce immeasurable morbidity and mortality for the cancer patient. They occur not only in the moribund patient, riddled with disease, but also in the otherwise well patient thought to be free of disease.

Brain metastases are felt to be derived from hematogenesis spread of microscopic tumor, and in most cases either a primary or secondary lung lesion can be identified. Common primary tumors that metastasize to brain include breast, melanoma, kidney, gastrointestinal, and non-Hodgkin's lymphoma. Their increased incidence is probably due to improved control elsewhere in the body. Brain metastases are the first manifestation of malignancy in 15% to 20% of patients. Some tumors, like small cell carcinoma of the lung, so commonly metastasize to the CNS that brain MR or CT is used in the staging process. Prophylactic whole-brain radiation therapy has been employed in this disease, decreasing the amount of symptomatic brain disease but not increasing overall survival.

Brain metastases usually appear as brightly enhancing lesions, which are multiple about 50% of the time. They are usually associated with considerable surrounding cerebral edema. Certain tumors have hemorrhagic tendencies and can mimic intracranial hemorrhages. Most notorious for this are choriocarcinoma, malignant melanoma, renal cell, and thyroid carcinoma. Overall the most common hemorrhagic brain metastasis is from a primary lung tumor. Controversy exists as to a posterior fossa predilection for metastases from abdominal and pelvic primaries.

Dexamethasone is the most common initial form of therapy. It is a corticosteroid and helps reduce surrounding edema and greatly improves symptoms in most patients. The initial dose is usually 16 mg/day in divided doses, but higher doses delivered intravenously are sometimes warranted in patients with severe or rapidly worsening symptoms. It is usually given in conjunction with an H_2-blocker or a stomach-coating agent to prevent some of the gastrointestinal side effects. Close monitoring for hyperglycemia is necessary, especially in diabetic patients and those on high doses of medications.

A recent study comparing the use of radiation therapy with or without surgical extirpation produced some interesting results in a select group of patients with singular brain metastases. Surgical removal followed by radiation therapy prolonged survival and decreased the likelihood of local recurrence and death due to neurologic disease. Though long-term survival at 90 weeks was not significantly improved, the duration and quality of survival in the short term were greatly improved. Obviously, treatment decisions need to be individualized. Surgery is a clear choice in those 15% to 20% of patients whose brain metastasis is the first sign of systemic cancer. It is probably also a treatment option in those patients with well-controlled or controllable systemic disease and a life expectancy of at least 6 months. It is also important to realize that surgery secures the diagnosis definitively. Not all patients with cancer and brain lesions have brain metastasis and its inherent dismal prognosis. Other pathologies have been found in up to 11% of surgically treated patients in this clinical situation.

The most common treatment of brain metastases is radiation therapy. It is used both alone or postoperatively in conjunction with corticosteroids in most patients. A typical dose is 3000 cGy delivered to the whole brain over ten fractions. Modifications in total dose and dose per fraction are indicated in patients with more indolent tumors who may survive to suffer the sequelae of this high-dose-per-fraction schema. More specific radiation portals may be in order for certain patients and for retreatment. The absolute necessity of postoperative radiation therapy is also being studied, as is the use of chemotherapy.

Anticonvulsants are indicated for those patients who present with a seizure. They are also probably appropriate for those patients with hemorrhagic lesions or metastases near the motor cortex. Drug toxicity of anticonvulsants can easily be confused with tumor progression or recurrence, and levels should be monitored. The commonly used anticonvulsant phenytoin interacts with dexamethasone metabolism, and levels may fluctuate. Seizures in these patients may be very difficult to control. A few infrequent minor seizures may have to be tolerated to avoid oversedation.

SPINAL METASTASIS

Although systemic cancer may metastasize to the spinal cord parenchyma, is does so in a small percentage of patients. The usual cause of neurologic damage to the cord is on the basis of epidural spinal cord compression. Melanoma and lung cancer are the most likely to metastasize to cord parenchymas (Fig. 19-4).

EPIDURAL SPINAL CORD COMPRESSION

Epidural spinal cord compression (ESCC) usually occurs in the cancer patient when metastatic bony tumors grow to invade the epidural space. The compression may be caused either by the expanding tumor mass or by bony fragments extruded into the spinal canal as a complication of a compression fracture from a tumor-ridden vertebral body. In the case of neurofibromatosis and lymphoma, compression is usually from encroachment of the neural foramina. It occurs in about 5% to 10% of cancer patients, and unrecognized and untreated in the early stages it can leave the patient with loss of sensation, mobility, and sphincter control below the level of the lesion. It is seen most commonly in patients with breast, lung, and prostate primaries and non-Hodgkin's lymphoma. It can occur from direct extension of abdominal and pelvic masses as well.

In 95% of patients, ESCC presents as back pain. It is usually gradual in onset and progressive over weeks to months. It can be localized, radicular, or referred. Radicular pain is usually unilateral when it involves the cervical or lumbosacral region. In the thorax it is usually bilateral and can feel like a tight band around the chest. It can be mistaken for or occur concomitantly with herpes zoster or shingles. The pain is likely to worsen with recum-

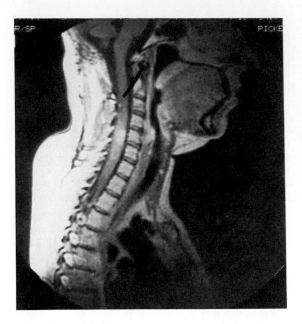

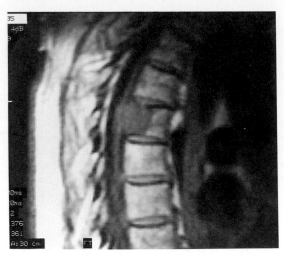

FIG. 19-5. Epidural spinal cord compression from breast cancer.

FIG. 19-4. Intramedullary metastasis from metastatic melanoma.

bency, requiring the patient to sleep in a chair. It is worsened by coughing or sneezing or other Valsalva's maneuvers.

The other signs and symptoms vary with the level of involvement. These include weakness, ataxia, autonomic dysfunction, sensory loss, a palpable bladder, and a Babinski sign. The presence of an ascending sensory level in a patient with back pain should be considered a medical emergency, especially when seen in the setting of weakness and reflex abnormalities. These patients should be evaluated with definitive neuroimaging studies on an emergent basis and be given large doses of intravenous corticosteroids, usually in the form of dexamethasone. MR has replaced myelography in many institutions since it is a noninvasive technique (Fig. 19-5). A problem with MR is that it usually has to be ordered for a specific spinal level. Treatment can be directed at one level, and the patient can then compress at an undiagnosed level that was asymptomatic earlier. Gadolinium can be useful to delineate lesions. Midsagittal screening views of the entire spine can be obtained. The clinician should not be comfortable with a report of a negative-screening MR; more specific views are usually war-

ranted. Myelography is an invasive procedure but can give a view of the entire spinal column. This allows for the formulation of radiation therapy treatment plans. CSF for cytology is also obtained at the same time. Lumbar puncture should not be performed routinely.

The evaluation of the patient with isolated back pain or minor or nonprogressive symptoms is more difficult. Plain films of the spine are positive in only 80% of patients. Bone scans can be useful as well, but epidural tumor may be present in a patient with a negative scan. A combination of plain films and bone scan may miss a small percentage of epidural tumor, and persistent symptoms should be persued with MR or myelography.

Symptoms of dyasthesias or cramping should not be taken lightly, and all sensory loss in the cancer patient should not be attributed to treatment-induced peripheral neuropathies. The diagnosis may be more difficult in these patients. Medial spread from lumbosacral or brachial plexus lesions to the epidural space are relatively common.

Treatment plan algorhythms have been derived to evaluate back pain in the cancer patient. These plans are useful in determining the timing and urgency of a patient work-up. It is always better to err on the side of the expeditious evaluation since prognosis for continued ambulation is dependent on the neurologic status of the patient at the institution of treatment. Symptoms may progress rapidly.

Radiation is the standard therapy for the treatment of epidural tumor. It should be instituted as soon as possible after the diagnosis of epidural tumor is made. Patients ambulatory at the beginning of treatment have a good chance of remaining so. Paretic patients have a 50–50 chance of ambulation after treatment, and plegic patients rarely walk after treatment. Reports of return of motor strength have been recorded as late as six months after treatment and pain control is usually better.

Corticosteroids are used if spinal cord compression is demonstrated or if there is a delay in diagnosis in patients in whom there is a high index of suspicion. They typically give great relief of symptoms. Care must be used to avoid side effects. This is especially important with impaired spinal cord function. Atonic bowel is prone to perforation, and enlarged catheterized bladders easily become infected. Bedsores can develop, and pneumonia is frequent in atelectatic lung. Laxatives, H_2-blockers, antiembolic stockings, and especially designed mattresses are useful in severely impaired patients.

Radiation therapy has proved to be as effective as a combination of surgery and radiotherapy for the majority of patients. Important exceptions exist. Surgery is indicated if the primary tumor is unknown and in patients with radioresistant tumors. Preoperative embolization of highly vascular tumors has been employed. It can be helpful for patients with posteriorly located lesions that are amenable to laminectomy. Lesions of the vertebral body probably deserve a vertebral body replacement if surgery is performed. Surgery in the patient with symptomatic tumor in an already treated field or who are worsening despite radiation can be useful. These are major surgeries and produce considerable morbidity. The decision to operate requires consideration of the patient's overall status.

LEPTOMENINGEAL TUMOR

Leptomeningeal tumor in those patients with systemic carcinoma is also called *meningeal carcinomatosis*. It occurs in about 5% of cancer patients and is more commonly diagnosed as treatment for systemic tumor improves. It is seen in patients with breast, lung, and melanoma primary tumors, but can be seen with virtually any carcinoma. It is also seen in the hematologic malignancies.

The symptoms may be that of increased intracranial pressure as the cancer cells impede flow through the ventricular system and produce hydrocephalus. Tumor cells gravitate to the base of the brain or to the cauda equina, where they produce symptoms of cranial nerve palsies or cauda equina symptoms of leg weakness and sphincter dysfunctions, respectively.

Diagnosis is made with a high index of suspicion. Gadolinium-enhanced MR is sometimes but not always positive. Initial lumbar puncture cytology is positive in about 50% of the cases. Cisternal puncture may increase the yield. It is generally accepted practice to perform up to three CSF analyses to increase the probability of a positive cytology. The presence of elevated CSF protein, lactate dehydrogenase (LDH) isoenzymes, beta-glucuronidase, $beta_2$-microglobulin, and glucophosphate isomerase may all be suggestive of meningeal tumor but are not specific. Alpha-fetoprotein and beta human chorionic gonadotropin are specific tumor markers useful in the diagnosis of germ cell tumors.

Corticosteroids may provide relief of symptoms. Radiation therapy can be used in areas of heavy tumor burden or to relieve CSF blockage. A limited amount of chemotherapy agents can be given intrathecally and may produce a short-lived response. The placement of an intraventricular catheter provides better drug delivery and alleviates the need for repeated lumbar punctures. Monoclonal antibodies have shown promise in the treatment of leptomeningeal tumor.

NONMETASTATIC COMPLICATIONS

PARANEOPLASTIC SYNDROMES

The term *paraneoplastic* refers to a variety of syndromes occurring more frequently but not always in patients with cancers that are not due to metastases or direct extension. They are rare, occurring in only about 1% of patients with cancer. Though the cause is unknown, autoimmune and viral etiologies have been hypothesized. The identification of unique antibodies in the serum of some of these patients has supported the autoimmune hypothesis. Specific antibodies have been identified in five of these syndromes, and oncoantigens (antigens common to both tumor and nervous tissue) have been identified as well.

The importance of these rare syndromes is that they occur and can be diagnosed before the diagnosis of tumor in about 50% of cases. This allows for earlier treatment and perhaps a better outcome.

Though there are many recognized syndromes, only a few of the most common will be discussed.

Paraneoplastic cerebellar degeneration (PCD) is the most common of these syndromes. It is usually seen in the setting of lung cancer, gynecologic tumors, and Hodgkin's disease. The symptoms of dizziness, ataxia, dysarthria, and nystagmus usually progress over weeks to months and then stabilize. It may occur with signs of more diffuse nervous system dysfunction. MR and CSF may be normal. Several different antibodies have been found to react to the cerebellar Purkinje cells, the affected cell. The most well characterized is the anti-Yo antibody. It has been found in the serum and spinal fluid of patients with PCD associated with gynecologic tumors. There is no known treatment, though immunosuppressive therapy and plasma exchange have been used.

The opsoclonus–myoclonus (OM) syndrome, with its almost continuous, multidirectional eye movement and jerk-like myoclonus, occurs in 2% of children with neuroblastoma, but 50 percent of patients with OM have neuroblastoma. These children are more likely to have less aggressive tumor histology. Symptoms may improve with the treatment of the tumor.

Paraneoplastic sensory neuropathy is a complication usually seen with small cell carcinoma of the lung. It may be associated with sensory ataxia and dropped reflexes. It also may be seen as part of a more diffuse dysfunction of the nervous system. The anti-Hu antibody has been identified in patients suffering from this syndrome in conjunction with small cell cancer of the lung. It has also been found in patients with small cell carcinoma of the lung with other neurologic symptoms and in patients without identifiable cancer.

Other paraneoplastic syndromes include the Lambert–Eaton myasthenic syndrome. Patients have symptoms of weakness that improve with repetitive movements. Electrodiagnosis is useful in establishing the diagnosis. There is a presynaptic abnormality with the release of acetylcholine. 3-4-Diaminopyridine is the treatment of choice; cholinesterase inhibitors, steroids, and plasma exchange may be useful.

Dermatomyositis and polymyositis have been reported to have varying correlations with cancer. The association is more striking in patients over 40 and usually occurs in carcinoma of the breast, lung, and ovaries and with gastric malignancies. A metastatic work-up should be done in these patients.

VASCULAR COMPLICATIONS OF CANCER

Cerebrovascular complications of cancer may be thrombic or hemorrhagic. They occur frequently and are sometimes secondary to therapy. Hemorrhagic complications are common in the lymphoreticular malignancies. The most common complication is a coagulopathy. This may be due to poorly controlled disease and thrombocytopenia, disseminated intravascular coagulation (DIC), or organ failure. It can be iatrogenically induced by chemotherapy and radiation. It can present with hemorrhage to the parenchyma, or to the subdural or subarachnoid space. It can also present as hemorrhage into a tumor mass. Spinal subdural hematoma can also occur, and care should be taken when performing a lumbar puncture in patients with low or falling platelet counts or in patients with abnormal bleeding parameters. Sinus thrombosis has been seen in cancer patients and can be associated with L-asparaginase. Subdural hematoma can be a complication of dural-based metastases. Multiple CNS infarcts may be secondary to nonbacterial thrombotic endocarditis.

COMPLICATIONS OF CANCER THERAPY

CHEMOTHERAPY

Corticosteroids are probably the most commonly prescribed drug in the cancer patient. They have a "laundry list" of side effects with which the clinician should be familiar, including hyperglycemia, gastrointestinal bleeding and perforation, and an increased susceptibility to infection and hypertension. The common neurologic complications include psychosis, myopathy, and dependence. A steroid withdrawal syndrome is now well recognized, with myalgias, arthralgias, and worsening of neurologic symptoms. Care should be taken with the withdrawal of corticosteroid therapy for this reason, and more importantly to avoid adrenal insufficiency secondary to prolonged suppression of the adrenal gland or hypothalamic-adrenal axis.

Methotrexate causes acute and delayed toxicities. The acute syndromes include aseptic meningitis and transverse myelitis when given intrathecally. Infection and spinal hematoma should be considered in the differential diagnosis respectively. Delayed toxicities include a stroke-like syndrome seen with high-dose intravenous therapy. A diffuse encephalopathy with leukoencephalopathy can be seen, especially when methotrexate is given after radiation therapy.

Cisplatin causes a peripheral neuropathy often presenting with numbness and tingling of the fingers and toes after a total dose over 400 mg/mm^2. The major effects are on the large sensory fibers and affect proprioception, at times affecting the patient's ability to walk. Pinprick and temperature sense is spared, but reflexes are diminished. Ototoxicity is also a feature and may be increased with irradiation. Generalized brain dysfunction is rare and must be separated from electrolyte abnormalities that sometimes occur with its usage, including hypocalcemia, hypomagnesemia, and water intoxication.

The vinca alkaloids, most often vincristine, cause a peripheral neuropathy. They usually affect the fingers and toes and cause dropped reflexes after several weeks of treatment. Autonomic neuropathy can also occur, including ileus, orthostasis, urinary retention, and impotence.

5-Fluorouracil and cytosine arabinoside (ara-C) can produce pancerebellar syndromes, especially when given in high doses. Procarbazine is a monamine oxidase inhibitor that interacts with other drugs, alcohol, and tyramine-containing foods. It may also produce an antabuse-like reaction with alcohol.

RADIATION THERAPY

BRAIN

The acute affects of radiation to the brain include headache, nausea, vomiting, somnolence, and worsening of neurologic defect. Corticosteroids help alleviate these symptoms, and most patients beginning radiation therapy should be given them. A similar syndrome can occur about 6 weeks after the end of therapy and sometimes is confused with tumor recurrence. An MR or CT is usually helpful to differentiate the two. This early-delayed radiation syndrome is usually responsive to steroids and usually remits spontaneously in 6 to 8 weeks. Late-delayed toxicities occur most commonly 1 to 2 years after radiation therapy. They can mimic the symptoms of tumor recurrence, and the MR may be confusing. Positron emission tomography may be useful. Biopsy or resection is diagnostic.

SPINAL CORD

It has been argued that there are no acute affects of radiation to the spinal cord. The early delayed ef-

fects usually occur several weeks after therapy, and patients sometimes feel a shock-like sensation when bending the neck (Lhermitte's sign). This effect is transient and does not predict delayed, permanent dysfunction. The late delayed effects include a myelopathy that may progress slowly months to years after radiation therapy. It may present asymmetrically, and recurrent tumor should be ruled out. The late effects may present with a flaccid weakness following pelvic irradiation, though other forms exist.

QUESTIONS AND DISCUSSION

1. A 50-year-old woman presents to a walk-in clinic where you are moonlighting when you are not on duty as an oncology fellow. She had an unexplained loss of consciousness while home alone. She woke with the taste of blood in her mouth. You determine that she probably had a seizure. She does not have a history of seizures, so you:

   A. Send her home and tell her to see her doctor if it happens again
   B. Send her home on phenytoin and tell her to see her doctor if it happens again
   C. Order a CT scan of the brain and tell her to see her doctor
   D. You ascertain that she is neurologically intact, check her for metabolic abnormalities and intoxications, order a CT or MR scan, and arrange for admission and appropriate follow-up

The answer is (D). Idiopathic epilepsy is not the most common cause of seizures in this age group. One needs to do a CT or MR scan to rule out intracranial pathology, and the patient needs to be followed to ascertain the etiology and arrange treatment of any possible lesion.

2. The patient's MR shows two ring-enhancing lesions, one in the right parietal lobe and one in the left occipital lobe. She is neurologically intact. You then:

   A. Start her on dexamethasone and an H$_2$-blocker
   B. Refer her to the oncology clinic
   C. Start her on phenytoin
   D. All of the above

The answer is (D). If the patient is clinically stable and there is minimal mass effect on the scan, you may be able to avoid admission but expeditious follow-up is warranted. Though not required in every case, anticonvulsants are indicated in this patient who presented with a seizure. You may also refer her to a neurosurgeon at this time if the situation warrants.

3. When the patient gets to clinic, your attending physician wants to know the patient's primary lesion. You would like to do a total body scan but instead you decide to be more selective this time. The most informative tests would include:

    A. Chest x-ray
    B. Mammogram
    C. Complete blood count, urinalysis, and liver function tests
    D. Stool guaiac
    E. All of the above

The answer is (E). Since most metastatic tumors come from primary or secondary lung tumors, a chest x-ray and perhaps even a CT is usually in order. Given the incidence of breast cancer in American women, a mammogram is a good choice as well. A breast nodule would be easier to biopsy than the brain. A complete blood count may disclose a lymphoreticular malignancy, a urinalysis may suggest renal cell cancer, and a stool guaiac may indicate a gastrointestinal tumor. Abnormal liver function tests may indicate primary or secondary liver disease.

4. The mammogram is positive. The diagnosis confirmed histologically. The radiation therapists are now happy that you have a tissue diagnosis and agree to start treatment with whole-brain radiation therapy. The patient tolerates the treatment well but comes to the clinic 6 weeks after therapy with symptoms of headache, fatigue, and generalized arthralgias. At first you are convinced that the radiation did not work. You decide to investigate other differentials. You order the post-treatment scan but you also order:

    A. Phenytoin level
    B. Serum calcium
    C. Electrolyte profile
    D. All of the above

The answer is (D). The increasing symptoms that the patient is experiencing can be expected as an early delayed complication of radiation therapy. They could also be due to early steroid withdrawal. Reinstituting the dexamethasone or increasing the dose with a more gradual taper will help the symptoms. Phenytoin toxicity could be a cause of the patient's somnolence, and phenytoin levels should be monitored. They will fluctuate with the changes in steroid dose and can be a cause of difficulties.

The patient's repeat scan is if anything improved, but the calcium is elevated. You suspect that this is part of the problem.

5. The patient is constipated as well. You would like to admit her to the in-house oncology service for hydration. As you sit with the patient waiting for transportation to take her to her room, you listen to her complaints. She claims to not have moved her bowels for a week; you also noticed that she had some difficulty walking into the office today. You examine the patient and find marked weakness in the proximal muscles in the lower extremities. Her sphincter tone is good, and she is not complaining of any new back pain. Your differential includes:

    A. Epidural tumor
    B. Steroid myopathy
    C. Leptomeningeal tumor
    D. All of the above

The answer is (D). Without progressive symptoms of back pain and with normal sphincter tone, the diagnosis is not clear. The most pressing of these differentials is epidural tumor, and this should always be promptly investigated. The symptoms could be rapidly progressive, and prognosis depends on prompt diagnosis and treatment. These symptoms could result from a steroid myopathy; if this is the case, you may reassure the patient that she will get better when the steroids are withdrawn. Leptomeningeal tumor should be considered, and a lumbar puncture may be in order if the MR is unrevealing. Hypercalcemia could be contributing to the constipation.

SUGGESTED READING

Black PMcL: Brain tumors (p. 1). N Engl J Med 324:1471, 1991

Black PMcL: Brain tumors (p. 2). N Engl J Med 324:1555, 1991

Bradley C, Selby P: In search of the unknown primary. Br Med J 304:1065, 1992

Davies-Jones GAB: Neurological manifestations of hematological disorders. In Aminoff MJ (ed): Neurology and General Medicine, p 187. New York, Churchill Livingstone, 1989

Delettre J-V, Posner JB: Neurological complications of chemotherapy and radiation therapy. In Aminoff MJ (ed): Neurology and General Medicine, pp 365–387. New York, Churchill Livingstone, 1989

Packer RJ, Finlay JL: Medulloblastoma: Presentation, diagnosis and management. Oncology 9:35, 1988

Portenoy RK, Lipton RB, Foley KM: Back pain and the cancer patient: An algorithm for evaluation and management. Neurology 37:134, 1987

Patchell RA, Tibbs PA, Walsh JW et al: A Randomized trial of surgery in the treatment of single metastases to the brain. N Engl J Med 322: 494, 1990

Posner JB: Paraneoplastic syndromes involving the nervous system. In Aminoff MJ (ed): Neurology and General Medicine, pp 341–364. New York, Churchill Livingstone, 1989

Neurologic Evaluation of Low Back Pain

Russell H. Glantz

The purpose of this chapter is to distinguish non-neurologic from neurologic causes of back pain. The physician must frequently answer whether back pain from disease of the spine and its surrounding structures has involved the nervous system by spinal cord or spinal root compression. The determination of neurologic involvement has specific prognostic and management implications.

The most common form of back pain is *spondylogenic*. This pain originates in the vertebral spinal column and associated soft tissue structures. These soft tissues are most frequently incriminated in the causes of back pain and include diseases of the associated tendons, muscles, joints, and, most importantly, intervertebral disks.

Vascular back pain may result from abdominal aneurysms and is often a deep-seated, boring lumbar pain. In addition, vascular insufficiency of the superior gluteal artery may give rise to buttock pain of a claudicant nature. These symptoms may even radiate down the leg. The pain of vascular insufficiency is, however, not aggravated by other stresses on the lumbar spine, such as bending, twisting, or stooping.

Viscerogenic back pain may result from retroperitoneal tumors or diseases of the kidneys or pelvic viscera. Backache, however, is rarely the sole symptom of a visceral disease. Furthermore, this pain is neither aggravated by activity nor relieved by rest. Patients with severe visceral pain frequently writhe around to obtain relief.

Primary neurogenic pain is caused by a disease of the nervous system, which is reflected as back pain. Some causes are neurofibromas, ependymomas, astrocytomas, and other lesions within the dural contents but outside the spinal cord itself. These conditions are uncommon, however, and it is beyond the scope of this chapter to discuss the differential diagnosis of all primary neurogenic back pains. The emphasis is placed instead on the accurate diagnosis of the more common causes of nerve root compression in the lumbar spine. A physician most frequently sees nerve root compression as a result of acute or chronic intervertebral disk degeneration.

ANATOMY AND PHYSIOLOGY

Each vertebra has three functional components: (1) the vertebral bodies, (2) the neural arches, and (3) the bony processes (spinous and transverse). The vertebral bodies are connected by the intervertebral disks, and the neural arches are joined by the zygapophyseal joints. The vertebral bodies are braced front and back by the anterior and posterior longitudinal ligaments (Fig. 20-1). The stability of the spine depends on two types of supporting structures: the ligamentous (passive) structures and the muscular (active) structures. Although the ligaments are strong, they alone cannot resist the enormous forces on the spinal column. Most of the stability is de-

270

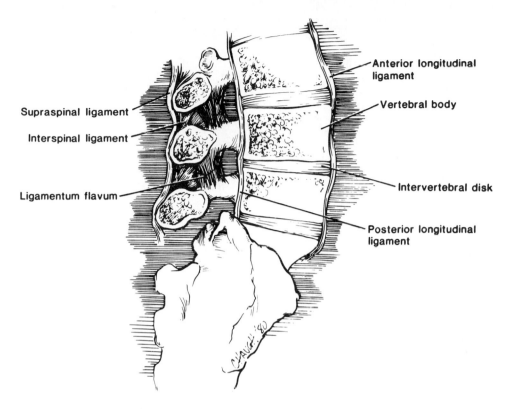

Supraspinal ligament

Interspinal ligament

Ligamentum flavum

Anterior longitudinal ligament

Vertebral body

Intervertebral disk

Posterior longitudinal ligament

FIG. 20-1. Anatomic landmarks of lumbosacral spine.

pendent on the reflex contractions of the sacrospinalis, abdominal, glutei, and hamstring muscles.

One of the most important anatomic features of the lumbar spine is the relationship that the neural elements bear to the bony skeleton and the intervertebral disks. The spinal cord ends at L1. From this point, all the lumbar, sacral, and coccygeal nerve roots run as distinct entities within the dural sac and exit through the lumbar, sacral, and coccygeal intervertebral foramina. The nerve roots course downward and outward. They cross the intervertebral disk and pass anterior to the superior articular facet, hugging the medial aspect of the pedicle before emerging into the intervertebral foramen. The nerve root, therefore, is vulnerable to compression by pathologic changes occurring at several points during its course down the spinal canal. The L4 root emerges between L4 and L5, in other words, *below* the vertebra that is numerically similar (Fig. 20-2). In the same way, the L5 root emerges

between L5 and S1. However, in syndromes caused by disk protrusion, an L4–L5 disk protrusion will usually compress the L5 root. This is because the more usual protrusion is posterolateral, and it catches the more medially placed downcoming root from a higher segment (Fig. 20-3). If a protrusion is far lateral, the L4 root is compressed in an L4–L5 syndrome; however, this situation is unusual. An L5–S1 protrusion generally implies an S1 root compressive syndrome. Similarly, an L3–L4 protrusion would give rise to an L4 root compressive syndrome, and an L2–L3 protrusion will cause an L3 root compressive syndrome. The anatomy is different in the cervical region, so that the root emerges above the vertebra from which it takes its name. The C6 root emerges between C5 and C6; the C7 root emerges between C6 and C7; the C8 root emerges between C7 and T1 (Fig. 20-2). The root, from this level downward, emerges below the vertebral from which it takes its name. *As a general rule*, for both cervical and lum-

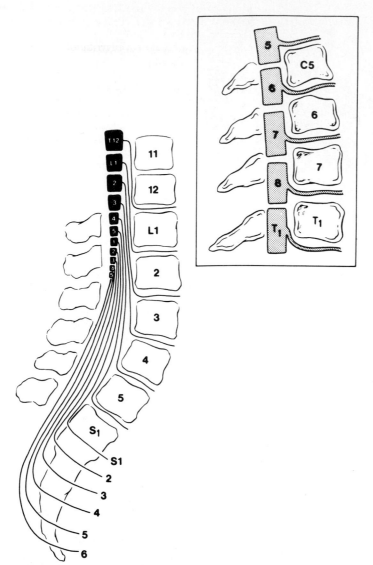

FIG. 20-2. Cervical (*upper right*) and lumbosacral (*lower left*) spine, showing the emergence of spinal roots.

bar compressive syndromes, the clinical lesion corresponds to the lower vertebral segment (C5–C6 = C6 syndrome, L5–S1 = S1 syndrome).

DIAGNOSIS

Back pain of non-neurogenic or neurogenic origin may be (1) local, (2) referred, or (3) radicular (or root).

Once a diagnosis is made in terms of these simple guidelines, the physician may focus on the differentiation between non-neurogenic causes (*e.g.*, spondylogenic, viscerogenic, or vascular) and neurogenic causes.

Local pain is caused by any pathologic process that irritates sensory endings in the back. Because nerve endings are irritated, it does not necessarily mean that the cause is primarily neurogenic. The final ex-

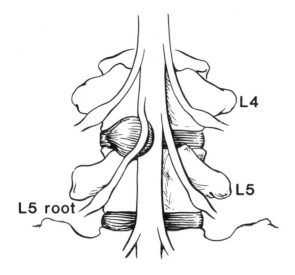

FIG. 20-3. Herniated disk at L4–L5 compressing the L5 rootlet.

pression of any pain, whatever the cause, has to be through nerve endings. Local pain may be due to the involvement of bone, muscle, ligaments, or periosteum. The pain is usually steady; it may be sharp or dull; and it is always felt in or near the affected part of the spine. The pain may change with a variation in position or activity. Firm tissue pressure in the region involved usually evokes tenderness and thus helps in localization. Most local pains fit generally into the spondylogenic category.

Referred pain may be projected from the spine into viscera and other structures lying within the area of the lumbar and upper sacral dermatomes. Referred pain may also be projected from the pelvic and abdominal viscera to the spine. Pain due to upper lumbar spine disease is usually referred to the anterior aspects of the thighs and legs. This pain may have to be distinguished from L3 radicular pain, which has a similar distribution. Pain from the lower lumbar spine is usually referred to the lower buttock and is due to an irritation of lower spinal nerves that activate the same pool of neurons as the posterior thighs and calves. The referred pain often parallels in intensity the local pain in the back, thus maneuvers that alter local pain have a similar affect on referred pain. This is not the case with lancinating radicular pain, which may shoot suddenly and may be unassociated with a maneuver that causes aggravation of local pain. Fur-

thermore, referred pain is rarely felt below the knees, whereas pain due to root irritation may spread into the calf or even the foot.

Radicular or root pain relates to an irritation or damage of neural structures by primary neurologic diseases or non-neurologic disease (*e.g.*, disks) and hence must be specifically distinguished from local or referred pain. The misdiagnosis of local or referred pain as radicular pain often results in unnecessary investigations and unwarranted treatment. Root pain has some of the characteristics of referred pain but differs in its greater intensity, distal radiation, circumscription to the territory of a root, and, very importantly, the factors that induce it. Typically, any maneuver that raises the pressure of the spinal fluid (with secondary pressure on nerve roots) usually aggravates radicular pain. Hence, coughing, sneezing, and straining at stool characteristically evoke this sharp radiating pain.

Most causes of root pain are due to nerve root compression by a herniated intervertebral disk. True neurologic causes of the same syndrome include neurofibromas, ependymomas, and cysts, and these may give rise to similar symptoms and signs. Furthermore, the root entrapment may be bony in etiology, as in spinal stenosis, but here the problem is asymmetrical and bilateral.

The symptoms of nerve root compression may present in three ways: (1) backache only, (2) pain resulting from the radiation only (sciatica), or (3) pain and backache together. The onset is frequently dramatic in the fully developed syndrome. There is a severe knife-like pain that is aggravated by any movement or valsalva maneuver (*e.g.*, sneezing or coughing). Most patients lie still in bed with legs flexed at the knees and hips. Some patients find a lateral decubitus position more comfortable. Not infrequently, patients will contort themselves into strange postures to alleviate their pain. A sitting position is frequently painful. Some patients with nerve root tumors, simulating radicular disk compression symptoms, find relief by walking around.

When examined, the patient's posture is characteristic. The lumbar spine is flattened and slightly flexed. The patient usually leans toward the side of his pain, and this action becomes more obvious when he is trying to bend forward. Symptoms may be improved by standing with the hip and knee slightly flexed and with the forced scoliosis to the sound side. This posturing diminishes any stretch on the sciatic nerve. Pain may be typically provoked by pressure over the involved vertebral spines and along the course of the sciatic nerve (sciatic notch, retrotrochanteric gutter, posterior surface of thigh, head of fibula). Pressure at one point may cause pain and tingling to radiate down the leg. It would be unusual not to find local vertebral spine pain when direct pressure is applied in a disk syndrome. Its lack, or the presence of symptoms with more lateral pressure, should cast some doubt on the diagnosis.

On further assessment of the degree of root involvement, it is important to test specifically for root tension. The two most useful tests are the straight leg-raising and bowstring signs (Figs. 20-4 and 20-5). The patient should be lying on a flat surface and the leg should be raised slowly. The knee must be fully extended. If the test is positive, pain will be produced in the back or the leg. Pain in the popliteal fossa produced by simple stretching of the legs does not signify a positive test. Two additional maneuvers add significance to straight leg raising: (1) aggravation of pain by forced dorsiflexion of the ankle at the limit of straight leg raising, and (2) relief of pain by knee flexion. Sciatic pain is almost always relieved by flexing the knee. The bowstring sign can also be another important indication of root compression. The straight leg-raising test is carried out to the point at which the patient experiences some discomfort. At this level, the knees are allowed to flex and the examiner allows the patient's foot to rest on his shoulder. The test demands sudden firm pressure applied to the popliteal nerve behind the knee. The reproduction of pain in the leg or in the back is irrefutable evidence of nerve root compression. As in the case of straight leg raising, local popliteal fossa pain does not indicate a positive result. These maneuvers aim to diagnose radicular pain but do not distinguish the specific causes of such pain (*e.g.,* disk or tumors).

Lesions of the fifth lumbar and first sacral roots are the most common. The former lesions usually give symptoms of pain in the hip, groin, posterior lateral thigh, lateral calf, and dorsum of the foot including the first to third toes. Paresthesias in this distribution may be of great diagnostic aid. There may be a weakness of dorsiflexion of the foot and great toe. The extensor hallucis (great toe extensor) is a powerful muscle and should not be overcome even in a slightly built or generally weakened patient. A weakness in this muscle is, therefore, very significant in the diagnosis of an L5 lesion. No reflex change will be present, the knee and ankle jerks being subserved by L2–L4 and S1, respectively.

Lesions of the first sacral root give rise to pain in the midgluteal region, the posterior thigh, the posterior calf to the heel, and the sole of the foot extending over to the dorsum and involving the fourth and fifth toes. Weakness, if present, involves the flexors of the foot and toes, the abductors of the toes, and the hamstring muscles. The ankle reflex is invariably decreased or lacking, and this finding forms an important diagnostic criterion in S1 root compression.

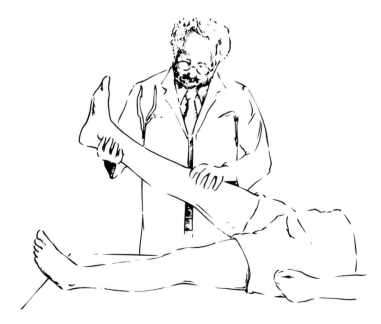

FIG. 20-4. Straight leg-raising sign. Note that the examiner maintains the knee in the extended position.

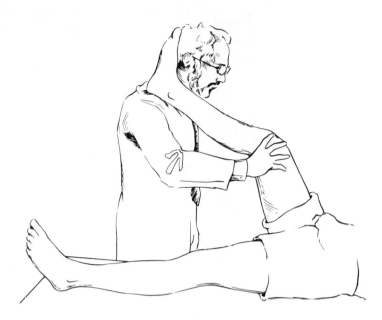

FIG. 20-5. The bowstring sign.

Symptoms of nerve root compression may be confined to back pain. In patients who have recurrent episodes, the presentations may be difficult on each occasion. For example, the patient may initially present with the complete syndrome, and subsequently, with back pain only. The physician, therefore, must take an accurate history when trying to formulate the anatomy of any particular pain complex. Root entrapment due to disk protrusion has mainly been discussed thus far. It is certainly the most common and is frequently the most dramatic type of pain. Chronic lumbar spondylosis (which is more insidious than disk degeneration) and osseous overgrowth may also cause nerve entrapment. Pain due to these latter causes is usually chronic and has a local and referred component. Typical back and radicular pain are lacking. There may, however, be appropriate neurologic signs (*e.g.*, loss of ankle reflex) indicating nerve root dysfunction.

SPECIAL INVESTIGATIONS IN DIAGNOSIS

Spine x-ray films will not diagnose disk disease, but they should be done in the initial work-up of all acute and chronic low back pain syndromes. This noninvasive test may reveal a tumor deposit, marked osteo-

phytosis with canal narrowing, or even inherent bony anomalies such as lumbarization or sacralization. At this point, the physician is faced with an array of more specialized and invasive tests in order to determine a specific abnormality of structure and function. Unless the physician has a reasonably clear clinical picture, these tests may be unnecessary and they may aggravate a patient's state because they are often uncomfortable. The nature of these tests is discussed first, and their individual indications are mentioned in the treatment section.

MYELOGRAPHY

Myelography is still an important procedure for localizing the exact site of disk herniation or ruling out the possibility of a nerve root tumor masquerading as a disk. Magnetic resonance imaging (MR) or computed tomography (CT) is almost always done first, and the current role of myelography is as a prelude to postmyelogram CT scanning. The myelogram itself often provides useful information as to which levels to scan (see later text). The flow of the injected dye (in the subarachnoid space) is impeded by an extruded disk or other space-occupying lesions; the lesion can thus be localized (Fig. 20-6). Nonionic water-soluble contrast media are

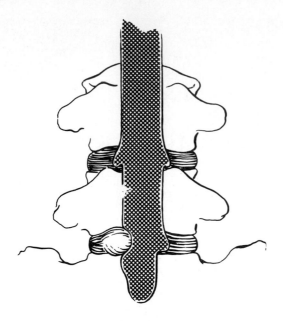

FIG. 20-6. Diagram depicting myelographic sign of indentation from extradural defect (speckled area represents dye column).

currently used. These are less neurotoxic, but occasional instances of cerebral cortical, meningeal, and radicular irritation have been reported. The outlines of the lower lumbar cord, the root sleeves, and extradural defects from disk disease (if present) are usually excellent. No disturbance in dye is produced if a lesion is very lateral and the result of the myelogram will be negative. In these instances, postmyelographic CT scanning will provide the diagnosis. When performing myelography, the physician must keep in mind that disk protrusion may occur in the asymptomatic patient. This finding is not uncommon and, therefore, the clinical findings remain paramount in order to use the radiographic findings accurately.

ELECTROMYOGRAPHY

Electromyography (EMG) is the only test that may reveal functional impairment. The aim of this test is to localize the level of root or nerve involvement and also to help distinguish nerve damage from non-

neurogenic disease, which may be the source of back pain. A normal muscle is silent at rest, but a denervated muscle gives rise to involuntary electrical discharges. These discharges take the form of fibrillation potentials or altered wave forms (positive waves). On voluntary contraction of a normal muscle, the motor unit potentials are biphasic or triphasic in form. With partial denervation, the quantity of motor units recorded is diminished and polyphasic potentials are seen (see Chaps. 2 and 12).

The paraspinal muscles are supplied by the posterior primary rami of the emerging lumbosacral roots. No electrical activity is seen in the paraspinal muscles in a normal person who is completely relaxed. The physician may sample the high lumbar, midlumbar, and low lumbar areas, thereby gaining a fairly accurate localization of proximal nerve damage. These findings can be corroborated with the results of needle studies on other muscles. For example, the gluteus medius and tibialis posterior muscles are almost purely innervated by L5. Conversely, the soleus muscle has almost a pure S1 innervation; therefore, finding denervation in gluteus medius, tibialis posterior, and low lumbar paraspinals without soleus denervation is strong evidence for L5 denervation. Similar inferences can be made with S1, L3, L4, and so forth.

The H reflex is a subtle electrical test of S1 function. The physician stimulates the afferent limb of S1 in the popliteal fossa and measures the time it takes to travel up the dorsal root, through the reflex arc, and back down the lower limb, eventually producing a contraction of gastrocnemius. This is equivalent to the ankle jerk, except that the stretching of the Achilles tendon is bypassed. The H reflex may elicit minor degrees of S1 root involvement before clear evidence of motor, reflex, and sensory dysfunction is clinically seen.

The EMG may also reveal root lesions at many levels, such as may be seen in lumbar spondylosis and stenosis with multilevel nerve root encroachment.

COMPUTED TOMOGRAPHY OF THE LUMBAR SPINE

One of the most important diagnostic advances has been the addition of CT scanning. With new-generation scanners and thin overlapping sections, this technique has provided the clinician with a noninvasive method of examining the spinal canal and surrounding structures. The ability to vary the window width and center allows all structures from dense bone to more lucent fat to be examined together or individually. It can be useful in accurately diagnosing a protruded disk (Fig. 20-7), and spinal stenosis from bony hypertrophy, congenital scarring, or masses can be demonstrated clearly (Fig. 20-8). Currently, CT scanning is used in a number of ways. It can either be used as an initial screening procedure or, as mentioned above, it is used after myelography to provide excellent detail, especially with more lateral pathology. As CT scanning technology advances, its interface with myelography will probably continue to change.

MAGNETIC RESONANCE IMAGING

Magnetic resonance imaging (MR) can show abnormalities of disk and bone as well as CT scanning (Fig. 20-9). At the time of writing this chapter, MR is not as widely available as CT scanning, and therefore many radiologists and clinicians have less experience with it. With more experience and changes in technology, MR could well become the preferred test in the future. The use of MR presently complements the aforementioned tests.

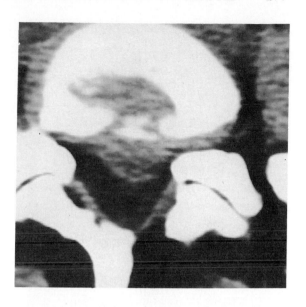

FIG. 20-7. Computed tomography scan of the lumbar spine showing prominent disk protrusion into the spinal canal.

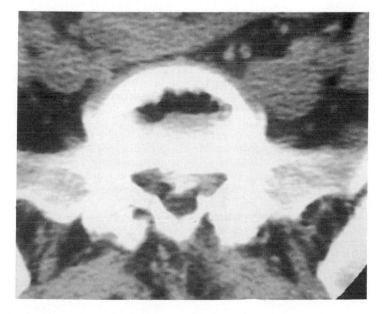

FIG. 20-8. Computed tomography evaluation of lumbar spine showing a markedly narrowed spinal canal as a result of protrusion of disk material as well as encroachment by bony hypertrophy and spurring. The vacuum disk phenomenon caused by disk degeneration is noted in the upper half of the picture.

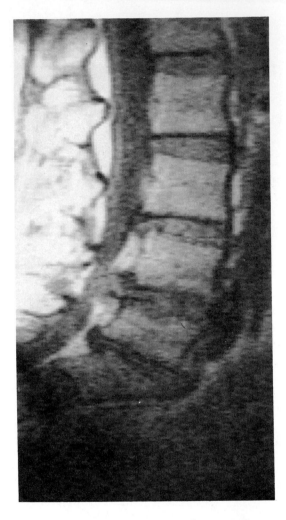

FIG. 20-9. Sagittal spinal cord magnetic resonance imaging showing evidence of extruded disk material between L4 and L5.

TREATMENT

The treatment of low back pain varies widely according to the severity of the syndrome. Initially, at least, the treatment of back pain from any cause is rest. This applies to pain that is caused by ligamentous, tendonous, muscular, or disk problems. However, when the neurologist examines a patient with nerve root compression due to a probable disk protrusion, the question of conservative *vs* operative therapy is always posed. The decision depends on the history and physical examination. There are only three absolute indications for laminectomy: (1) marked muscular weakness pertaining to a nerve root or roots, (2) progressive neurologic deficit despite absolute bed rest, and (3) bladder or bowel dysfunction. The relative indications for operative intervention are (1) pain unrelieved by complete bed rest, and (2) recurrent episodes of severe pain and sciatica.

The hallmark of conservative management is complete bed rest. Traction is indicated only if severe pain persists despite 48 hours of bed rest and analgesia. If after 48 hours, the patient is comfortable, he may then carefully get up to use the toilet. In many instances, the bed rest can be carried out at the patient's home, where he is comfortable and in familiar surroundings. If, however, adequate home facilities are lacking, the patient should be admitted to the hospital. The patient should lie on a firm mattress if available. A bedboard is unnecessary and, in some instances, may even increase the level of discomfort that the patient experiences. While in bed, the patient should be placed in a position such that the hips and knees are flexed to a moderate and comfortable degree. The amount of bed rest recommended by physicians varies, but most physicians require the patient to spend 1 to 2 weeks in bed, with 4 weeks being the maximum amount of time. Patients previously received 6 weeks of bed rest. However today, such a length of time spent in bed may be financially disastrous, especially since there is no guarantee of recovery.

The intelligent use of drug therapy is an important adjunct during the period of conservative therapy. Because diminution of inflammation around the degenerated disk is the primary aim of therapy, an anti-inflammatory drug should be used. There are many classes of nonsteroidal anti-inflammatory drugs currently available, and no one drug has been clearly shown to be better than another with respect to treatment of low back pain. During the weeks of therapy, the stomach should be coated with food or milk in order to prevent gastric irritation. Some patients who fail to respond to these drugs may obtain dramatic relief from a short course of systemic steroids.

If there is a prominent amount of paravertebral muscle spasm, which may be present especially in the acute phase, a muscle relaxant may be therapeutically effective. A drug such as cyclobenzaprine hydrochloride (Flexeril) may be tried.

Although the anti-inflammatory drugs also have an analgesic action, this latter effect might not be sufficient, and additional pure analgesia might be required, especially in patients with severe pain. Narcotics should only be used if the symptoms are extreme. The use of non-narcotic analgesia is more preferable.

In the subacute phase of the disease, as the patient is recovering and his pain is disappearing, lumbar flexion exercises should be started. These exercises were first described by Williams, and their overall aim is to reduce the lumbar lordosis and strengthen the lumbosacral area of the spine. In practice, these exercises should not be started sooner than about 3 weeks after the initiation of conservative therapy. The exercises should be started gently and should be discontinued immediately if a flare-up of symptomatology appears.

However, if the patient fulfills either the absolute or relative criteria for surgery, the aforementioned diagnostic procedures should be undertaken to localize the problem. One or more of these tests can be done, depending on the clinical picture. For example, for a patient with a clear-cut unilateral radicular syndrome, a CT, MR scan showing a disk protrusion appropriate to the patient's symptoms may be the only test required. On the other hand, in another instance a combination of EMG, MR, CT, or myelography and postmyelography depends on the particular clinical situation and the personal preferences of the treating physician.

QUESTIONS AND DISCUSSION

Answer *true* or *false* to each of the following statements.

1. The most common cause of low back pain is nerve root compression from disk protrusion.

The answer is false. The most common cause of low back pain is spondylogenic: This includes bone, muscle, tendon, and disk abnormalities. Thus, although disk abnormalities are frequent, secondary nerve root compression is less common. The neurologist, however, is frequently consulted about whether nerve compression exists or not.

2. The L1 nerve root emerges between L1 and L2.

The answer is true. The nerve root exists below the vertebra from which it takes its name in the thoracic, lumbar, and sacral regions. In the cervical

region, the root emerges *above* the vertebra with which it is associated numerically. For example, the C2 root emerges between C1 and C2. However, disk lesions that compress roots clinically follow the lower vertebrae for both cervical and lumbar areas.

3. Tingling or numbness on the lateral aspect of the leg extending to the great toe signifies an S1 root lesion.

The answer is false. This sensory distribution strongly suggests an L5 lesion. Supportive evidence would be weakness of the great toe extensor. An S1 lesion usually causes numbness of the posterior calf and sole and also a diminution of the ankle jerk.

4. The H reflex is an electrically obtained equivalent of the ankle reflex.

The answer is true. The H reflex tests the same reflex as the ankle jerk. However, stimulation of the Achilles tendon is bypassed in this case. When ankle reflex diminution is equivocal, the prolongation of the electrical H reflex may be useful especially in the diagnosis of S1 root lesions.

5. In a patient who displays clinical symptoms of nerve root compression, myelography should be performed to localize the lesion.

The answer is false. Surgery should be considered if there is a marked muscle weakness or a progressive neurologic dysfunction in a particular root distribution. A myelogram should be considered at this point. Root entrapment symptoms by themselves are not necessarily indications for myelography or surgery.

SUGGESTED READING

Adams RD, Victor M: Principles of Neurology, 4th ed. New York, McGraw-Hill, 1989

Glantz RH, Haldeman S: Other diagnostic studies: Electrodiagnosis. In Frymoyer JW (ed): The Adult Spine: Principles and Practice. New York, Raven Press, 1991

Heithoff KB, Herzog RJ: Computed tomography (CT) and enhanced CT of the spine. In Frymoyer JW (ed): The Adult Spine: Principles and Practice. New York, Raven Press, 1991

Herzog RJ: Magnetic resonance imaging of the spine. In Frymoyer JW (ed): The Adult Spine: Principles and Practice. New York, Raven Press, 1991

Sleep Disorders

Ružica Kovačević-Ristanović

Sleep is a subject that has fascinated physicians and the public since antiquity. A search for a "sleep center" in the brain has demonstrated the complexity of the sleep process, the multiplicity of structures involved in sleep, and the reciprocal interactions necessary for the initiation and maintenance of this behavior.

The structures found to facilitate sleep are the basal forebrain (*i.e.*, preoptic area of the hypothalamus), the area surrounding the solitary tract in the medulla, the dorsal raphe nuclei, and the midline thalamus. Structures found to facilitate waking are the ascending reticular activating system of the pons and the midbrain and posterior hypothalamus. The functions of these structures appear to be modulated by serotonin, catecholamines, acetylcholine, and other neurotransmitters. Two antagonistic systems, aminergic and cholinergic, are suggested by Hobson and McCarley to be involved in the control of alternating sleep stages. The aminergic and cholinergic systems are also involved in the process of cortical activation of arousal. The discovery of the involvement of different neurotransmitters in different stages of sleep has raised the possibility of more specific treatments of sleep disorders. The important clinical, diagnostic, and therapeutic features of some sleep disorders are described in this chapter. Useful guidelines for diagnosis and therapy are also presented, although there are few universally accepted treatments for common sleep complaints.

SLEEP ARCHITECTURE

Since the work-up of many patients with sleep disorders will involve the use of a sleep laboratory, it is important to understand the tests available and the parameters measured. A portion of the sleep recording, referred to as a polysomnogram (PSMG) of a normal subject, is shown in Figure 21-1. Three basic parameters are needed to define the stage of sleep: an electroencephalogram (EEG), an electrooculogram (EOG), and an electromyogram (EMG). The normal EEG of an alert, resting subject with closed eyes shows an 8-Hz to 12-Hz posterior activity known as alpha. Two major sleep stages are distinguished: nonrapid eye movement (NREM) and rapid eye movement (REM) sleep. Electroencephalographically, NREM sleep is composed of four stages: Stage 1 sleep is a stage of NREM sleep that directly follows the awake state. An EEG shows a low voltage tracing of mixed frequencies predominantly in the theta band with alpha activity less than 50%, vertex sharp activity, and slow eye movements. Stage 2 sleep is a stage of NREM sleep that is characterized by the presence of sleep spindles (12 Hz to 14 Hz) and K-complexes against a relatively low voltage, mixed frequency background. High-voltage delta waves may constitute up to 20% of Stage 2 sleep. Stage 3 of NREM sleep is defined by at least 20% and not more than 50% of the period consisting of EEG waves less than 2 Hz; if more than 50%

William J. Weiner and Christopher G. Goetz, eds. *Neurology for the Non-Neurologist*, Third Edition. Copyright © 1994, 1989 by J. B. Lippincott Company. Copyright © 1981 by Harper and Row Publishers, Inc.

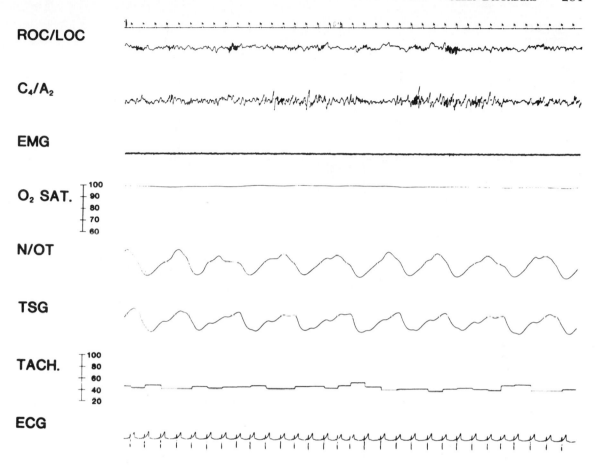

ROC/LOC

C₄/A₂

EMG

O₂ SAT.

N/OT

TSG

TACH.

ECG

FIG. 21-1. A typical eight-channel polysomnogram recorded from a normal adult male in stage 2 of NREM sleep. Electro-oculogram (ROC/LOC) recorded from right outer canthus referred to left outer canthus; electroencephalogram (EEG) (C_4/A_2) recorded from the right central lead referred to the right mastoid; electromyogram (EMG) recorded from the submental musculature; arterial oxygen saturation (O_2SAT) transduced by an ear oximeter; nasal and oral airflow (N/OT) recorded by a thermocouple mounted in a plastic respiratory mask; thoracic movement (TSG) recorded by a strain gauge; heart rate recorded by a cardiotachometer; electrocardiogram (ECG) recorded from V_5 referred to the left mastoid.

of the period contains such slow waves, it represents Stage 4 NREM sleep. Both Stages 3 and 4 are often combined into a Stage 3 or 4 NREM because of the lack of documented physiologic differences between the two stages. This sleep usually appears only in the first third of the sleep period (Fig. 21-2).

REM sleep alternates with the NREM sleep at about 90-minute intervals in adults and 60-minute intervals in infants. The EEG pattern during REM sleep resembles Stage 1 sleep but is accompanied by rapid eye movements. In addition, EMG activity is low. There is a general activation of the autonomic system, with a higher average respiratory rate, heart rate, and blood pressure and, more importantly, much more pronounced variability throughout the REM period. In about 80% of awakenings

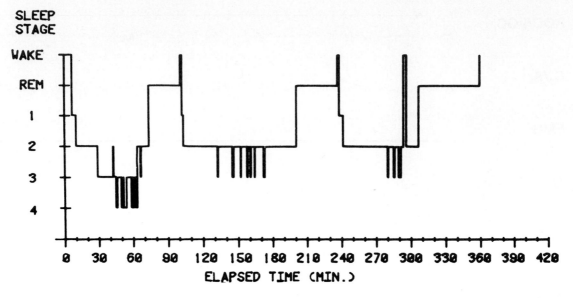

FIG. 21-2. The sleep architecture of a normal adult man. The progression of EEG stages of sleep demonstrates a concentration of Stages 3 and 4 within the first half of the sleep period. Episodes of REM sleep occur at approximately 90-min intervals, and the majority of REM appears within the latter half of the sleep period. Waking arousals are few.

from REM sleep, people recall vivid dreams compared to only 5% of awakenings from NREM sleep. However, in about 60% to 80% of awakenings from NREM sleep, people may recall thought-like fragments. Population studies have shown that the percentage of time spent in each stage varies with age and sex. Figures 21-1 and 21-2 represent a sleep PSMG and architecture plot from a normal adult.

NEUROCHEMICAL ASPECTS OF SLEEP

Attempts to understand the neurochemistry of sleep are important for practical reasons because of the underlying hope that better sleep-promoting and sleep-inhibiting compounds can be synthesized if the systems on which these drugs act are defined. Most current treatments for "sleep disorders" do not relate to the known neurochemical substrates for sleep. Of more immediate concern is the attempt to comprehend the myriad effects on sleep of currently used medications (both those used to alter sleep and those employed for an unrelated pur-

pose). Although serotonin was postulated to represent the transmitter governing NREM sleep, it appears that a complex interaction of serotonin, catecholamines, and acetylcholine is necessary for a modulation of the sleep–wake cycle. In addition, long-acting hormones or peptides have been isolated in some species and have been considered to represent a "hypnogenic factor." The demonstration of vasoactive intestinal peptide in the suprachiasmatic nucleus was considered to imply its role in the control of circadian rhythmicity. Their effects on humans have not yet been defined.

SLEEP ABNORMALITIES

The new International Classification of Sleep Disorders divides the primary sleep disorders into (1) the *dyssomnias*, or disorders that produce a complaint of either insomnia or excessive daytime sleepiness, and (2) the *parasomnias*, or disorders that intrude or occur during sleep but do not produce a primary complaint of insomnia or excessive daytime sleepiness. The dyssomnias are further subdivided into *extrinsic, intrinsic*, and *circadian sleep disorders*. This distinction puts stress on the major cause of either insomnia or hypersomnolence being either within the body (intrinsic) or outside the body (extrinsic). Both primary sleep disorders are separated from the medical–psychiatric sleep disorders. Future advances in understanding of the pathophysiology of sleep disorders will improve classification of sleep disorders along pathologically oriented lines.

INSOMNIA

Among intrinsic sleep disorders, disturbances such as psychophysiologic insomnia, sleep state misperception, restless legs syndrome, and idiopathic insomnia produce primarily a complaint of insomnia. Similarly, many extrinsic sleep disorders such as inadequate sleep hygiene, environmental sleep disorder, altitude insomnia, adjustment sleep disorder, limit-setting sleep disorder, food allergy insomnia, hypnotic-dependent sleep disorder, and alcohol-dependent sleep disorder are likely to be accompanied by insomnia. Among circadian rhythm sleep disorders, delayed sleep phase syndrome is associated with a complaint of sleep onset delay, while advanced sleep phase syndrome is accompanied by a complaint of an early awakening. In general, the pattern of insomnia may be primarily (1) difficulty falling asleep (sleep onset delay), (2) early morning arousal (premature awakening with inability to fall asleep again), or (3) sleep fragmentation (repeated awakenings).

Insomnias can generally be transient (less than 3 to 4 weeks) or chronic (more than 3 to 4 weeks) in duration. Multiple factors can trigger transient insomnia, including life stress, brief illness, rapid change of time zones, drug withdrawal, use of central nervous system (CNS) stimulants, and painful conditions. An individual can usually recover rapidly. Such insomnia is experienced by everyone.

Chronic insomnia may be lifelong. It is usually related to chronic psychophysiologic arousal, psychiatric disorders, use of drugs and alcohol, and other medical, toxic, and environmental conditions; however, it may also represent a "primary" sleep disorder in the form of sleep apnea syndrome, alveolar hypoventilation syndrome, sleep-related (nocturnal) myoclonus, and "restless legs."

SLEEP ONSET DELAY

Sleep onset delay is a common problem and probably accounts for most patients who present with a complaint of insomnia. It is usually due to psychogenic causes. Sleeplessness may develop from a continued association with stimulating practices and objects at bedtime. Such patients sleep better away from their bedrooms and usual routines. A conditioned internal factor may also develop in the form of apprehension about unsuccessful and excessive efforts to sleep. Conscious efforts to fall asleep result in CNS arousal. These patients consider themselves "light sleepers." They often have multiple somatic complaints such as back pains, headaches, and palpitations that lead to occasional abuse of alcohol, barbiturates, and minor tranquilizers. The sleep of such patients in the sleep laboratory is usually good, because the conditioning factors that are active at home are reduced in the laboratory. Multiple specific psychiatric illnesses associated with anxiety, such as personality disorders (*e.g.*, anxiety and panic disorders, hypochondriasis, obsessive-compulsive disorders), and schizophrenia can also be associated with sleep onset difficulty.

Drugs can also compromise the initiation of sleep. When obtaining the history, the physician should inquire specifically about possible precipitants of drug-induced insomnia. In addition to steroids and dopaminergic agents, xanthine derivatives (*e.g.*, caffeine and theophylline) may cause sleep disruption. A frequently overlooked class of agents is the beta-adrenergic agonists, such as terbutaline and phenylethylamine derivatives (used as stimulants, appetite suppressants, and decongestants). If such medications are taken late in the day, and in increasing amounts because of the development of tolerance, they can easily cause sleep onset delay, as well as sleep fragmentation and "lightening" of sleep. Such inadequate sleep provokes daytime symptoms including sleepiness, which is responsible for a further increase of ingestion of the drug in order to promote alertness.

In addition to the psychological and drug causes of sleep onset delay, patients who have a disturbed circadian rhythm may have the same sleep complaint. In delayed sleep phase syndrome, patients naturally fall asleep at 2 AM to 3 AM or later. They cannot fall asleep if they go to bed at conventional times. If they must then get up for a job or school at 6 AM, they will be sleepy in the morning because they did not get enough sleep. They, however, have no trouble going to sleep and getting full rest if they can go to bed late and sleep until mid-day. A change in life-style and chronotherapy can correct this problem. Likewise, chronotherapy may help patients who have irregular sleep–wake patterns and who sleep for short and variable periods of time throughout 24 hours. These people often cannot fall asleep at conventional times because they have napped recently. A final category of sleep onset difficulties is pseudoinsomnia, in which patients feel that they do not rest; however, these patients do obtain good quality sleep when they are monitored in the sleep laboratory.

Most patients affected by sleep onset delay do not require drug treatment for therapy. Specifically, a delayed sleep phase syndrome and an irregular sleep–wake pattern should be treated by chronotherapy in a regional Sleep Disorder Center. With this therapy, the patient receives an individually designed sleep schedule to correct his sleep onset delay and the patient gradually attains a desired sleep onset time and normal quality sleep.

Counseling appears to play an important role in the therapy of sleep disorders. If the physician spends some extra time talking with the patient, he is sometimes rewarded by the revelation of useful historical items. Some patients who complain of insomnia may actually be attempting to discuss problems that they find difficult to raise, such as impotence, marital discord, or alcoholism in a family member. The complaint may be resolved, if attention is given to these problems, regardless of whether sleep behavior is actually altered.

Sleep hygiene includes setting a fixed hour for retiring each night, eliminating daytime naps, avoiding caffeine-containing beverages or anxiety-producing activities at night, and assuring that the bedroom is quiet, dark, and comfortable. Because patients may neglect to think of over-the-counter preparations as drugs, mentioning the need to avoid sympathomimetic substances may prove fruitful.

The effects of behavioral therapies have been reviewed by Williams and Karacan. Only a few practical points need to be reviewed here. Techniques that attempt to increase relaxation, either through biofeedback or more conventional learning paradigms, may be valuable if they are aimed at a specific physiologic disturbance. For example, a patient whose PSMG indicates a large amount of muscle activity prior to falling asleep might benefit from EMG biofeedback. These techniques will generally require the facilities of a sleep laboratory. Attempts at operant and classic conditioning as aids in treating insomnia have also had some limited success. A widely accepted behavioral modification technique (stimulus control) is especially useful in correcting maladaptive association of arousal with bedtime routine.

Sleep-promoting medications can be used in the management of insomnia; however, their use must be considered carefully. These medications are most helpful in situations in which their use is self-limited, such as acute hospitalization, or as part of a more comprehensive program of sleep hygiene. In the latter regard, they may allow the physician time to explore the roots of the sleep disturbance more thoroughly.

The choice of a sedative agent is dictated primarily by the duration of clinical sedation; ideally, the hypnotic–sedative effect should cease by the time the patient arises. An effective hypnotic drug should decrease sleep latency and increase the total sleep time.

The value of a hypnotic depends on the balance of its efficacy and side effects. The efficacy is defined by its ability to induce and maintain sleep, and directly depends on the drug's dose, absorption, and duration of action. Thus, an efficacious hypnotic is rapidly absorbed and has duration of action consistent with the sleep period (usually around 8 hours). Ideally, such hypnotic has no adverse effects. However, hypnotics with duration of action that exceeds the sleep period usually lead to residual sedation during daytime. In contrast, use of short-acting hypnotics in doses higher than required is often associated with possible rebound insomnia and anterograde amnesia as major adverse effects. Dependence is also an undesirable possibility with the use of hypnotics. This possibility can be minimized by the intermittent use of low doses, together with limited duration of drug intake and gradual withdrawal in the event the continuous treatment has been given for more than a month. Furthermore, an ideal hypnotic should decrease nocturnal awakenings and should also improve daytime alertness. The available drugs have a surprisingly heterogeneous set of effects on sleep architecture.

Although almost all agents employed as hypnosedatives will suppress REM sleep when given in sufficiently large quantities, two patterns of effects are seen at lower doses. Barbiturates, chloral hydrate, anticholinergics, tricyclics, and ethanol demonstrate REM suppression, whereas most benzodiazepines decrease Stages 3 and 4. Flurazepam, triazolam, and tryptophan have minor effects on sleep architecture. All of these agents appear to decrease sleep latency and reduce the number of spontaneous awakenings. Although the drugs that have the least effect on sleep architecture may offer a theoretical advantage in the therapy of insomnia, there is no clear demonstration that they induce "better" sleep.

Data on commonly used sleep promoting medications and some miscellaneous agents are summarized in Table 21-1. Sleep latency is decreased, except where indicated. There is seldom a reason to use more than a single agent in the treatment of insomnia. A failure to obtain an adequate response on the first night does not imply a need to increase the dosage immediately; a trial of at least 2 or 3 nights is indicated. Sleep induction is related to the rate of absorption. Flurazepam is absorbed rapidly and temazepam is absorbed slowly. Sleep mainte-

nance is related to dosage and half-life. The timing of the intake of the medications is, therefore, important. Hypnotics with longer half-lives (lasting more than 24 hours) show increased efficacy with 2 or 3 nights of administration, but they also show increased residual daytime effects. Some benzodiazepines produce persistent long-acting metabolites and cause definite impairment in alertness, motor performance, and cognitive function in the morning. Flurazepam (Dalmane) produces a "hangover effect." When the initial therapy is unsuccessful, changing classes of medications may be useful. A barbiturate (with REM suppressant ef-

TABLE 21-1. Commonly Available Hypnosedative Drugs

MEDICATION	DOSAGE*	EFFECTS ON SLEEP ARCHITECTURE
Barbiturates		
Amobarbital	200 mg	Decreases REM; increases REM latency
Heptobarbital	400 mg	Decreases REM
Pentobarbital	100 mg	Decreases REM; increases REM latency
Phenobarbital	100 mg	Decreases REM
Secobarbital	100 mg	Decreases REM
Amobarbital and secobarbital (Tuinal)		Decreases REM
Ethanol	100 ml	Decreases REM, first half of night
	200 ml	Decreases REM, entire night
Benzodiazepines		
Chlordiazepoxide	50 mg	Decreases Stage 4
Diazepam	10 mg	Decreases Stage 4
Flurazepam	15 mg	Slight decrease REM and Stages 2 and 4
	30 mg	Slight decrease Stages 3 and 4
Lorazepam	2 mg	Decreases REM
Oxazepam	10 mg	Increases REM
Triazolam	0.1–1 mg	Decreases REM
Tricyclics		
Amitriptyline	50 mg	Increases Stage 1; decreases REM
Desipramine	50 mg	Increases Stage 4; decreases REM
Doxepin	25 mg	Increases Stage 4; decreases REM
Imipramine	50 mg	Increases Stage 4; decreases REM
Nortriptyline	25 mg	Increases Stage 4; decreases REM
Protriptyline	5 mg	Increases Stage 4; decreases REM
Miscellaneous		
Chloral hydrate	500–1500 mg	No significant effect
Diphenhydramine	50–100 mg	Decreases REM
Glutethimide	500–1000 mg	Decreases REM
Meprobamate	400–800 mg	No significant effect
Methaqualone	300 mg	No significant effect
Triclofos	1000 mg	No significant effect
Tryptophan (L-form)	1–10 g	Normal sleep architecture
	10 g	Decreases REM

*Dosages are suggestions for initial therapy only and will depend on usual factors influencing a patient's tolerance to medication.

fect), for example, may be useful when a benzodiazepine fails. L-tryptophan is no longer in use because of its removal from the market due to occurrence of a potentially fatal condition, eosinophilia–myalgia syndrome, presumably related to its use. Due to the intrinsic "tapering" effect of compounds with long half-lives, rebound and/or withdrawal phenomena appear to be unlikely; when they do occur, such effects are delayed in onset and are relatively mild. On the other hand, there is a much higher likelihood of rebound or withdrawal effect after abrupt discontinuation of short half-life hypnotics. Dose tapering is appropriate when short half-life hypnotics are discontinued.

In the last decade, benzodiazepines have almost completely replaced barbiturates. The choice of drug for sleep onset insomnia and sleep maintenance insomnia will be different (e.g., triazolam [Halcion] vs temazepam [Restoril]). A new benzodiazepine, estazolam, was recently introduced.

Onset of action after oral dose depends on rapidity of absorption from the gastrointestinal tract. For instance, the capsule preparation of temazepam is very slowly absorbed from the gastrointestinal tract, with peak concentration reached on the average of 2 to 3 hours after dosing. The duration of action of a single dose of benzodiazepine hypnotic depends on distribution, in which the drug is circulated to other sites (such as adipose tissue), where it exerts no pharmacologic activity; and on elimination and clearance. With repeated administration at a fixed dosing rate, a drug will accumulate in plasma and brain until a steady state is reached. More than 90% of time necessary to reach a steady-state condition depends only on the drug's elimination half-life. For a drug such as triazolam with a very short elimination half-life, accumulation will be complete within 1 day; that is, the mean plasma concentration will be no higher after multiple days of therapy than after the first day. At the other extreme is a drug such as flurazepam, with its principal active metabolite desalkylflurazepam. This compound has a very long elimination half-life; 2 weeks or more of long-term treatment will be necessary for a steady state to be attained. The rate of drug disappearance following discontinuation after long-term treatment will mirror the rate of accumulation; that is, the longer the elimination half-life, the more time will be needed for the drug to disappear. A potential benefit of accumulating a benzodiazepine is that persistence of drug at the receptor sites throughout each 24-hour dosing interval increases the likelihood of a daytime anxiolytic effect, a po-

tential benefit for patients with both anxiety and insomnia. For short half-life hypnotics such as triazolam, on the other hand, increased daytime anxiety has been reported in some studies, possibly attributable to wide fluctuations in plasma and receptor-site concentrations between doses. Pregnant women, alcoholics, and sleep apneics should not be given hypnotics, except in low doses and only in special circumstances. Preference for benzodiazepines over barbiturates is based on the former's lower toxicity (less respiratory and cardiac depression) and less marked tolerance rather than on its superior hypnotic effect. The prescribing of hypnotics to children is not recommended, except for rare use in the treatment of night terrors or severe somnambulism. Benzodiazepine metabolism varies and is largely age-dependent. The elimination half-life of diazepam in healthy men may increase three- to four-fold from 20 years of age to 80 years of age. The elimination of hypnotics is decreased in elderly people who might have a low renal glomerular filtration rate, a reduced hepatic blood flow, and a decreased activity of hepatic drug-metabolizing enzymes. Benzodiazepine dosage should be halved in the elderly, and even then daytime functioning may be impaired significantly.

The choice of hypnosedatives for elderly patients with sleep onset delay, especially when they are acutely hospitalized, is complicated by the risk of a paradoxical excitation at nighttime ("sun-downing"), which may be precipitated or exacerbated by medication. Although diphenhydramine has been useful in many of these patients, there is a risk of increasing their confusion because of its anticholinergic effect. These problems can be minimized by adjunctive measures, such as leaving a light on in the patient's room, and by frequently reorienting the patient to the unfamiliar surroundings. A family member may occasionally be required to stay with the patient.

In patients with early morning awakening, sedative therapy is usually accompanied by an unacceptable degree of morning sedation ("hang-over"). If the patient's work-up suggests that depression is the cause of or contributes to the disorder, tricyclic antidepressants appear to offer the best results and should be the initial form of therapy. Although an improvement in sleep often precedes an improvement in mood, changes of affect should determine the end point in therapy.

The withdrawal from sedative drugs, especially barbiturates, is potentially the most dangerous of drug withdrawals and should be carried out in a hospital setting. Although guidelines for this procedure are beyond the scope of this discussion, some comments are in order. The dose of the drug should be gradually reduced if a large quantity was being employed routinely. These agents should never be discontinued abruptly (except in the rare case of hypersensitivity reactions). In addition to rebound insomnia and irritability, hallucinations are common, and hyperthermia due to increased physical activity may be life threatening. Abrupt barbiturate withdrawal is one of the commonest causes of status epilepticus. Most of these problems can be corrected by adequate attention to fluid and electrolyte balance and by adequate sedation; however, they can all be prevented if the withdrawal process is done slowly.

Due to the intrinsic "tapering" effect of long half-life compounds, rebound and/or withdrawal phenomena appear to be unlikely; when they do occur, such effects are delayed in onset and are relatively mild. On the other hand, there is much higher likelihood of rebound or withdrawal effect after abrupt discontinuation of short half-life hypnotics. Dose tapering is appropriate when a short half-life hypnotics are discontinued.

A new benzodiazepine, estazolam, was recently introduced. Estazolam in a dose of 2 mg remains an effective hypnotic for at least 6 weeks of continuous administration with no evidence of clinically significant tolerance. It improves sleep latency and total sleep time, reduces the number of nocturnal awakenings, and improves both depth of sleep and sleep quality in adults with chronic insomnia.

Zolpidem is another new hypnotic, a benzodiazepine receptor ligand structurally unrelated to benzodiazepines (omega 1-selective nonbenzodiazepine hypnotic). It has a mean elimination half-life of 3.5 to 5.1 hours (mean 4 hours). In young adults zolpidem leads to marked increase in slow wave sleep with reduction of Stage 2. No change in REM sleep occurs. In the middle-aged there was a reduction of awake time, increase of Stage 2 NREM sleep, without changes of REM sleep. Food and Drug Administration approval for marketing of zolpidem in the United States is pending. Zopiclone is a cyclopyrrolone compound, another new hypnotic that is chemically unrelated to benzodiazepines. Enhanced binding of gamma-aminobutyric acid (GABA) to the GABA-chloride ionophore complex occurs to a lesser extent with zopiclone than with benzodiazepines. Recently, a separate site of cyclopyrrolones on the benzodiazepine receptor complex has been identified. Zopiclone has a half-life of 5 hours and no long-acting metabolites. Its use is accompanied by an increase of NREM sleep without REM sleep reduction. Rebound phenomena have not been shown consistently. Zopiclone is not yet available in the United States.

Although many of these drugs, especially the benzodiazepines, have been marketed with emphasis on their short duration of action, many have long-acting active metabolites. This is often a problem in the patient who experiences a decrement in liver function. Sedative effects are additive and may convert what would have been a mild metabolic encephalopathy into a coma days after the initiation of treatment.

EARLY MORNING AWAKENING

This problem can be seen in numerous clinical settings. Endogenous depression is characterized by a typical premature awakening and an inability to fall asleep again, with variable sleep onset disturbance depending on the individual's component of agitation. A key polysomnographic finding is shortened REM sleep latency, which is considered by some experts to be a biologic marker of depression, in addition to an increased intensity of REM sleep. Deep (delta) NREM sleep is also reduced; this is a relatively nonspecific feature. In contrast, bipolar depression is frequently associated with hypersomnia; however, this state is again accompanied by a shortened REM latency and reduced Stages 3 or 4 NREM sleep. The onset of sleep is delayed and sleep is short in mania and hypomania. Insomnia may precede all other symptoms of depression, and restoration of sleep may be the first sign of recovery. Obviously, treatment consists of an appropriate use of antidepressants.

Advanced sleep phase syndrome is occasionally responsible for a complaint of early morning awakening and, as such, may mimic a typical pattern of sleep disturbance seen in depression. It is seen fairly frequently in elderly patients as well as in some young adults. There are few and relatively experimental treatments for this condition, including either reverse chronotherapy or exposure to light in the evening and light deprivation in the morning. Either treatment requires the skills of experts in the Sleep Disorder Centers.

Drug-induced early morning awakening may occur with the use of some short-acting benzodiazepines, such as oxazepam (Serax) or lorazepam (Ativan). They are almost completely inactivated by a conjugation in the liver, and they have few residual morning aftereffects. Patients who drink alcoholic beverages prior to sleep may develop early morning awakening, apparently related to an increase in REM sleep ("REM rebound") after the alcohol is metabolized. An underlying psychiatric problem should be considered, as in any patient with an alcohol-related problem. Therapy involves a slow withdrawal of the causative agent.

SLEEP FRAGMENTATION

If a patient's major complaint is frequent awakenings at night, it often signals the presence of a primary sleep disorder, specifically sleep apnea or nocturnal myoclonus. Multiple medical conditions can also interfere with sleep maintenance, but a psychiatric etiology is a less likely explanation for this complaint.

In sleep apnea, sleep disruption is due to cessation of breathing during sleep apnea and subsequent frequent awakenings associated with an occasional gasping for air or a choking sensation. In most cases, it is predominantly central sleep apnea occurring during NREM, as well as REM sleep. Patients usually report daytime "tiredness," but they do not take naps.

Insomnia sometimes results from alveolar hypoventilation which, in adults, may be secondary to conditions such as massive obesity, chronic obstructive pulmonary disease, myopathy, cordotomy, or lesions involving structures that control sleep. Primary alveolar hypoventilation is usually reported in infants and is associated with a further worsening of hypercapnia and hypoxemia in sleep. Treatments of sleep-induced respiratory impairments are discussed in the section on disorders of excessive somnolence.

Sleep-related (nocturnal) myoclonus is a condition in which insomnia is associated with the occurrence during sleep of periodic episodes of repetitive and highly stereotyped leg muscle jerks. They are consistently followed by a partial arousal. Patients are often unaware of the movements at night; rather, they report frequent nocturnal awakenings and unrefreshing sleep. A history from a bed partner is important, because they usually provide accurate description of the movements. Insomnia can be also associated with so-called "restless legs" syndrome when the patient has disagreeable deep sensations of creeping inside the calves whenever sitting or lying down, causing an almost irresistible urge to move the legs, and thus interfering with the sleep onset. Almost all patients with the "restless legs" syndrome also have sleep-related (nocturnal)

myoclonus. The most widely accepted and successful treatment is obtained by the use of clonazepam.

Secondary causes of sleep fragmentation include various nocturnal behavioral disruptions: for example, parasomnias such as bruxism (teeth grinding). Furthermore, gastroesophageal reflux with regurgitation, heartburn and dyspepsia, nocturnal angina, sleep-related asthma, nightmares, and cluster headaches may all cause a serious insomnia due mainly to severe sleep fragmentation. Other multiple medical and neurologic conditions can be associated with this form of insomnia, including CNS infections, head traumas, nocturnal epilepsy, fibrositis syndrome, cardiovascular disorders, pulmonary disease, any painful condition, toxic conditions, endocrine disease, such as hyperthyroidism, and Addison's disease. In these patients, treatment of the underlying disorder is expected to alleviate the sleep disturbance and thus obviate the need for hypnotics. Hypercortisolism (especially iatrogenic hypercortisolism) should be considered if sleep fragmentation is prominent. Parkinsonian patients receiving therapy with levodopa (or levodopa-carbidopa [Sinemet]) are also subject to this complaint. Daytime napping is frequently reported. The response to hypnosedatives and tricyclics is unpredictable. The avoidance of dopaminergic drugs after supper is helpful for many patients.

SLEEP DISORDERS ASSOCIATED WITH HYPERSOMNOLENCE

Included in this category are intrinsic and extrinsic sleep disorders as well as parasomnias and disorders associated with medical–psychiatric disorders. The chief symptoms of this group of disorders include an inappropriate and undesirable sleepiness during waking hours, decreased cognitive and motor performance, an excessive tendency to sleep, unavoidable napping, an increase in total sleep over 24 hours ("true" hypersomnia), and a difficulty in achieving full arousal on awakening. This diagnosis should, in a strict sense, be reserved for patients who have a demonstrable tendency to fall asleep in the waking state when sedentary or who have sleep "attacks." There may also be diminished alertness in waking, described by the term *subwakefulness*. In all of the cases presenting with these symptoms it is important to separate excessive daytime somnolence from less specific symptoms of fatigue, malaise, or depression.

The major causes of excessive daytime sleepiness are sleep apnea syndrome (43%), narcolepsy (25%), and insufficient sleep.

SLEEP APNEA

A potentially lethal condition, sleep apnea is a basic abnormal breathing pattern during sleep and is defined as a cessation of airflow at the level of the nostrils and the mouth, lasting for at least 10 seconds. Apneas are subdivided by type:

1. Obstructive or upper airway apnea is secondary to a sleep-induced obstruction of the airway (Fig. 21-3).

2. Central or diaphragmatic apnea is secondary to decreased respiratory muscle activity.

3. Mixed apnea combines both phenomena; it usually starts as a central apnea (with no respiratory effort) and develops into an obstruction later.

Obstructive or central apnea predominates in each patient.

Obstructive sleep apnea seems to be due to the concentric pharyngeal collapse during inspiration and

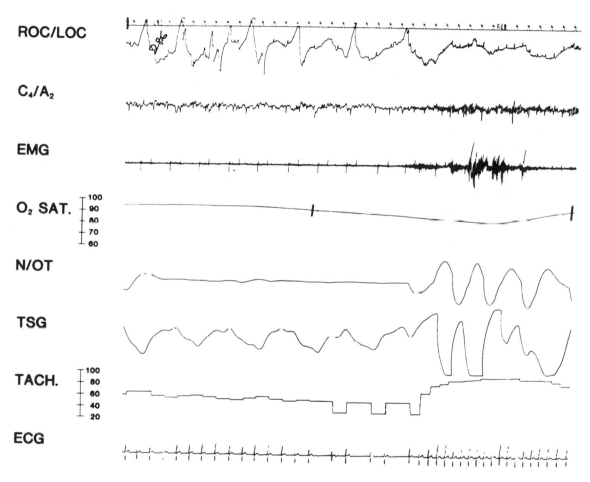

FIG. 21-3. Obstructive apnea. During the REM stage, airflow ceases for 21 sec while unsuccessful respiratory effort continues, indicating obstruction of the upper airway. Oxygen saturation falls to 81%. Immediately prior to the resumption of ventilation, the ECG demonstrates second-degree A-V block. When ventilation occurs, rhythm appears in the EEG and tachycardia is evident in the ECG.

is not due to an active musculature contraction. Contributing factors may include:

1. Abnormal anatomic relationships among the muscular or bony structures of the naso-, oro-, or hypopharynx (*e.g.*, a short thick neck, macroglossia, a relatively small hyoid bone, or a narrow pharynx)
2. Inappropriate involuntary respiratory control of the pharyngeal and diaphragmatic muscle tone
3. Increased compliance of the pharyngeal walls, especially fatty or redundant pharyngeal and submucosal folds
4. The amount of inspiratory, intraluminal negative pressure

Clinical symptoms usually include snoring, persistent daytime sleepiness, tiredness and fatigue, unrefreshing sleep attacks, deterioration of memory and judgment, early morning confusion, automatic behavior at times (*i.e.*, amnestic attacks), serious morning headaches, personality changes, and a generally depressed outlook. Although many patients with obstructive sleep apnea are moderately overweight, morbid obesity is present only in the minority. Waking respiratory functions are usually within normal limits. Hypertension is present in about 40% of the patients at the time of diagnosis. Alveolar hypoventilation, associated with an elevated waking $PaCO_2$, occasionally accompanies obstructive sleep apnea. Increased $PaCO_2$ of 45 mmHg or higher has been reported in 23% of obese patients with obstructive sleep apnea. Marked cyclic sinus arrhythmia appears during sleep and apnea. This rhythm pattern is characterized by progressive sinus bradycardia during apnea (heart rates of less than 30 beats/min are not uncommon) with an abrupt reversal and sinus acceleration at the onset of ventilation. Second degree atrioventricular (AV) block, prolonged sinus pauses, limited runs of ventricular tachycardia, and paroxysmal atrial tachycardia episodes also occur. Furthermore, systemic and pulmonary artery pressures rise in association with obstructive apneas. On the other hand 22% to 30% of patients with systemic hypertension were found to suffer from obstructive sleep apnea. Although both conditions are also more frequent in males and obese people, the association of hypertension and obstructive sleep apnea seems to be independent of obesity. When episodes of apnea occur in rapid succession, pressures do not return to baseline but show a stepwise increase.

In contrast to patients with obstructive sleep apnea, patients affected predominantly by *central sleep apnea* are older (*i.e.*, they have a mean age of 63 *vs* 46); they mainly complain of sleep fragmentation; they are not overweight; and they have less pronounced oxygen desaturation and a more moderate hemodynamic impact. There is no definite sex distribution. Central sleep apnea is not a single disease entity but is likely the result of any one of a number of processes that yield instability of respiratory control. Two groups of patients were identified on the basis of the daytime ventilation. Nonhypercapnic patients were described as "idiopathic hyperventilators" with low or normal awake PCO_2 and exaggerated hypercapnic ventilatory responses. Hypercapnic patients demonstrated CO_2 retention and blunted hypercapnic ventilatory responses. In general, all apneas are more frequent with increasing age and following alcohol or sedative drug intake.

Both central and obstructive sleep apnea can be a complication of another medical or neurologic disorder. These disorders include brain-stem infarction, lateral medullary syndrome, bulbar poliomyelitis, medullary neoplasms, syringomyelia and syringobulbia, olivopontocerebellar atrophy, Alzheimer's disease, encephalitides, Jakob–Creutzfeldt disease, postencephalitic parkinsonism, cervical cordotomy, neuromuscular disorders affecting intercostal muscles and the diaphragm like myasthenia gravis, higher cervical spinal poliomyelitis, Guillain–Barré syndrome, limb–girdle dystrophies, and especially myotonic dystrophy. Hypoventilation and daytime drowsiness are prominent in all these disorders.

Of special interest is a development of a "postpolio syndrome" years after the acute stage of poliomyelitis. It starts with fatigue, new muscular weakness, musculoskeletal pain, and dysphagia. During sleep patients experience central and obstructive sleep apnea, which is worse during REM sleep because of the combined REM sleep–induced atonia and abnormal motor (phrenic) output caused by medullary dysfunction. Poliomyelitis can also cause atrophy of respiratory accessory muscles and thoracoabdominal muscles, leading to severe chest deformity such as kyphoscoliosis. Furthermore, impairment of cranial motor nerves (hypoglossal, facial, and trigeminal) may affect adversely tongue and other upper airway muscles. As a consequence, all types of apneas may occur. These patients are vulnerable to develop respiratory failure with acute respiratory infection and may require assisted ventilation in intensive care units until the infection is controlled. Predominantly obstructure sleep apnea may result from enlarged tonsils (an especially important factor in the etiology of sleep apnea and snoring in children), myxedema, micrognathia and other facial or mandibular abnormalities, platybasia, neck infiltration secondary to Hodgkin's disease and lymphoma, acromegaly, and familial or acquired dysautonomia (usually mixed central and obstructive sleep apnea).

An evaluation of the patient suspected of having sleep apnea syndrome includes not only a history obtained from the patient but also (and most important) a history obtained from the bed partner. A physical examination should concentrate on blood pressure, evidence of right heart failure, abnormal facial, neck, and skeletal or muscle configuration. The ear, nose, and throat examination is of prime importance. Pulmonary function studies may be necessary to investigate for primary hypoventilation during the waking state and responsiveness to CO_2 stimulation. These studies should be followed by an all-night polysomnographic study, which is essential for an accurate diagnosis and an estimation of the severity of oxygen desaturation. The severity of sleep apnea, defined by the so-called apnea-hypopnea index (*i.e.*, the number of episodes per hour of sleep), the degree

of oxygen desaturation, and the presence of significant arrhythmias will be derived from sleep study and will guide future treatment (Fig. 21-4). The treatment of sleep apnea syndromes depends on the associated abnormality, which may become treatable once it is defined.

Pharmacologic approaches including acetazolamide, theophylline, naloxone, medroxyprogesterone, and clomipramine have not been studied systematically on large numbers of subjects. The only widely used drug is protriptyline, which may exert a beneficial effect in an occasional patient with obstructive sleep apnea. Its effect may be due to reported direct action on the upper airway's muscle tone. A recent crossover unblinded trial of protriptyline and fluoxetine suggests equal effectiveness of either drug, with about 30% to 50% of patients showing improved oxygenation during sleep.

A number of studies suggest that the administration of oxygen may be a useful method of treating central sleep apnea, although the mechanism by which oxygen administration reduces central apneic events has not been established. It is hypothesized that the potential destabilizing influence of the hypoxic ventilatory response on respiratory control may

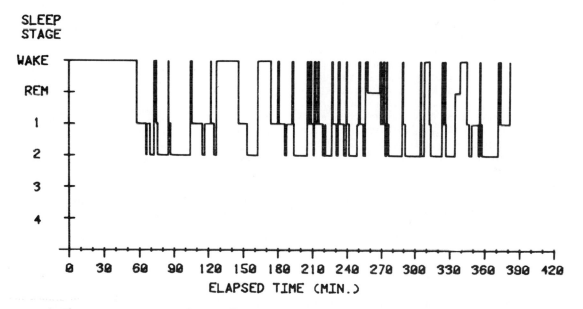

FIG. 21-4. The sleep architecture of an adult man with obstructive sleep apnea syndrome. Stages 3 and 4 are lacking; frequent waking arousals occur, which fragment the sleep cycle; REM sleep is much reduced as a proportion of the sleep period; and REM periodicity is abolished. The majority of the sleep period consists of NREM Stages 1 and 2.

in fact be counteracted by the administration of oxygen. However, in some cases hypercapnia and the frequency of obstructive sleep apnea may increase. The most widely used treatment of obstructive sleep apnea is Nasal continuous positive airway pressure CPAP, which acts by establishing a "pneumatic splint" to the upper airway. The key element of its effect is that it causes elevation of the pressure in the oropharynx, thus reversing the transmural pressure gradient across the oropharyngeal airway.

Nasal CPAP is the only treatment as effective as tracheostomy. The major reasons for CPAP failure are poor compliance due to social or cosmetic reasons, and nasal obstruction. Some patients whose apneas are eliminated with CPAP continue to have nonapneic desaturations, especially during REM sleep. Usually, these patients are obese, with chronic obstructive pulmonary disease (COPD) in addition to sleep apnea. In such situations supplemental oxygen may be beneficial. The benefits derived from oxygen treatment should be polysomnographically verified.

Bilevel positive airway pressure (BiPAP) offers an effective alternative to patients who are uncomfortable while expiring against high pressures delivered by CPAP. This device allows independent titration of expiratory and inspiratory airway pressure and has been very helpful in cases of comorbid obesity, intrinsic lung disease, and chest deformity.

One of the major general measures in treatment of sleep apnea is weight loss. Along these lines abstinence from alcohol and avoidance of sedative-hypnotic drugs and beta blockers are advocated. Sometimes, correction of nasal obstruction can result in significant reduction of sleep apneas. Adenoidectomy, tonsillectomy, and surgical correction of the maxillofacial anomalies will abolish apneas. Patients with serious mandibular deformities can undergo surgical procedures of maxillary, mandibular and hyoid bone advancements, but a significant number of failures occur, primarily in patients with the most severe mandibular deficiency.

Attempts to promote uvulopalatopharyngoplasty (UPPP) as an alternative surgical treatment of sleep apnea have not been successful. Multiple studies indicate at best a variable success rate, ranging from 33% to 70%. The success rate may improve somewhat, provided selection of patients is based on the determination of the level of obstruction prior to the surgery. Cessation of snoring following UPPP is expected, because structures generating the sounds of snoring are surgically removed. This may be misinterpreted as a sign of apnea cure,

while apneas may persist despite disappearance of snoring. The use of prosthetic devices focuses on the nasopharyngeal inlet and position of the base of the tongue. The only two devices tested in a sleep lab for their effectiveness are a tongue-retaining device (TRD) and Snore-Guard (Snore-Guard, Hayes & Meade, Inc., Albuquerque, New Mexico). TRD is most effective in patients demonstrating positional apnea who are not excessively obese. For some positional apneics, just training them to sleep on their sides may represent an effective cure.

NARCOLEPSY

Narcolepsy is defined as a syndrome consisting of excessive daytime sleepiness and abnormal manifestations of REM sleep. The latter includes frequent sleep-onset REM periods, which may be subjectively appreciated as hypnagogic hallucinations, and dissociated REM sleep inhibitory processes: cataplexy and sleep paralysis. The appearance of REM sleep within 10 minutes of sleep onset is considered evidence for narcolepsy. In narcolepsy the patient falls asleep in the midst of activities, although most people will stay awake during animated conversation, walking, eating, or coitus.

Although sleep attacks are characteristic of this disease, excessive sleepiness is equally disturbing (i.e., a permanent impairment of vigilance or wakefulness, that can be profound between attacks). Both represent primary symptoms of narcolepsy in addition to cataplexy. Sleep attacks usually last about 15 minutes. The patient awakens refreshed and there is a definite refractory period of 1 to 5 hours before the next attack in such patients. Cataplexy is a sudden decrease or abrupt loss of muscle tone that is either generalized or limited to particular muscle groups. Cataplexy ranges from weakness in the muscles supporting the jaw, or a sense of weakness in the knees, to a complete muscular weakness causing the patient to slump to the floor, unable to move. Cataplectic attacks are characteristically initiated by laughter, surprise, outbursts of anger, or a feeling of exaltation. These attacks generally last for only a few seconds or as long as 30 minutes.

Auxiliary symptoms of narcolepsy include sleep paralysis, which occurs while the patient is falling asleep or waking from sleep. Consciousness is preserved and it is accompanied by an intense feeling of fear. Hypnagogic hallucinations also occur at the onset of sleep or on awakening, and they are usually frightening. Automatic behavior is sometimes reported as "blackouts," and is a reflection of severe sleepiness. Nocturnal sleep is also disturbed with frequent awakenings, frequent sleep-onset REM periods, and vivid dreams.

The diagnosis of narcolepsy is based on (1) a normal physical examination, (2) a normal routine EEG, (3) the Multiple Sleep Latency Test showing a mean sleep latency of 5 minutes or less, and (4) sleep onset REM periods. Narcolepsy is familial and transmission seems to be autosomal dominant with variable penetrance. HLA typing may become diagnostically useful in view of a report by Langdon and associates that all narcoleptics are DR2 positive.

In some patients, successful treatment involves only improved sleep hygiene: obtaining adequate sleep at night, regulating sleep phase, maintaining a regular daily schedule of bedtime and rising time, and therapeutic naps. Most patients, however, will need CNS stimulants. These stimulants primarily include dextroamphetamine, methylphenidate, and pemoline. Cataplectic attacks respond to imipramine or protriptyline. Patients refractory to previous treatments may sometimes require the use of monoamine oxidase (MAO) inhibitors. HLA typing of narcoleptic patients revealed that almost 100% of Orientals and Caucasians have HLA-DR2 and DQw1 antigens, whereas the prevalence of these antigens in the general population is between 20% and 40%. The association of HLA-DR2 and narcolepsy in blacks is not that strong, but the DQw1 association has been identified in almost 100% of cases reported in the literature. This HLA-DR2 link to narcolepsy is the strongest association of any HLA type with human disease, and it may represent a genetic marker for the disorder, indicating possible presence of a "narcolepsy-susceptibility" gene on chromosome 6. The idea, based on these observations, that there may be an immunologic basis for narcolepsy has not yet been substantiated.

Modafinil (an alpha-adrenergic agent), mazindol (an imidazole derivative), and selegiline (an MAO-B inhibitor) improve daytime alertness and may have fewer side effects than amphetamines, but none have been shown to be more effective than amphetamines in treating narcolepsy. The improvements observed with the use of L-tyrosine, codeine, or propranolol have not been documented in controlled trials. When sleep fragmentation represents one of the major complaints, judicious use of short-acting hypnotics once or twice per week may be helpful. The improvement of nocturnal sleep with gamma-hydroxybutirate did not result in demonstrable improvement of diurnal symptoms. The use of amphetamines produces common adverse effects like restlessness, agitation, tachycardia, dizziness, and psychotic episodes. Stimulants may all be associated with dependence. Pharmacologic approaches are generally not entirely satisfactory, and many patients benefit from social support provided by groups like the American Narcolepsy Association. Idiopathic CNS hypersomnolence is a condition resembling narcolepsy, but without sleep-onset REM periods, cataplexy, or auxiliary symptoms. The treatment with stimulants is usually less effective.

INSUFFICIENT SLEEP

Insufficient sleep is a frequent cause of daytime somnolence. The individual is voluntarily, but often unwittingly, chronically sleep deprived. Although this relationship may seem self-evident, most of the patients are unaware that their chronic sleep deprivation is responsible for their continuous excessive sleepiness. When these individuals obtain adequate sleep, their complaint of somnolence during the day disappears.

Various other medical and medicinal causes of excessive daytime somnolence deserve mention. Sedative-hypnotics, anticonvulsants, antihypertensives, antihistamines, and antidepressants are common causes. A withdrawal from stimulants may also give rise to severe sleepiness. Multiple medical and toxic conditions may be associated with drowsiness: hyperglycemia (prior to ketoacidosis or nonketotic coma), hypocortisolism, hypoglycemia, hypothyroidism, panhypopituitarism, hepatic encephalopathy, hypercalcemia, renal insufficiency, vitamin B_{12} deficiency, chronic subdural hematoma, encephalitis, intracranial neoplasm (primary or secondary), meningitis, or post-trauma. Hypersomnolence is a misnomer in many of these conditions since more often a state of obtundation occurs. There are also two rare periodic disorders of excessive sleepiness: (1) Kleine—Levin syndrome, characterized by recurrent periods of extended sleep, megaphagia, sexual disinhibitions, social withdrawal if awake, and (2) menstruation-associated hypersomnia, a period of sleepiness during a patient's menstrual period. No changes in behavior were observed in this syndrome.

PARASOMNIAS

Parasomnias include a heterogeneous group of behavioral disturbances that occur only during sleep or are exacerbated by sleep. They do not have a common pathophysiologic mechanism. Certain conditions may represent disorders of arousal because they occur with the emergence of partial arousal from delta sleep. They are present usually in children and include sleepwalking (somnambulism), sleep terror (pavor nocturnus, incubus), and sleep-related enuresis. There is often a concurrence of more than one of these disorders in the same child, and a hereditary predisposition to parasomnias has been noted. Somnambulism in children is not considered to be caused by psychological factors, although its persistence into adulthood represents a serious problem and may be associated with diverse forms of personality disturbance and psychopathology. Most children grow out of this condition between the ages of 7 and 14. Most somnambulistic episodes last a few seconds to a few minutes. It is important to protect patients against injury by installing safety rails at the head of stairways, or by placing locks on windows. In cases of frequent sleepwalking, diazepam may reduce the episodes, probably through the suppression of delta sleep. The usual dose is 5 mg to 10 mg at bedtime. Sleep-related enuresis is involuntary micturition beginning usually during deep NREM sleep in an individual who has or should have gained voluntary waking control of the bladder. In contrast to this idiopathic nocturnal enuresis, symptomatic enuresis is due to urogenital or other diseases and is generally less benign. Idiopathic enuresis as well as somnambulism tend to disappear by late childhood or adolescence, probably representing a phenomenon of delayed maturation. At 5 years of age, 15% of boys and 10% of girls are enuretic. With regard to treatment, tricyclic antidepressants, specifically imipramine 10 mg to 25 mg q.h.s., is valuable. Conditioning with a buzzer and pad is the most successful modality of treatment for the enuresis.

A night terror is an arousal from NREM sleep accompanied by a piercing scream or cry and behavioral manifestations of intense anxiety indicating autonomic arousal—mydriasis, perspiration, piloerection, rapid breathing, and tachycardia. Morning amnesia for the episode is a rule. By contrast, a nightmare is an arousal from REM sleep with the recall of a disturbing dream, accompanied by anxiety and much less prominent autonomic arousal. The awakened patient is momentarily oriented and alert.

REM sleep behavior disorder (RBD) is a parasomnia characterized by vigorous motor activity in response to dream content, instead of atonia, often resulting in an injury. One-third of people with RBD have a demonstrable underlying neurologic disorder. Most of the cases are, however, idiopathic and tend to occur in the elderly. Transient RBD has been seen in association with acute drug intoxications and withdrawal states. Clonazepam is the drug of choice for treatment of RBD.

Withdrawal from alcohol, amphetamines, and hypnotics at the time of the REM rebound is frequently a cause of nightmares. Parasomnias also include a cluster headache and the related (but more chronic) condition of paroxysmal hemicrania. Cluster headaches occur in REM sleep and may be related to an increased cerebral blood flow during REM sleep. About 45% of patients with seizure disorders have seizures mainly during sleep. Generalized seizures are markedly activated by NREM sleep; specifically, generalized tonic–clonic seizures are most common during Stages 1 and 2 NREM sleep. Focal seizures may occur during NREM and REM sleep. Prolonged EEG monitoring may be necessary in some difficult cases when a diagnosis of epileptic vs nonepileptic episodic behavior is needed.

Other parasomnias that may occur in childhood as well as in adulthood include bruxism (teeth grinding), head banging (jactatio capitis nocturna), abnormal swallowing, and painful penile erections. Whether these conditions require a polysomnographic evaluation and treatment depends entirely on the persistence of the symptoms and the degree of the patient's disability. Bruxism affects up to 15% of children. This condition may contribute to periodontal disease and temporomandibular joint dysfunction.

USE OF SLEEP LABORATORIES FOR EVALUATION OF NONSLEEP-RELATED COMPLAINTS

The examination of nocturnal penile tumescence during sleep represents a useful tool for the evaluation of impotence. Sleep-related erections are always abnormal in cases of organic impotence. Impotence is more likely to be psychogenic in nature if sleep-related erections are normal. Attention should be paid to a careful drug history, because many drugs have the potential to cause an impairment of erectile mechanisms.

QUESTIONS AND DISCUSSION

1. A 23-year-old man presents with the chief complaint of "narcolepsy." His history indicates the presence of sleep attacks, cataplexy, sleep paralysis, and hypnagogic hallucinosis for the last 4 years. He states he has never been treated for the disorder and recognized his problem from reading about narcolepsy in a magazine. The neurologic examination is normal. The physical examination reveals a nervous man with a heart rate of 102 beats/minute but otherwise normal vital signs. The remainder of the physical examination is normal. A routine complete blood count (CBC), SMA-25, ECG, and chest x-ray film are normal. A thyroid battery is within normal limits. Management at this point would consist of:

   A. Prescription of d-amphetamine, 5 mg three times daily
   B. Administration of d-amphetamine in combination with a tricyclic antidepressant
   C. Routine all-night PSMG
   D. Urine screening for amphetamine metabolites
   E. Scheduling for a series of daytime naps in the sleep laboratory

The correct answer is (D). Our usual practice is to screen the urine for amphetamine metabolites before doing a more involved study. It is usually a bad sign to have a patient who knows the classic symptoms of narcolepsy and maintains he has never been diagnosed or treated. In most cases of narcolepsy, excessive daytime sleepiness and sleep attacks are initial symptoms of the disease, whereas associated symptoms develop later. A patient with all components of the syndrome early in the course of the disorder is suspicious. Once urine samples are known to be "clean," all-night polysomnography and nap studies are useful in establishing the diagnosis. If a patient is suspected of covert stimulant use, a prolonged period of abstinence should be documented before assuming that an REM-onset sleep episode is narcolepsy (since the same pattern may appear as part of stimulant withdrawal). Empirical therapy with stimulants is a practice that should be avoided.

2. A 36-year-old schoolteacher is referred for an evaluation of excessive somnolence. The patient states that he feels extremely drowsy unless he is actively involved in a novel behavior. The problem has been present for at least 3 years but seems to be getting worse. He has fallen asleep at the wheel of his car twice in the last 6 months. He denies a significant history of alcohol ingestion and is not taking medications. The physical examination reveals a large (1.6 m, 82 kg) individual with normal vital signs. The physical and neurologic examinations are normal. When you walk out of the room to answer a call, you return and find the patient sleeping. A routine blood count reveals a hemoglobin (Hb) of 17.2%, with normal indices and white blood cell count. Biochemical screening is normal. A routine ECG is normal. Thyroid hormone levels and cortisol determinations are unremarkable. A reasonable differential diagnosis at this point would include:

   A. Sedative drug abuse
   B. Narcolepsy
   C. Sleep apnea
   D. Depression
   E. Idiopathic hypersomnia

   Which of the following studies might be of value in evaluating these possibilities?

   A. EEG
   B. Computed tomography of the head
   C. Brain scan
   D. All-night PSG with respiratory and cardiac monitoring
   E. Urine drug screen
   F. Diagnostic psychiatric interview
   G. A series of daytime naps in the sleep laboratory
   H. An empirical trial of d-amphetamine without additional testing

This is a fairly typical history—it lacks the important details that would help in clarifying the diagnostic possibilities, that is, history of snoring, cataplectic episodes, or episodes of sleep paralysis, episodic amnesia, morning headache, or a family history of a similar problem. Any of the possibilities could be entertained from this history. The patient's weight and sex make sleep apnea statistically more likely, but sedative drug abuse is too frequently a cause of this symptom to overlook it as a possibility. Our usual approach is to screen for sedatives, then to proceed with an all-night PSG, with respiratory and cardiac monitoring. If the results are negative, daytime naps are studied the following day to exclude narcolepsy. The studies in answers (A), (B), and (C) are rarely of any value in evaluating these patients. In this particular case, an all-night PSG documented the presence of a severe obstructive sleep apnea with associated cardiac arrhythmias. The elevated red blood cell count appeared to be a secondary complication of nocturnal apnea.

3. A 71-year-old man is receiving levodopa–carbidopa for Parkinson's disease. After 2 years of therapy he complains of severe insomnia and daytime somnolence. By history he awakens at 2 AM each night and cannot return to sleep before 4 AM. He falls asleep at 11 PM with no difficulty. Each day he finds it necessary to take one or two 1-hour naps. The patient's wife complains that the patient often awakens the household during the night with loud screams. The patient is not aware of this behavior and denies any abnormal dreams. This history reflects:

    A. Probable dementia in association with Parkinson's disease
    B. Psychotic depression
    C. A side effect of chronic dopaminergic therapy
    D. An unrelated sleep disorder

Management would include:

    A. Administration of a hypnosedative before retiring
    B. Antidepressant therapy
    C. All-night sleep study
    D. Discontinuation of antiparkinsonian medications
    E. Restriction of antiparkinsonian medications, avoiding administration in the evening.

The answer (C) is correct. Although there is some debate on the relationship of dementia to sleep disruption in this patient group, symptoms usually clear when dopaminergic therapy is stopped. In most cases, continued therapy is necessary, and in these patients, avoiding drug administration after 6 PM often improves the insomnia and daytime napping. Nightmares in patients receiving levodopa appear to arise out of Stage 2 sleep, and patients are frequently amnestic for the episodes. Hypnosedatives and antidepressants are unpredictable in their response in these patients and frequently exacerbate the complaint. In most cases answer (E) seems to be the most appropriate.

4. You are consulted by a 23-year-old man who described episodes of "amnesia." On several occasions he has found himself at various locations with no recollection of having traveled to them. He recollects being at another location hours before; his memory for previous events is good, and he denies any other symptoms preceding the attack. Observers have seen him during an episode, and he appeared distracted but carried on social conversations appropriately and on one occasion drove a car without incident. He appears relatively stable, and attacks occur in situations that seem devoid of any emotional importance. The patient does not drink. The neurologic examination is normal. A sleep-deprived nasopharyngeal EEG without sedation is read as normal, though it is noted that drowsiness is followed quickly by the onset of low-voltage fast activity. Biochemical studies including a 6-hour glucose tolerance test are all normal. A CT scan is normal. Empirical therapy with phenytoin 100 mg three times daily leads to worsening of the symptoms. Your differential diagnosis at this point should include:

    A. Hysterical seizure state
    B. Narcolepsy–cataplexy syndrome
    C. Somnambulism
    D. Recurrent transient global amnesia
    E. Sleep apnea syndrome
    F. Psychomotor seizure disorder
    G. Amnestic migraine

The appropriate answers are (B) and (E). The episodes described are typical of "automatic behavior" syndrome. This behavioral abnormality is associated with the appearance of "microsleep" episodes which electroencephalographically are Stage 1 sleep. Sleep apnea and narcolepsy are associated with this disorder. Although the diagnosis of psychomotor seizures is difficult to rule out on the basis of a normal EEG, the adverse response to empirical anticonvulsants is more typical of an "automatic behavior" syndrome. Transient global amnesia presents a similar clinical picture but is an entity restricted to late middle life; frequent recurrences are unusual in this syndrome. Somnambulism is a similar phenomenon but is more frequent in childhood and arises from a period of normal sleep. It is usually a Stage 4 sleep event. Psychiatric disorders are frequently present in adults with somnambulistic disorders.

Amnestic migraine may produce recurrent amnestic episodes but usually does so in the presence of more typical migrainous episodes. There is some question of whether this disorder represents a *sui generis* or the coexistence of two phenomena in a single individual.

Hysterical seizure states are rarely characterized by global amnesia and are usually situationally related.

Appropriate management in this case would include an all-night PSMG followed by the Multiple Sleep Latency Test the next day as well as a routine 16-channel EEG. A careful history taking directed specifically toward cataplexy, daytime napping, and snoring, nocturnal apnea would help in a differentiation of the underlying condition. Treatment with amphetamine is usually not entirely successful. Sedative-hypnotics, anticonvulsants, and diazepam usually cause worsening of the symptoms. In patients with sleep apnea of any cause, proper medical or surgical management has been reported to alleviate this symptom complex.

SUGGESTED READING

Aldrich MS: Narcolepsy. N Engl J Med 323:389, 1990

Bootzin RR, Nicassio PN: Behavioral treatments for insomnia. In Hersen M, Eisler R, Miller P (eds): Progress in Behavior Modification. New York, Academic Press, 1978

Byerley B, Gillin JC: Diagnosis and management of insomnia. Psychiatr Clin North Am 7:773, 1984

Cartwright RD, Ristanovic R, Diaz F et al: A comparative study of treatments for positional sleep apnea. Sleep 14:546, 1991

Cartwright DR, Samelson FD: The effects of nonsurgical treatment for obstructive sleep apnea. JAMA 248:705, 1982

Dement WC: Rational basis for the use of sleeping pills. Int Pharmacopsychiatry (Suppl 2)17:3, 1982

Diagnostic Classification Steering Committee: International Classification of Sleep Disorders: Diagnostic and Coding Manual. Rochester, MN: American Sleep Disorders Association, 1990

Dickson RI, Blokmanis A: Treatment of obstructive sleep apnea by uvulopalatopharyngoplasty. Laryngoscope 97:1054, 1987

Fletcher EC, DeBehnke RD, Lovoi MS et al: Undiagnosed sleep apnea in patients with essential hypertension. Ann Intern Med 103:190, 1985

Fletcher EC, Munafo DA: Role of nocturnal oxygen therapy in obstructive sleep apnea. Chest 98:1497, 1990

Gottlieb GL: Sleep disorders and their management: Special considerations in the elderly. Am J Med 88 (Suppl 3A):29S, 1990

Guilleminault C: Narcolepsy 1985. Sleep 9(Vol 1, Pt 2):285, 1986

Guilleminault C, Stoohs R, Quera-Salva M-A: Sleep-related obstructive and nonobstructive apneas and neurologic disorders. Neurology 42 (Suppl 6):53, 1992

Hanly PJ: Mechanisms and management of central sleep apnea. Lung 170:1, 1992

Hobson JA: Sleep: Order and disorder. Behav Biol Med 1:1, 1983

Hudgel DW: Mechanisms of obstructive sleep apnea. Chest 101:541, 1992

Kupfer JD, Thase EM: The use of the sleep laboratory in the diagnosis of affective disorders. Psychiatr Clin North Am 6:3, 1983

Mahowald MW, Schenk CH: REM sleep behavior disorder. In Kryger MH, Roth T, Dement WC (eds): Principles and Practice of Sleep Medicine, pp 389–401. Philadelphia, WB Saunders, 1989

Parkes JD: Sleep and Its Disorders. Philadelphia, WB Saunders, 1985

Pierce MW, Shu VS: Efficacy of estazolam: The United States clinical experience. Am J Med 88(Suppl 3A):6S, 1990

Roth T, Roerhs TA, Stepanski EJ et al: Hypnotics and behavior. Am J Med 88 (Suppl 3A):43S, 1990

Schmidt–Nowara WW, Meade TE, Hays MB: Treatment of snoring and obstructive sleep apnea with a dental orthosis. Chest 99:1378, 1991

Westbrook PR: Sleep disorders and upper airway obstruction in adults. Otolaryngol Clin North Amer 23:727, 1990

Williams RL, Karacan I: Sleep Disorders: Diagnosis and Treatment. New York, John Wiley, 1978

Eye Signs in Neurologic Diagnosis

James A. Goodwin

This chapter is intended as a survey of visual signs and symptoms that are of use for localization and etiologic diagnosis in neurologic disease. The organization of the chapter reflects both anatomic and functional classifications, and in all cases the close relation between anatomic and physiologic details and a practical clinical diagnosis is drawn. This chapter includes a discussion of the afferent or sensory visual system, the pupillomotor and the oculomotor systems. The localizing value for lesions of the cerebral hemispheres, brain stem, spinal cord, and peripheral anatomic pathways provided by an examination of these visual systems is emphasized.

AFFERENT (SENSORY) VISUAL SYSTEM: SENSORY OR MOTOR?

It seems so simple to refer to a part of the visual system as afferent, and another as efferent or ocular motor, but the two parts must function together to such an extent that the separation is artificial, although useful in a practical sense.

Man is a *foveate* animal, which means that the retina is not equipotential throughout; it is specialized for high-resolution vision in a small central area called the *fovea* or pit. The special architecture of the retina at the fovea and the immediate surrounding region, the *macula lutea* (so-called because of its concentration of yellow pigment), underlies its capacity to resolve fine detail in the visual scene.

The general structure of the retina is such that groups of photoreceptors are connected by way of bipolar cells to a ganglion cell that provides input to the central nervous system (CNS) by way of its axon. This basic arrangement is complicated by a host of horizontal interactions mediated by other cells in the retina.

Light captured by one of the photoreceptors within a receptive field can only signal to the ganglion cell that a visual event has occurred within its receptive field, not where in the field the photon has been captured. Thus, in areas of the retina where receptive fields are large—many hundreds of photoreceptors connected to a single ganglion cell—the capacity for fine spatial resolution is poor, whereas at the fovea, where there are only a few photoreceptors in the receptive field of a ganglion cell, the spatial resolution is very fine. Two tiny spots of light may be close together and still signal two separate ganglion cells at or near the fovea, and the nervous system has therein a mechanism for encoding their duplicity. The same two spots in the periphery would both be likely to fall within the receptive field of a single ganglion cell, where their duplicity could not be registered. Because there were two spots, the encoded brightness would be greater than if only one spot were present; however, information on the spatial array of the spots would be lost.

William J. Weiner and Christopher G. Goetz, eds. *Neurology for the Non-Neurologist*, Third Edition. Copyright © 1994, 1989 by J. B. Lippincott Company. Copyright © 1981 by Harper and Row Publishers, Inc.

The individual who wishes to see something clearly must, therefore, bring the image of the object onto the fovea (an act that involves the oculomotor system interacting with the afferent system in an intimate way). The afferent system must have the capacity to perceive that a potentially interesting object exists in the peripheral visual field. The afferent system must then provide coordinates for the motor system to bring the eye from its original position to a new position in which the image to be examined will be on the fovea. There are stages in this process that are neither clearly visual (afferent) nor motor (efferent), but are in between. Our concepts of sensory and motor are inadequate in this gray zone between taking information in and putting it out in the form of executive or motor commands. This activity possibly takes place somewhere in the higher-order visual centers of the occipitoparietal convexity. Bilateral lesions in this region produce a clinical syndrome in which there is an unraveling of the afferent and the efferent command structure. Balint called it *optic ataxia*, and the syndrome now bears his name. Patients who have *Balint's syndrome* have special difficulty in directing their gaze in an orderly manner to scan or *palpate* an extended visual scene. The world is perceived as a fragmentary and disordered array of images, none organically articulated in a meaningful way. This perceptual difficulty can be shown to accompany a disorder of motor scanning behavior. The patient acts as though the coordinates by which to direct his gaze have been scrambled. As an example, these patients lose the orderly *scan path* used by normal viewers to investigate a human face, with many fixations on areas of high information such as the eyes, nose, mouth, and brows. Instead, these patients shift their line of gaze aimlessly, often fixing on low information areas such as an ear or a bit of hair. They fail to conceive of the object as a human face in the course of this random scanning. It can be shown that the basic afferent functions—visual acuity and field—are normal as routinely tested. Although large scenes are improperly synthesized, small objects that can be encompassed in a single fixation are recognized correctly. These patients should be tested with pictures of objects that can be shown in both small and large versions to demonstrate this special difficulty of spatial synthesis with preserved visual acuity and visual field. Visual field testing may be particularly difficult in these patients because of their inability to simultaneously perceive two points in the field. When they are aware of the central fixation point, they fail to respond to the peripheral target; however, when they lose the fixation point, they can see the peripheral target with near-normal sensitivity. This facet of the disease has been called *simultanagnosia* or *amorphosynthesis*.

These brief introductory remarks on the shady limits of the sensory and motor visual systems serve to promote a sense of mystery about vision. This is certainly appropriate at these limits and at every stage of visual processing. Even the retina is poorly understood in all its physiologic aspects. The neural signal that is conducted to the lateral geniculate body is highly processed even at this early stage. We are only beginning to learn the complexity of visual disorders that originate from retinal disease.

The more usual disorders of the afferent visual system and the standard office methods for testing them will now be examined. The following discussion is aimed at the practicalities of office or bedside testing without further discussion of the controversies that might be involved. The information can be considered *safe* in that it has been in common clinical usage for a long time and has proved its reliability for localizing and etiologic diagnosis.

TESTING VISUAL ACUITY

Visual acuity as tested with *Snellen's optotypes* is probably the best-known and most widely used visual examination. It is important to realize, however, that some conditions are poorly characterized by visual acuity testing. These conditions are diseases in which the early manifestations involve a loss of the peripheral visual field. Glaucoma and papilledema are notable examples. Even total hemifield defects do not degrade the visual acuity unless they are bilateral, thus all the hemianopic disorders from lesions behind the optic chiasm cannot be adequately characterized by acuity testing.

In neuro-ophthalmology, a reduction of central visual acuity is an important sign of optic nerve disease. The fact that visual acuity is also degraded by several other conditions unrelated to nerve function is unfortunate for diagnostic purposes. An optical blur from improper refraction is a common one, but clouding of the ocular media by corneal opacity, cataract, or by blood or other debris in the vitreous is also a consideration. In addition, visual acuity is reduced by *amblyopia ex anopsia*, which is the practically permanent visual defect that accompanies childhood strabismus or early life anisometropia (unequal refractive error in the two eyes). The differential diagnosis of poor visual acuity also includes retinal disorders that affect the macula (another broad category of diseases).

All the clinical features of a case are important to establish a diagnosis of optic nerve disease as the cause of reduced visual acuity. Once the diagnosis is established, visual acuity is the most useful and the most universally used test for following the course of optic nerve disease. Visual field examination is also useful in this regard and must be used as a complement to acuity determination in the follow-up of optic neuropathies.

The ophthalmologist usually measures acuity in an *examination lane*, a long testing room in which letters of calibrated size are projected on a screen that the patient views. The original letters were made to be viewed at a distance of 20 feet, but the economics of office building construction have led to modifications. The commercially available projection devices can be made to project the letters small enough to make a valid test at viewing distances as short as 10 feet, and mirrors can be used to test a patient in even more cramped conditions.

An optical supply company representative should be consulted for instructions on how to set up a regular eye lane in an office. Nonophthalmologists will probably not wish to purchase an expensive projection system for occasional use; however, inexpensive wall-mounted reading charts are available for use at various reading distances from 10 to 20 feet. Adequate lighting must be provided, and standard ceiling fluorescent lights are usually sufficient.

TESTING VISUAL ACUITY ON THE NEAR CARD

Most nonophthalmologists, including neurologists, internists, and family physicians, test visual acuity on a *near card*, which is intended for viewing at 14 inches—a comfortable reading distance. The distance from eye to card should be measured if the near card is the only acuity measurement used. Once the examiner gets used to the distance, he can usually judge it without measuring.

Some other features need attention in order to make the near card approximately equivalent to a formal testing lane. The light must be sufficient and should be provided either by good fluorescents from the ceiling or by a bright lamp that can be positioned to illuminate the card without shining into the patient's eyes. This is not difficult to provide in one's office, but I have found that hospital beds are seldom well lighted. It is best to carry a bright handlight that provides illumination even for bedside testing. The best handlights are the *Finoff heads*, which are angled bulb carriers that attach to the battery handle of the ophthalmoscope. Penlights seldom stay bright, and most have uneven zones of illumination. The handlight is especially useful for testing near-card acuity, because the beam can be positioned to indicate which set of letters you want the patient to read. The handlight should not be held too close, however, because the diminished contrast of the *spotlighted* letter makes it difficult to see. It is best to create an elliptical zone that illuminates one entire line of letters by shining the handlight onto the card from one side. Oblique illumination also eliminates glare from the surface of the card.

Proper refraction is mandatory regardless of the method used to test visual acuity. Reduced acuity from needing glasses is of no neurologic interest and creates a great deal of confusion on hospital charts. A brief discussion of lenses and refraction follows. A basic understanding of these optical principles is useful for anyone planning to do visual acuity testing or a field examination, even though the nonophthalmologist will not actually be doing refractions.

LENSES AND REFRACTION

Light travels in a straight line through a homogeneous refractive medium such as air, glass, transparent plastic, or water. When light encounters an interface between refractive media of different density, its path is bent. A sheet of plate glass with flat parallel surfaces does not, however, alter the path of entering light. Light rays are bent as they enter the glass from air, but they are bent back to an equal degree as they go from the glass into air on the other side (Fig. 22-1*A*). Flat (plano) glass does not alter the *vergence* of light.

A glass wedge bends light rays toward the base (Fig. 22-1*B,C*), but parallel entering rays remain parallel on exit. These pyramids are useful optical devices called *prisms* that are often used to measure eye deviation by shifting images to meet the line of sight of a deviated eye. Wide-based prisms bend light more than narrow-based ones (Fig. 22-1*B* and *C*), and quantitative units called *prism diopters* can be used to measure this degree of deviation. The patient views a small light while the examiner introduces prisms of increasing power in front of one eye. The patient specifies the amount of eye devia-

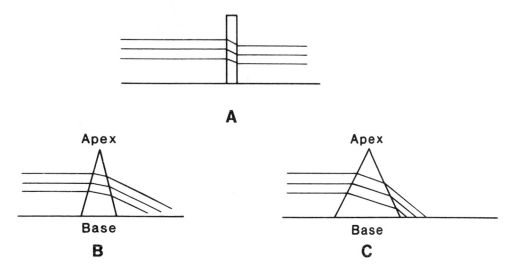

A

Apex

Base

B

Apex

Base

C

FIG. 22-1. (*A*) The path of light through flat (plano) glass. Parallel rays entering from the left, exit parallel to the right and the *vergence* of light is not changed. (*B*) A *prism* bends light toward its base (down in the figure). Parallel rays remain parallel, and the vergence of light is not changed. (*C*) A "stronger" prism has a broader base and a less acute angle at the apex. It bends light more drastically than the "weaker" prism in *B*.

tion by telling the examiner when the false image from the deviating eye overlies the centered (foveated) image from the other eye—the power of the prism needed to do this provides the measure of deviation.

Lenses are defined as refractive objects that *change the vergence of light*: Light rays that enter parallel will be nonparallel when they emerge at the other side. A *convex* lens causes *convergence* of light rays and is called a *positive* or *plus* (+) lens; an upright image is created at the focal plane behind the lens, or on the side opposite the object, and is called a *real* image (Fig. 22-2*A*). A *concave* lens produces a *divergence* of light rays and is called a *negative* or *minus* (−) lens; the object is imaged inverted at the focal plane in front of the lens, or on the same side as the object, and is termed a *virtual* image (Fig. 22-2*B*). Figures 22-2*A* and *B* illustrate parallel rays of light from an infinitely distant *point* source of light rather than rays emanating from an object with dimensions. They do not illustrate the upright or inverted quality of images. *Cylindrical* lenses act as lenses in one plane and as plano or flat nonlenses in a plane orthogonal to the first plane (Fig. 22-2*C*). A *plus* (+) *cylinder* converges light rays in its plane of power

and a *minus* (−) *cylinder* diverges rays in this plane. A person whose natural optical system—the cornea, lens, and vitreous—creates a focused image of an infinitely distant point on the fovea is *emmetropic* (Fig. 22-3*A*).

Ametropia refers to a significant deviation from emmetropia. A near-sighted person, or *myope*, brings the image of a distant point to focus in front of the retina (Fig. 22-3*B*) and needs a concave or diverging lens to move the focal point of an infinitely distant point *back* to the retina (Fig. 22-3*D*). A *hyperope*, or far-sighted person, creates a focused image of an infinitely distant point behind the retina (Fig. 22-3*C*) and needs a convex or *converging* lens to move the focal plane *forward* to the surface of the retina (Fig. 22-3*E*). The natural optical system of a person with *astigmatism* has varying power in different planes and requires a *cylindrical* lens to correct the aberration. This is not illustrated in Figure 22-3.

Once a person has achieved the focus of distant objects, either naturally or through spectacles or contact lenses, he must alter the power of the crystalline lens of the eye to maintain focus for objects nearer than infinity. Specifically, the *plus* (+) *power*

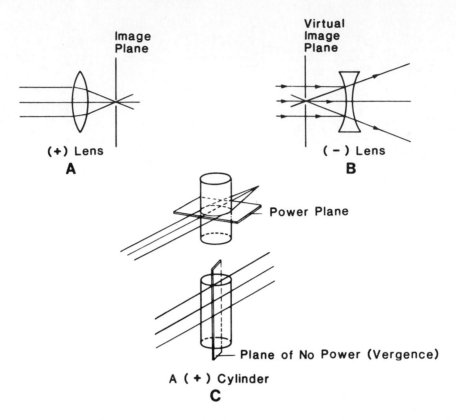

FIG. 22-2. Lenses alter the vergence of light. (*A*) A convex or "plus" lens converges light rays to a focal point in the *image plane* on the side opposite the light source which is the *object plane*. (*B*) A concave or "minus" lens causes *divergence* of light rays. A "virtual" image is formed on the same side of the lens as the source of light rays in the object plane. (*C*) Light rays converge through a "plus" or convex cylinder in the *power plane (upper figure)* and remain parallel as they pass through the cylinder in a plane orthogonal to the power plane (*lower figure*).

of the eye's crystalline lens must be increased to focus on objects near the eye. This is done by contracting the ciliary muscle, which increases the convexity of the lens. This process is called *accommodation*. The power of accommodation is lost progressively with age; when a person reaches his mid-forties he needs an additional *plus* lens to correct for this normal condition, which is called *presbyopia*. Emmetropes (normal focus for distant objects), as they become presbyopes, usually require reading glasses that they take off for distant viewing (the images of distant objects are blurred to the emmetrope wearing his reading glasses). Those individuals who must constantly look from near to far in the course of daily activities, require *half eyes* (*i.e.*, those narrow glasses that ride low on the nose) or they have to acquire bifocals with no correction in the upper segment. Moderately near-sighted (minus distance refraction) presbyopes may simply take off their distance glasses to read at 14 inches—this is what near-sighted means. Highly near-sighted people have their natural focus at distances shorter than 14 inches. Although they can see clearly at such a distance, they usually find it too close for comfortable reading. These people may have bifocals in which the lower segment is still

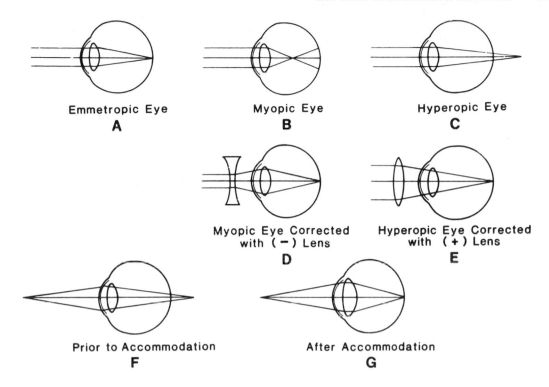

Emmetropic Eye
A

Myopic Eye
B

Hyperopic Eye
C

Myopic Eye Corrected
with (−) Lens
D

Hyperopic Eye Corrected
with (+) Lens
E

Prior to Accommodation
F

After Accommodation
G

FIG. 22-3. (*A*) An emmetropic eye in which an infinitely distant point source of light is imaged on the retina by the natural refractive media of the eye (cornea, aqueous, lens, vitreous). (*B*) A myopic eye in which an infinitely distant point source of light is imaged in front of the retina. (*C*) A hyperopic eye in which an infinitely distant point source of light is imaged behind the retina. (*D*) A myopic eye corrected with a minus lens. The lens superimposes divergence on the overconverged light rays and moves the focal plane back to the retina. (*E*) A hyperopic eye corrected with a plus lens. The lens superimposes convergence on the overdivergent light rays and moves the focal plane forward to the retina. (*F*) A point source of light near the eye produces divergent rays entering an emmetropic eye as in *A*. Without the act of accommodation, the refractive power of the eye is unchanged and the rays are brought to a focal plane behind the retina. In (*G*) the crystalline lens has become more convex or has increased its plus power by virtue of ciliary muscle contraction. The near source of divergent rays is now imaged on the retina because of the added convergent power that results from the act of *accommodation*.

minus, but less minus than the upper segment. The relative *plus* power needed for near vision is added arithmetically to the distance refraction.

This information will help the nonophthalmologist to make sure that the patient is optimally corrected for an assessment of visual acuity, either in a distance lane or on the near card. Reading glasses or the bifocal segment should always be used by the presbyopic patient when testing is done on the near card. The poor acuity that results from uncorrected presbyopia is not interesting in a neurologic assessment and creates great confusion when it is noted in the patient's chart without regard to the state of refraction. Visual acuity tested at a distance of 10 to 20 feet will require the distance correction for an ametrope. The patient should be asked to put on his distance correction or, if he has bifocals, to be sure that he is looking through the top part. The lower segment of the bifocal generally contains the *"near add,"* which refers to the additional plus power for reading distance.

PINHOLE

Those not wishing to trust themselves with the vagaries and complexities of optics can depend on the *pinhole*. The pinhole, known since the earliest days of the camera obscura, was the earliest focusing device. The hole is small enough to admit only the central rays from the object, eliminating the divergent rays that would not reach focus in the image plane. Of course, this has the disadvantage of admitting only a fraction of the light and thus creates a dim image. Most significant refractive errors can be bypassed, however, by having the patient read through a pinhole placed in front of the eye, approximately where a spectacle lens would sit. The hole should measure about 2 mm in diameter and can be made in a card with a pin, or purchased as a manufactured item made of plastic with numerous holes in an array. This arrangement makes it easier for the patient to find the chart through one of the holes.

TECHNIQUE OF TESTING AND RECORDING VISUAL ACUITY

Most of the technique issues have been already covered. Near-card acuity is done at 14 inches for most printed cards, but the card should be checked for this information. Instructions are usually printed somewhere on the card. As mentioned, the light should be good, and a *standardized* lighting condition in the office is preferable if the near card is to be the only method of testing. The best refraction for a near card must be used. This usually means reading glasses or the bottom segment of bifocals for the presbyope. The recording of the results is now discussed.

Ophthalmologists have a convention in which they record near-card acuity using *Jaeger*, which is a printer's notation system—J$_1$ print is equivalent to 20/25, for instance. The near cards usually show both Jaeger and Snellen fractions, thus one can choose which type one is going to use. A notation should be made of the reading distance that was used so that the test conditions can be reproduced. A notation should also be made of the optical conditions that were used (*e.g.*, the "patient's bifocal segment," if the exact refractive correction is not known or "with pinhole" if that is how the test was performed).

The Snellen fraction is not really an arithmetic fraction, although it is sometimes expressed as a decimal equivalent. For instance, 20/40 can be written as 0.5, and 20/20 would be 1.0. An acuity of 20/40 means that the patient reads at 20 feet (the numerator) that which a normal person could read at a viewing distance of 40 feet (the denominator). The definition of 20/20 as normal visual acuity was made by population studies; however, this definition is too liberal. The 20/20 figures are calibrated so that at the retina the image of each letter measures (subtends) 5 minutes of arc and the width of each stroke is 1 minute of arc. Since the retina is on the back surface of a sphere, an angular measure is more convenient than a lateral or tangent measure (*e.g.*, millimeters of height or width).

OPTIC NERVE DISEASE AND VISUAL ACUITY

It was mentioned earlier that hemianopia does not degrade visual acuity. Any disorder that is constrained to affect only one half of the visual field will leave the patient with 20/15 vision on the eye chart as long as there is no coexisting condition that diminishes visual acuity. One corellation is that if any half of the fovea is functionally intact, then the resolving power of the fovea is not disturbed. Let us explore the anatomic implications of this axiom and the contrary rule that visual acuity is commonly affected by optic nerve diseases.

The functional midline in the retina is an imaginary vertical line drawn through the center of the fovea—the *vertical hemianopic midline*. Ganglion cells to either side of this line send axons through the optic nerve in an intermingled array without any systematic segregation of axons that arise from nasal or temporal ganglion cells. It is not until the axons reach the chiasm that there is a systematic separation of nasal fibers that cross the chiasm and temporal fibers that go through the chiasm uncrossed. Because of this, optic nerve diseases most often affect afferent units on both sides of midline and thereby degrade visual acuity. Quantitation of visual acuity is an important aspect of assessing either the response to treatment or the natural course of an optic nerve disease.

VISUAL FIELDS

Analysis of visual fields provides another key to localizing a diagnosis in the CNS. First, certain principles are emphasized, because they pertain to field defects that accompany lesions at all locations. Some particulars that relate to lesions at specific locations are then outlined.

GENERAL FEATURES

MONOCULAR *VS* BINOCULAR DEFECTS

Field defects limited to one eye suggest a lesion anterior to the optic chiasm, whereas binocular defects, when caused by a single lesion, localize to the visual pathways at, or behind, the optic chiasm.

Of course, bilateral multiple lesions anterior to the chiasm can give binocular field defects; however, for this discussion we are concerned primarily with signs of localizing value for single lesions.

LOCATION IN THE VISUAL FIELD

The location of defects in the visual field provides at least broad information regarding the responsible lesion. Central scotomas are associated with a wide variety of optic nerve lesions but are especially characteristic of optic neuritis, compressive optic neuropathy, and toxic-metabolic optic neuropathy. Nasal quadrant defects are associated commonly with glaucoma, a degenerative condition of the optic nerve head in which ganglion cell axons at the upper and lower poles of the nerve head are preferentially lost. Temporal defects, usually binocular, are characteristic of chiasmal compression. Homonymous hemianopic defects, which are on the same side in both eyes, characterize lesions anywhere from the optic tract to the calcarine cortex.

These broad principles of locale within the visual fields can be used for an analysis of confrontation fields. Confrontation field data usually lack precision as to the shape and density of the defect, but one can generally determine which quadrants are involved and whether or not a central or paracentral defect is present. The technique of confrontational visual field testing is now considered.

SHAPE OF THE VISUAL FIELD DEFECT

The shape of the defect corresponds to the morphology of the fiber bundles in the afferent pathways. This morphology is unique for each part of the CNS, and the details for each part are discussed in the particular sections on each locus. The shape of the defect is thus one of the most important features of the visual field.

DENSITY OF THE FIELD DEFECT

The density or severity of light sensitivity loss in the field defect gives some indication of the etiology. This is not as fine a distinction as some of the other features; however, vascular lesions, especially infarctions, generally produce dense or severe defects. Tumors, in particular the slowly growing ones, tend, on the other hand, to produce field defects of lesser severity, because the tissue is more likely to be affected in a graded manner.

CONGRUITY OF THE VISUAL FIELD DEFECT

For a single lesion behind the chiasm, congruity refers to the degree to which the density and extent of the defect are similar in the two eyes. This has a practical meaning only for subtotal homonymous field defects. Total hemianopsia is often associated with complete tract lesions as well as with complete calcarine infarctions; total hemianopsia has no localizing value apart from placing the lesion behind the chiasm.

In order to understand congruity, it is necessary to imagine the overlapping fields of the two eyes, a condition effected by the binocular fusion of the foveal representations of the two eyes (Fig. 22-4). Within the binocular field, every point in visual space is registered by a particular ganglion cell in each eye (an example is point AB in Fig. 22-4). If the lesion occurs in a portion of the afferent pathways where there is little tendency for the axons from these two ganglion cells to lie adjacent to one another, then there is a good chance that one axon (A) may be affected without the other (B). In this case, a defect of visual field function will be produced in one eye but not in the homologous area of field of the other eye.

Lesions of the optic tract characteristically produce incongruous field defects; a monocular hemianopsia is one extreme case. In the optic tract, the ganglion cell axons serving receptive fields for the homologous points in visual space are not necessarily adjacent to one another. Hence, a disease process may affect the axon from one eye serving a particular point in binocular visual space without affecting the axon for the homologous point in visual space from the other eye. Axons A and B are shown separate from one another in the left optic tract in the midportion of Figure 22-4.

The calcarine cortex, area 17 of Brodmann, is organized so that the axons from homologous

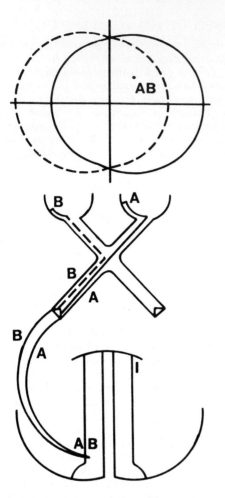

FIG. 22-4. A diagrammatic representation of the binocular visual fields and the afferent fibers serving a point in binocular visual space, point *AB* in the upper figure. A hypothetical photoreceptor, *A* in the right eye and *B* in the left eye, connects with the central nervous system by way of a ganglion cell axon from each eye, also labeled *A* and *B*, respectively. The ganglion cell axon from the right eye crosses in the chiasm (point *AB* is in the temporal field of that eye), while that from the left passes through to the ipsilateral optic tract (point *AB* is in the nasal field of that eye). Each ganglion cell axon synapses in the left lateral geniculate body and second-order neuron axons continue in the geniculocalcarine radiations to the occipital cortex, area 17 in the bottom figure (see text for further explanation).

points in space—here the axons are those of lateral geniculate cells—project to the same column of cortical cells. A cortical disease will, therefore, affect the visual fields of the two eyes in exactly the same way, producing congruous defects.

Lesions in the geniculocalcarine pathways produce an intermediate degree of congruity, thus this feature is much less reliable in determining the anteroposterior position of lesions than is the case with tract and cortex lesions. The geniculocalcarine projections A and B are shown in Figure 22-4 as being separate anteriorly, near the geniculate body. They converge progressively as they near their point of entry into the calcarine cortex.

SLOPE OF THE VISUAL FIELD DEFECT

The slope of a visual field defect refers to the amount of lateral increase in the defect's size with a reduction of stimulus visibility. A steeply sloping region changes little in horizontal dimension with a major reduction in stimulus visibility. A gently sloping area of defect becomes much larger with reduced visibility. A gentle slope thus denotes a region of transition between a severe dysfunction and a milder dysfunction in the visual pathways. The marginal area of field, which is sensitive enough to see the more visible target but which is reduced in sensitivity and unable to see the less visible target, is what constitutes the sloping region. *Slope denotes change*. Vascular lesions that are healing and tumors that are advancing will have a dense core of total dysfunction surrounded by an area of relative dysfunction, probably related to tissue compression and edema. This gradual transition to normal function in afferent pathways brings about the gentle slope to the visual field defect. Old vascular lesions in which the dense core of infarcted tissue remains, but in which the surrounding pathways have returned to normal sensitivity, are characterized by a steeply sloped transition from a defective to a normal field. The defect in Figure 22-5A is gently sloping in the right lower quadrant, typical of a fresh infarct or hemorrhage with surrounding edema. The defect in Figure 22-5B is steeply sloping in the same region, as would be expected of an old infarct in which the necrotic zone leaves a field defect of absolute density, but in which the transition to normal function is abrupt. The slope is only readable in subtotal hemianopsias in which there is some sparing of either upper or lower sectors. The slope should also be analyzed only along the margin of the defect, where there is the opportunity of transi-

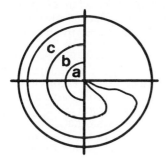
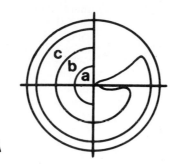

A

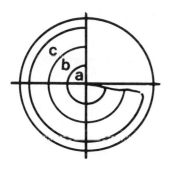
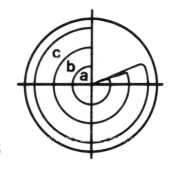

B

FIG. 22-5. In (A) a *gently sloped* right homonymous upper quadrant defect is illustrated. The extent of field defect for isopters *a* and *b* is greater than for *c* in the right lower quadrant. In (B) a *steeply sloped* defect is shown. The extent of all isopters is the same. The defects in A and B are also *incongruous*.

tion to normal across a gradient (*i.e.*, adjacent to the spared sector). There is almost always an abrupt transition at the vertical hemianopic midline, because here the lesion has produced maximal effects in the involved half field and has no opportunity of causing any defect in the other half field because the other half is served by the opposite cerebral hemisphere. The transition at the vertical midline is *always* steep, thus no information is provided on the tempo of the lesion.

TOPICAL FEATURES OF THE VISUAL FIELDS

RETINA AND OPTIC NERVE

Figure 22-6 indicates the arrangement of ganglion cell axons in the retina and optic nerve. Bundles of axons coming into the optic nerve from all sides follow a converging course from ganglion cells widely distributed in the retina. On the nasal side of the optic disk the bundles have a straight trajectory in the form of a wedge with the apex at the optic nerve head. Accordingly, interruption of a nasal retinal bundle gives rise to a wedge-shaped visual field defect with the apex at the *physiologic blind spot*. This normal blind spot in the visual field corresponds to the optic nerve head, where there are no photoreceptors. The papillomacular bundle occupies most of the temporal side of the optic nerve head. Because of this, ganglion cells in the periphery of the retina on the temporal side of the fovea must send their axons in an arcuate course around the papillomacular bundle to gain access to the optic nerve at the upper and lower poles.

Embryologically, the fovea started out at the margin of the retina. With development, an invagination carried the fovea toward its final position near the optic nerve with final fusion of the upper and lower halves of the retinal margin that formed the invagination. The embryonic discontinuity between the upper and lower halves in the temporal retina persists, however, as the *temporal raphe* extending from the fovea to the temporal margin of the retina.

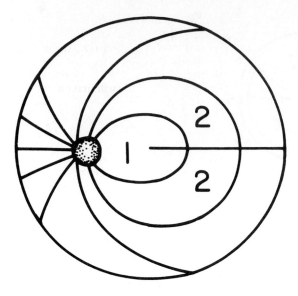

FIG. 22-6. The arrangement of retinal ganglion cell axons in a left eye fundus. Region 1 is the *papillomacular bundle* serving foveal function. Region 2 is the *arcuate bundle* or *Bjerrum region*, where ganglion cell axons from the temporal retinal periphery arch over the massive papillomacular bundle.

This means that all the ganglion cells immediately above the raphe must send their axons into the upper pole of the disk via the upper arcuate region, while all the ganglion cells below the raphe are constrained to send their axons into the lower pole via the inferior arcuate region. This forced discontinuity provides for arcuate visual field defects with an abrupt transition to normal at the *nasal horizontal midline*—the famous *nasal step*. It is typical of glaucoma to produce these arcuate defects with nasal steps; they were described long ago by Bjerrum and are still referred to by his name.

The location and shape of visual field defects are potent indicators of the site of an optic nerve lesion but also give some indication as to etiology. Ischemia of either the retina or the optic nerve tends to produce upper- or lower-half field defects that "respect" or have a sharp border along the horizontal midline of the visual field. These are called *altitudinal* field defects and can be thought of as extended arcuate bundle defects in which the temporal quadrant is affected as well as the nasal quadrant. Since

there is no *retinal raphe* serving the temporal quadrant, the reason for the sharp border at the horizontal midline must be sought in the patterns of vascular supply.

The reason for altitudinal-type field defects is intuitive for the case of inner retinal infarction, since the retina is supplied by an upper and a lower primary branch of the central retinal artery and selective branch occlusion may occur (*branch retinal artery occlusion [BRAO]*). The altitudinal quality of visual field defects in ischemia of the optic nerve (*acute anterior ischemic optic neuropathy [AION]*) is more difficult to understand, however, since the anterior optic nerve is supplied by an array of arterioles that stem from an anastomotic vascular circle just behind the globe—the *circle of Zinn and Haller*. This arterial circle is in turn supplied by a variable number (two to five) of *short posterior ciliary arteries* that supply the nerve head and the adjacent vascular choroid layer of the eyeball. It has been suggested that sectoral infarction of the optic nerve head occurs when there is critically low perfusion in the ciliary distribution and a watershed zone between adjacent posterior ciliary—choroidal territories cuts across the optic nerve head. The orientation of these watershed zones does not always conform to an upper- or lower-half distribution, and this seems to leave the stereotyped altitudinal character of the resulting visual field defects unexplained.

Another common optic neuropathy is *optic neuritis* of the demyelinating type, which is strongly, but still enigmatically, associated with multiple sclerosis. We used to teach that the most common type of visual field defect in optic neuritis is the central scotoma, a roughly circular area of low visual sensitivity centered on the fixation point. The scotoma may be large enough to engulf the physiologic blind spot, and then it is called a *centro-cecal* scotoma. The recently concluded *Optic Neuritis Treatment Trial (ONTT)* in which 448 patients with optic neuritis were randomly assigned to different treatment groups provided a unique opportunity to study the visual field and other clinical characteristics of the disease. Among affected eyes at onset, 48.2% had diffuse field loss, but among those with focal defects (the remaining 51.8%) the commonest pattern was *altitudinal* in 15%. The investigators concluded that the morphology of field loss is an unreliable criterion upon which to differentiate optic neuritis from ischemic optic neuropathy. Differentiating features include pain exacerbated by eye movement, subacute evolution, and visual field abnormalities in the fellow eye in patients with optic neuritis. Features suggestive of AION include more acute onset, lack of pain, and upper- or lower-half swelling of the optic disk with flame hemorrhages.

OPTIC CHIASM

Axons from ganglion cells on either side of the retinal hemianopic midline, which run a mingled course in the optic nerve, separate for the first time at the optic chiasm (Fig. 22-7A). This divergence of pathways is the anatomic feature that creates the *hemianopic midline* and determines the existence of field defects that *respect* the midline (*i.e.*, the lateral half-field defects that denote lesions at and behind the optic chiasm).

Fibers from the inferior retina (*i.e.*, the upper temporal visual field) loop forward in the opposite optic nerve as they cross the midline. A lesion at the posterior end of one optic nerve will first encounter these inferonasal fibers of the other eye at the chiasm junction, which creates a distinctive combination of field defects in the two eyes (Fig. 22-7B1). The field defect ipsilateral to the lesion is any of those typical for optic nerve disease—a central

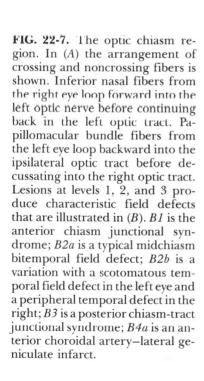

FIG. 22-7. The optic chiasm region. In (*A*) the arrangement of crossing and noncrossing fibers is shown. Inferior nasal fibers from the right eye loop forward into the left optic nerve before continuing back in the left optic tract. Papillomacular bundle fibers from the left eye loop backward into the ipsilateral optic tract before decussating into the right optic tract. Lesions at levels 1, 2, and 3 produce characteristic field defects that are illustrated in (*B*). *B1* is the anterior chiasm junctional syndrome; *B2a* is a typical midchiasm bitemporal field defect; *B2b* is a variation with a scotomatous temporal field defect in the left eye and a peripheral temporal defect in the right; *B3* is a posterior chiasm-tract junctional syndrome; *B4a* is an anterior choroidal artery–lateral geniculate infarct.

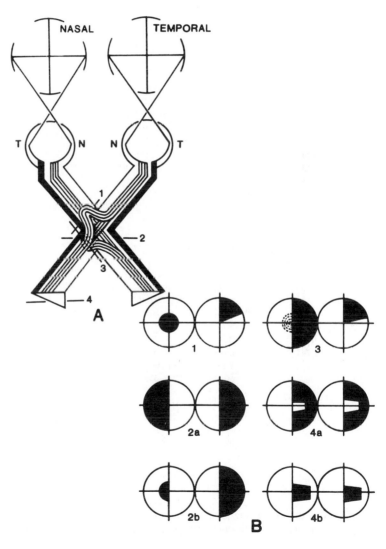

scotoma or other nerve fiber bundle defect. In the opposite eye there will be a midline respecting upper temporal defect, or "pie in the sky" defect according to J. Lawton Smith. This is the *anterior junctional syndrome* of the chiasm.

Some fibers from the nasal retina, especially papillomacular bundle fibers, loop backward in the ipsilateral optic tract before crossing. Thus, a lesion at the junction of the posterior chiasm and optic tract will produce a characteristic *posterior junctional syndrome* of the chiasm (Fig. 22-7*B3*). The basic defect is a homonymous hemianopsia contralateral to the lesion. *Homonymous* means that the hemifield defect is on the same side in both eyes. A left tract lesion, for instance, gives rise to a right-sided field defect in either eye—the defect is in the nasal half field of the left eye and is also in the temporal half field of the right eye. As the tract lesion spreads anteriorly and encounters the posterior chiasm, the first chiasmal fibers affected are those from the ipsilateral nasal retina that loop back into the tract before crossing. These fibers serve central vision because the papillomacular bundle crosses relatively posterior in the chiasm. Thus, in the ipsilateral eye there is the nasal *hemifield* defect that is part of the homonymous pair, plus some loss of *central temporal field* secondary to the involvement of the posterior looping nasal retinal fibers. The field defect thus involves both sides of the foveal field in the ipsilateral eye and reduces the visual acuity, whereas the purely hemianopic defect in the temporal field of the opposite eye leaves acuity normal, in accord with the aforementioned axioms.

The typical central chiasmal defects will now be considered. Most symptomatic lesions of the chiasm are tumors, and most of these encounter the chiasm from below. *Chiasmal compression is most often accompanied by bitemporal visual field defects.* The crossing fibers are apparently least able to tolerate mass effects, probably because they are *tethered* across the middle, whereas the uncrossed fibers are free to splay out over the mass. However, nine and a half times out of ten, compression of the chiasm will first cause midline-respecting temporal field defects in both eyes. This can involve any combination of central (scotomatous) defects and peripheral defects in the two eyes. The most common variations for chiasmal field defects are demonstrated in Figure 22-7*B2a* and *B2b*.

LATERAL GENICULATE BODY

Two highly characteristic field defects caused by vascular lesions of the lateral geniculate body are shown in Figure 22-7*B*. Frisen has provided elaborate detail on the dual vascular supply of the geniculate by the *anterior choroidal* and the *lateral (posterior) choroidal* arteries. Anterior choroidal artery occlusion can be associated with upper and lower quadrant homonymous defects that spare a rectangular area along the horizontal midline (Fig. 22-7*B4a*). Lateral choroidal artery occlusion has been associated with a rectangular homonymous scotoma along the horizontal midline, sparing the upper and lower quadrants (Fig. 22-7*B4b*)—the exact complement of the other geniculate syndrome.

GENICULOCALCARINE RADIATIONS

Figure 22-8 illustrates how the axonal outflow from the lateral geniculate radiates within the deep white matter of the cerebral hemispheres. These radiations form a thin band just external to the lateral ventricle. They take the form of a ribbon that is broad in the vertical plane but very thin in the horizontal plane (Fig. 22-8*A* and *B*). Thus, lesions must extend deep into the white matter to encounter the geniculocalcarine radiations.

Parietal lobe lesions encounter the upper radiations on the way to the upper bank of the calcarine cortex (area 1 in Fig. 22-8*B*) and cause inferior quadrantic homonymous visual field defects. Temporal lobe lesions interfere with the anterior looping fibers that are destined for the lower bank of the calcarine cortex (area 3 in Fig. 22-8*B*) and produce upper quadrantic homonymous field defects. The anterior temporal contingent of fibers in the geniculocalcarine radiations is called *Meyer's loop* after Adolph Meyer who described them.

CALCARINE CORTEX

A semifinal way-station in the afferent system is the primary visual cortex, area 17 of Brodmann on the mesial surface of the occipital lobe. The localization of lesions can be very precise here, owing to the sometimes restricted nature of the lesions. Small infarcts from branch occlusions of the calcarine artery may produce exceedingly localized, but always congruous, homonymous field defects.

There are two basic axes of localization: from anterior to posterior in the calcarine cortex, and from lip to depth of the calcarine fissure (Figs. 22-8 and 22-9). The anteroposterior dimension translates to an axis from center (fixation point) to periphery in the visual fields (Fig. 22-8*C*). The fixation area is represented at the posterior end of the calcarine cortex, a portion of which wraps around

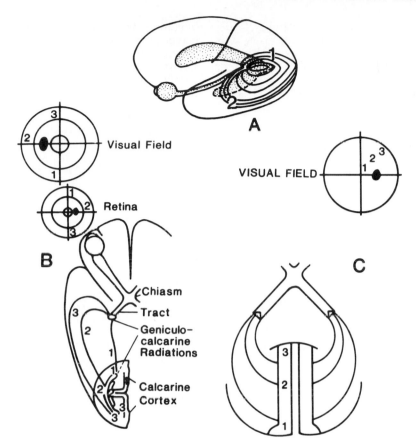

FIG. 22-8. (*A*) Lateral view of the brain showing the geniculocalcarine radiations emanating from a focal point deep to the lateral ventricle (the location of the lateral geniculate body) and fanning out to occupy the parietal and temporal lobes on the way to the calcarine cortex. The anterior looping contingent in the temporal lobe is called *Meyer's loop.* (*B*) Diagram of the geniculocalcarine radiations in a mixed horizontal and coronal section of the brain (*lower figure*) together with a diagram of the left eye retina (*middle figure*) and corresponding left eye visual field (*upper figure*). The numbers correlate lesion locations in the lower figure with affected retinal and visual fields in the middle and upper figures, respectively. (*C*) A horizontal section through the calcarine cortex is depicted in the lower figure with successive zones from the left occipital pole to the anterior end of the left calcarine cortex numbered 1 through 3. Corresponding zones in the right visual field are shown in the upper figure. The fixation area is represented at the occipital pole, and the periphery of the visual field is represented at the anterior end of the calcarine cortex (see text and Fig. 22-9 for further details).

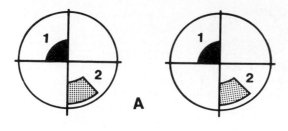

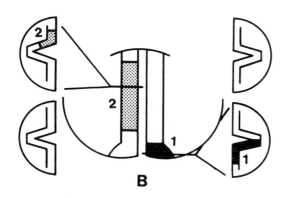

FIG. 22-9. Two practice field defects are depicted in *A*. The corresponding localization in the calcarine cortex is shown in *B* both in the horizontal plane (*central figure*) and in the coronal plane (*lateral figures*).

onto the convexity of the occipital pole. The periphery of the visual field is represented at the anterior end of the calcarine fissure, near the splenium of the corpus callosum.

Sparing of the visual field, either at the center or at the far periphery, is a useful sign that localizes a homonymous hemianopsia to the occipital cortex.

Central Sparing, or Sparing of Fixation

Many hemianopsias result from an infarction of calcarine cortex with occlusion or stenosis of the posterior cerebral artery. The occipital pole receives a collateral blood supply from the middle cerebral artery and may be spared when the flow in the posterior cerebral artery reaches a critical status, and infarction occurs in the more anterior portions of the calcarine cortex.

Testing for this spared circle around fixation can best be done at the tangent screen, or even on a wall, as long as a vertical line through the fixation point can be drawn or imagined. The problem with eliciting fixational sparing is the fact that patients often shift their gaze a few degrees to either side of fixation, and the examiner cannot always see these little eye movements. Of course, the whole hemianopic midline will shift with the angle of gaze, and the patient may then seem capable of perceiving test objects a little way into his hemianopic field.

The examiner should use two vertically aligned test spots to avoid mistaking this refixation for *central sparing*. One spot is placed in the hemianopic field even with the fixation point and the other is held either above or below the first one. Most real central sparing measures between 5° and 15° radius, thus vertical separation of the two spots by 15° or 20° should be sufficient. The spots are brought from the hemianopic to the seeing field, keeping them vertically aligned. The patient is asked to call out "one" or "two" when he first sees any test spot, depending on how many spots he sees. Under these test conditions, if the patient says "two," there has been a shift of the whole hemianopic midline; if the patient says "one," then the central target has fallen into a circular area of real central sparing whereas the other (above or below) is still in a hemianopic field.

Sparing of the Unpaired Temporal Crescent

The nasal field (with a maximum extent of 60°) is smaller than the temporal field (with a maximum extent of 75° to 80°) in both eyes. Therefore, with binocular fusion, there is a large area of binocular field, beyond which is a crescent of 20° or so in which the temporal field of one eye has no corresponding nasal field of the other—this is the *unpaired temporal crescent*. Posterior cerebral lesions, basically those in the occipital lobe, may spare the anterior fibers of the geniculocalcarine radiations and the anterior calcarine cortex, leaving some preserved peripheral field in an otherwise dense and complete homonymous hemianopsia. If the extent of preserved periphery is all beyond 60° of eccentricity, there will be no corresponding nasal field spared in one eye, and the spared crescent of field will exist only in the eye with the temporal field on the side of the hemianopsia.

Imagine a right occipital lesion and a dense left homonymous hemianopsia. There is some sparing of the unpaired crescent. This means that the left eye, which has its temporal field on the left (the side of the hemianopsia) will perceive objects in the far periphery, but the right eye (with nasal field toward the hemianopic side) will have no peripheral sparing.

This sparing of the unpaired crescent is an important sign of occipital localization in hemianopsias. It can be detected most consistently with confrontation techniques. I have seen several patients with *total* homonymous hemianopsia by perimetry who can perceive hand motion in the far temporal periphery of the one eye but not in the nasal periphery of the other. When testing for this, the patient should cover one eye at a time and the examiner should extend his arm beside and just behind the patient's head on the side of the patient's hemianopsia. The examiner should bring his hand forward, wave it up and down, or wiggle his fingers. This motion can be a more potent stimulus for the far visual periphery than light.

The other important dimension for occipital localization is a series of sectors extending from the *lip* of the calcarine fissure, which faces the opposite occipital cortex across the interhemispheric fissure, to the *depth* of the calcarine fissure. The corresponding visual field dimension is a series of pie-shaped sectors extending from an apex at fixation to a broader base at the periphery. The sector abutting the *vertical hemianopic midline* corresponds to the *lip* of the calcarine cortex, and the sector abutting the *horizontal midline* corresponds to the *depth* of the calcarine cortex. Intermediate field and tissue sectors lie between these limits. The upper bank (lip to depth) serves the inferior homonymous field quadrant, and the lower bank (lip to depth) serves the superior quadrant. Thus, we have a dimension that extends all the way around one half of the visual field from the upper vertical midline through the horizontal midline to the lower vertical midline in a series of pie-shaped sectors. The more sectors you divide the pie into, the more pieces you have, and the finer the localization. At the cortex this dimension flows from the inferior lip of one (right or left) calcarine cortex by way of the depth of the calcarine fissure to the upper lip.

Once the location of the pie-shaped sector has been established, then localization within the sector should be established along the dimension from fixation to periphery, which is from occipital pole to anterior calcarine cortex.

An exercise in calcarine cortex localization is shown in Fig. 22-9. Two small field defects, one in the left upper quadrant, the other in the right lower, are depicted in Figure 22-9. A horizontal section through the calcarine cortex is flanked on either side by coronal sections in Figure 22-9B. Consider first lesion 1. It extends to fixation, but not far into the periphery; thus, in the horizontal section, it is represented at the pole with little anterior extension. It occupies a series of pie-shaped sectors all the way from the vertical midline to the horizontal midline. In the coronal section to the right, the lesion extends all the way from the inferior lip to the depth of the calcarine cortex. The lesion must be in the inferior bank because the field defect is in the upper quadrant.

The reader should try to map the lesion that would accompany field defect 2 in Figure 22-9A before reading on or looking at the answer in Figure 22-9B. Set up the cortical diagrams as in Figure 22-9B and draw in the lesion.

The field defect caused by lesion 2 does not extend to fixation or to the periphery; hence, the lesion is in the middle of the calcarine cortex in the horizontal section, extending neither to the pole nor to the anterior end. The field defect occupies pie-shaped sectors abutting the inferior vertical midline but not extending all the way to the horizontal midline. The lesion, therefore, is in the upper bank of the left calcarine cortex; it involves the lip but does not extend all the way to the depth of the calcarine fissure.

It is fun to draw these diagrams and take them to the radiologist as you read the computed tomography (CT) scan or the magnetic resonance imaging (MR) results. Small cortical lesions can often be identified that were radiographically questionable without the iron clad visual field correlation.

CONFRONTATION VISUAL FIELD EXAMINATION

Many patients must be tested with confrontation techniques because their overall condition and lack of mobility preclude formal testing. Bedside methods are most practical for physicians other than ophthalmologists.

Confrontation test results must be used in a special way, however, because they do not have the specificity or the quantitative detail of well-done perimetry. Nonetheless, confrontation results can indicate the proper direction for a further workup and may thereby save a great deal of time and expense.

This method is called *confrontation* because the examiner stands in front of the patient and presents targets while he watches the patient's eyes. Fixation is a problem, as with all field testing, thus the examiner must have a method for monitoring this. It is best always to start with the right eye, because it will be easier to remember the sequence of findings and to relate them to the correct side when recording the results.

Ask the patient to cover his left eye with the palm of his left hand, and be sure that the fingers are all the way up onto the forehead so that no peeking is possible between them. To peek is human. . . . The examiner faces the patient and closes either eye. The patient is asked to fix his gaze on the examiner's open eye so that the examiner can see small deviations of the patient's eye and can thereby accurately monitor fixation.

The presentation of targets follows. The best initial test is *finger counting*. Although form resolution is the key function of the fovea, motion detection is performed with great sensitivity by the peripheral visual system. A waving motion of the hand or a wiggling of the fingers is, therefore, the grossest stimulus one can present to the periphery. This means that peripheral field function must be almost gone before a field defect to motion detection will be present. Motion, then, is too gross a stimulus to be sensitive, and thus it is not the ideal screening test. Form detection, on the other hand, is poorly done by the periphery. Thus, finger counting, which requires spatial analysis of a stationary form, is a sensitive test for peripheral dysfunction—it will be abnormal with only minor reduction of field function.

Fingers should be presented *en face* to the patient. Obviously, the patient must be able to see all the fingers to make it a valid test, and if you orient your hand so that all the fingers are lined up one behind the other from the patient's perspective, he will be unable to count them.

The test can be done quickly. All that is necessary is to present enough combinations of fingers to be sure the patient is not succeeding by guesswork. Combinations should include all fingers, one, two, or none—it is difficult to present three fingers because of the way that the tendons in our hands are arranged. Present the combination once in each of the four quadrants and then go around again in a random sequence of quadrants. Two presentations for each quadrant should be sufficient. If errors are made, then more presentations may be required to be sure whether an apparent defect is real.

Some quantitation of confrontation fields is possible, although it will never match formal quantitative perimetry. If the fingers are counted in all quadrants there may still be a field defect. First, some

defects are scotomata occupying only the central 10° to 20° field. Finger counting will often miss these defects. Second, the degree of peripheral defect may be so minor that fingers are still adequately counted.

Color perception is a sensitive, though subjective, measure of visual field dysfunction. It is common for patients to report that colors are less vivid in defective field areas—they seldom mention this, but they will agree to it when specifically tested. Present a fairly large bright red object in the four quadrants and ask the patient if there is any difference in the *redness* of the object in any field. *Desaturation* is the term applied to a subjective loss of color intensity in the defective field. Patients may report that the reds are shifted to a darker amber color, or bleached toward a lighter, pinkish, or yellowish color; however, in either case, the stimulus is perceived as *less red*. Try to avoid the term *brightness*, because it is a separate parameter of visual function and should be tested separately. If color saturation is lost in a quadrant, the boundaries should be explored by moving the test red object and by asking the patient to indicate quickly if it becomes redder. The most important area to screen is the vertical midline. To do this, two red spots, one on either side of the midline, may be presented either above or below the examiner's eye (*i.e.*, the fixation point), and the patient should be invited to compare the redness of the two spots. This may bring out a difference across the midline that the patient was unable to describe by viewing the spot sequentially in different quadrants. The examiner should then present one red spot as a stationary target in the normal quadrant and he should move the other spot horizontally from the defective field. The patient is told to indicate immediately when the two spots become equal in redness, and the examiner determines if this transition corresponds to the vertical hemianopic midline. The location of the midline is easily sensed by the examiner: It is an imaginary vertical line through the examiner's line of sight to the patient's eye.

If the patient has trouble counting fingers in a defective field, then other stimuli can be presented to determine the relative density of the defect. Moving fingers or a waving hand is a grosser stimulus than stationary fingers. If motion is not detected, a bright light may be moved within the defect and its margins plotted to light.

Thus, we can imagine a hierarchy of stimuli by which to grade the density of a visual field defect. From most intense to least, this hierarchy of stimuli is ordered as follows:

1. Moving light
2. Moving hand or fingers
3. Finger counting
4. Subjective judgment of color saturation

Using the hierarchy, one can even derive information on the relative slope of the defect. Consider a patient who is unable to perceive light or hand motion in the upper right field; who is able to see movement; but who is unable to count fingers in the lower right field. This finding would indicate a hemianopsia that is denser in the upper than in the lower quadrant; in other words, there is a sloping defect with a transition from an upper to lower field.

PUPILLARY SYSTEM

The eye has many structures and functions that are analogous to those of a camera, and the eye shares some common optical requirements with the latter. Among them is the capacity to limit the amount of light entering the optical system; this is a function of the adjustable camera diaphragm. The iris of the eye is essentially an opaque diaphragm with an adjustable central opening (*i.e.*, the pupil). Diameter adjustments are accomplished by coordinated action of the concentrically arranged sphincter muscle together with a set of radially oriented dilator fibers. The sphincter is a 1-mm-wide band of smooth muscle surrounding the pupillary margin. The radial fibers, also smooth muscle, originate at the iris root near the limbus of the cornea and insert within the collagenous substance of the iris near the pupil and the sphincter muscle. Although the sphincter is innervated by the parasympathetic nervous system and the dilators are innervated by the sympathetic system, the two muscle groups function together as an organized unit; that is, when the sphincter is activated, the dilators are concomitantly inhibited at the CNS level. There is always a resting tonus in both systems—they are in a state of mutual opposition when the pupil is at rest. Of the two groups, however, the sphincter is stronger and tends to dominate the equilibrium determining pupil size at average levels of illumination. This is in accordance with the common observation that anticholinergic sphincter inhibitors, such as tropicamide (Mydriacyl), are much stronger pupil dilators than are sympathomimetics such as phenylephrine.

EXAMINATION OF THE PUPILS

PUPIL SHAPE

Under normal circumstances, the entire sphincter–dilator network functions in a coordinated manner and the pupil margin remains round as diameter changes occur. There are pathologic states, however, in which an altered function in the CNS brings about a circumferentially unequal contraction and dilatation of the pupil. Wilson called this condition *corectopia pupillae* or *ecotopic pupil*. This condition might involve either unequal segmental sphincter contraction or independent activation of a small sector of the dilator fibers. Irregular pupils are, however, more commonly the result of direct iris muscle damage, as in trauma or infection in the eye.

PUPIL SIZE AND REACTIVITY

The diameter of the pupil at any particular time reflects the coordinated activity of the sphincter and the dilator systems. As already mentioned, the former is the stronger of the two but can be overcome in the presence of a massive increase in dilator tone caused by activation of the sympathetic system. The adequate sensory stimulus for activating the sphincter is light falling on the retina, whereas "psychosensory" inputs cause dilator activation by way of the sympathetic nervous system. Pupil size tends to be small in infants, with progressive enlargement through early childhood, and eventual return to a smaller diameter in the elderly.

In a fixed ambient light, the pupils constrict as the subject becomes drowsy, and they dilate with arousal or startle. Fear and anxiety are thus commonly associated with larger-than-average pupils for a particular light level. Dilator system activation resulting from anxiety can even inhibit the pupil's contraction in response to light. When testing pupil function, it is common to obtain only a small response to the first series of light stimuli. The amplitude of contraction usually increases as the patient becomes less fearful and more relaxed with the situation. One should never conclude that the pupils are nonreactive or sluggish until several stimuli have been delivered and the patient has been put *at ease*, if possible. This anxiety-related fixity of the pupil seldom lasts more than 20 or 30 seconds under usual conditions.

Pharmacologic agents can obviously cause prominent effects on the size of the pupil. This subject is too vast for review, but some examples are worthy of mention. Glutethimide (Doriden) is a sedative–hypnotic drug that is sometimes the causative agent in drug overdose cases. In toxic doses, it characteristically causes widely dilated, unreactive pupils. Opiates generally cause small pupils, as do sedative drugs. Therefore, in coma resulting from an overdose with opiates, barbiturates, and other sedative hypnotics (except glutethimide), pupils that are widely dilated should raise suspicion of anoxic damage to the CNS secondary to respiratory suppression. The effects of atropinic substances introduced directly into the eye are discussed later. Systematically administered sympathomimetics can cause widely dilated pupils, but this is seldom observed clinically. Such a finding has been occasionally referred to in patients taking levodopa for treatment of Parkinson's disease. Pupillary dilatation occurs with the systemic administration of amphetamines, most commonly in the setting of drug abuse. The size of pupils in all of these situations, however, may reflect the psychic state of the patient due to factors other than the presence of pharmacologically active substances in the system. Furthermore, the examiner must have considerable experience to know the range of expected pupil sizes among normal persons in the usually varying sorts of illumination in which patients are examined. The light intensity in the examination area is uncontrolled in most cases, thus judgments about pupil size are often unreliable. Fortunately, in most cases, anisocoria or asymmetry of pupil diameter is more important for a diagnosis than is absolute pupil size.

TECHNIQUE OF PUPIL EXAMINATION

Every physician should take time to define a certain reproducible type of lighting in which he will always carry out his pupil examination. He will then build up a personal log of experience by which to assess whether a particular patient's pupils are abnormally large or small. The ideal area is one that can be both brightly and dimly illuminated in a standard way. Bright light causes relative activation of the sphincter system and can enhance anisocoria resulting from parasympathetic (*i.e.*, third cranial nerve) system lesions. Similarly, dim light shifts the balance of tone to the sympathetically innervated dilator systems and may serve to uncover anisocoria caused by Horner's syndrome. The anisocoria in ocular sympathetic lesions may not be detected in bright light.

Thus, it can be appreciated that the degree of anisocoria, or the *difference* between diameters of the pupils in defined dim and bright light is important in pupil diagnosis. Approximately 15% of normal individuals have anisocoria of up to 1 mm

without any lesion in either the sympathetic or parasympathetic systems. The difference in size remains the same in bright and dim lighting, which serves to distinguish this *physiologic anisocoria* from pathologic states.

The light reaction is usually observed with the patient in a dim room. Contraction of the sphincter is brought about by exposing each eye to bright light from a focal source for periods of 0.5 to 2 seconds at a time. The most commonly used source is a penlight, but any bright light that can be directed into one eye at a time will do. Penlights tend to become dim rapidly and also to flicker because of cheap on–off switches. The Finoff head is an angled carrier that attaches a halogen bulb to the battery handle of the ophthalmoscope. It provides a bright, steady light source that is ideal for testing the pupil. It is a small accessory that is easy to carry in the examining bag along with the ophthalmoscope and otoscope.

Light delivered to one eye causes equal contraction of both pupils. The *direct* light response refers to pupil constriction in the eye stimulated, and the *consensual* response is that which occurs when the eye opposite the observed pupil is illuminated.

The contraction of the pupils to *near* stimulation should be approximately as brisk and extensive as that to light. This contraction is best elicited by having the patient attempt to focus on his own thumb held about 2 cm or 3 cm from his nose. The resulting proprioceptive cues, together with common narcissistic tendencies, make this a more compelling target for *near effort* than any external object, even the examiner's finger. Simple *awareness of near* is said to be an effective stimulus for activation of the neurally linked *near triad*—pupillary constriction, lens accommodation (increase of diopteric power to focus at close range), and convergence of the optic axes (to maintain binocular fusion on a near object). There is often pupil constriction even if the patient does not make any convergent eye movements or accommodative changes in the lens of the eye.

FORMAT FOR REPORTING THE PUPIL EXAMINATION

The notation "Pupils equal, round, regular, and reactive to light and accommodation (PERRLA)" is best avoided in all cases except in an examination under battlefield conditions, in which the main distinction to be drawn is between the living and the dead. Obviously, all cases do not demand the same intensity of systematic examination of the pupil, thus abbreviated and extended formats are warranted. A good brief form follows:

PUPILS	SIZE (MM)	RESPONSE TO LIGHT	AFFERENT DEFECT?
RE	6	Brisk	None
LE	6	Brisk	

The *near reaction* has not been discussed. It is generally unnecessary to examine the near response if the light response is normal. The important *light-near dissociated* pupils, which are discussed later, involve a failure of the light reaction with preservation of the near response (never the reverse).

OVERVIEW OF CENTRAL PUPILLARY PATHWAYS

The importance of the pupil in neurologic diagnosis rests on the fact that structures determining pupil size and motility occupy extensive portions of the CNS in addition to the circuitous pathways of the peripheral ocular sympathetics in the head and neck. Lesions in widely separated portions of the anatomy will thus lead to specific disorders of pupil function.

The cerebral hemispheres probably contribute to pupil tone, although (for practical purposes) the hemispheres do not have localizing pupillary significance, because lesions and irritative states at this level do not produce any reliable changes in the pupils. It is useful to envision the pupillary motor systems as reflex arcs analogous to those in the spinal cord. Each system (parasympathetic and sympathetic) has an afferent side and a motor side to its reflex arc, which is similar to the situation at the segmental level. The optimal afferent stimulus, however, is different in the two systems. This is discussed later on in more detail, however, the parasympathetic system basically involves a reaction of the pupil to light on the retinas, whereas the dilator system functions in response to *psychosensory* inputs.

The afferent arc of the parasympathetic reflex is mediated by way of inputs from the retina to the midbrain, where connections exist with the Edinger–Westphal subgroup of the third cranial nerve nucleus. The motor side is mediated by way of axons of the Edinger–Westphal nucleus passing in the third cranial nerve to the ciliary ganglion, where synapses with the postganglionic fibers are found. These postganglionic fibers form neuro-

muscular junctions with the pupillary sphincter muscle.

Within the sympathetic system, the afferent arcs come from ascending sensory pathways with collaterals into the brain stem and diencephalic reticular formation. Inputs from the cerebral hemisphere are not anatomically well defined, but probably feed into the descending reticular system, perhaps at the hypothalamic level along with other limbic-diencephalic interfaces. The efferent side is mediated by way of descending pathways within the brain stem and spinal cord, which then make contact with a preganglionic neuron, the cell body of which is in the intermediolateral cell column of the spinal cord. The preganglionic and postganglionic fibers for the sympathetic system follow a complex pathway through the head and neck to reach the iris dilator fibers.

This brief overview will serve to emphasize that there is a tremendous diversity of sensory inputs to the pupil systems. These afferent pathways, together with pupillomotor efferent pathways, occupy an extensive and functionally critical portion of the nervous system.

PARASYMPATHETIC PUPIL SYSTEM (LIGHT REFLEX)

The parasympathetic system provides a mechanism for reflex adjustment of pupil size in response to the amount of light entering the eye. This serves to maintain the image quality by limiting excessive quantities of light, and it also increases the depth of focus while reducing spheric aberration of the eye's optics. The same optical phenomena occur in a camera when the aperture (f-stop) of the diaphragm is reduced.

Figure 22-10 is a diagrammatic representation of the afferent and efferent sides of the reflex pupillary pathway for light. Changes of luminous intensity in the environment normally enter the system through both eyes simultaneously. However, for purposes of clarity, we have chosen to illustrate the more usual mode of clinical testing in which a light is introduced selectively into one eye. In this diagram, the flashlight is directed at the right eye, and the photoreceptors of the right retina are activated. Through several intermediate neurons in the retina, excitation is conveyed to the retinal ganglion cells, the axons of which constitute the optic nerve. An important aspect of this system is the fact that when light is introduced into one eye, both pupils constrict to an equal degree. The extent of pupil-

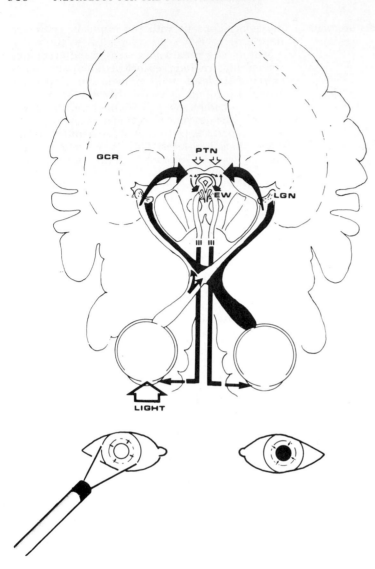

FIG. 22-10. Pathways for the parasympathetic light reflex. The upper portion of the figure illustrates afferent pathways from the retina of the right eye to both sides of the midbrain by way of the hemidecussation at the chiasm. Afferent fibers of retinal ganglion cells leave the optic tracts anterior to the lateral geniculate bodies and innervate pretectal nuclei (PTN, *open arrows*). Closed triangles just below the superior colliculi in the midbrain section indicate neurons of the *pretectal nuclei*. Pathways from either PTN innervate the Edinger–Westphal (EW) nuclei bilaterally, constituting a second hemidecussation in the afferent side of the reflex arc. The outflow pathways from the Edinger–Westphal nuclei are in the third cranial nerves to the ciliary ganglion, where a synapse occurs with postganglionic neurons (not shown) that innervate the iris sphincter muscle. The inset below illustrates that both pupils constrict to an equal degree when light is applied to one eye as a consequence of the twin hemidecussations in the afferent pathways.

lary constriction was once considered to be greater on the side of the light stimulus, but pupillographic studies have disproved this contention. The anatomic substrate for a bilateral symmetrical pupil constriction with monocular stimulation will become clear on inspection of this diagram. Figure 22-10 shows that when the right eye is stimulated, the optic nerve carries impulses to the optic chiasm where the fibers originating nasal to the macula (serving temporal fields) cross, and the fibers origi-

nating temporal to the macula (nasal fields) pass undecussated in the ipsilateral optic tract. At some point anterior to the termination of these fibers in the lateral geniculate nuclei (LGN), a collateral pathway leads to the pretectal region of the midbrain just ventral to the collicular plate. Neurons in this pretectal nuclear (PTN) region are indicated in Figure 22-10 by triangle symbols (open arrows, PTN). Right eye stimulation produces bilateral activation of pretectal nuclei because of the hemidecussation at the chiasm. Some of the pretectal neurons send axons across the midline to the opposite Edinger–Westphal nucleus, whereas others send fibers to the ipsilateral nucleus (Fig. 22-10). Thus, there are crossing fibers at two levels in the afferent system to explain the observed symmetrical pupillary contraction when light stimulates one eye.

The efferent arm of the light reflex is generally considered to begin with cell bodies in the Edinger–Westphal nucleus, a subunit of the third cranial nerve (oculomotor) nuclear group. The third cranial nerve innervates quite a number of extraocular muscles as well as the pupils, and the architecture of its nucleus is complex (Fig. 22-11). For the moment, we will consider only the pupillomotor fibers that exit from the midbrain within the third cranial nerve, bound for the orbit. The upper left-hand inset of Figure 22-11 shows the location of pupillary fibers within the nerve—they are depicted as the black band at the periphery of the nerve trunk.

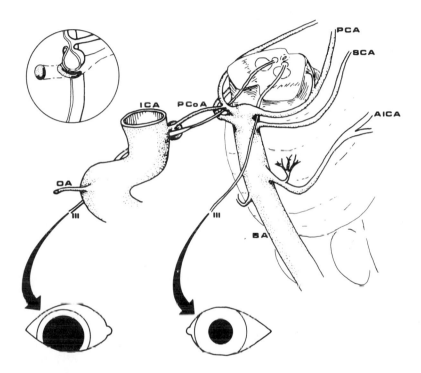

FIG. 22-11. The third cranial nerve is depicted in relation to an aneurysm of the right posterior communicating artery (PCoA). The main body of the figure illustrates the anatomical relationship of the right third cranial nerve to the posterior cerebral artery (PCA) and the superior cerebellar artery (SCA) as the nerve exits from the brain stem and crosses the subarachnoid space. It also illustrates the close relationship between the nerve and the internal carotid artery (ICA) at its junction with the PCoA more anteriorly. The figure shows that an aneurysm of the PCoA at its origin from the ICA is in an ideal position to compress the third nerve. The upper left-hand inset shows the relationship of an aneurysm to the passing third nerve. Note that the pupillary parasympathetic fibers, indicated by a solid black band, are peripherally placed and especially vulnerable to sudden enlargement of the aneurysm or to breach of the nerve surface by localized hemorrhage. The lower inset indicates a typical aneurysmal type right third nerve palsy. The right eye is abducted and depressed with maximum pupillary dilatation. (BA = basilar artery; OA = ophthalmic artery; AICA = anterior inferior cerebellar artery)

This is important in the diagnosis of third cranial nerve lesions, because the peripheral pupillomotor fibers are vulnerable to the effects of external compression by aneurysms (Fig. 22-11).

Within the orbit, the parasympathetic fibers synapse with postganglionic cell bodies in the ciliary ganglion. The postganglionic fibers enter the anterior segments of the eyes as the *long posterior ciliary* nerves and form neuromuscular junctions with the pupillary sphincter muscle. The synaptic neurotransmitter at the ciliary ganglion level and at the neuromuscular junction is acetylcholine. The transmitter at the pretectal level and at the Edinger–Westphal nucleus is unknown. Pharmacologic manipulation of the cholinergic neuromuscular junction at the eye is important in the diagnosis of pupil sphincter paralysis.

CLINICAL DISORDERS OF THE PARASYMPATHETIC PUPILLARY SYSTEM

Relative Afferent Pupillary Defect (Marcus Gunn)

A quantitative neural signal that varies with the amount of light entering the eyes is conveyed by retinal ganglion cell axons to the pretectal nuclei, where it is translated into a motor command for the appropriate pupil size and is relayed by way of the third cranial nerve to the irides of both eyes. The system functions as if there were a fixed relationship between the amount of light entering the two eyes and the neural code for the resultant pupil size. Anything that reduces the amount of light entering will cause the pupils to attain a larger diameter, all other stimuli remaining equal. This can be demonstrated by covering one eye of a subject and by noting that the uncovered pupil dilates slightly. Both pupils are dilating, but the pupil under cover cannot be seen. This type of observation led Marcus Gunn to describe the *relative afferent pupillary defect* (RAPD), which is now routinely tested by the *swinging flashlight* technique. Marcus Gunn's original observation, made in 1904, was that covering an eye with an optic nerve lesion caused relatively little dilatation of the pupil, because almost all the light-induced signal was coming to the midbrain from the opposite eye. As the cover was switched to the normal eye, however, the pupils would dilate strikingly, because all the light information was now coming from the eye with the defective afferent function. This *variance* of pupil size with alternating occlusion when one of the eyes is providing most of the brightness signal was the basis for the *swinging*

flashlight test. Rather than alternately covering each eye as Marcus Gunn did, the RAPD is now tested by illuminating each eye separately with a focal light source. Both pupils dilate as the light is swung to the defective eye, and both pupils constrict as it is swung to the normal eye. The test is best done in the dark, and only the eye illuminated by the flashlight can be seen at any one time. The unseen fellow eye, however, is undergoing the same pupillary constriction and dilatation that you are observing in the illuminated eye. The swinging flashlight technique provides a sensitive means of comparing afferent function in the two eyes. If one eye is totally blind, and the other has normal visual acuity and fields, the difference in magnitude of the direct light reflex between eyes will be evident without the swinging flashlight technique. The test becomes useful when the difference in direct light reflex between the eyes is less, in which case observation of the extent and velocity of pupil constriction may seem the same when either eye is stimulated alone. Nonetheless, a clear difference is usually apparent when either eye is stimulated alternately.

Under the best circumstances, an afferent pupillary defect is easy to detect, even when small. However, certain variances of pupil function among normal individuals sometimes makes interpretation of the swinging flashlight test difficult. The presence of a Marcus Gunn pupil, or RAPD, indicates a lesion in the afferent pupillary reflex arc between the eye and the midbrain, although the type of lesion is not directly specified by the test.

One should not conclude, however, that the RAPD has no specificity as to the cause of visual loss in the defective eye. Cataracts and other opacities in the ocular media do not produce a significant RAPD even with a major visual loss. This is probably true because such opacities *diffuse* light within the eye and degrade the visual image but do not significantly reduce the total quantity of light that reaches the retina. A visual loss resulting from opacities in the media of the eye is not generally a major diagnostic problem. The opacities are easily seen on ophthalmoscopic examination. There is greater difficulty in distinguishing among macular lesions, optic nerve lesions, and childhood amblyopia. In any of these cases, the fundus appearance may not give a clue as to which is causing the visual loss. Although macular lesions usually cause an observable change in the optic fundus, the findings may be subtle and may even require adjunctive examinations, such as fluorescein angiography, to demonstrate them.

The usefulness of the afferent pupillary defect in this type of situation lies in the relationship between the degree of afferent defect and the degree of visual dysfunction. In the presence of a minimal functional impairment (nearly normal visual acuity and fields), a prominent afferent pupil defect signifies a high probability that the lesion is in the optic nerve. A macular lesion must produce a more extensive visual loss than an optic nerve lesion to result in an equivalent RAPD.

Thus, if the visual acuity is severely impaired from a macular lesion, there may be a fairly prominent RAPD, and the test is specific for optic nerve lesions mainly when visual impairment is minor. The same is true of amblyopia, in which case a severe reduction of visual acuity is sometimes accompanied by a small afferent pupil defect; however, none is present with moderate amblyopia. *The specificity of the afferent pupillary defect is poorer in patients with major visual loss than it is with relatively normal vision.*

The afferent pupil defect is decisive in evaluating functional or hysterical visual loss. Most commonly, the differential diagnosis falls between hysteria and optic neuropathy behind the globe (retrobulbar neuropathy), because the fundus is normal in both cases.

If a patient has vision worse than 20/40 in one eye and normal vision and fields in the other eye, and there is no RAPD, it is reasonably safe to conclude that the problem is functional. A problem exists if a person has reduced acuity in one symptomatic eye and an asymptomatic peripheral field defect in the other eye. The peripheral field loss may be sufficiently great as to balance the central visual loss in the symptomatic eye, in which case there will be no RAPD. The swinging flashlight technique is a comparative test that uses the fellow eye as an internal control. The phenomenon that has been called Marcus Gunn pupil should, therefore, be referred to as the *relative* afferent pupillary defect. *It is important to keep in mind that the absence of an RAPD in a patient with symptomatic reduction of vision in one eye is a useful sign of hysteria or malingering only if one has detailed information on the visual function in the fellow eye.*

Occasionally, there is confusion between the Marcus Gunn pupil and *hippus*, which is a random, often rhythmic pupillary oscillation that can be observed in many normal individuals during steady illumination of the eyes. The term *hippus* is usually reserved for those pupils that oscillate with large amplitude; almost every pupil has small sinusoidal oscillations of size with steady illumination. High-amplitude oscillation is a curiosity, but not a disease—there are no currently accepted disease associations with the phenomenon. It often complicates the interpretation of the swinging flashlight test, however, because there can be an interaction between the rhythm of flashlight alternation and that of the spontaneous pupil fluctuation. The examiner sometimes swings the light between the eyes in such a way that a false afferent defect is produced on one side or a real afferent defect is negated by the pattern of alternation. To avoid this problem, the examiner should probably swing at *different rhythms* during a single examination, including at least one trial of very slow alternation, changing eyes every 3 to 5 seconds. During the steady illumination of each eye, the examiner can observe whether there is significant hippus; if there is, the results should be interpreted carefully. An apparent afferent defect that is not seen with most alternation rates may be spurious.

A person can see his own pupil oscillate by his sense of the brightness of the stimulus light, which brightens as the pupil widens and dims as the pupil contracts. When you shine a light in your own eye, the pupil first *constricts* and then slightly *dilates*. This is normal *early release* and does not in itself indicate an afferent defect; many normal pupils behave in this manner, although others assume a new smaller size with illumination and do not redilate. This early contraction and slight redilatation should be equal in amplitude between eyes to qualify as a normal variant. If there is significant early release, the swinging flashlight test should be done at slow alternation rates to let the new steady-state pupil size be expressed before changing eyes.

A pupil that dilates straight away when it is illuminated, without *any* early constriction, strongly indicates a Marcus Gunn pupil. However, an afferent defect may only be manifest in lesser early constriction in one eye than the other during the swinging flashlight test. It is not necessary for *all* early constriction to be abolished in mild degrees of unilateral optic neuropathy. The asymmetry of pupil behavior is the important feature to look for.

Preganglionic Ocular Parasympathetics (Third Cranial Nerve Lesions)

The diagnosis of third cranial nerve lesions based on an abnormal eye position with weakness of the extraocular muscle is discussed in a later section. In this section, we will concern ourselves with the involvement or sparing of the *pupil* in oculomotor nerve lesions, because a good deal of clinically important information revolves around this issue. Since the large studies of lesions involving third, fourth, and sixth cranial nerves were published from the Mayo Clinic in the 1950s and 1960s, the importance of the pupil in etiologic diagnosis of third cranial nerve lesions has been recognized. In these studies, and in subsequent clinical investigations, it has become well established that paralysis of the pupillary sphincter is the rule in third cranial nerve lesions resulting from aneurysms (Fig. 22-11). Conversely, older patients who develop third cranial nerve palsies on the basis of presumed microvascular occlusive disease within the nerve itself seldom have major pupillary involvement. A rather high proportion of patients in this latter category have a history that would favor accelerated atherosclerosis, diabetes mellitus, or hypertension. Such a background history is often not present in a person who develops a presumed microvascular third nerve palsy, and the lack of these factors should not rule out the diagnosis. These "medical" lesions tend to improve and most often make a nearly full recovery within 3 to 6 months.

Although there are only a few pathologic studies of third cranial nerve ischemia, consistent morphologic changes have been observed. The lesion is dominated by demyelination in the acute stages, and the lesion shrinks with fibrosis in the late "recovery" stages. In both the acute and chronic phases there is relatively little, if any, disruption of axons as they pass through the lesion. This correlates well with the usual clinical outcome in which complete or nearly complete recovery of function occurs over several months.

Since axons are not disrupted, there is no opportunity for the development of *aberrant* or *misdirected regeneration* of fibers in the late stage of recovery. This contrasts with the outcome when the third cranial nerve is damaged by a hemorrhage from aneurysms in which there is often a loss of axonal continuity. A fairly high incidence of *aberrant regeneration* tends to be seen in the late stages of recovery. The most commonly observed clinical manifestation of this is an inappropriate contraction of the levator palpebrae muscle together with activation of either the medial rectus or inferior rectus on attempted adduction or depression of the eye. This causes the striking appearance of lid elevation as the affected eye moves inward (adduction) or downward (depression). These phenomena are caused by a misdirection of axons that had been destined originally for one of the extraocular muscles but

which on regrowth attain the wrong channel in the peripheral portion of the nerve and end up at the wrong muscle.

Both the *medical* third cranial nerve palsies and those caused by aneurysms tend to present acutely with considerable pain in the eye and orbit at the onset. One tends to accept painful third cranial nerve palsy caused by aneurysms without much need for explanation. The cause of pain in microvascular occlusive lesions, however, is not readily apparent. On close examination, the cause of pain in the presence of aneurysms is not entirely explained. Although there is often evidence for enlargement of an aneurysm prior to the occurrence of small hemorrhages into the nerve, this is by no means always the case. Whether or not the aneurysm has enlarged, it is always possible that a direct irritation of pain carrying afferent pathways from the artery wall at the site of the aneurysm is responsible for the pain. The important point is that pain is characteristic of both aneurysmal third cranial nerve lesions and of those secondary to ischemia within the nerve substance. The criterion of pain should, therefore, not be used to make a diagnosis of intracranial aneurysm.

The importance of making a differential diagnosis prior to angiography is that the group of patients with an intraneural lesion caused by small-vessel disease carries a high risk for angiographic procedures, whereas in this group the angiogram does not lead to any beneficial therapy. It is, therefore, optimal to avoid angiography in those patients who stand to suffer most from it and who do not need it. Fortunately, sparing of the pupil is sufficiently reliable evidence of a *medical* cause so that most of these patients can be managed without angiography.

Although this seems simple and clear-cut in abstract discussion, the evaluation of individual cases presents ambiguities. Since all biologic phenomena tend to fall along continua rather than on all-or-none fashion, it is not surprising that this occurs in relation to pupillary involvement with third cranial nerve lesions. The safest statement that can be made is that in aneurysm-induced third cranial nerve palsies, the pupil is strongly involved, whereas in microvascular lesions the pupil is *relatively* spared. This means that the degree of pupillary involvement in relation to the degree of extraocular muscle involvement is the critical factor. There is little difficulty in diagnosis when a person presents with a total involvement of all extraocular muscles, including complete ptosis, and the pupil is only slightly larger than that of the other eye and remains reactive to light. This would be the profile of a clear-cut *medical* third cranial nerve palsy. Unfortunately, some patients present with *partial involvement of the extraocular muscles*, and then, even though the pupils are normal, or nearly so, it is difficult to exclude an aneurysm. Newer radiographic methods such as intravenous (IV) or intra-arterial digital subtraction angiography, rapid sequence CT with bolus IV contrast injection (*i.e.*, a type of angiogram), or duplex scanning methods all have the capacity to visualize larger aneurysms. There is presently no definitive test except standard angiography, and some patients with non-aneurysmal third cranial nerve palsies have to be studied using this invasive technique when the characteristics of the cranial nerve involvement are not definitive.

Pupillary involvement in other third cranial nerve–compressive lesions such as meningioma, pituitary adenoma, and nasopharyngeal carcinoma is much less predictable. The onset and course of the third cranial nerve dysfunction may be the most valuable clue to the presence of one of these other compressive lesions. The onset is generally much less explosive than that resulting from aneurysms or microvascular infarctions. Furthermore, the lesions caused by aneurysm or infarction are usually complete within hours or days, whereas the level of pupillary and extraocular muscle dysfunction with neoplasms tends to be slowly progressive over weeks or months.

It would seem practical to undertake a small-scale work-up on each patient in whom the diagnosis of a microvascular infarction of the third cranial nerve may be considered. Laboratory screening, especially for diabetes, may be followed by CT or MR of the sella turcica, ethmoid, and sphenoid regions, depending on the degree of suspicion. If the patient is hypertensive and diabetic and in the mid- to late sixties, it may be appropriate to stop tests after the blood studies. If the patient is without risk factors for accelerated atherosclerosis, or is under the age of 55 or even 60, it is wise to proceed to a CT scan with special attention to the parasellar and posterior orbital areas. Angiography remains the definitive test for an aneurysm.

Herniation Syndromes. Supratentorial masses large enough to herniate the medial temporal lobe over the tentorium cerebelli bring pressure to bear against the midbrain and third cranial nerve, which results in pupillary dilatation. Once the stage of third cranial nerve dysfunction has commenced in the course of the transtentorial herniation syndrome, there is often only a matter of minutes or hours until irreversible brain damage occurs. This is clearly a medical emergency. As with more distal third cranial nerve lesions—caused by aneurysms, infarcts, and tumors—the pupillary involvement is on the *motor* side of the reflex arc. Although it is axiomatic that a lesion on the afferent side of the reflex arc does not cause anisocoria, lesions on the motor side of the arc do so routinely. It is also the rule that a lesion in the efferent pupillary pathway will result in a sluggish pupillary response to either direct or consensual light stimulation on the involved side. It is thus always possible to distinguish an afferent pupillary lesion from one at or distal to the Edinger–Westphal nucleus in the third cranial nerve complex. In the latter instance the neural message from the midbrain is not conducted on one side only, whichever eye is being stimulated with light.

Depending on the location of the supratentorial mass lesion causing herniation, one can distinguish *central* and *lateral herniation syndromes.*

Central herniation, caused by lesions near the midline, commonly in the parasaggital regions, tends to present with symmetrical pupillary paralysis in both eyes. In these cases the entire substance of the diencephalon and midbrain are shifted downward, with a tendency for bilateral dysfunction from the onset. It is not uncommon for both pupils to be small and sluggishly reactive in the early stage of central herniation. The *lateral herniation syndrome* occurs in conjunction with laterally placed supratentorial masses, commonly in the temporal lobe itself. The third cranial nerve findings tend to be unilateral until the final stages of global midbrain dysfunction.

In both central and lateral herniation syndromes there is a sufficient disruption of function in the ascending reticular activating system that the patient is usually obtunded by the time that pupillary signs emerge. The end stage of both central and lateral herniation is bilateral pupillary paralysis, which is accompanied by large nonreactive pupils, probably caused by severe ischemia, often with a hemorrhage in the midbrain and pons. At this stage, it is usually not possible to determine whether the antecedent herniation was of the central or the lateral type.

It is worthy of repeated emphasis that the patients who are in the midst of cerebral herniation syndrome do not present to the office or hospital complaining of pupillary dilatation, or of anything else for that matter. They are usually severely obtunded by the time that the pupillary phenomena have begun. Gradual somnolence and outright stupor evolve during the earlier *diencephalic* phase of herniation, when the level of functional compromise is at the thalamus, above the midbrain level.

Confusion often occurs when an ostensibly healthy, alert patient presents to the emergency room complaining of a dilated pupil. This is not a rare presentation. This clinical presentation must, therefore, be dealt with effectively in the emergency ward, and a firm differential diagnosis of the *monosymptomatic dilated pupil* is important for all emergency room physicians to keep in mind.

POSTGANGLIONIC PARASYMPATHETIC LESION (ADIE'S SYNDROME, TONIC PUPIL, AND VARIATIONS)

Adie's Pupil

In 1932, Adie published findings concerning a group of generally healthy young women who presented with a unilaterally dilated pupil. He found that the affected pupil had a peculiar *tonic* light reaction: it responded slowly to light stimulation and had a more brisk, although still pathologically slow, response to near-vision effort. The pupil seemed totally fixed or unresponsive to light in the usual examination setting in which the patient was placed in a dim environment and a bright light flashed into either eye briefly (Fig. 22-12). When the patient was observed in a bright environment for several minutes, the "tonic" pupil would gradually decrease in diameter. When the environment was dimmed again, the normal pupil would dilate briskly and the "tonic" pupil would remain small for several minutes, although it would redilate slowly given enough time.

The absolute diameter of the affected pupil, therefore, depends on the *immediate past light experience* of the individual: a "tonic" pupil at a particular time may be smaller or larger than the normal pupil depending on the ambient illumination and the immediate past illumination. It is important to keep this in mind, because the Adie's pupil is usually described in textbooks as a pathologically large pupil. The average diameter of an Adie's pupil generally decreases as months and years go by. These pupils tend not to recover their normal function once the "tonic" state has begun. An old Adie's pupil is often small and does not dilate in dim light over any period of time.

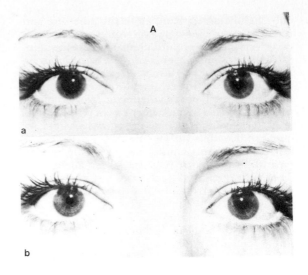

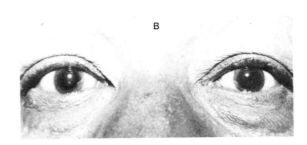

FIG. 22-12. The isolated unilaterally dilated pupil. (*A*) Adie's syndrome: *a.* the right pupil is widely dilated and unreactive to light. There is no ptosis or extraocular muscle weakness. *b.* The right pupil constricted to a greater extent than the left after instillation of "weak" 1/8% pilocarpine in either eye. (*B*) Atropinized pupil. The right pupil was widely dilated and fixed to light. It failed to constrict on instillation of "strong" 4% pilocarpine.

Adie observed that there was a high incidence of areflexia in his group of patients. Many had lost all of their deep tendon reflexes, although others retained some reflexes in a patchy manner. The etiology of this syndrome has never been elucidated; it remains an *idiopathic dysautonomic state.*

The presence of normal deep tendon reflexes does not rule out the diagnosis, because a significant percentage of patients have normal reflexes, at least when the syndrome first presents, and the features of the pupil syndrome do not distinguish between those with reflex loss and those without. Any of the limb reflexes may be diminished, and asymmetrical loss is found in nearly half the patients. The reflexes generally become less active as time passes, although in some patients they become a little more brisk (Thompson et al, 1979).

Aside from simply noticing the large pupil in the mirror, occasionally symptoms lead the patient to be indirectly aware of the problem. The pupil normally limits the amount of light entering the eye by reacting to variations in ambient illumination. When too much light enters the eye, it creates the sensation of *glare*. Furthermore, the large pupil alters the optics of the eye toward a state in which there is a *shallower depth of focus* and an increased *spheric aberration*. This tends to cause a sensation of blurred vision in both bright and dim environments. The accommodative mechanism is also affected in Adie's syndrome: The change in diopteric power (convexity) of the lens to *accommodate* for near vision takes many minutes to occur and then the focus remains for many minutes after the patient has shifted his gaze from a near to a distant object. Vision from the affected eye will, therefore, be blurred for the first few minutes of any near-vision effort and will remain blurred for several minutes as the patient subsequently attempts to use his eyes for distant viewing. The tonic accommodation with a sustained effort at near vision occasionally causes a *ciliary spasm*, which is manifested as pain in the eye, usually in the vicinity of the brow and inner canthus during close work.

The patient with an Adie's pupil is completely alert without any of the CNS signs that accompany transtentorial herniation. Nonetheless, many patients with Adie's syndrome are subjected to needless cerebral angiography, often as an emergency procedure.

The *tonic pupil* is caused by a postganglionic parasympathetic lesion. Some authors believe that this is a viral infection of the ciliary ganglion; however, no definitive data exist as to the cause of the lesion. The lesion is in the postganglionic parasympathetic system, because there is *denervation supersensitivity* to cholinergic substances. This seems to follow the same principles as denervation supersensitivity in skeletal muscle that has lost its direct innervation. Normally, the muscle can be activated only through its motor end plate; however, 4 or 5 weeks after an acute loss of direct nerve supply, the functional

muscle and plate begins to expand until nearly the entire sarcolemmal membrane becomes responsive to circulating or experimentally applied acetylcholine. This procedure forms the basis of a definitive test for Adie's pupil. Since acetylcholine is unavailable as a pharmaceutical solution, the physician can choose another direct-acting cholinergic such as *methacholine chloride (Mecholyl)* or *pilocarpine* for the test. The physician must select a solution that is too weak to cause a normally innervated sphincter muscle to contract. For these purposes $1/8\%$ pilocarpine is ideal, because it will not cause a significant contraction of a normally innervated sphincter muscle.

The normal pupil serves as an internal control in this test. One drop of $1/8\%$ pilocarpine is placed in either eye, and a second drop is applied 10 minutes later. The pupil size is measured approximately 40 to 60 minutes from the first application. In most cases, the Adie's pupil will become smaller than the fellow pupil under the influence of this weak solution of pilocarpine, thus demonstrating the presence of *denervation supersensitivity*. This is categorically different from the failure of a contraction to weak pilocarpine that characterizes the dilated pupil of an intracranial third cranial nerve lesion, in which case the postganglionic innervation is intact. Preganglionic lesions of the intracranial third nerve result in a dilated pupil, but there is no denervation supersensitivity and the pupil does not constrict in the presence of $1/8\%$ pilocarpine.

One can, therefore, distinguish the Adie's pupil from the dilated pupil caused by aneurysms, transtentorial herniation, and intracranial mass lesions that directly compress the third cranial nerve. The dilated pupils caused by all of these central lesions, together with all normal (nondilated) pupils, will remain the same size after the instillation of a weak pilocarpine solution. There is seldom great difficulty in distinguishing Adie's syndrome from compressive lesions of the third cranial nerve, even without pharmacologic tests. The intracranial lesions that compromise function in the third cranial nerve generally cause clinical findings related to the extraocular muscles in addition to the pupil. Some cases of intracranial aneurysms that cause isolated pupillary involvement have been documented. In these rare instances the extraocular and lid muscles become involved shortly after the pupil, and there are often subtle lid and ocular motility findings even when the pupil seems to be involved in isolation. My experience has not included any aneurysms that caused enough denervation sensitivity of the pupil to cause a clearly positive weak cholinergic test. The reader should be aware that the differential value of weak cholinergic testing is being scrutinized.

Up to this point we have been discussing the diagnosis of the unilateral denervated pupil in which the normal fellow pupil is used as an internal control. Bilateral denervation occurs in autonomic neuropathies such as occurs in diabetes mellitus. Both pupils are affected in these cases, and thus one pupil cannot serve as a control for the other. In testing for bilateral denervation, the pilocarpine solution must be weak enough that it will not cause *any* constriction of normal pupils. For this type of test 1/16% pilocarpine is recommended. If there is any contraction of either pupil, denervation can be diagnosed without reference to the other pupil.

Atropinized Pupil

The second major category of patients who present to the emergency room with an isolated large pupil is that of postsynaptic sphincter blockade by atropinic substances. The old term "bella-donna" (alkyloid), indicating atropine and its congeners, derives from the use of these agents by women (donna) who wanted to enhance their beauty (bella). It was once considered attractive for one's eyes to appear as bottomless pools, and this was accomplished by dilating the pupils. This seldom adequately accounts for the situation today. Basically two groups of people end up with atropinics in one eye—those who do so accidentally and those who put the drug in the eye willfully. The first category includes those people whose work involves the use of atropine, such as nurses, other paramedical personnel, and those who manipulate plants. Many plants have naturally occurring atropinics in the sap and on the surfaces of stems, leaves, and roots. The willful application of atropine to one eye is less easy to understand. In many cases such a person will present to the emergency room with a large pupil and a history of either blurred vision or headaches, as though there were some secondary gain attached to the frequent sequel of cerebral angiography. It stretches the imagination to assume that all these patients are aware of the relationship between pupil size and cerebral herniation syndromes. Some of the patients, though, are medical personnel who are aware of the relationship and its medical implications. It must be concluded that certain individuals are motivated to seek invasive diagnostic procedures, and the physician must be prepared to rule out CNS causes of the dilated pupil in these cases. This is easily done by the instillation of a strong solution (4% to 6%) of pilocarpine in each eye. A strong solution of pilocarpine is a potent cholinergic activator of the iris sphincter that produces a pinpoint pupil in normal eyes. Of additional importance is the fact that 6% pilocarpine will also constrict all pathologically denervated pupils including the postganglionic parasympathetic lesions of Adie's syndrome and the preganglionic third cranial nerve lesions. The only condition that will cause a failure of the pupil to constrict to 6% pilocarpine is a postsynaptic receptor blockade at the sphincter muscle—atropinization. If the pupil is large because of iris trauma or infection, with muscle atrophy or synechiae causing an adhesion to the lens capsule, there will also be a failure of constriction; however, this situation should not present a diagnostic problem because the anterior segment appears abnormal. It may require slit lamp biomicroscopy of the anterior segment to observe iris damage or lens capsule adhesions, and an ophthalmologic consultation should be obtained if this is considered a possibility.

The use of strong pilocarpine, therefore, unequivocally segregates those with a large pupil caused by lesions or pharmacologic blockade at the iris sphincter from normal persons and from those with large pupils caused by intracranial lesions of all types. There are few diagnostic procedures in medicine for which such a claim can be made!

It is theoretically possible for an aneurysm or other mass to compress the third cranial nerve in such a way as to cause isolated paralysis of the pupil. The pupillary fibers are superficial in the subarachnoid portion of the nerve and might be selectively disrupted by any lesion that compresses the nerve. Such a presentation is rare, and only a few cases have been documented. In most of these cases the extraocular muscles and levator palpebrae are affected within days of isolated pupillary involvement. I have found that subtle, often fluctuating lid and ocular motor signs are present in patients who are said to have isolated pupil dilatation caused by aneurysms. A carefully repeated examination often gives evidence that leads to the proper diagnosis of these cases. Any patient with a dilated pupil that contracts to strong pilocarpine must, therefore, be observed carefully because there may be a serious intracranial cause such as an aneurysm.

OCULAR SYMPATHETIC SYSTEM

The sympathetic system produces a dilator tone in opposition to the iris sphincter. The dilator system functions by way of a reflex arc just as the sphincter system does; however, the afferent arm is much less circumscribed than that of the light reflex, which probably accounts for the fact that the sympathetic system is often not thought of as a reflex circuit.

Afferent stimulation along pain and temperature pathways from the spinal cord generally causes pupil dilatation that is abrupt in onset and lasts on the order of 20 to 60 seconds. More sustained dilatation often attends mental states involving fear, anxiety, or surprise. Since the sympathetic afferent pathways are anatomically ill defined, especially at rostral levels of the CNS, the subsequent discussion will focus on efferent sympathetic pathways.

Anatomic studies have shown sympathetic fiber degeneration in the upper brain stem after experimental lesions in the hypothalamus. These degeneration studies document widely dispersed fiber tracts in the upper midbrain and diencephalon but no reliably demonstrated pathways in the pons and medulla. The descending system is most likely, therefore, a polysynaptic one, even though in clinical usage it is referred to as *"the central neuron"* in the chain leading to the iris dilator.

Clinical studies have documented that dorsolateral lesions throughout the brain stem often produce ocular sympathetic dysfunction ipsilaterally, whereas medial and ventral lesions do not. This is the basis for the widely accepted view that the polysynaptic descending system is dorsolaterally disposed in the brain stem. This pathway continues into the spinal cord to the C8 through T2 segmental levels, where the "central" fibers synapse with cells in the intermediolateral gray horns; this zone between C8 and T2 is commonly known as the *ciliospinal center of Budge and Waller.* The central pathways through the cervical spinal cord are located superficially (near the pia) in the lateral columns. The preganglionic cells from the ciliospinal center send axons to the *paravertebral sympathetic ganglion chain* by way of the C8–T2 ventral roots. These preganglionic fibers travel upward in the sympathetic chain through the *stellate* (combined upper thoracic and lower cervical ganglion) and the *middle cervical* ganglion. They synapse with postganglionic cells in the *superior cervical ganglion,* which is usually found high in the neck, often under the angle of the mandible. This means that the common lesions that cause ocular sympathetic palsy (Horner's syndrome) interfere with preganglionic fibers as they course through the upper thorax. Virtually all the lesions producing postganglionic sympathetic dysfunction are intracranial and intraorbital in location, since the superior cervical ganglion is so near the base of the skull.

The postganglionic axons at first travel in the adventitia of the carotid artery. Those supplying vascular and sweat gland structures in the lower face travel with external carotid branches, whereas the ocular sympathetics and those serving vasomotor and sudomotor function for the forehead go with the internal carotid into the middle cranial fossa. A contingent of ocular sympathetic fibers takes a "side path" through the otic ganglion in the middle ear. This apparently explains the occasional occurrence of Horner's syndrome with middle ear infections. The main ocular sympathetic pathway, however, follows the carotid artery through its *siphon* region, and then joins the *first division (ophthalmic)* of the *trigeminal nerve,* which carries it into the orbit. A sympathetic contingent passes through the parasympathetic ciliary ganglion, constituting the so-called sympathetic root of the ganglion, but no sympathetic synapses occur there. In the orbit, the ocular sympathetics innervate the iris dilator muscles together with small smooth muscles in the lids, which contribute to upper lid elevation and lower lid depression. Defective contraction of these sympathetically innervated *Muller's muscles* causes a low-grade ptosis or a descent of the upper lid. Less well recognized, however, is the fact that the weakness of Muller's muscle in the lower lid causes the latter to elevate. Upper lid ptosis and elevation of the lower lid together cause a narrowing of the *palpebral fissure.* This contributes to an illusion that the involved eye is displaced backward in the orbit, the so-called "apparent enophthalmos" that has been described with Horner's syndrome. It used to be stated that the enophthalmos was real in Horner's syndrome; however, only frogs have a sympathetically innervated muscle that normally holds the eye forward in the orbit, the weakness of which allows the eye to move backward. Thus, the enophthalmos in Horner's syndrome is truly *apparent*—an illusion caused by the narrowed palpebral fissure.

Sympathetic fibers serving the skin of the forehead just above the brow travel with the nasociliary branch of the first or ophthalmic division of the trigeminal nerve. With postganglionic sympathetic lesions, a triangular patch of altered vasomotor tone and decreased sweating may present just above the brow extending to the midline.

CLINICAL DISORDERS OF THE OCULAR SYMPATHETICS

The defective function of the sympathetically innervated Muller's muscle in the upper lid results in the minor degree of ptosis that occurs typically in

Horner's syndrome. The position of the upper and lower lids and thereby the width of the palpebral fissure is determined by the relative tone in the orbicularis muscle, which closes the lids, compared with the tone of the levator palpebrae plus Müller's muscles, which open the eyes. The levator palpebrae, a striated muscle innervated by the third cranial nerve, provides most of the upper lid's elevation, whereas Müller's muscle produces some upper lid elevation and lower lid depression. Thus, the levator and Müller's muscle work together and in opposition to the orbicularis muscle, which encircles the palpebral fissure. When assessing lid position, one must be careful of illusions crated by asymmetrical skin folds, by altered position of the eye in the orbit (extraocular muscle palsies and strabismus), and even by anisocoria. The observer's eye uses all of these landmarks for assessing where the lid margin is expected to fall and whether its position is the same in the two eyes. Eyelid position and the relation of lid margins to landmarks such as skin folds is often asymmetrical for various non-neurologic reasons. It is useful, therefore, to measure the distance between a central corneal light reflex and the upper and lower lids, respectively, and also to compare these for symmetry between eyes. This reflex, produced when a point source of light such as a penlight or handlight is directed toward the eyes from a position in front of the patient, does not move appreciably with a variation in eye position as long as it still falls on the cornea.

A pitfall that occurs not uncommonly is the false diagnosis of a facial or seventh cranial nerve palsy caused by apparent widening of one palpebral fissure (orbicularis oculi weakness) when the fissure is really narrowed on the other side from an ocular sympathetic lesion. This error is more likely to occur if the normal range of facial asymmetry produces an apparent flattening of the nasolabial fold on the side of the wider palpebral fissure and if the pupillary meiosis is minimal or lacking in the ocular sympathetic palsy. Pharmacologic pupil testing can be a useful arbiter in this setting.

Etiologic Diagnosis in Horner's Syndrome

The most common ocular sympathetic palsies one encounters are those caused by an interruption of preganglionic fibers in relation to lesions of the lung apex and the neck. The bulk of these lesions are malignant tumors, often primary in the lung, or metastases to cervical nodes that can complicate a wide variety of carcinomas, lymphomas, and leukemias.

Some of these cases of preganglionic Horner's syndrome will be secondary to trauma and will usually include penetrating neck wounds and root involvement in spinal injuries. These cases should be obvious from the history and physical findings. Inflammation, caused by suppurative infections and granulomatous diseases such as sarcoidosis or tuberculosis in cervical lymph nodes, is an occasional nonmalignant cause for preganglionic ocular sympathetic palsy.

Central nervous system (*e.g.*, of the hypothalamus) lesions are an uncommon cause of Horner's syndrome. They are almost always recognizable by the associated cranial nerve, cerebellar, and sensorimotor long tract findings. A classic example is *Wallenberg's lateral medullary syndrome*, which is usually caused by an occlusion of one vertebral artery with an infarction in the distribution of the *posterior inferior cerebellar artery*. The attendant dorsolateral medullary lesion produces a syndrome that includes ocular sympathetic palsy along with facial numbness ipsilateral to the lesion, pain and temperature loss in the contralateral extremities, vertigo, dysphagia, and dysarthria. This typical central lesion is distinct from the usually isolated, frequently asymptomatic Horner's syndrome that accompanies preganglionic peripheral lesions.

Postganglionic ocular sympathetic palsy is commonly associated with pain in the ipsilateral orbit and eye. In the early part of this century, a Norwegian ophthalmologist named Raeder reported this combination of pain, meiosis, and ptosis as a *"paratrigeminal"* syndrome with a localizing value for mass lesions in the middle cranial fossa. All four of his patients had, in addition to ocular sympathetic palsy, findings referable to the ipsilateral cranial nerves III through VI, either singly or in combination. During the past two decades there has been an increasing awareness of patients with painful ocular sympathetic palsy without demonstrable middle fossa mass lesions. These patients often have histories of episodic retrobulbar and orbital pain that in many cases is typical of *cluster* or *histamine headache*. The ocular sympathetic lesion comes about during a cluster of headaches and sometimes resolves spontaneously after the cluster has ended, although it sometimes remains as a permanent sequel. This benign condition, which is considered a migraine variant, has acquired the name *Raeder's paratrigeminal syndrome, type II*. The patient must have no objective neurologic deficit of cranial nerves III through VI in order to qualify for this benign diagnosis; the presence of cranial nerve findings strongly favors the presence of a middle fossa lesion. It has been speculated that in type II Raeder's syndrome, the postganglionic ocular sympathetic fibers are affected by edema in the wall of the carotid artery. Vascular wall changes, probably including edema, are presumed to occur during severe migrainous episodes. The exact sequence of events leading to the ocular sympathetic palsy in this setting is, however, unknown.

Figure 22-13 presents the ocular findings in a man 46 years of age who had frequent episodes of steady intense pain in the left orbit. Each headache lasted 45 to 60 minutes and occurred daily, often at predictable times. These findings had been present for 2 weeks prior to the examination. He had had similar bouts of frequent headaches in previous years. These headaches lasted 1 to 3 weeks at a time. During this symptomatic period, however, a physician had noted left ptosis and meiosis of which the patient was unaware. The neurologic examination was otherwise completely normal. This was a typical case of type II Raeder's syndrome with a presumed migrainous etiology. We will discuss the pupillary pharmacologic aspects of this diagnosis later.

Pharmacologic Work-Up of Ocular Sympathetic Lesions

The objectives of pharmacologic testing in the sympathetic system are two-fold. In some cases one wishes simply to document the presence or absence of an ocular sympathetic lesion without regard to further localization. A typical example would be a case of isolated anisocoria or isolated ptosis in which the evidence is insufficient for the reliable diagnosis of a sympathetic lesion. The second objective of pharmacologic diagnosis is identifying the level of involvement (pre- or post-ganglionic) in a case in which one is reasonably certain an ocular sympathetic lesion exists.

There is great practical value in segregating patients with Horner's syndrome into those with preganglionic and those with postganglionic lesions. The group with preganglionic lesions has a high incidence of malignant disease requiring extensive investigation, whereas the group with post ganglionic involvement has primarily benign causes (usually a vascular headache).

The physiologic basis of clinically useful pharmacologic tests is noradrenergic transmission at the iris dilator neuromuscular junction where the sympathetic postganglionic axon terminals contact the

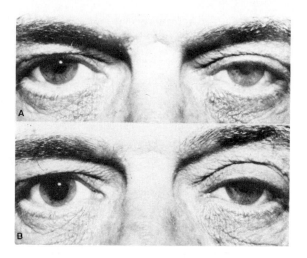

FIG. 22-13. Left ocular sympathetic lesion with ipsilateral orbital headache of migraine type (Raeder's syndrome type II). (*A*) The asymmetrical position of the upper lid margin with respect to the overlying skin fold is the most prominent feature of this man's ptosis. The relation of the lid margin to the iris and globe is relatively symmetrical between eyes. (*B*) The left pupil failed to dilate on instillation of 1% para-OH-amphetamine, indicating a postganglionic ocular sympathetic lesion.

muscle cells. The drugs of greatest clinical usefulness are the *indirect-acting sympathomimetics: cocaine* and *para-OH-amphetamine (Paredrine).*

These schemes for clinical usage have been worked out primarily by Thompson and coworkers (1971). Transmission in the sympathetic system at the superior cervical ganglion is cholinergic, but there are no clinically useful diagnostic tests for evaluating the function at this level.

At the postganglionic axon terminal, norepinephrine (NE) is maintained in storage vesicles by metabolically active processes. The bound vesicular NE is in equilibrium with a pool of unbound NE in the vesicle and in the cytoplasm of the nerve terminal. A small portion of the vesicular pool is released as each nerve action potential arrives along the postganglionic cell axon. The released NE interacts with specific receptors on the dilator muscle membrane causing a contraction. As in other adrenergic systems, the effect of the released transmitter is terminated by a metabolically active reuptake from the neuromuscular junction into the postganglionic nerve terminals. Cocaine exerts its primary effect by *blocking reuptake* at this stage. This potentiates pupil dilator tone due to ongoing tonic neural activity and neurotransmitter release in the ocular sympathetic efferents. Failure of this potentiation in the presence of ocular sympathetic lesions at all levels is useful evidence for Horner's syndrome. The reason that cocaine fails to dilate pupils with central and preganglionic sympathetic dysfunction is related presumably to the fact that the tonic release of NE at the postganglionic terminal is reduced, even with these proximal lesions, so that the blockage of NE reuptake has little effect compared to the normal other eye. A positive cocaine test is defined as failure of the pupil to dilate on the side of the lesion with dilatation of the fellow pupil, which is used as an internal control. Cocaine is a weak dilator, thus if neither pupil enlarges, the test must be considered uninterpretable and should be ignored.

Para-OH-amphetamine not only blocks reuptake of naturally released NE but promotes the release of any stored NE from the postganglionic axon terminals into the neuromuscular junctions at the iris dilator muscles. This means that regardless of the level of ongoing neural activity in the system, if the postganglionic cell and its terminals at the dilator muscles are intact, para-OH-amphetamine will release the stored NE and will then block its reuptake, both of which bring about pupillary dilatation. Para-OH-amphetamine, unlike cocaine, will thus dilate the pupil in the presence of both central and preganglionic Horner's syndrome. Only a pupil with the loss of postganglionic sympathetic fibers and the stored NE at their terminals will fail to dilate in response to para-OH-amphetamine. This is the basis of the localizing value of the para-OH-amphetamine test (Fig. 22-13). It is used primarily to differentiate postganglionic lesions (pupil will not dilate) from preganglionic lesions (pupil will dilate), because central lesions are usually not a problem for localizing diagnosis on account of the associated neurologic findings. Obviously, one must be sure that an ocular sympathetic lesion exists before using par-OH-amphetamine because this test will "miss" the central and preganglionic lesions by shortcircuiting the neural chain and causing release of the NE stored at the postganglionic terminal, even though the level of spontaneous release was diminished because of the more proximal lesion. Para-OH-amphetamine should, therefore, be reserved for the localization of an ocular sympathetic lesion and not for the identification of the lesion. An exception may be a case in which one suspects only a postganglionic deficit, as for instance in a patient with orbital pain plus ptosis and meiosis. A note of caution is in order at this point. Some patients have pain in the orbit ipsilateral to *preganglionic* ocular sympathetic lesions caused by trauma in the neck. The pathogenesis of this condition is obscure, but it often responds favorably to propranolol (Inderal) with relief of pain. The important point for this discussion is that one should not conclude *a priori* that the sympathetic lesion is postganglionic because of concomitant orbital pain or frontotemporal headaches. If the para-OH-amphetamine test is negative, a cocaine test should be done on another day.

The para-OH-amphetamine and cocaine tests should be done prior to any manipulations that might disrupt the corneal epithelium, because any breach of corneal integrity can lead to an unequal drug absorption in the two eyes and false-positive or false-negative test results. Thus, corneal reflex testing, ocular pressure measurements (tonometers usually operate through pressure on the cornea), and use of any other topical ophthalmic agents should be done on a separate day, or at least after the completion of sympathetic testing. The usual protocol is instillation of one drop of either *cocaine 10% solution* or *para-OH-amphetamine 1% solution* in each eye with a second dose 10 minutes later. The pupil size in standard dim illumination is measured before the first drop and 60 minutes after this dose. An increase in the amount of anisocoria is a positive test result. In other words, selective failure of the involved pupil to dilate *as much as* the normal eye after an adequate interval is the criterion for a positive test.

Determining the Age of the Lesion

Since malignant disease is such a prominent feature of recently acquired preganglionic ocular sympathetic lesions, it can be helpful to document that a newly observed Horner's syndrome is actually of long standing so that an extensive work-up for carcinoma can be avoided. The history is usually not helpful, since most patients are unaware of the lesion. The best way to prove that the lesion is not new is to inspect old photographs, which might reveal the ptosis and perhaps even anisocoria.

If the iris of the eye with Horner's syndrome is blue and the other is brown, one can establish that the lesion was probably present at birth, or at least during the first year of life. A sympathetic lesion, if present early in life, prevents the development of ipsilateral iris chromatophores in a person who is genetically destined to have brown eyes. This condition is known as *heterochromia iridis*. The lesion will not be manifest if both eyes are blue.

ARGYLL–ROBERTSON PUPIL

A good deal of confusion literature has accumulated concerning the pupillary manifestations of CNS syphilis, most notably that pertaining to the so-called Argyll–Robertson pupillary phenomenon. The original report by Argyll–Robertson appeared in 1896 under the title: *Four Cases of Spinal Myosis; with Remarks on the Action of Light on the Pupil.* The thrust of the report centered on the association between spinal cord disease and the peculiar observation of very small pupils that failed to constrict to light but were still capable of response on *near viewing effort.* Argyll–Robertson noted that although most of the patients had ophthalmoscopic evidence of mild optic atrophy, their vision was not significantly impaired. That is, of course, crucial because a person who is blind from optic nerve disease will have pupils that do not respond to light, but which constrict normally to near effort. In this setting, a dissociation between the light and near responses would have no specificity in itself. The differential diagnosis would simply be that of the optic neuropathy. Argyll Robertson was puzzled by the meiosis that he felt must have been caused by an involvement of the ciliospinal nerves by the spinal disease. When this classic observation was first made there was no serologic or other method by which the spinal disease could be ascribed to neurosyphilis. In fact, syphilis was not mentioned in the discussion, and only one of the four cases was noted to have previously had syphilis.

In subsequent years, the link between "locomotor ataxia," now called *tabes dorsalis*, and syphilis came to be well recognized and Argyll–Robertson's sign attained common usage as a powerful diagnostic sign of neurosyphilis. It was noted to be present in 60% to 84% of tabetics and in up to 50% of patients with dementia paralytica or general paresis of the insane.

Much controversy has occurred concerning whether the *meiosis* should be considered essential to the definition of the Argyll–Robertson pupil.

The problem arose with the observation that diseases other than syphilis can be associated with pupils that are fixed to light, but which constrict on near effort in patients with normal vision. This has been reported in a wide variety of disorders, including difficult-to-understand entities such as alcoholism, myotonic dystrophy, and diabetes mellitus. The phenomenon seems easier to accept as specific for the disorder when linked with mid-brain lesions such as infarcts, hemorrhages, tumors, and encephalitis lethargica, all of which can produce destructive lesions in parts of the brain stem and spinal cord that are known to participate in pupil function. Most of these nonsyphilitic light-near dissociated pupils "or" Argyll–Robertson-like pupils are not meiotic, being of average size or larger, and this serves to distinguish the syphilitic from the nonsyphilitic cases. It would certainly be a wonderful universe if a differential diagnosis could be so simple and reliable! Irene Lowenfeld has shown by an exhaustive review of the literature and by extensive personal observations that the absolute size of the pupil does not definitely discriminate between syphilic and nonsyphilitic Argyll–Robertson pupils. Lawton Smith has shown that moderately large light-near dissociated pupils occur in many tabetics and paretics, thus one cannot rule out syphilis in this setting if a work-up fails to reveal an alternative cause. Fortunately, the situation is rendered somewhat academic by the availability of reliable and sensitive serologic markers for past syphilitic infection (*e.g.*, FTA-Abs and others), tests that usually remain positive for the life of the patient.

The anatomic pathology leading to the Argyll–Robertson pupillary phenomenon must still be considered problematic. It is difficult to imagine a single locus in the nervous system at which the afferents from the retina to the pupillomotor centers (midbrain tectum and Edinger–Westphal nucleus) would be involved together with fibers or centers that oppose the mydriatic tone of the sympathetic system. Kerr (1968) reviewed pathologic studies indicating that syphilis tends to produce a superficial demyelination, or *subpial encephalopathy* throughout the neuraxis. He postulated that, in neurosyphilis, subpial demyelination of the superficial pretectal area would affect the light reaction, whereas lesions of the lateral columns just under the pia at the cervical level could produce meiosis by interfering with the descending central sympathetic pathways, the combined lesions resulting in the full Argyll–Robertson syndrome.

In summary, the Argyll–Robertson pupil sign is manifest as a variable meiosis, but more crucially by fixity of the pupil to light stimulation with preserved ability to constrict on near-viewing effort (accommodation) in a patient with normal or near-normal vision. This is most commonly bilateral but may be unilateral when first observed, often becoming bilateral as months or years pass. The phenomenon is frequently associated with neurosyphilis, particularly tabes dorsalis and general paresis, but may occur with all sorts of destructive lesions, suitably situated. Observation of the Argyll–Robertson pupil in a patient should first prompt a serologic investigation and an appropriate history to establish or preclude past syphylitic infection. If such infection can be ruled out, a workup for structural lesions, in particular at the midbrain or diencephalic area, should be undertaken.

OCULAR MOTILITY IN NEUROLOGIC DIAGNOSIS

The importance of eye movements for daily visual activity is perhaps intuitively obvious. Humans are "foveate" animals, meaning that their sharp or high-resolution vision resides in a small area (2° to 3°) of visual field surrounding the fixation point. The *fixation point* can best be defined as the point in external space at which one is looking. The *object of regard* is then projected on the *fovea centralis* of the retina, where high-resolution vision is served. Perception is acute outside of the central few degrees of field *motion*; however, the resolution of fine spatial details declines rapidly toward the periphery. In order to adequately perceive an extended visual scene (as in daily viewing), therefore, one must "palpate" the environment by moving the fovea from point to point while compiling and storing a central image or engram of the scene. Accordingly, the eye movement system has developed in close association with the sensory or afferent visual system. This is reflected in the anatomy of the ocular motor system, particularly at the cerebral hemisphere level, where major intra- and interhemispheric connections link the so-called *frontal eye fields* (area 8 of Brodmann, just anterior to the primary motor strip) with occipital visual centers. This is of practical significance, because lesions in the cerebral hemispheres often produce a diagnostically useful alteration of ocular motility.

We will begin our survey with the *supranuclear* organization of eye movement and then discuss the *final common pathway* for the accomplishment of eye movements—the third, fourth, and sixth) cranial nerves, including their nuclei in the brain stem and their connections with the individual extraocular muscles. The emphasis of this review is on the *supranuclear* organization, because this area is rich in diagnostically useful signs that are only beginning to be outlined in medical textbooks. The characteristics of third, fourth, and sixth cranial nerve lesions and of primary disorders of the eye muscles are also discussed.

SUPRANUCLEAR ORGANIZATION OF EYE MOVEMENTS

FUNCTIONAL ORGANIZATION

As indicated in the preceding discussion, it is important to bring images of objects in the visual environment onto the retinal fovea where a clear neural representation can be generated. This process of *foveation* is the central issue for the various supranuclear eye movement control systems. In general terms, one must be able to move the eye so as to bring the image of the *object of regard* onto the fovea and then keep it there despite both object movement in space and head movement—these are unavoidable conditions of daily viewing. The control networks that serve these functions are the saccade system, the pursuit system, and the vestibulo-ocular system, each with a specific anatomic arrangement in the cerebral hemispheres, brain stem, and cerebellum.

All of the supranuclear systems are concerned with *conjugate* eye movements, meaning that the visual axes of the two eyes remain parallel during the movement. Dysconjugate eye movements indicate a disorder at or below (peripheral to) the third, fourth and sixth cranial nerve nuclei, or the pathways joining these nuclei.

Saccade System

The saccade system generates high-velocity ballistic movements, or *saccades*, by which we foveate the elements of a stationary but large or extended visual scene. An adult scans a scene in a highly organized way, extracting data from the highest information areas but directing relatively few saccades to nonspecific or uninformative areas in the display. This efficient palpatory behavior is highly learned: It develops progressively during infancy. The efficiency of ocular scanning is often degraded in the presence of cerebral lesions, particularly those associated with dementia, but this type of eye movement alteration is not accessible to bedside examination. It requires elaborate equipment to record exactly where on a visual scene the eyes are fixed at any particular time. Obviously, this type of ocular motor behavior has organizational elements that encompass the highest levels of whole brain function. We will focus, however, on the motor aspects alone, because they can be observed directly at the bedside.

Lesions in the frontal lobes most commonly interrupt saccade function selectively. The system is represented also at the brain-stem level where "burst" cells deliver high levels of innervation to oculomotor neurons and produce the high-velocity eye movements characteristic of saccades. The cerebellum also participates in the saccade system: Lesions here are associated with abnormal saccade characteristics such as low velocity or altered metrics (both overshoot and undershoot).

The parameters by which we can measure saccadic eye movement performance include *latency*, *velocity*, and *metrics* or *accuracy*.

The average normal human being takes about 200 msec to generate a refixation eye movement or saccade to a new target presented in his visual periphery. The time required for each saccade varies widely, but most saccades occur between 180 and 250 msec. This latent interval includes time for the visual stimulus in the peripheral field to travel along afferent pathways to the cerebral cortex where the spatial coordinates of the object to be foveated are turned into motor commands or vectors that have both direction and amplitude specifications. This computation of vectors and passage of the efferent commands to the brain stem require additional time. It has also been postulated that the system works by way of intermittent data samples rather than a continuous intake of afferent data. Thus, if a novel visual stimulus occurs just after a sample is taken, it will have to wait for the next sampling interval, which may be 40 to 50 msec later, before entry into the system. This would explain much of the latency variability observed for the generation of individual saccades. The real story is much more complex, however, and there is considerable controversy as to whether saccade vectors are calculated in an intermittent or continuous sampling way. It is also unclear at present whether saccade motor com-

mands can be modified as the eyes are in motion during a saccade. Under ordinary circumstances saccades behave as a *ballistic* movement—as with a thrown ball, the saccade trajectory is not modifiable after the movement begins. Under special test circumstances, however, some individuals are capable of modifying the saccade trajectory in midflight. These special features of some saccades in normal patients have not yet been adequately explained by existing models of brain-stem circuitry.

Saccades have characteristic peak velocities that bear a direct relationship to the size of the eye movement in normal persons. Larger saccades are faster than smaller ones, but it is impossible to perceive these subtle velocity variations by direct observation of the eyes in flight. Fortunately for diagnosis, pathology in the saccade system often slows refixational eye movements sufficiently that the movements are easily perceived as slow by direct inspection. The best way to observe this is by asking the patient to redirect his gaze to stationary points right and left of primary gaze. A major reduction in saccade velocity generally indicates cerebellar or brain-stem disorders, although minor slowing that usually requires electronic eye movement measurement to document can accompany cerebral hemisphere pathology, particularly if it involves the frontal lobes.

Another aspect of saccade abnormality is *dysmetria*, in which there is an altered excursion amplitude—the eyes either fall short of their goal (*hypometric saccades*) or overshoot the target (*hypermetric saccades*). When saccades are hypometric, the eyes achieve the target by a series of small saccades (usually three or more). This gives the movement a "jerky" or ratchet-like quality that is easily observed. It is useful to count the number of saccades necessary for the eyes to achieve a target 25° or 30° to either side of center (*primary gaze*). Normal persons often require two and occasionally three saccades, but a patient who consistently uses three or more saccades to make a 30° refixation can be considered abnormal. It is easier to be sure that saccade hypometria is significant if the number of saccades used for refixation to one side of primary gaze differs markedly from the number required to make an equal distance excursion to the other side.

Overshoot or *hypermetric* saccades are also easily observed. The eyes overshoot and attain the target by way of a series of decreasing amplitude reversals, each of which overshoots to a smaller degree than the preceding one. Each corrective saccade is separated from the last by the normal obligatory intersaccadic interval of approximately 200 msec. This gives the movement a discontinuous quality as opposed to a smooth to-and-fro pendular appearance.

In the acute stages of vascular lesions—infarctions or hemorrhages—of one frontal lobe, the eyes are usually deviated tonically to the side of the lesion because of the suddenly unopposed tonic influence of the normal hemisphere. It can be deduced from this that the normal tonus of a particular hemisphere, and perhaps of the frontal eye field specifically, brings about contralateral eye movements. This *contraversive* functional orientation is also observed in the disordered saccadic behavior that accompanies chronic frontal lobe lesions. In these cases, after the tonic eye deviation of the acute stage wears off and the patient is able to deviate the eyes fully in both directions, there remains a subtle disorder in which saccades directed away from the side of the lesion are *hypometric*. As an example, a patient with right frontal lobe infarction will have trouble looking volitionally to the left. During the first 4 or 5 days after the acute event, his eyes may be strongly deviated to the right, sometimes along with a forceful head and even torso deviation in the same direction. He will gradually be able to direct his gaze further to the left, and finally, full deviation will be possible. He may also require an abnormally long latency before initiating leftward eye movements during the acute stages. This directional latency effect must be distinguished from bidirectional increased latency, which may represent an altered mental function rather than a specific disorder of the saccade system. In the chronic stages of this right hemisphere vascular lesion, leftward refixations may continue to evoke numerous hypometric saccades, while normometric single saccades are generated for rightward refixations.

This contraversive organization is peculiar to the saccade system, because the *pursuit* system operates in an *ipsiversive* mode, controlling eye movements toward the hemisphere that is active. This fact of opposing functional orientation in the saccade and pursuit systems at the cerebral hemisphere level greatly enhances the diagnostic usefulness of eye signs related to these subsystems.

Pursuit System

The task of the pursuit system is the maintenance of a target on the fovea with motion of the target in space. If the viewer's head remains stationary, the tracking of a moving target is achieved by matching the angular velocity of the eyes turning in the orbits to the angular velocity of the target moving across visual space.

The visual system is oriented about the retinas, which are on the spherical back surfaces of the eyes, and angular measurements in degrees or minutes of arc are more convenient than the tangent measure, which would have to include the distance traveled in the frontal plane and the distance of that plane from the viewer in order to define the appropriate pursuit eye movement. The pursuit movement would also be awkward to specify in tangent measure because it involves a rotation about a vertical axis rather than translational movement in a flat plane.

The normal behavior of the pursuit system can be specified as the *gain (G)*:

$$G = I/O$$

I is the input or target velocity in visual space (deg/sec) and **O** is the output, in this case pursuit eye velocity (deg/sec). Normal tracking involves a gain of 1.0 such that the eyes stay on the target as it moves.

The most frequently observed abnormality of pursuit is subnormal gain in which the eyes fall progressively behind the target. The examiner cannot perceive the velocity of a patient's pursuit movements by inspection. Fortunately, the visual system will not tolerate the error that develops as the eyes fall behind the target, and an easily observed saccade is generated as soon as the eye is sufficiently far behind to generate a *position error* signal. Thus, low-gain pursuit is interrupted by a series of *catch-up saccades* aimed at refoveating the target. These inserted saccades occur rhythmically, since it requires about the same amount of time to generate the necessary position error throughout the course of the pursuit movement. Normal pursuit is smooth with no inserted saccades. *Low-gain pursuit is indicated to the observer by the presence of rhythmic saccades rather than the slowness of the pursuit movement itself.*

This pursuit abnormality, which I think is best referred to as *low-gain pursuit with catch-up saccades*, has engendered various descriptive names including *saccadic pursuit*, and even *cogwheel pursuit* in patients with Parkinson's disease. This movement should not, however, be linked to the pathophysiology of parkinsonian cogwheeling. The saccadic pursuit of Parkinsonism is the manifestation of low gain in the pursuit system with a relatively normal saccade function so that forward saccades achieve refoveation during defective tracking. This does not differ from low-grain pursuit in other pathologic conditions.

The pursuit system is highly susceptible to degraded function, and bidirectional low-gain pursuit may be a nonspecific abnormality in various clinical settings in which the finding has no localizing value. Fatigue and the effects of many drugs bring about bidirectional symmetrical low-gain pursuit. Bidirectional low-gain pursuit is common in the elderly and has little prognostic or localizing value.

Unidirectional low-gain pursuit, however, is highly specific for a lesion of the horizontal gaze pathway on one side. The pursuit function in the cerebral hemisphere is *ipsiversive* and a unidirectional defective pursuit suggests a lesion of the parieto-occipital convexity on the side toward which pursuit is low gain, that is, a right-sided posterior hemisphere lesion will cause low-gain pursuit with catch-up saccades rightward, but will leave leftward pursuit unaffected.

Large hemisphere lesions may involve both saccade and pursuit functions, in which case there will be hypometric saccades in one direction (opposite the lesion) and low-gain pursuit in the other (toward the lesion). Low-gain pursuit can also be observed as part of the supranuclear conjugate gaze disorder that accompanies lesions of the rostral pons and midbrain, usually in conjunction with altered saccade parameters, but here the saccades and pursuit are defective in the same direction.

A fundamental distinction must therefore be made between cerebral hemisphere and brain-stem conjugate gaze syndromes. At the cerebral level the direction of the saccade abnormality (contraversive) is opposite to the direction of the pursuit abnormality (ipsiversive), whereas at the brain-stem level both are ipsilateral to the lesion side. Clinical evidence tells us that the saccade control pathways cross somewhere caudal to the diencephalon but rostral to the pons, whereas the pursuit pathways either do not cross at all, or they cross and recross such that their functional direction is ipsilateral to the disordered hemisphere at the brain-stem level. We have published a case in which a small hematoma at the posterior thalamus resulted in contraversive hypometric saccades and ipsiversive low-gain pursuit with catch-up saccades. This indicates that the hemisphere bidirectionality is preserved as far caudal and as deep as the thalamus. This may indicate that the pursuit and saccade pathways both operate by way of the ipsilateral frontal eye field outflow through the thalamus. Alternatively, the pursuit system may have pathways in the corona radiata separate from the saccade system outflow, but these may funnel through the same region in the thalamus as the frontal system. Clinical evidence does not as yet discriminate between these two possibilities. The fact that some frontal lesions are associated with an ipsidirectional pursuit defect in conjunction with a contraversive saccade disorder supports the idea of a pursuit system outflow by way of a common frontothalamic brain-stem pathway. The repeated observation of frontal lesions with isolated contralateral saccade disruption and normal pursuit weigh against a common pathway. Further clinical observations are required to specify more precisely how this might operate.

Saccade *vs* Pursuit Testing

Proper testing means the separate elicitation of saccade and pursuit-type eye movements. The examiner should stand about 1 meter in front of the patient.

Visually guided saccades are tested by asking the patient first to look at the examiner's nose and then to look at an object about 30° to either side of the midline. Appropriately placed objects will be provided if the examiner holds his arms semiextended (elbows about 90° flexed) with hands slightly in front of his own facial plane. The patient should keep his head stationary in a straight-ahead position during this type of testing to avoid introducing vestibulo-ocular components. The patient is asked to refixate his gaze from the examiner's nose to one of his hands, then back to his nose, and finally to his other hand. It is often useful to wiggle the fingers of the hand toward what you want the patient to look at as an added stimulus for a *visually guided* saccade.

The clinical setting sometimes suggests the need to test for saccades without visual targets. This has to do with the ability to imagine coordinates for the saccade system and can be selectively defective in some cases of higher cortical function abnormality with diffuse or widespread lateralized hemisphere lesions. In this case, simply ask the patient to "*look left*" or "*look right*" without providing any target.

A selective examination for *pursuit system* defects involves providing a slowly moving target for the patient to view. One can infer that pursuit function is pathologic if the normally smooth following or pursuit eye movement is interrupted by a series of "jerky" appearing saccades. The target should not be moved too rapidly, since the pursuit system in normal persons falls behind when target velocities reach 40° to 50°/second, producing saccadic pursuit at faster target speeds. A target excursion that carries the patient's eyes from extreme right to extreme left gaze should take about 5 seconds.

Vestibulo-ocular System

The vestibulo-ocular system maintains the fixation of objects in visual space in the presence of head movement. The afferent arm of this reflex is initiated by acceleration receptors in the inner ear. A mathematical *integration* is performed on the acceleration data by virtue of the mechanics of the semicircular canal and cupula, and information on *head rotational velocity* in space is supplied to the vestibular nuclei by way of the eighth cranial nerve. The information is relayed from there to the brain-stem gaze centers, where slow eye movements with velocity equal to and direction opposite head rotation are generated. For instance, if the head rotates rightward at 10°/second, there is a leftward eye movement at 10°/second, thus the external world remains fixed on the fovea. The operation of this system, like that of the pursuit system, is conveniently expressed as "*gain*," that is, eye movement velocity divided by head rotation velocity in degrees per second. Naturally, a gain of 1.0 is needed to maintain foveation with head rotation. It turns out, however, that the vestibulo-ocular reflex does not supply the entire eye movement drive, since in total darkness the gain of this system falls to about 0.6 in normal persons. This means that the vestibulo-ocular reflex normally works together with the pursuit system, which optimizes function, since the vestibuloocular reflex has no retinal feedback by which to monitor its performance and keep its output accurate. Any inappropriate velocity drive from this "open loop" vestibulo-ocular system is adjusted by the "closed-loop" pursuit system, which receives direct retinal afferent feedback for fine control of the foveal position on the visual environment.

The key symptom of pathologic underactivity in the vestibulo-ocular reflex is *oscillopsia*, which is an illusory sense of movement in the visual environment as the head moves. This is a direct consequence of foveal slippage engendered specifically by head movement. The illusion ceases when the head is immobile. Vertigo, another common symptom of vestibular disorders, is often present when the head is still, although it is usually aggravated by head movement. Vertigo is a rotational illusion that is often accompanied by rhythmic oscillopsia as a consequence of nystagmus, in which case the rhythm is probably imposed by the regular fast phases of the nystagmus.

Nystagmus is defined as a repetitive bidirectional or multidirectional ocular oscillation in which the slow-phase movement is the pathologic one. When caused by vestibular disease, the nystagmus is created by tonic imbalance or *bias* in the vestibular subsystems on either side of midline, including the central connections and the peripheral labyrinthine apparatus. Tonic vestibular system imbalance passes a tonic directional bias to the brain-stem gaze centers, which causes the eyes to drift toward the side with reduced activity. The tonic influence of each side is *contraversive* and a lesion creates underactivity of the ipsilateral system, with relative overactivity of the opposite system. The unopposed contraversive tone of the system opposite the lesion imposes eye drift toward the lesion side. This drift is checked by rhythmically occurring saccades in the opposite direction. The ensemble effect is rhythmic jerk-type nystagmus with slow-phase movements toward the side with the lesion and fast phases away from the lesion. This nystagmus is *rhythmic* because the slow phase drift is constant velocity, determined by the degree of bias or imbalance between the two lateral vestibular subsystems, and the corrective saccades occur whenever a certain fixed amount of retinal position error between the object of regard and fovea occurs.

The vestibular disorders are discussed in other chapters. This discussion is meant to provide the basis for understanding the more important ocular motility aspects of vestibular function.

BRAIN-STEM ORGANIZATION OF EYE MOVEMENT CONTROL: THE FINAL COMMON PATHWAY

Zones within the tegmental reticular formation in the brain stem serve to combine the various eye movement commands and to present an integrated set of final motor commands to the ocular motor nuclei. The *pontine paramedian reticular formation (PPRF)* refers to the zone surrounding the seventh nerve nucleus on either side of midline in the pontine tegmentum. This area is specialized for integration of horizontal eye movement commands. The *rostral interstitial nucleus of the medial longitudinal fasciculus (riMLF)*, the *interstitial nucleus of Cajal (iC)*, the *nucleus of Darkschewitsch (nD)*, the *nucleus of the posterior commissure (nPC)*, and the adjacent portions of the *mesencephalic reticular formation* probably perform similar integration of commands for vertical eye movement and pass the final innervation pattern to the nuclei of the third and fourth cranial nerves.

Commands for saccades and pursuit come down to the brain stem by way of the supranuclear eye movement pathways outlined above. In addition, the vestibular nuclei in the medulla and the flocculi and noduli of the cerebellum provide vestibular inputs to both the horizontal eye movement system in the PPRF and to the vertical eye movement zones of the mesencephalic reticular formation, primarily the riMLF and iC.

VERTICAL GAZE

The organization of the vertical eye movement system is complex and is not completely understood. The riMLF appears to contain primarily burst neurons that generate vertical saccades, whereas cells of iC, nD, nPC, and MRF carry the fully assembled burst-tonic firing pattern needed to perform saccades, and pursuit and vestibulo-ocular movements, and to hold the eyes in eccentric positions of gaze. Nuclei at the pontine and medullary levels are important in the control of vertical eye movements. Bilateral lesions of the *medial longitudinal fasciculus* (MLF), which carries complex ascending influences from vestibular nuclei and PPRF gaze centers, abolish vertical pursuit and vestibulo-ocular reflex movements but spare saccades. Thus, the riMLF apparently has functional connections with the cerebral hemispheres independent of supranuclear pathways that operate by way of the PPRF. Although vertical saccades are spared with bilateral lesions of the ascending pathways, the eye position signal is abolished and gaze paretic nystagmus occurs with up and down gaze effort.

For all practical purposes there are no clinical disorders in which vertical gaze palsy is caused by cerebral hemisphere disease. Brain-stem structures classically thought to mediate vertical gaze are situated in the midbrain tectum and pretectal areas. In this region, lesions commonly cause upward and downward gaze palsies along with certain other classic features, the constellation of which constitute the *midbrain pretectal syndrome*, also referred to as the *periaqueductal gray matter syndrome*, or *Parinaud's syndrome*. It is sometimes referred to as the *syndrome of Koerber and Salus*, who documented similar findings in a patient with a mass lesion in the sylvian aqueduct itself, whereas Parinaud described the findings related to pinealomas compressing the midbrain pretectum from the outside. The same clinical constellation results from infarction and hemorrhage involving these same anatomic structures as intrinsic lesions. The syndrome to be described is, therefore, of localizing value but does not provide evidence for a specific etiology in a particular case. For this, the tempo of evolution and the regression of signs and symptoms, along with other clinical details, are needed.

Aside from vertical gaze palsy, the common features of midbrain pretectal lesions include pupillary paralysis with unequal pupils that are sometimes large and sometimes small, convergence–retraction nystagmus, and variable degrees of ptosis or pathologic lid retraction. Retractory nystagmus is characterized by rhythmic backward movement of the globes into the orbits in a nystagmus-like cycle.

In conjunction with globe retraction there may be convergence movements of the two eyes with respect to one another. This constitutes the classic convergence–retraction nystagmus of midbrain pretectal lesions.

HORIZONTAL GAZE

Efferents from the PPRF on one side connect with large motor cells in the ipsilateral sixth nerve nucleus for abduction of the ipsilateral eye, and with small cells in the same nucleus which in turn connect by way of the MLF with the opposite medial rectus subnucleus of the third nerve for adduction of the contralateral eye. Thus, a contraversive (opposite direction) saccade command from one hemisphere descends to the opposite side PPRF, then to the abducens nucleus for both abduction of the eye ipsilateral to the active PPRF and adduction of the opposite eye—this produces conjugate gaze contralateral to the hemisphere issuing the command, ipsilateral to the activated PPRF.

Figure 22-14 illustrates schematically the brainstem and hemisphere pathways that participate in conjugate leftward gaze. Beginning at the right cerebral hemisphere, we can follow the path through the deep cerebral white matter and diencephalon to the midbrain, where a proposed crossing occurs just caudal to the third cranial nerve nucleus. This route continues to the PPRF on the left side of the brain stem, probably in the basis pontis. A synapse occurs here with PPRF neurons, which, in turn, make a relay to the ipsilateral sixth cranial nerve nucleus. Activation of the sixth nerve (abducens) nucleus causes abduction of the left eye. It is clear that conjugate leftward gaze will require coordinated adduction of the right eye, thus the next step is a requisite connection between the small cell population of the left abducens nucleus and the right third cranial nerve nucleus, specifically the medial rectus subnucleus. This connection is served by a paired bundle of fibers that run throughout the

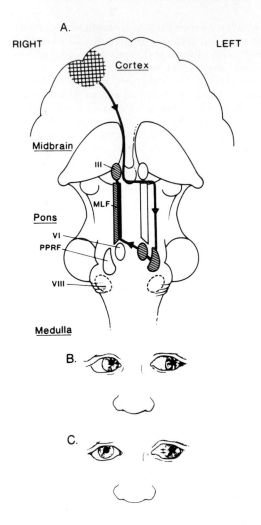

brain stem dorsally and just on either side of midline: the MLF.

These multidirectional systems are admittedly difficult to follow; however, it will make more sense if you trace the steps carefully from level to level and you work out the directions for yourself.

MEDIAL LONGITUDINAL FASCICULUS AND "INTERNUCLEAR OPHTHALMOPLEGIA"

Up to this point our discussion has concerned only disorders that bring about *conjugate* disorders of gaze; that is, if one eye fails to deviate leftward, the other eye also fails in the same direction and to an equal degree. Thus, the eyes in all these lesions remain *"straight"* with parallel visual axes when viewing objects at a distance. For simplicity we will ignore the case of near-object viewing with convergence of the visual axes, because it is irrelevant for most neurologic diagnoses. After the supranuclear organizational systems supply input to the PPRF for horizontal eye deviation, the neural information must be conveyed to the motor nuclei of the third cranial nerve (medial rectus subgroup for adduction) and the sixth nerve (lateral rectus nucleus for abduction) as outlined above. This relay is performed by the MLF, and lesions of this *internuclear* connection cause *internuclear ophthalmoplegia (INO)*.

Lesions affecting the MLF cause failure of the adducting eye to move, whereas the abducting eye deviates laterally to its full extent. This striking pattern of dysconjugate eye movement is called *internuclear ophthalmoplegia* because the lesion in effect disconnects the sixth and the third cranial nerve nuclei by causing a failure of neural conduction in the internuclear pathway, the MLF.

In addition to failure of the eye on the side of the MLF lesion to adduct, there is usually "dissociated" monocular nystagmus of the abducting other eye in cases of INO. This peculiar monocular nystagmus can be either transitory (one or two beats) or sustained. The clinical importance of diagnosing the MLF syndrome is its exquisite localizing value for lesions deep in the substance of the brain-stem tegmentum. This general area in the brain stem contains the ascending reticular activating system,

FIG. 22-14. (*A*) Semischematic diagram of the brain-stem pathways and centers that serve horizontal conjugate gaze. Multisynaptic pathways from the right frontal cortex decussate in the midbrain and form synapses in the left *pontine paramedian reticular formation (PPRF)*, which relays innervation to two cell populations within the sixth cranial nerve nucleus. The large cells in the nucleus send axons to the lateral rectus muscle to abduct the left eye. The small cell population gives rise to a pathway that decussates and ascends in the contralateral *medial longitudinal fasciculus (MLF)* and makes synaptic contact with cells of the medial rectus subnucleus of the third cranial nerve complex. This pathway gives rise to coordinated adduc-

tion of the right eye to complete the act of conjugate leftward gaze as illustrated in *B*. A lesion in the MLF causes *internuclear ophthalmoplegia*, which is characterized by a failure of adduction of the ipsilateral eye during attempted conjugate gaze as illustrated in *C*. The abducting eye often manifests dissociated or monocular nystagmus.

which is necessary for alert consciousness, along with several adjacent cranial nerve nuclei and various ascending and descending sensory and cerebellar pathways. Therefore, the isolated occurrence of an MLF syndrome in an alert individual without other brain-stem signs or symptoms suggests the presence of a discrete lesion. For practical purposes in the adult this is caused by either small *demyelinating plaques* of multiple sclerosis or by tiny *infarctions* due to small vessel disease, which occur mainly in hypertensive patients past 60 years of age, the *lacune*. An MLF syndrome is occasionally encountered as a result of trauma, and in children it can be the first sign of a brain-stem glioma (astrocytoma).

Differentiating between multiple sclerosis and lacunar infarction can be a problem, because in either, the lesions tend to evolve acutely or subacutely and then resolve slowly over a period of days or weeks. Some generalizations can be helpful, however. The patient with an MLF lesion caused by multiple sclerosis will most often be less than 40 years of age, whereas the group at risk for lacunae are generally over 60 years of age. It has been said that a bilateral MLF lesion favors multiple sclerosis, because there is nothing to limit a plaque at the anatomic midline, whereas vascular lesions are often limited to one side by the margins of the vascular territory of a particular paramedian penetrating branch of the basilar artery.

The clinical appearance of internuclear ophthalmoplegia can be mimicked in most details by myasthenia gravis. There are certain patients with this condition in whom there is a failure of adduction in one eye with dissociated nystagmus of the other eye. It is theoretically interesting that the dissociated, unilateral nystagmus of internuclear ophthalmoplegia is also present in myasthenia, which is, of course, a peripheral disorder. The mechanisms that cause the dissociated nystagmus in MLF lesions are not understood. The practical offshoot is that any patient presenting purely with findings of an MLF lesion, either unilateral or bilateral, without other brain-stem signs or symptoms should have an edrophonium chloride (Tensilon) test as part of the work-up. If the disorder of eye motility is caused by myasthenia, it will clear dramatically during the time the edrophonium chloride is in effect.

EYE MOVEMENT DISORDERS WITH NUCLEAR AND INFRANUCLEAR LESIONS

Lesions of the oculomotor (third), trochlear (fourth), and abducens (sixth) nerve nuclei and

their outflow pathways produce disconjugate eye movements. The pattern of movement disorder is highly characteristic of the cranial nerve involved and serves to localize the disorder. The medial recti cause adduction of the eye, whereas the lateral recti cause abduction or outward rotation of the eye. The anatomy and physiology of the vertically acting muscles are more complicated.

Elevation and *depression* are the terms applied to upward and downward rotations of the eyes about a horizontal axis. The term *torsion* has been applied to rotation of the globe about an anteroposterior axis. *Intorsion* refers to the rotation of the 12:00 meridian of the iris inward, toward the nose, and *extorsion* refers to the rotation of this reference point outward toward the ear. The names *incyclodeviation* and *excyclodeviation* have also been applied to torsional movements.

The superior and inferior recti function, respectively, as elevators and depressors of the globe when the eye is in abduction. The inferior and superior obliques serve as respective elevators and depressors when the eye is in adduction. The torsional component for each of these muscles comes into play when the optical axis is not in alignment with the axis of pull for the particular muscle (Table 22-1).

THIRD CRANIAL NERVE PALSIES

The third cranial nerve innervates the medial rectus, superior rectus, and inferior oblique muscles, along with the pupil sphincter and the levator palpebrae that elevates the upper eyelid. The third nerve originates in a rostrocaudally elongated group of subnuclei clustered in the midbrain just rostral to the level of the fourth cranial nerve nucleus. The architecture of this nuclear group has been the subject of intensive study over the years. The most widely accepted anatomic scheme is that of Warwick, which is represented in a stylized view in Figure 22-15. Warwick conceived of the subnuclei as col-

TABLE 22-1. Muscle Action by Position

MUSCLE	POSITION	
	Adduction	*Abduction*
Superior rectus	Intorsion	Elevation
Inferior rectus	Extorsion	Depression
Inferior oblique	Elevation	Extorsion
Superior oblique	Depression	Intorsion

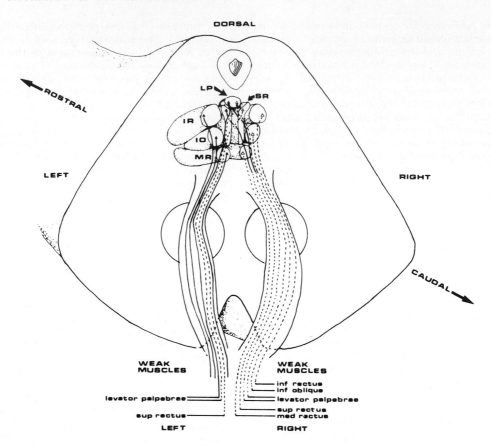

DORSAL

ROSTRAL

LP   SR

IR

IO

MR

LEFT   RIGHT

CAUDAL

WEAK
MUSCLES

WEAK
MUSCLES

inf rectus
inf oblique
levator palpebrae
levator palpebrae
sup rectus
med rectus
sup rectus

LEFT   RIGHT

FIG. 22-15. A cross section through the midbrain showing the third cranial nerve nuclear complex. The subnuclei extend in rostrocaudally oriented columns as depicted in this three-dimensional representation modeled on Warwick's schemata. The letters superimposed on each nuclear group indicate the muscle innervated as follows: LP—levator palpebrae; SR—superior rectus; IR—inferior rectus; IO—inferior oblique; MR—medial rectus. A right *nuclear* third nerve lesion is illustrated. Open triangles and dotted lines indicate lesioned neurons and their axons. Filled triangles and solid lines denote normal neurons and their axons. All of the outflow to the right third nerve is lesioned. Crossed outflow from the right SR and LP subnuclei gives rise to paresis of contralateral eye elevation and ptosis. The left ptosis is partial since there is still ipsilateral (uncrossed) outflow from left LP subnucleus to the left LP. The crossed pathway from left LP subnucleus to right LP is affected at the axonal level as the fibers course through the damaged right third nerve complex (transition of solid lines to dotted), thus right ptosis is complete. The contralateral elevator palsy and ptosis thus distinguish *nuclear* nerve palsy from *fascicular* palsy in which the findings are limited to the ipsilateral eye.

umns of cells in elongated arrangement along the rostrocaudal dimension. Axons from the more dorsally situated subnuclei pass through the middle and inferior columns of cells on their way to the point of exit from the ventral aspect of the midbrain near the cerebral peduncles. The nuclei for the inferior rectus, inferior oblique, and medial rectus muscles send axons only to the ipsilateral third cranial nerve. The subnucleus for the levator palpebrae (caudal central nucleus) is a midline structure and sends axons to both nerves. The superior rectus subnucleus sends axons only to the contralateral third nerve trunk. These anatomic details lead to clinical rules by which one can determine whether a lesion is in the third nerve trunk or at the level of the nucleus. Figure 22-15 is set up to illustrate the effects of a right third nerve nuclear lesion. The filled triangles and solid lines indicate uninterrupted neurons from the left subnuclei. The open triangles and dotted lines represent neurons that are affected by the lesion in the right third nerve nucleus. Lesioned neurons include those with cell body damage in the affected nucleus, and others with damage primarily to the axons as they pass through the lesioned nucleus. Note that with destruction limited to the right side of the nucleus, there is a complete disruption of outflow to the right third cranial nerve. In addition, fibers coming from the *left* superior rectus and levator palpebrae subnuclei are shown as solid lines changing to dotted lines indicating axonal disruption as they pass through the right-sided lesion. This is a necessary consequence of the fact that fibers flow through the other nuclear subgroups and are almost always involved in clinical lesions such as infarction or hemorrhage limited to one side. There is also a disruption of fibers crossing the midline from the defective right side to the left third cranial nerve trunk. These fibers serve the levator palpebrae (bilateral outflow) and the superior rectus (contralateral outflow) muscles on the left. This leads to the rule that nuclear lesions on one side cause partial bilateral ptosis and failure of elevation of both eyes. The contralateral ptosis is usually incomplete because there are some intact fibers to the levator contralateral to the nuclear lesion supplied by noncrossing neurons in the normal side of the caudal central nucleus.

Nuclear lesions are caused primarily by small infarctions secondary to occlusion of the medial penetrating vessels from the basilar artery. On rare occasions small hemorrhages in this area may cause nuclear third cranial nerve palsies. More ventral lesions in the brain-stem substance may cause a disruption of the *fibers* emerging from the third cranial nerve nuclei along with contralateral hemiplegia caused by the involvement of the cerebral peduncle (Weber's syndrome). The characteristics of these *fascicular* third nerve lesions are the same as any distal lesion, affecting only the axons of one nerve.

An important third nerve lesion is caused by aneurysms of the posterior communicating artery that involve the nerve trunk as it passes near this vessel at its junction with the supraclinoid portion of the internal carotid artery near the cavernous sinus. Figure 22-11 illustrates semidiagrammatically the anatomy of the third nerve course in relation to the posterior cerebral artery, the superior cerebellar artery, and the posterior communicating artery. This figure illustrates an aneurysm of the posterior communicating artery at its origin from the internal carotid. The inset shows an aneurysm in cross section with its relationship to the adjacent third cranial nerve. The pupillary fibers from the Edinger–Westphal subnucleus are shown as a black band at the periphery of the nerve. The fact that aneurysms commonly produce dilatation of the pupil on the side of the third nerve lesion was discussed previously. Figure 22-11 shows that the right eye is slightly abducted and depressed on account of a weakness of the medial rectus, superior rectus, and inferior oblique muscles, with unopposed tone in the lateral rectus and superior oblique muscles.

The third nerve is often involved in lesions of the cavernous sinuses, commonly in conjunction with the other cranial nerves that pass in this structure, namely the fourth (trochlear), the sixth (abducens), and the first two divisions of the fifth (trigeminal). The most commonly encountered lesions in this area are inflammatory diseases of unknown etiology, aneurysms of the subclinoid internal carotid artery, and tumors. Granulomatous or primarily lymphocytic inflammation in the cavernous sinus and superior orbital fissure is known as the *Tolosa–Hunt syndrome*. It is manifest primarily by *painful ophthalmoplegia* and nearly always improves with steroid treatment. This relatively benign inflammatory disease must be distinguished, however, from other infiltrating lesions such as lymphomas and carcinomas, which may also respond transiently to steroid administration. Meningiomas of the medial sphenoid ridge and pituitary tumors expanding laterally from the sella can also involve the cranial nerves within the cavernous sinuses. Mucocele of the sphenoid and ethmoid sinuses can, on rare occasions, also present in this way.

The subject of "medical" third cranial nerve palsy, referring to a microvascular occlusion with infarction in the nerve trunk has already been discussed in the pupil section. Since the infarction is often limited to the center of the nerve and the pupillary fibers occupy the periphery, the rule for diagnosis of this type of lesion is *sparing of the pupil*.

FOURTH CRANIAL NERVE PALSIES

The trochlear nerve innervates the superior oblique muscle. Lesions affecting this cranial nerve produce a failure of the eye to depress in adduction with consequent vertical diplopia. With a right fourth cranial nerve palsy, the vertical diplopia would typically increase in gaze to the left (adduction of the right eye) and in downward gaze (into the field of action of the superior oblique). Since the superior oblique contributes to intorsional tone in primary gaze, the image from the involved eye is tilted. An astute patient with a right fourth nerve palsy may tell you, for instance, that the false image of a horizontal edge is not only below the image from the left eye but is also tilted with respect to the latter. Some patients develop a habitual head tilt, presumably to compensate for this torsional imbalance. A person with a right fourth cranial nerve palsy would tend to tilt his head to the left to bring the extorted eye back to the vertical position. The sound left eye can then increase its intorsional tone to make the two eyes parallel in the plane of rotation around the optic axis (anteroposterior axis). Since some intorsional tone can be contributed by the superior rectus, this muscle may be called into play to overcome the intorsional weakness caused by the fourth cranial nerve palsy. If, for instance, the examiner tilts the head of a person with right fourth nerve palsy to the right, even more intorsion than normal is required. The superior rectus is recruited in an effort to maximize intorsional power. This causes further inappropriate elevation of the right eye, because the primary effect of superior rectus contraction is an elevation of the eye.

This is the basis for the Bielschowski test for a fourth nerve palsy. The patient is directed to gaze straight ahead, and the head is then tilted to the right and to the left, making sure that there is no vertical deviation away from primary gaze. If the degree of elevation of the eye on the side of the cranial nerve palsy increases as the head is tilted *toward the side of the palsied muscle*, the test is positive.

The fourth cranial nerve is unique in that it exits from the brain stem dorsally and crosses to the other side before encircling the brain stem on the way to the cavernous sinus. This renders it particularly susceptible to trauma in which forces are brought to bear on the dorsal midbrain. This usually occurs in the setting of severe head trauma in which the brain stem is forced downward and is angulated backward by a sudden shift of supratentorial structures. The dorsal midbrain and both fourth nerves are impacted in the crotch of the tentorium cerebelli, and both nerves tend to be contused together. Because of bilateral injury to the ascending reticular formation, the patient is usually unconscious for a protracted period of time after the injury, following which he complains of vertical double vision. On examination, one finds relative elevation of the right eye in left gaze and relative elevation of the left eye in right gaze. This reversal of vertical deviation indicates bilateral fourth cranial nerve palsies.

Unilateral fourth nerve palsy sometimes follows minor head trauma. There is reason to believe that many of these represent "*decompensation*" of long-standing or congenital fourth nerve palsies that were never previously symptomatic. Exactly how this comes about is unclear, but it is important to ask these patients to bring in childhood photographs to search for head tilt that would indicate a congenital condition.

Fourth cranial nerve palsies can occur secondary to intraneuronal microvascular disease as seen in elderly patients, often associated with diabetes and long-standing hypertension. These are presumably similar to the type of third and sixth cranial nerve palsies that one encounters in this same group of patients. The diplopia tends to improve over several weeks or months following the onset. Tumors in the region of the midbrain tectum can also occasionally present with fourth cranial nerve palsies.

SIXTH CRANIAL NERVE PALSIES

The abducens nucleus is medial and dorsal at the pontomedullary juction. Its axons course almost directly ventral and exit from the pons near the midline. The large cells of the abducens nucleus innervate the lateral rectus muscle, while a small cell population innervates the contralateral medial rectus subnucleus of the oculomotor complex (third cranial nerve) by way of the MLF.

The abducens nucleus is activated by input from the ipsilateral PPRF leading to coordinated abduction of the ipsilateral (to the active PPRF) eye and adduction of the contralateral eye; this yoked deviation of both eyes is horizontal *conjugate gaze*.

Figure 22-16 illustrates a patient with weakness

of the right lateral rectus due to a sixth cranial nerve palsy. Note that in primary gaze the eyes are slightly crossed or convergent (esodeviated). This is caused by the unopposed tone of the medial rectus that is acting without the normal tonic innervation of the weak lateral rectus muscle. In left gaze the eyes are parallel, but in right gaze there is a clear-cut failure of right eye abduction. In this case it is the right eye that is deviating inward in primary gaze, and it is the right lateral rectus muscle that is weak. Be aware, however, that in primary gaze the right eye might be used for fixation of the target, with deviation of the *left* eye, even with a weak *right* lateral rectus muscle. Which eye the patient chooses for fixation is a matter of habit that may not be disrupted by muscle paresis, even if the weakness is profound. There is also a strong tendency to fixate with the eye that has better vision.

The degree of esodeviation in primary gaze may be different depending on which eye is fixing. *Primary deviation* refers to the angle that results from fixation with the "good" eye. *Secondary deviation* results from fixation with the paretic eye and it is larger than primary deviation. In primary gaze, the bad eye is "struggling" to abduct the eye even to the midposition against the tone of the medial rectus, and a great deal of rightward innervation is required by the right eye. According to Hering's law of equal innervation, the yoked medial rectus of the opposite (left) eye will also get this large amount of innervation and will adduct a great deal, creating a large angle esotropia. When the nonparetic left eye is fixing, a standard quantity of rightward innervation is required, and a lesser deviation results from the failure of the right eye to abduct completely.

This difference between primary and secondary deviation is a good clue to the presence of *muscle paretic* deviation, as opposed to deviation caused by *squint* or childhood *strabismus* in which the deviation remains the same whichever eye is fixing. Fixation with one or the other eye can be forced by occluding the fellow eye and then by quickly uncovering it to observe the degree of deviation of the covered eye before fixation is shifted.

As with the third and fourth cranial nerves, sixth cranial nerve palsies can occur on the basis of microvascular lesions in hypertensive and diabetic patients, in which case the abduction deficit tends to improve over a 3- to 6-month period. In addition, the sixth cranial nerve is susceptible to all of the local lesions that one could imagine in the pons, including hemorrhage, infarction, demyelination, and neoplasia (*e.g.*, pontine glioma in childhood; metastatic tumor, reticulum cell sarcoma in adults). The sixth nerve may also be involved in inflammatory and infiltrating lesions of the cavernous sinuses, as already mentioned, or of the leptomeninges (*e.g.*, carcinomatous meningitis, chronic or acute infectious meningitis). In addition to these standard lesions, the sixth cranial nerve is susceptible to stretching and distortion in a way that the other cranial nerves are not. This phenomenon results in the so-called *false localizing* sixth cranial nerve palsy in which the failure of abduction in one eye or both accompanies lesions that are remote from the sixth cranial nerve or its muscle, the lateral rectus. This occurs most commonly with raised intracranial pressure. Sixth nerve palsy has also been documented occasionally as a transient phenomenon following lumbar puncture. The pathophysiology in these cases is unclear, although presumably a transient shift of the brain stem secondary to cerebrospinal fluid pressure gradients is sufficient to cause the problem. The susceptibility of the sixth nerve to small brain-stem displacement may be based on the fact that it is fixed on one end at its emergence from the pons and at the other end, at its entry point into the cavernous sinus—Dorello's canal in the petrous tip. The sixth nerve is between the proverbial rock and a hard spot.

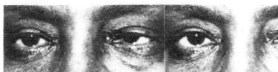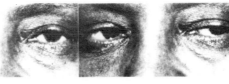

FIG. 22-16. Right lateral rectus palsy. In primary gaze (*center*) the eyes are slightly inturned with respect to one another (esodeviated). In right gaze (*left figure*) the angle of esodeviation increases as the right eye fails to abduct fully. In left gaze (*right figure*) the visual axes are parallel.

WEAKNESS OF INDIVIDUAL EXTRAOCULAR MUSCLES

In the preceding sections we have referred to a weakness of the muscles innervated by the third, fourth, and sixth cranial nerves and to lesions of these cranial nerves as though they were synonymous. This type of thinking should be avoided when one first encounters a patient with a weakness of one or several of these muscles. Disorders of muscle may mimic a lesion in any of these cranial nerves. Myasthenia gravis and thyroid eye disease are frequent offenders because they have a tendency to affect one or several extraocular muscles of one eye, or an asymmetrical array of muscles in both eyes. The level of the lesion may be difficult to determine when the nerve in question innervates only one muscle. In the case of the third cranial nerve, however, it should be easy to distinguish peripheral muscle disorders from those caused by an involvement of the cranial nerve. It is generally held that a lesion in the nerve trunk or at the nuclear level will involve, to some degree, all of the muscles within the distribution of the third cranial nerve. Isolated weakness of a superior rectus, or an inferior oblique, or a medial rectus muscle should engender suspicion that the disorder is peripheral, in the muscle or the terminal orbital branches of the third nerve, rather than in the more proximal intraorbital or intracranial portion of the nerve. Although isolated medial rectus weakness is caused most commonly by an MLF lesion, the involvement of an inferior oblique or a superior rectus in isolation should immediately lead one to suspect that the disorder is in the orbit or in the muscles themselves. Myasthenia gravis and thyroid eye disease should both be considered as the most likely etiologies. Myasthenia gravis can mimic INO (an MLF lesion) in all its aspects, including the dissociated monocular nystagmus of the abducting eye. An edrophonium chloride test is therefore warranted in cases in which there are no brain-stem signs or symptoms other than the ocular motility disorder of INO. Masses and infiltrating diseases within the orbit may affect one or the other of the muscles in the third cranial nerve group, but in these cases orbital signs (*e.g.*, proptosis, lid edema, and conjuctival chemosis) should be evident.

QUESTIONS and DISCUSSION

1.　A 58-year-old man presents with a history of pain in the left orbit. He denies diplopia. The pain is described as intense and "boring" in quality without throbbing. He has no previous neurologic or ophthalmologic history. You have been monitoring him for 5 years for fairly well-controlled adult-onset diabetes mellitus treated with diet restriction alone.

There is a complete left ptosis and the left eye is externally rotated (exodeviated) and depressed (deviated downward, hypodeviated). The pupil is 8 mm and fixed to light (direct stimulation). The patient is able to elevate and depress the eye through only about 10% of the expected range. There is no adduction past midline, but the left eye abducts fully. Your differential diagnosis includes:

A. Myasthenia gravis
B. Thyroid eye disease
C. Third cranial nerve (oculomotor nerve) palsy secondary to diabetes mellitus
D. Third cranial nerve palsy secondary to a tumor in the left cavernous sinus
E. Third cranial nerve palsy due to an intracranial "berry aneurysm"

You would order the following:

A. Carotid angiography
B. Skull series
C. Tomograms of the sella turcica region
D. Nothing

Course

As it happens, the patient leaves town because of a family crisis and is away for the next 3 months. When he returns, he is able to open the left lid almost completely, although ptosis is still easily observed. Elevation and depression of the globe are more complete, and he can now adduct the left eye through about 70% of normal range. On adduction and attempted depression (downward rotation), however, there is a peculiar "staring" appearance to the left eye in that the lid elevates further than its resting position with eyes straight ahead. You now conclude:

A. The danger is over.
B. Despite no change in diabetic management the lesion has begun to improve, thus no further intervention is warranted.
C. There is an "aberrant regeneration" of fibers.
D. You feel that because there has not been a complete recovery, an aneurysm should be ruled out.

Starting with the first office visit, one can make an educated guess as to the cause of the patient's clinical picture. The problem is not myasthenia gravis, because the pupil is involved (internal ophthalmoplegia) as well as the extraocular muscles (external ophthalmoplegia). Thyroid eye disease must be considered in a patient with external ophthalmoplegia; however, ptosis and pupillary involvement in this condition is rare, if it occurs at all. The combination of ptosis, dilated pupil, and weakness of medial, superior, and inferior recti, and inferior oblique reliably establishes the diagnosis of third cranial nerve (oculomotor nerve) palsy. It is left to decide what is the most likely cause. The differential diagnosis should include (C), (D), and (E) in the first question.

The primary physician is commonly required to make the basic and important decision as to whether a particular patient's third cranial nerve palsy is "medical" or "surgical." Medical third cranial nerve palsies are common in the age-group past 55 years and are generally thought to represent ischemic lesions in the substance of the cranial nerve caused by insufficiency of vasa nervora. The scant available pathologic material relating to "medical" third cranial nerve palsies shows that healed lesions are characterized by fibrosis and acute lesions by demyelination. *Axons are not disrupted* to any appreciable degree in early or late lesions, which accounts for the recovery of function within a few months and which underlies the fact that aberrant regeneration does not occur late in the course. The ischemic lesion is also restricted to the center of the nerve trunk, which is the anatomic basis for another characteristic feature of "medical" third cranial nerve palsies—*the pupil is relatively spared.* Anatomic studies have shown that the pupillary (sphincter) fibers run in the periphery of the nerve, which is spared from the more centrally distributed ischemia.

These ischemic lesions are commonly associated with long-standing hypertension or diabetes mellitus but can occur without these systemic risk factors for atherosclerosis, in which case the cranial nerve palsy is, by default, called *idiopathic*, although they are probably based on arteriosclerosis in patients over 60 years of age. These palsies generally clear within 3 to 6 months, and persistence of the deficit beyond this time calls for a further diagnostic work-up.

Surgical third cranial nerve palsies are most commonly caused by *berry aneurysms*, particularly those that originate from the junction of the posterior communicating artery and the internal carotid artery. Observations at surgery or autopsy suggest that small bleeds from the aneurysm break into the parenchyma of the nerve, causing disruption of axons as well as local demyelination. This characteristically causes pupillary dilatation with little or no light reaction, because the superficially placed pupillary fibers are disrupted. This pupillary finding is the most reliable differential diagnostic feature to separate *medical* (ischemic) from *surgical* (aneurysms) third cranial nerve palsies, at least early in the course of the disease. Sparing of the pupil is most reliable as an indicator of "medical" third nerve palsy when the external ophthalmoplegia is complete. With partial external ophthalmoplegia, one must strongly consider angiography to make the distinction, even with relative sparing of the pupil. This is certainly true if the patient is under 60 years of age.

The disruption of axons caused by aneurysmal leakage into the nerve sets the stage for the misdirection of regenerating axons during the recovery phase. As an example of this, fibers destined originally for the medial or inferior rectus are sometimes misdirected to the levator palpebrae. Consequently, when the patient attempts to look down or to adduct the eye, the lid elevates.

Tumors compressing the third cranial nerve also cause pupillary involvement, but less frequently than do aneurysms.

This patient, therefore, has compelling evidence in favor of an aneurysm as the cause of his cranial nerve palsy, even though he is diabetic. One should be highly suspicious of this finding at the first office visit, because the pupil was large and fixed to light. After enough time has elapsed for the regeneration of axons and misdirection (aberrant regeneration) to occur, the finding of lid elevation on adduction and downward rotation of the eye further supports the diagnosis of an aneurysm or a tumor as opposed to an ischemic cause.

The best answers for the first question would, therefore, be (D) and (E). One would be justified in ordering carotid angiography in this case. If this study is negative for aneurysm, it may become necessary to order tomograms of the sella region in search of a meningioma or other tumor in the cavernous sinus or superior orbital fissure area. The angiogram or a routine CT scan is likely to reveal such a lesion, but may not if the lesion is an *en plaque* meningioma, in which case bony erosion or hyperostosis may require thin-section CT with bone windows to be visualized.

The answer to the third question is clearly (C). Response (D) is correct, but for the wrong reason.

2. An 18-year-old girl is brought in by her mother on account of her complaint that she had transiently gone blind in the right eye. The episode occurred in school and lasted 20 minutes. She noted that the right half of a large word on the blackboard seemed to be missing and that "everything seemed to be shimmering and wavy." She is in good general health, and the physical as well as neurologic examinations are normal. Useful questions you could ask include:

   A. Where were you the night before this happened?
   B. Did you cover the right or left eye to see if the vision changed?
   C. Did you develop a headache during or after these visual symptoms?
   D. Do you get sick headaches or sinus headaches?

Which of the following tests would be most appropriate for a work-up of this patient?

   A. Cerebral angiography
   B. Pneumoencephalography
   C. Carotid duplex examination
   D. CT scan with enhancement or MR
   E. Visual-field examination
   F. Reassurance and a follow-up visit in 1 month or sooner should symptoms recur

Choices (B), (C), and (D) are potentially rewarding in the first part of this question. Patients, even those with reasonable intelligence, often fail to make a simple test of whether a visual defect exists in one or both eyes. People conceptualize vision as a unitary experience and are unaware of binocularity in daily life. As part of this unity of experience, many patients are unwilling to comprehend the concept of a homonymous field defect and doggedly stick to the contention that they lost vision in the right eye when, in fact, they experienced a right homonymous hemianopsia.

Careful consideration of this patient's history indicates an inability to see the right half of a word written on the blackboard. This finding was experienced with both eyes open and must, therefore, represent a homonymous binocular loss of vision even though the patient's natural reaction was to ascribe the symptom to a loss of vision in the right eye.

It would be comforting in this case to elicit a history of left temporal throbbing headache, because this would almost undeniably label this patient's symptom complex as a *classic migraine*. It is important to realize, however, that many migraine patients have typical migrainous aura without a subsequent headache. A previous history of severe throbbing headaches with nausea, vomiting, diaphoresis, diarrhea, and vertigo would also identify the individual as one who is prone to *common migraine*. Such persons may occasionally have classic episodes (with aura) interspersed among common migraine attacks without aura. Patients with common migraine will often deny that they have migraine, because they ascribe their recurring, often unilateral frontal throbbing headaches to "sinus infections."

Choices (C), (D), and (E) would certainly be practical and justifiable noninvasive procedures for the second part of this question. Aside from migraine, which this patient almost certainly has, one should consider the less likely diagnosis of occipital arteriovenous malformation with small volume bleeding or transient steal syndrome and ischemia of the visual cortex, giving rise to the evanescent visual symptoms. Contrast-enhanced CT scan and MR (D) should identify the vast majority of such lesions.

My personal choice when confronted with this patient, however, would be to give reassurance that the syndrome is common and would not be expected to produce any serious complications. Teenagers are often easily frightened by diagnostic procedures and may actually develop a functional overlay when confronted with the apparent seriousness of their condition engendered by a flurry of complex and dramatic examinations. The statistical chances of missing a significant structural lesion are small. Return visits are advisable, however, to assure against missing progressive symptoms and to provide confidence on the part of the patient and family that they are not being abandoned. In treating patients who suffer from headaches, this sense of ongoing commitment is more important than the type of medicine prescribed.

3. A 38-year-old man presents with a 2-week history of frequent severe headaches in the right orbital area. The pain is steady and "boring" in character and severe, but lasts only 40 to 60 minutes. It tends to occur two to three times daily and can be anticipated regularly at 10 PM usually just after the patient retires. On examination, there is right ptosis and meiosis but no other physical or neurologic findings. Work-up should include:

A. Carotid angiography

B. CT scan including sphenoid and ethmoid paranasal sinuses

C. Instillation of 1% para-OH-amphetamine in either eye

D. Instillation of 4% cocaine in either eye

The most reliable indicator of a postganglionic lesion is failure of the pupil to dilate on instillation of 1% para-OH-amphetamine. Para-OH-amphetamine, like cocaine, blocks the reuptake of norepinephrine into the presynaptic sympathetic nerve terminals in the iris. In addition, however, it causes the release of any existing presynaptic norepinephrine stores. This means that, regardless of a lesion in the oculosympathetic preganglionic or central pathways, para-OH-amphetamine will release stores of norepinephrine and cause pupillary dilatation. Failure of dilatation, therefore, establishes the presence of a postganglionic oculosympathetic neuron lesion in which the normal stores of transmitter are pathologically absent.

Raeder, a Norwegian ophthalmologist, described patients with painful oculosympathetic palsy and space-occupying lesions of the middle cranial fossa. All his patients also had findings referable to one or more of the third through sixth cranial nerves, and he put forth this combination as diagnostic of middle fossa masses. This original, or *Type I*, form of Raeder's syndrome has now been separated from a benign, probably migranious form, referred to as *Type II*.

The original description of *Raeder's syndrome Type II* included seven patients with *painful* oculosympathetic palsy. All patients had unilateral brief steady headaches that conformed to the pattern of *cluster* or *histamine* headache, but they also had an ipsilateral oculosympathetic syndrome. None had findings of third, fourth, or sixth cranial nerve dysfunction. Lawton–Smith's concept that these patients with Raeder's Type II have a form of migraine with secondary sympathetic involvement has come to be widely accepted. The patients are generally middle-aged, and men predominate. There must be no associated cranial nerve palsy, and the headache history should be typical of the cluster pattern. The oculosympathetic lesion should also be documented as *postganglionic* using the para-OH-amphetamine test. The theory is that the sympathetic lesion is caused by edema in the adventitia of the carotid siphon as a consequence of frequent and severe vascular headaches.

The diagnosis of Raeder's syndrome Type II relieves the physician of the obligation to consider the patient to be a cancer suspect.

4. A 62-year-old man presents for a routine examination. He has no head or neck symptoms, but an examination reveals 1 mm to 2 mm of left ptosis. In the examining room, however, the pupils are noted to be equal in size at 3 mm. The patient denies awareness of the lid droop and denies head or neck trauma. A reasonable work-up would include:

A. Chest roentgenogram

B. Sputum cytology with AFB smear and culture

C. Examination of the pupils in a dim room

D. Instillation of 1% pilocarpine in either eye

E. Instillation of 4% cocaine in either eye

F. Instillation of 1% para-OH-amphetamine in either eye

G. Nothing

H. Ask for old full-face photographs

I. Observation of iris color

The most serious concern on first observing a patient with Horner's syndrome is the possibility of cancer, which is one of the most common causes of an acquired ocular sympathetic lesion in the adult. Apical carcinoma of the lung (Pancoast Ca) is a common type that causes Horner's syndrome, but any neoplasm infiltrating cervical lymph nodes can present this way. Most often the patient is unaware of a change in his facial appearance, because the degree of ptosis is small and the onset is insidious without visual or other symptoms. The most practical approach is to determine (1) whether ptosis is actually due to oculosympathetic dysfunction, and (2) the age of the lesion.

Grimson and Thompson (1975) reviewed pharmacologic testing in Horner's syndrome with a logical approach to diagnosis. They found that the use of a weak direct-acting sympathomimetic (1:1000 epinephrine) was unreliable in clinical diagnosis. Four percent cocaine blocks the reuptake of norepinephrine into presynaptic terminals at the iris and causes pupillary dilatation in the normal eye. In the presence of Horner's syndrome, the release of norepinephrine is reduced and a reuptake block fails to dilate the pupil as much as it does in the fellow eye, which is used as a control. The cocaine test is useful to identify an oculosympathetic lesion in patients with ptosis and minimal or no anisocoria.

A simple preliminary approach is to observe the eyes for anisocoria in a dim an environment as possible consistent with adequate visualization of the pupils. In bright light the iris (parasympathetic) sphincter dominates pupil size and can overcome minor asymmetry of tone in the radially oriented, sympathetically innervated dilator muscles. The sphincter relaxes in a dim light and anisocoria, due to weakness of the pupil dilator muscles on the side of the oculosympathetic lesion, may become apparent.

Obviously, if the ptosis has been present for several years, carcinoma can be ruled out almost categorically as the cause. An examination of old photographs will often settle the issue without an expensive work-up by demonstrating the ptosis to be long-standing and unchanged over the years. Furthermore, an oculosympathetic lesion arising before birth, and perhaps in the first 1 to 2 years of life at the latest, will cause failure of iris chromatophores to develop. If the patient has one brown iris contralateral to the ptosis and a blue iris ipsilateral, the Horner's syndrome can be identified as ancient.

If the lesion cannot be documented as old and stable, a work-up for carcinoma of the lung or carcinoma metastatic to cervical nodes could be undertaken. This presumes that there is no history of stroke or of head or neck trauma to explain the lesion. If the first round of tests is negative it is important to follow the patient closely for emergence of signs or symptoms of underlying carcinoma. Frequent chest roentgenograms or CT scans with attention to apical regions are usually necessary. MR will probably be the preferred method for examining the upper chest and neck.

SUGGESTED READING

Asbury AK, Aldridge H, Hershberg R et al: Oculomotor palsy in diabetes mellitus: A clinicopathologic study. Brain 93:555, 1970

Boniuk M, Schlesinger NS: Raeder's paratrigeminal syndrome. Am J Ophthalmol 54:1074, 1962

Daroff RB, Hoyt WF: Supranuclear disorders of ocular control systems in man. In Bach-y-Rita P, Collins CC, Hyde JE (eds): The Control of Eye Movements, p 175. New York, Academic Press, 1971

Daroff RB, Troost BT, Leigh RJ: Supranuclear disorders of eye movements. In Glaser JS (ed): Neuro-Ophthalmology, 2nd edition, pp 299–323. Philadelphia, PA, J.B. Lippincott Co., 1990

Giles CL, Henderson JW: Horner's syndrome: An analysis of 216 cases. Am J Ophthalmol 46:289, 1958

Glaser JS, Bachynski B: Infranuclear disorders of eye movement. In Glaser (ed): Neuro-Ophthalmology, 2nd edition, pp 361–418. Philadelphia, PA, J.B. Lippincott Co., 1990

Goldstein JE, Cogan DG: Diabetic ophthalmoplegia with special reference to the pupil. Arch Ophthalmol 64:592, 1960

Grimson BS, Thompson HS: Drug Testing in Horner's Syndrome, Vol 8, pp 265–270. St. Louis, CV Mosby, 1975

Hayreh SS: In vivo choroidal circulation and its watershed zones. Eye 4:273, 1990

Hayreh SS: The ophthalmic artery: III. Branches. Br J Ophthalmol 46:212, 1962

Keltner JL, Johnson CA, Spurr JO et al: Baseline visual field profile of optic neuritis: The experience of the Optic Neuritis Treatment Trial. Arch Ophthalmol (in press)

Kerr WL: The pupil: Functional anatomy and clinical correlation. In Smith JL (ed): Neuro-Ophthalmology, Vol 4, pp 49–80. Hollendale, FL, Huffman, 1968

Leigh JR, Zec DS: The Neurology of Eye Movement. Philadelphia, FA Davis, 1983

Rucker CW: The causes of paralysis of the third, fourth and sixth cranial Nerves. Am J Ophthalmol 61:1294, 1966

Rucker CW: Paralysis of the third, fourth, and sixth cranial nerves. Am J Ophthalmol 46:787, 1958

Smith JL: Raeder's paratrigeminal syndrome. Am J Ophthalmol 46:194, 1958

Thompson HS, Bourgon P, Van Allen MW: The tendon reflexes in Adie's syndrome. In Thompson HS (ed): Topics in Neuro-Ophthalmology, pp 104–113. Baltimore, Williams & Wilkins, 1979

Thompson HS, Mensher JM: Adrenergic mydriasis of Horner's syndrome: Hydroxyamphetamine test for diagnosis of postganglionic defects. Am J Ophthalmol 72:472, 1971

Weber RB, Daroff RB, Mackey EA: Pathology of oculomotor nerve palsy in diabetics. Neurology 20:835, 1970

CHAPTER 23

Central Nervous System Infections

Larry E. Davis

Central nervous system (CNS) infections can be caused by viruses, bacteria, fungi, and parasites, but bacteria and viruses are the most common. Infectious agents enter the body by way of the gastrointestinal tract, respiratory tract, or following skin inoculation (animal or insect bite). The organism sets up the initial site of replication in the gastrointestinal tract, respiratory tract, or subcutaneous/muscle/vascular tissue. The majority of organisms then reach the CNS by way of the bloodstream, but occasional organisms reach the brain by way of peripheral nerves or by direct entry through adjacent bone from infected mastoid or air sinuses.

In spite of the many infections we develop during our lifetimes, few organisms ever reach the brain. Important protective systems include the reticuloendothelial system (which efficiently removes bacteria and viruses from blood), cellular and humoral immune responses (which destroy organisms from the blood and primary site of infection), and the blood–brain barrier (which prevents entry of organisms into the brain or cerebrospinal fluid [CSF]). Organisms that do enter the brain or CSF from blood generally do so by infecting endothelial cells of the cerebral blood vessels (many encephalitis viruses), by penetrating the blood–CSF barrier in the choroid plexus or meninges (many bacteria) or by occluding small cerebral blood vessels with infected emboli from the heart or lung (brain abscess organisms). Once the invasion has occurred, the brain and CSF have less immune protection than the rest of the body. The CSF has about 1/200th the amount of antibody as blood, and the brain lacks a lymphatic system and has few white blood cells in normal CSF. Thus, individuals who develop a brain or meningeal infection often die without antimicrobial intervention.

Inflammation of the meninges or brain is the hallmark of CNS infection. Inflammatory cells are seen in the meninges, in perivascular spaces, or around an abscess. The inflammatory lymphocytes show specific immune activity against the infectious agent.

The signs and symptoms of a CNS infection depend on the site of the infection and not the organism. The organism determines mainly the time course of the infection. In general, the time course to develop CNS signs for viruses is hours to 1 day; for aerobic bacteria it is hours to a few days; for anaerobic bacteria, tuberculosis, and fungi it is days to weeks; and for parasites and *Treponema pallidum* (syphilis) it is weeks to years. Follow these steps to diagnose and treat CNS infections:

- Determine the site of infection
- Determine the class of organism (*e.g.*, bacteria, virus)
- Begin initial treatment
- Determine specific etiology and antimicrobial sensitivities and modify treatment if necessary
- Watch for and treat complications

William J. Weiner and Christopher G. Goetz, eds. *Neurology for the Non-Neurologist*, Third Edition. Copyright © 1994, 1989 by J. B. Lippincott Company. Copyright © 1981 by Harper and Row Publishers, Inc.

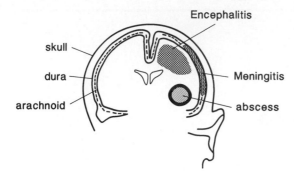

FIG. 23-1. Coronal section of head demonstrating locations of three major central nervous system infections.

There are three major sites where infections occur in the nervous system: diffusely in the meninges (meningitis), diffusely in the brain (encephalitis), and locally in the brain (abscess) (Fig. 23-1). Although patients may develop infections at other sites such as epidural abscess and subdural empyema, this chapter will focus on the most common infections.

MENINGITIS (INFECTION OF MENINGES)

A variety of viral, bacterial, fungal, parasitic, chemical, and neoplastic agents may cause inflammation of the meninges. These patients all have common clinical features:

- *Early features*: Prodromal illness, fever, headache, stiff neck, relative preservation of mental status, no focal neurologic signs, no papilledema
- *Later features*: Seizures, stupor and coma, cranial nerve palsies, deafness, focal neurologic signs

Clinical findings that suggest meningitis rather than encephalitis include stiff neck, relative preservation of mental status, lack of focal neurologic signs, and no papilledema. The time course of the meningitis may give clues as to its etiology. Viral meningitis is hyperacute, and patients develop acute symptoms and signs over a few hours. Patients with bacterial meningitis develop an acute illness over hours to 1 day. Patients with fungal meningitis

or tuberculous meningitis develop symptoms over days to 2 weeks.

COMMON LABORATORY FINDINGS

In blood, the white blood cell count is usually elevated, as is the erythrocyte sedimentation rate. The CSF exam is the key to the diagnosis of meningitis, ascertainment of the class of infecting agent, establishment of the etiologic agent, and determination of antimicrobial sensitivities (Fig. 23-2). Viral, bacterial, tuberculous, and fungal infections of the meninges have differing CSF profiles (Table 23-1). CSF culture determines the etiology of the infection as well as antimicrobial sensitivities. In general, cultures for bacteria take 1 to 3 days, for tuberculosis and fungi 1 to 6 weeks, and for viruses days to 3 weeks. Rapid diagnosis of bacteria can be made by Gram stain of CSF sediment and by testing CSF for common bacterial antigens. The Gram stain will detect bacteria in CSF sediment in over three-fourths of patients with acute bacterial meningitis and often gives clues for initial antibiotic treatment. Latex agglutination antigen tests are commercially available to detect *Hemophilus influenzae*, *Streptococcus pneumoniae*, *N. meningitidis*, and group A beta-hemolytic streptococci. Antigen tests have about the same sensitivity as the Gram stain.

VIRAL MENINGITIS

Enteroviruses (echoviruses and Coxsackie viruses) are the most common cause of viral meningitis. Less common causes include herpes simplex virus type 2, mumps virus, and human immunodeficiency virus. Viruses often can be isolated from CSF early in the meningitis. Treatment of viral meningitis is usually symptomatic and may include analgesics for the headache and antiemetics for nausea and vomiting. Hospitalization is often not required, but the patient should be observed at home by a responsible individual. The prognosis of viral meningitis is excellent, and most patients fully recover within 1 to 2 weeks.

ACUTE BACTERIAL MENINGITIS

Aerobic bacteria, both gram-positive and gram-negative, cause meningitis mainly in young children, in the elderly, and in the immunosuppressed. *H. influenzae*, *S. pneumoniae* and *N. meningitidis* are the most common offending bacteria. Unlike viral

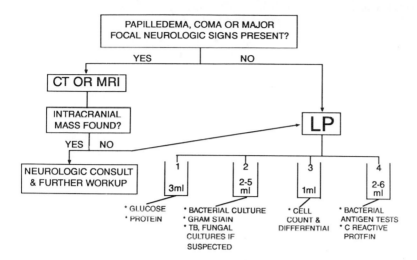

FIG. 23-2. Flow diagram for lumbar puncture and cerebrospinal fluid tests in suspected bacterial meningitis. With permission from Davis LE: Acute bacterial meningitis. In Weiner WJ (ed): Emergent and Urgent Neurology, p 139. Philadelphia, JB Lippincott, 1992.

meningitis, patients with bacterial meningitis will progress to death if untreated with antibiotics. Therefore, prompt diagnosis and treatment are essential. If bacterial meningitis is suspected, the lumbar puncture becomes an emergency procedure (Fig. 23-2). In general, it is not necessary to perform a computed tomography (CT) or magnetic resonance imaging (MR) scan before the lumbar puncture unless the patient is comatose, has focal neurologic signs, or has papilledema. The presence of these signs suggests the possibility of a space-occupying lesion and increased intracranial pressure. If there is to be a significant delay before the neuroimaging can be obtained, broad-spectrum antibiotics may be given before the lumbar puncture. One should always obtain a blood culture, as it

is positive in about 60% of patients with bacterial meningitis.

The key to treatment of acute bacterial meningitis is the prompt administration of appropriate antibiotics. *General principles involved in the use of antibiotics include the following: (1) The antibiotic should be given early in the clinical course; (2) the bacteria must be sensitive to the antibiotic; (3) the antibiotic must cross the blood–brain barrier and achieve sufficient CSF concentrations to kill the bacteria; and (4) a bacteriocidal antibiotic is preferable to a bacteriostatic antibiotic.* Once the diagnosis of bacterial meningitis is made, one should begin treatment with a broad spectrum antibiotic, which can be later modified when antibiotic sensitivities become available. The choice of an antibiotic for initial treatment depends on several fac-

TABLE 23-1. Spinal Fluid Profiles in CNS Infections

	OPENING PRESSURE	WHITE BLOOD CELLS	PROTEIN	GLUCOSE	BACTERIA OR FUNGAL CULTURE
Epidural abscess	N or sl ↑	0–20 (lymphs)	N or sl ↑	N	Negative
Subdural empyema	↑	10–1,000 (polys)	sl ↑	N	Negative
Viral meningitis	N or sl ↑	20–1,000 (lymphs)	sl ↑	N	Negative
Bacterial meningitis	↑	50–10,000 (polys)	↑	Low	Positive
Fungal or tuberculous meningitis	↑	50–10,000 polys & lymphs	↑	Low	Positive
Meningovascular syphilis	N or sl ↑	10–1,000 lymphs	↑	N	Negative
Brain abscess	↑	0–10 lymphs & polys	N	N	Negative
Viral encephalitis	sl ↑	10–200 lymphs	N or sl ↑	N	Negative

N = normal; sl ↑ = slight increase; ↑ = increased.

tors: age of patient, immune status of patient, predisposing medical conditions, results of CSF Gram stain, presence of positive CSF bacterial antigen tests, knowledge of the types of drug-resistant bacteria in the community, and knowledge of whether the patient is allergic to any antibiotic. Table 23-2 gives common initial antibiotic regimens for newborns, children, and adults.

There is increasing evidence that administration of corticosteroids shortly before or at the start of antibiotic treatment may minimize complications of the meningitis. Dexamethasone (0.15 mg/kg intravenously every 6 hours for 2 to 4 days) is the most common regimen. If corticosteroids are administered, one should ensure that the etiologic agent is quickly identified. If the meningeal infection is treated with incorrect antimicrobial drugs, administration of corticosteroids will make the infection worse.

In general, the CSF becomes sterile 1 to 2 days after antibiotic treatment. The fever usually disappears within a few days but may persist for up to 2 weeks. CSF abnormalities such as pleocytosis, elevated protein, and depressed glucose may persist

TABLE 23-2. Common Initial Antibiotic in Bacterial Meningitis Therapy While Awaiting Antibiotic Sensitivities of Infecting Bacteria

SETTING	THERAPY (IV IN DIVIDED DOSES)
Newborn	Ampicillin, first week of life: (50–100 mg/kg/day), 1 week to 1 month: (150–200 mg/kg/day) plus Gentamicin (dose to be determined by renal function) or Ceftriaxone (100 mg/kg/day)
2 months–adult	Ampicillin (300–400 mg/kg/day) plus Chloramphenicol (50–100 mg/kg/day) or Ceftriaxone (100 mg/kg/day)
Endocarditis, penetrating skull injury, or infected intraventricular device	Nafcillin (150–200 mg/kg/day) or Methicillin (250–300 mg/kg/day) plus Gentamicin or vancomycin (dose to be determined by renal function)

for several weeks. Dead bacteria may be seen on Gram stain of CSF for several days.

Even if the patient is promptly treated with appropriate antibiotics, serious complications may still develop. Seizures develop in about one-third of patients. The seizures usually occur early in the meningitis and seldom recur after the hospitalization. Causes of seizures in meningitis include cerebral cortex irritation from bacterial toxins or meningeal inflammation, CNS vasculitis, brain infarction, high fever, and hyponatremia from SIADH coupled with excess fluid administration. Treatment of the seizures is usually with phenytoin. At discharge, the anticonvulsant can be discontinued. Focal neurologic signs develop in up to 25% of patients. These include cranial nerve palsies, especially cranial nerves VIII (deafness) and VI and III (diplopia). Brain damage resulting in hemiparesis, ataxia, aphasia, or visual loss may also occur. CT or MR of the head is often helpful in the evaluation of these complications and may demonstrate cerebral or cerebellar infarction, brain necrosis, subdural hygromas, or mild ventricular dilatation. Hydrocephalus, subdural empyema, and brain abscess occur but are uncommon.

Mortality from bacterial meningitis ranges from 5% to 25%, depending upon the infecting bacteria, the age-group, and the predisposing illness. In surviving children, 15% have language disorders or delayed language development, 10% mental retardation, 10% hearing loss, 5% visual impairment, 5% weakness or spasticity, and 3% seizures.

Some bacterial meningitis requires chemoprophylaxis of immediate family members and close contacts because of their increased risk of developing meningitis. In *N. meningitidis* meningitis, treatment of all close contacts is indicated. If the organism is sulfa-sensitive, sulfadiazine (0.5 g to 1 g twice daily orally for 3 days) should be given. If the organism is sulfa-resistant or of unknown resistance, rifampin (600 mg for adults or 10 mg/kg for children twice daily orally for 2 days) is given. If the patient has *H. influenzae*, type B meningitis, chemoprophylaxis is indicated for children less than 4 years of age who have been in close contact with the patient and not previously vaccinated with the *H. influenzae* vaccine. Rifampin (10 mg/kg twice daily orally for 4 days) is usually given. All close contacts should be observed carefully for the next week.

SPIROCHETE MENINGITIS

Bacterial meningitis from spirochetes produces a chronic infection. In Lyme disease (*Borrelia burgdor-*

feri) and neurosyphilis (*T. pallidum*), a chronic meningitis can cause headaches, cranial nerve palsies (especially cranial nerve VII), and occasionally brain infarctions from thrombosis of cortical blood vessels (meningovascular syphilis). Years later, the spirochetes invade the brain to cause a low-grade encephalitis (general paresis or CNS Lyme disease). The CSF contains a lymphocytic pleocytosis, elevated protein, and usually normal glucose level. Spirochetes are seldom isolated from CSF, and the diagnosis is made by serologic tests (CSF–VDRL or Lyme antibody titers). Work-up for subacute meningitis is given in Table 23-3. Treatment is with high-dose penicillin or, alternately, ceftriaxone for several weeks.

TUBERCULOUS AND FUNGAL MENINGITIS

These patients usually develop a subacute meningitis with the onset of CNS signs developing over days to weeks. These infections occur most often in individuals who are malnourished, debilitated, or immunosuppressed. Although initial entry is usually by way of the lungs, less than 50% will have an active pulmonary infection at the time of the meningitis. Culture of the CSF is the key to establishing the etiology. Since tuberculous or fungal organisms may be in low concentrations in the CSF, one should culture 5 ml to 10 ml of CSF on several occasions. Treatment of tuberculous meningitis usually requires administration of three drugs (rifampin, isoniazid, and pyrazinamide) for 2 months followed by rifampin and isoniazid for another 7 months. Most

TABLE 23-3. Evaluation of subacute meningitis

Skin tests: intermediate purified protein derivative tuberculin test (PPD) and anergy skin tests

Serum antibody serologic tests: brucella, syphilis, toxoplasmosis, coccidioides, Lyme disease, and human immunodeficiency virus

CSF studies: opening pressure, cells, glucose, protein, IgG Gram stain, acid-fast stain, India ink, cytology, VDRL, coccidioides, and Lyme disease antibody tests and cryptococcal antigen test

Cultures for bacteria, brucella, tuberculosis, and fungi: CSF cultures repeated ×3, blood, urine, sputum or gastric aspirate, bone marrow biopsy, lesion biopsy

Computed tomography or magnetic resonance imaging

Chest x-ray

patients with fungal meningitis are treated with amphotericin B for weeks to months. In patients with cryptococcal meningitis, flucytosine is often added. Complications are similar to those seen in acute bacterial meningitis. Mortality rates range from 20% to 50% depending on the organism and predisposing factors. Survivors may be left with neurologic sequelae similar to those seen in acute bacterial meningitis.

ENCEPHALITIS (DIFFUSE BRAIN INFECTION)

The majority of infectious agents that cause encephalitis are viruses that reach the brain by way of a hematogenous route. Once the virus reaches the brain parenchyma, a widely disseminated infection of neurons and glia ensues. Neuronal necrosis and lysis of glial cells result in secondary cerebral edema. The inflammatory response includes perivascular cuffing with inflammatory cells and infiltration of lymphocytes and macrophages into the adjacent brain parenchyma. The invading immune response often terminates the infection, but the patient may be left with permanent neurologic sequelae.

CLINICAL FEATURES

Acute encephalitis is a febrile illness characterized by the abrupt onset of headache and mental obtundation. Other common features include seizures, which may be generalized or focal, hyper-reflexia, spasticity, and Babinski signs. Occasional patients develop hemiparesis, aphasia, ataxia, limb tremors, and blindness. Patients often have a prodromal illness, which varies with the infectious agent and can include parotitis (mumps virus) or fever, malaise, and myalgias (togavirus). Encephalitis differs from meningitis primarily because patients with encephalitis develop prominent mental changes and a minimal or absent stiff neck.

LABORATORY FINDINGS

The electroencephalogram (EEG) is always abnormal and usually shows diffuse bilateral slowing with occasional seizure activity. A lumbar puncture in a patient with early encephalitis will have an opening pressure that is normal or slightly elevated. The CSF contains five to several hundred WBC/mm^3

(predominantly lymphocytes). CSF glucose is normal, while CSF protein is mildly elevated. Bacterial and viral cultures are usually sterile. Early in the course of encephalitis, the CT scan may be normal while the MR scan shows areas of cerebral vascular permeability. Later, both scans may demonstrate areas of necrosis or hemorrhage.

ETIOLOGIES

Viruses cause more than 90% of cases. Worldwide, togaviruses (arboviruses) are the most common cause. Since togaviruses require a vector (mosquito or tick), togavirus encephalitis occurs primarily in the summer and fall, when the vectors are prevalent. Togavirus encephalitis often occurs in clusters or epidemics. In the United States, herpes simplex encephalitis is slightly more common than togavirus encephalitis. Herpes simplex virus is a latent infection in most individuals, and herpes simplex encephalitis occurs sporadically year round. The remainder of causes are usually due to bacteria (*T. pallidum*, *B. burgdorferi*) or parasites (toxoplasmosis or falciparum malaria).

The diagnosis of viral encephalitis is usually made by serologic tests. Since most togaviruses produce a systemic viral infection before producing the viral encephalitis, immunoglobulin M antibodies to the virus are often present early in the encephalitis. The IgM-antibody-capture enzyme linked immunoabsorbent assay (MacELISA) can be used to detect togavirus antibodies during the first few days of the encephalitis. Acute and convalescent serum titers can be determined for many viruses. A fourfold increase in antibody titer is usually diagnostic. Unfortunately, serologic tests have not been useful in establishing the diagnosis of herpes simplex encephalitis. At present, a brain biopsy with isolation of herpes simplex virus or detection of viral antigen from the brain sample is required to firmly establish the diagnosis. Experimental studies using the polymerase chain reaction to detect herpes simplex viral nucleic acid in CSF appears promising and eventually may replace the brain biopsy.

Treatment of encephalitis varies with the infectious agent. With the exception of herpes simplex virus encephalitis, no antiviral treatment is available. All patients require excellent symptomatic care to minimize complications. If seizures develop, anticonvulsants are indicated. If increased intracranial pressure develops from vascular engorgement and cerebral edema, treatment may require hyperventilation or the administration of mannitol.

Use of corticosteroids is controversial. In patients with herpes simplex encephalitis, treatment with acyclovir significantly improves outcome. Acyclovir should be administered early in the encephalitis course. Current recommendations are to give 30 mg/kg/day of acyclovir that is divided into three doses per day for at least 10 days. The drug should be intravenously delivered slowly over 1 hour to prevent renal toxicity. Drug complications include transient renal failure, thrombophlebitis, and elevations of serum liver enzymes.

Prognosis of encephalitis depends on the infectious agent. Patients with mumps meningoencephalitis and Venezuelan equine encephalitis have an excellent prognosis. Patients with western equine, St. Louis, and California encephalitis usually have a good prognosis (2% to 10% mortality). Occasional patients may be left with dementia, seizures, or focal neurologic deficits. Patients with eastern equine, Japanese B, and Murray Valley encephalitis have mortality rates from 20% to 40%. Patients with herpes simplex encephalitis who are treated with acyclovir have a 20% mortality rate, and 55% are left with some neurologic sequelae. Rabies encephalitis is fatal.

BRAIN ABSCESS (FOCAL INFECTIONS OF THE BRAIN)

While viruses tend to cause diffuse brain infections, most bacteria, fungi, and parasites cause localized brain disease. Brain abscesses may arise by direct extension from other foci of infection within the cranial cavity (mastoiditis and sinusitis), from infections following skull fracture or craniotomy, or as metastasis carried by the blood from infections elsewhere in the body. The infection usually begins as a localized encephalitis with focal softening, necrosis, and inflammation. As the process continues, fibroblasts proliferate at the edges, forming a capsule wall. A variable amount of cerebral edema surrounds the lesion. If the etiology is bacterial or fungal, the space-occupying lesion slowly expands. If untreated, the brain mass is lethal. Parasites such as cysticercosis usually stop growing after they reach about 10 mm to 15 mm in size.

CLINICAL FEATURES

Symptoms from localized brain infections typically are subacute in onset. Early symptoms include headaches, lethargy, intermittent fever, and focal or generalized seizures. Focal neurologic signs may develop depending upon the site of lesion. Thus, lesions in the frontal cortex may produce hemiparesis, while lesions in the occipital cortex cause homonymous visual defects. As the mass expands, increased intracranial pressure becomes more pronounced. Psychomotor slowing, lethargy, and confusion increase. Papilledema and a sixth-nerve palsy may be seen. Focal neurologic signs become more prominent. Eventually, brain herniation and death occur as a result of the expanding mass.

LABORATORY FINDINGS

CT and MR scans are extremely helpful in diagnosing brain abscesses. The CT scan usually demonstrates a lesion with a low-density necrotic center, a well-developed contrast-enhancing capsule, and surrounding cerebral edema (Fig. 23-3). A somewhat similar picture is seen on MR scan. Administration of gadolinium will cause the capsule wall to enhance. The EEG is often abnormal, usually producing localized slowing (delta waves). A lumbar puncture is seldom helpful in establishing the diagnosis and may be contraindicated since it increases the risk of brain herniation.

ETIOLOGIES

Anaerobic bacteria are found in over one-half of brain abscesses. Anaerobic streptococci and *Bacteroides fragilis* are common organisms. Occasionally, multiple bacteria are found in abscesses. Brain abscesses following head trauma or neurosurgery may contain *Staphylococcus aureus*. *Nocardia asteroides* may cause a fungal brain abscess.

Treatment of brain abscesses usually entails appropriate antibiotic therapy and surgical drainage. Broad-spectrum antibiotic treatment is usually given as soon as the clinical diagnosis is made. The antibiotics should be selected for effectiveness against all likely pathogens as well as for their ability to penetrate brain abscesses and surrounding brain parenchyma. Broad-spectrum antibiotic treatment often includes penicillin G (20 to 30 million units/day) and chloramphenicol (4 g to 6 g/day). This combination is active against most anaerobic bacteria and many aerobic bacteria. Additional drugs that penetrate brain abscesses and have proved clinically useful include metronidazole, ampicillin, vancomycin, cefotaxime, and trimethoprim–sulfamethoxazole. Antibiotics should be administered intra-

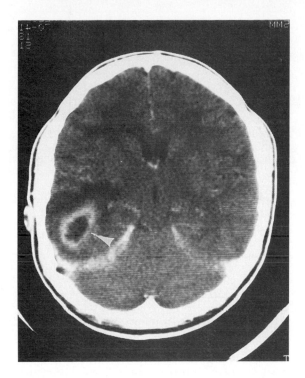

FIG. 23-3. Computed tomography scan with contrast demonstrating a brain abscess in the posterior temporal lobe. Arrow shows the enhancing capsule with necrotic center. There is some low-density surrounding edema.

venously, and treatment is normally continued for 6 to 8 weeks. Because the most immediate threat from brain abscesses is the mass effect, surgical aspiration of pus often alleviates the increased intracranial pressure. The simplest method is aspiration of the pus using a CT-guided stereotactic technique. The pus should be Gram stained and cultured for anaerobic and aerobic bacteria, fungi, and tuberculosis. If the brain abscesses are multiple or deep, they may be treated only with broad-spectrum antimicrobial agents. However, careful clinical observations and repeated CT scans are needed to determine whether the abscess continues to expand. If expansion occurs, neurosurgical intervention is required, as rupture of the brain abscess into the ventricles or brain herniation is usually fatal.

Corticosteroids may be necessary initially to control cerebral edema. However, corticosteroids should be used cautiously and tapered rapidly, as the corticosteroids may interfere with capsule formation and host defenses against the organism.

PROGNOSIS

Mortality from brain abscesses ranges from 30% to 65%, with the lower rates for patients who receive combined therapy with antibiotics and surgery. About 50% of survivors have neurologic sequelae, including seizures and focal neurologic deficits.

QUESTIONS AND DISCUSSION

1. Western equine encephalitis:

   A. Occurs sporadically all year
   B. Is contagious to others for about 1 year
   C. Begins with a severe headache and stiff neck
   D. Produces widespread death of glia and neurons
   E. Is best treated with acyclovir

The correct answer is (D). Western equine encephalitis virus is an arbovirus that is transmitted to man from the bite of infected mosquitoes during the summer and early fall. While meningitis begins with a headache and stiff neck, encephalitis usually begins with marked changes in mental status. The virus infects both glia and neurons, producing widespread cell death. Western equine encephalitis virus is not present in urine, saliva, or stool. Therefore, the patient is not contagious and does not need isolation. Acyclovir works as an antiviral drug only against viruses of the herpes family such as herpes simplex. Thus, current treatment is symptomatic and the prevention of severe increased intracranial pressure.

2. In a brain abscess, the best way to establish the etiology is to:

   A. Isolate bacteria from CSF
   B. Detect specific bacterial antigen in CSF
   C. Identify bacteria in CSF by Gram stain
   D. Isolate bacteria from abscess pus
   E. Isolate bacteria from blood or urine

The correct answer is (D). In a brain abscess, the bacteria are surrounded by a capsule and confined to the pus. Therefore, the CSF does not contain any bacteria or bacterial products. In a few patients, the blood may contain the bacteria if the organism

reached the brain from a bacteremia. Thus, patients with a brain abscess from an acute bacterial endocarditis may have a *S. aureus* bacteremia. The only certain method of isolating the bacteria causing the abscess is to culture the pus. This can be done by stereotactic aspiration of the pus or from a craniotomy and direct surgical aspiration or drainage. The pus should be cultured for anaerobic and aerobic bacteria, fungi, and tuberculosis.

3. In a right anterior frontal lobe brain abscess, the main signs and symptoms that the patient develops are due to:

   A. Increased intracranial pressure
   B. Inflammation of adjacent meninges
   C. Disruption of thalmofrontal tracts
   D. Destruction of frontal eye fields
   E. Compression of the anterior corpus callosum

The correct answer is (A). Brain abscess produces signs and symptoms by two major mechanisms. If the abscess is located in a critical area of the brain, such as the motor cortex, localized signs develop. The second mechanism is through mass effect. As the abscess expands in size, the mass effect increases intracranial pressure. Increased intracranial pressure causes headache, lethargy, and psychomotor slowing. Eventually, the increased pressure causes brain herniation and death.

4. Treatment of tuberculous meningitis requires multiple drugs. The combination that is often given is isoniazid plus:

   A. Streptomycin and para-aminosalicylic acid (PAS)
   B. Chloramphenicol and para-aminosalicylic acid (PAS)
   C. Rifampin and para-aminosalicylic acid (PAS)
   D. Rifampin and pyrazinamide (PZA)
   E. Ethionamide and ethambutol

The correct answer is (D). Rifampin, isoniazid, and pyrazinamide cross the blood–brain barrier well and are effective against *Mycobacterium tuberculosis*. PAS poorly crosses the blood–brain barrier, and chloramphenicol has weak activity against *M. tuberculosis*. Ethionamide and ethambutol are second-line drugs against *M. tuberculosis*. The Centers for Disease Control recommends that rifampin, isoniazid, and PZA be given for 2 months and then rifampin and isoniazid continued for another 7 months. Streptomycin is active against *M. tuberculosis* and crosses the blood–brain barrier. It is often added if isoniazid or rifampin drug resistance is suspected. Streptomycin is potentially toxic and can cause cochlear and vestibular hair cell damage, resulting in hearing loss or imbalance.

5. Enterovirus meningitis:

    A. Is transmitted by a mosquito bite
    B. Can be treated with acyclovir
    C. Follows a prodrome of cramps and diarrhea
    D. Causes cranial nerve palsies in 10% of patients
    E. Is the most common cause of aseptic meningitis

The correct answer is (E). In the United States, enterovirus causes about 75% of cases of viral meningitis and the majority of aseptic meningitis cases. The virus is transmitted to the gastrointestinal tract from infected water. Most patients develop an asymptomatic gastrointestinal infection. In occasional patients, a viremia occurs that spreads virus to the meninges. No antiviral drugs are available in treatment, but the clinical course is benign, with over 99% making a complete recovery.

SUGGESTED READING

Anderson NE, Willoughby EW: Chronic meningitis without predisposing illness: A review of 83 cases. Q J Med 63:283, 1987

Connolly KJ, Hammer SM: The acute aseptic meningitis syndrome. Infect Dis Clin North Am 4:599, 1990

Davis LE: Acute bacterial meningitis. In Weiner WJ (ed): Emergent and Urgent Neurology, pp 135–158. Philadelphia, JB Lippincott, 1992

Davis LE, Reed WP: Infections of the central nervous system. In Rosenberg R (ed): Comprehensive Neurology, pp 215–287. New York, Raven Press, 1991

Kaplan K: Brain abscess. Med Clin North Am 69:345, 1985

Leonard JM, DesPrez RM: Tuberculous meningitis. Infect Dis Clin North Am 4:769, 1990

Whitley RJ: Viral encephalitis. N Engl J Med 323:242, 1990

Neurologic Emergencies

John A. Difini
Lisa M. Shulman

Neurologic emergencies are frequently encountered in the practice of medicine and, if unrecognized, they may rapidly progress to a permanent neurologic disability or death. The topics included in this chapter represent the more common and treatable conditions with which all health care professionals should be familiar.

STATUS EPILEPTICUS

Status epilepticus (SE) has been defined as a seizure lasting for more than 30 minutes, or intermittent serial seizures lasting for more than 30 minutes without return of consciousness. Although the term *status epilepticus* is most commonly associated with generalized tonic–clonic convulsive SE, in fact, this definition applies to any seizure type. The seizures may be generalized or partial (focal), convulsive or nonconvulsive. Accordingly, the clinical manifestations of SE are extremely variable and run the gamut from acute confusional states, psychiatric disturbances, episodes of aphasia, and focal sensorimotor deficits to tonic–clonic convulsions with loss of consciousness. A high index of suspicion is required to make a diagnosis of nonconvulsive SE and therefore an electroencephalogram (EEG) should routinely be a part of the work-up of the acute onset of altered mental status.

While isolated case reports of neurologic impairment following nonconvulsive SE are present in the literature, significant morbidity and mortality are generally associated with generalized tonic–clonic convulsive SE. Various studies over the last 20 years have reported the mortality from SE ranging from 8% to 50%. With better recognition and experience, the mortality rate has improved and now is generally accepted as 10%. Brain damage in generalized convulsive SE is a consequence of the excessive neuronal excitation (so-called excitotoxicity) as well as the systemic complications of prolonged convulsive activity. The overall incidence of morbidity and mortality from SE is related to the aforementioned two factors, as well as to the underlying acute insult that precipitated SE.

The systemic manifestations are the sequelae of airway compromise, ventilatory failure, and excessive motor activity. Hypoxemia, respiratory acidosis, metabolic acidosis, hyperthermia, and, less commonly, rhabdomyolysis and fracture–dislocations have occurred. Laboratory investigations commonly demonstrate a peripheral leucocytosis, an acidotic pH, and a mild cerebrospinal fluid (CSF) pleocytosis.

The medical approach to SE must always take into account the underlying etiology of the prolonged seizure activity. It is important to remember that the majority of patients who present with SE do not have a history of epilepsy. Although treatment is initially directed at the control of the seizures, in

William J. Weiner and Christopher G. Goetz, eds. *Neurology for the Non-Neurologist*, Third Edition. Copyright © 1994, 1989 by J. B. Lippincott Company. Copyright © 1981 by Harper and Row Publishers, Inc.

certain instances aggressive medical or surgical intervention is necessary. The three most common precipitating factors for SE are withdrawal from anticonvulsive medications, alcohol withdrawal, and cerebrovascular disease, which are each responsible for approximately one-fifth of the cases. Metabolic disorders such as hyponatremia, hyper- or hypoglycemia, hypocalcemia, hepatic failure, and renal failure account for 10% to 15% of the cases reported. Other recognized etiologic conditions are anoxia, hypotension, infectious disorders (meningitis, abscess, encephalitis), tumors, trauma, and drug overdosage.

The general principles that guide a plan that will minimize the morbidity and mortality associated with SE are early diagnosis, early intervention, a standard protocol to follow, and the prompt identification and management of underlying medical and surgical conditions. The fundamental step of recognition and diagnosis is often the greatest stumbling block. Ambulance staff and emergency room nursing and medical personnel must be educated to recognize the protean manifestations of seizure activity. Documentation of the time of onset of seizure activity is essential. The slowing or cessation of overt epileptic activity can be misleading. The observation and documentation of a gradual return of consciousness over the ensuing minutes is of paramount importance. Delays in diagnosis can often be traced to faulty communication among the staff members in attendance. It is well recognized that the longer generalized convulsive status continues, the more difficult it is to control and the greater the possibility of irreversible brain injury.

Following the diagnosis of SE, the immediate response must be a timely and organized treatment plan in order to achieve the following objectives: basic life support, termination of SE, prevention and treatment of complications of SE, identification of the cause of SE, and prevention of the reoccurrence of SE (Table 24-1). The first steps are taken to assess vital signs and evaluate oxygenation. An oral airway is inserted and nasotracheal suction is performed if necessary. The need for oxygen therapy is evaluated by both clinical examination and arterial blood gas determination. Intravenous (IV) access is the next priority, and the establishing of two separate IV lines will optimize the patient's management. A second access not only serves as a backup in the event of dislodging of the first IV line but also will be useful for the delivery of glucose, medications, and fluids aside from the needs of anticonvulsant therapy. Simultaneously, sufficient

venous blood is drawn to evaluate for a complete blood count, electrolytes, glucose, calcium, magnesium, blood urea nitrogen, liver function tests, anticonvulsant drug levels, toxicology screen, and ethanol level. An IV bolus of 50 ml of 50% glucose and thiamine 1 mg/kg is administered as soon as the IV access is established. Electrocardiographic (ECG) monitoring is instituted immediately, and vital signs are checked regularly throughout the treatment protocol. Electroencephalographic monitoring should begin at the earliest possible opportunity.

Specific treatment in order to terminate seizure activity is begun with the infusion of IV lorazepam administered at a rate of 2 mg/minute (0.1 mg/kg) to a maximum dose of 5 mg. Alternatively, IV diazepam may be given at a rate of 2 mg/min until seizures stop or to a total of 20 mg. When available, lorazepam is preferable to diazepam, as it has a significantly longer duration of action against SE. Infusion of the benzodiazepine is immediately followed by IV phenytoin 20 mg/kg at a rate no faster than 50 mg/minute. Phenytoin must be delivered in normal saline as it will precipitate in a glucose solution. ECG and frequent blood pressure monitoring are essential. If hypotension or bradycardia develops, the rate of administration can be decreased or the infusion can be held until the vital signs stabilize. IV phenytoin should never be delivered by an automatic infusion pump to an unattended patient. If seizures are not controlled, a repeat bolus of phenytoin at 10 mg/kg can be administered.

If seizures persist, elective endotracheal intubation is recommended at this point (if not done prior to this) before starting the IV infusion of phenobarbital. Phenobarbital is administered at a rate of 50 mg to 100 mg/minute until seizures stop or to a loading dose of 2 mg/kg. Phenobarbital is a potent anticonvulsant and in combination with phenytoin is effective in controlling SE in the majority of cases. Unfortunately, it is also associated with significant degrees of respiratory depression and sedation. Therefore, the use of phenobarbital increases the risk of complications for the patient. In addition, postictal assessment of the patient's cognitive status is hindered by the long half-life of this drug.

When treatment is delivered in a timely and organized manner, the aforementioned medications can be administered within 1 hour. In the majority of cases SE will be treated successfully at this point. However, if the seizures continue, begin IV pentobarbital with a loading dose of 2 mg to 3 mg/kg initially and then a continuous infusion of a solution of 100 mg/500 ml. Titrate the infusion rate in order

TABLE 24-1. Management of Generalized Status Epilepticus

OBJECTIVES	TIME FRAME	INTERVENTION
Basic life support	0–5 minutes	1. Recognition of SE.
		2. Assessment of vital signs and oxygenation.
		3. Insert oral airway and administer oxygen if necessary.
		4. Establish two intravenous lines for clear venous access.
		5. Draw venous blood for evaluation of CBC, electrolytes, glucose, calcium, magnesium, BUN, LFTs, anticonvulsant levels, toxicology screen, and ethanol level.
		6. Draw arterial blood for evaluation of ABG.
		7. Begin ECG and EEG monitoring.
	6–9 minutes	Administer IV bolus of 50 ml of 50% glucose and thiamine 1 mg/kg.
Termination of SE	10–30 minutes	1. Infuse IV lorazepam at a rate of 2 mg/min (0.1 mg/kg) to a maximum dose of 5 mg or infuse IV diazepam at a rate of 2 mg/min until seizures stop or to a total of 20 mg.
		2. Immediately follow with the infusion of IV phenytoin 20 mg/kg at a rate no faster than 50 mg/min. If seizures persist, infuse another bolus of 10 mg/kg of phenytoin.
		3. Monitor blood pressure, ECG, and respirations.
	31–60 minutes	1. If seizures persist, perform elective endotracheal intubation
		2. Infuse IV phenobarbital at a rate of 50–100 mg/min until seizures stop or to a loading dose of 20 mg/kg.
	1 hour	1. If seizures still persist begin IV pentobarbital with a loading dose of 2 mg/kg followed by a continuous infusion of a solution of 100 mg/500 ml until an isoelectric EEG is obtained.
		2. Maintain an isoelectric EEG pattern for 4 hours and then gradually taper the infusion rate over 12–24 hours.
		3. Repeat the procedure if clinical seizure activity or electrical epileptiform activity is observed.
Prevention and treatment of complications of SE	Throughout	1. Monitor vital signs regularly.
		2. Monitor patient's volume status.
		3. Maintain airway and suction as necessary to prevent aspiration.
		4. Review laboratory information promptly and intervene without delay.
Identification of cause of SE	Throughout	1. Obtain history from relatives and friends.
		2. Review medical records when available.
		3. Obtain CT of the head.
		4. Lumbar puncture, when indicated.
		5. Initiate IV antibiotic coverage when any suspicion of meningitis exists.
Prevention of reoccurrence of SE	Following cessation of seizure activity	1. Continue to closely monitor anticonvulsant levels.
		2. Initiate daily therapy with appropriate anticonvulsant medications.
		3. Educate patient and family to ensure compliance with medication regimen.

to depress the background EEG to isoelectric for 4 hours. After this time, the infusion rate is gradually decreased. If epileptiform discharges reappear on the EEG or clinical seizures reoccur, repeat this procedure. If epileptic activity is terminated, the pentobarbital may be tapered over 12 to 24 hours. Careful attention to prevention and management of complications of SE is ongoing throughout the treatment protocol. Hypertension, hyperthermia, and acidosis are consequences of persistent seizure activity, and effective control of SE will reverse these problems. Hypotension is not a direct consequence of SE, and the possibilities of anticonvulsant medication effects, volume depletion, the sequelae of multiple trauma, or coincident cardiovascular disease must be considered and treated appropriately. The potential risks of rhabdomyolysis, aspiration pneumonia, or traumatic injury at the onset or during seizure activity must be recognized.

The management of SE cannot be separated from the exigency of identifying the underlying cause. Obtaining historical information from relatives or friends accompanying the patient or review of old medical records may reveal a pattern of noncompliance with medication or a recurrent history of alcohol binging and withdrawal. Reports of the recent onset of neurologic deficits or a history of systemic disease with elevated temperature raise the index of suspicion in new areas and will guide your evaluation. Computed tomography (CT) of the head is obtained, with and without contrast (if renal function and allergies permit), to exclude the possibilities of neoplasm, cerebrovascular infarction, intracerebral hemorrhage, or traumatic injury. Following CT, lumbar puncture is often indicated and evaluation of CSF often reveals a moderate pleocytosis (up to 150 white blood cells) and an increase in CSF protein (up to 100 mg/dl) caused by the persistent seizure activity. Nonetheless, if there is any suspicion of meningitis, antibiotic therapy should be promptly begun and appropriate cultures sent for evaluation.

Following the successful treatment of SE, careful attention to serum anticonvulsant levels and the initiation of a daily dosing schedule of either an effective single anticonvulsant medication or a combination of anticonvulsants will help to prevent a reoccurrence of seizure activity. In the coming years, the development of new anticonvulsant medications as well as the introduction of new classes of drugs that may prevent the toxic consequences of excessive neuronal activity hold promise for continuing to reduce the morbidity and mortality of SE.

MYASTHENIC CRISIS

Myasthenia gravis is an autoimmune disorder mediated by the binding of antibody to the postsynaptic acetylcholine receptor of striated muscle. Neuromuscular transmission is impaired, resulting in weakness and fatigability of voluntary muscles. Classically, a diurnal variation in strength is noted, which is stronger in the morning and weaker at night. Diplopia or ptosis is the initial symptom in about half of the cases. Dysphagia, chewing difficulty, nasal speech, and regurgitation of fluids are the presenting features in one-third of patients, reflecting the involvement of bulbar musculature. Proximal extremity weakness, without bulbar or ocular involvement, is the least common presentation and is easily misdiagnosed.

A myasthenic crisis occurs when muscle weakness interferes with vital functions such as breathing and swallowing. Emergency intervention is then required. The mortality rate remains approximately 6%, with cardiac complications and aspiration pneumonia being the leading causes of death. A crisis may be precipitated by infection, emotional stress, hypokalemia, thyroid disease, or, rarely, certain drugs (Table 24-2). A crisis may also be caused by overmedication with anticholinesterase agents, the so-called cholinergic crisis. A cholinergic crisis may sometimes be heralded by an increase in muscarinic symptoms such as abdominal colic and diarrhea, with more severe muscarinic signs such as vomiting, lacrimation, hypersalivation, and miosis indicating impending danger. The differentiation of myasthenic from cholinergic crises may be more academic than practical, however, because when faced with a patient whose respiratory function is severely compromised, the emergency management is the same—protection of the airway and maintenance of adequate ventilation. Medication adjustments and discussion of precipitating factors may be done after the patient is safe in the intensive care unit (ICU) and on a mechanical ventilator.

TABLE 24-2. Drugs That May Exacerbate the Weakness of Myasthenia Gravis

Aminoglycoside antibiotics
Quinine
Cardiac antiarrhythmics (*e.g.*, quinidine, procainamide, propranolol, lidocaine)
Polymyxin
Colistin

It is rare for a crisis to be the first manifestation of myasthenia gravis. It is our policy to hospitalize any known myasthenic patient who complains of shortness of breath or difficulty swallowing, preferably in an intensive care setting. Frequent monitoring of the vital capacity is important, with endotracheal intubation performed when the vital capacity is less than 800 ml or if dysphagia is so severe that there is a serious risk of aspiration. Oral anticholinesterase agents are stopped in all patients and are withheld for 48 hours even if cholinergic crisis is not suspected. This is justified because an increased response to these drugs may occur after this "drug holiday," and often less medication may be needed once resumed. Treatment begins with a shorter-acting drug, neostigmine (Prostigmin), 0.5 mg intramuscularly (IM) or 15 mg per nasogastric tube every 2 to 3 hours using the vital capacity or muscle strength as a guide to dosage titration. Once the optimal dose of neostigmine is found, the switch to the longer-acting agent, pyridostigmine (Mestinon), can be made. Approximately four times the neostigmine dose is required every 3 to 4 hours. Corticosteroids may also be helpful in ending myasthenic crisis, but they should be used cautiously in the presence of infection. It should be kept in mind that steroids can initially worsen weakness and result in respiratory failure, particularly in the first few days after being instituted. Since the employment of steroids is usually required for several weeks or more after the crisis situation has passed, a better approach is alternate-day steroid therapy to minimize long-term side effects. Prednisone 100 mg, or its equivalent, is given on alternate days, with a gradual taper beginning only after the patient's status is clearly stabilized, usually several weeks after the crisis is over. Some authors favor giving high-dose IV corticosteroids on a daily basis early in the course before switching to alternate-day prednisone therapy. Plasmapheresis has been advocated by many as an adjunct therapy in myasthenic crisis. This modality is directed at removing the acetylcholine receptor antibody that causes myasthenia gravis. The effects of plasmapheresis alone are only temporary and may not occur for several days. IV immunoglobulin, 400 mg/kg daily for 5 consecutive days, is advocated by some as adjunctive treatment for myasthenic crisis; this treatment has not yet been evaluated in controlled clinical trials.

Any infection may precipitate a crisis, and an infectious source should be sought and treated aggressively in any patient presenting in crisis. Many myasthenic patients are iatrogenically immunosuppressed and are thus highly susceptible to infection. If an infection is suspected, empiric therapy with broad-spectrum antibiotics is started at once after cultures have been sent. The change to more specific drugs is then made when the cultures' sensitivities are available. The aminoglycosides are known to interfere with neuromuscular transmission but may be used when necessary. Chest roentgenogram, blood, urine, and sputum cultures on all myasthenic patients presenting with exacerbation should be routinely checked. In addition, a diligent search for infections is required in elderly or steroid-treated patients who may not manifest the usual systemic signs of infection.

ANEURYSMAL SUBARACHNOID HEMORRHAGE

Aneurysmal subarachnoid hemorrhage (SAH) occurs as a result of the rupture of a saccular (or berry) aneurysm related to a defect of the media or intima of the blood vessel wall. There are approximately 25,000 cases of aneurysmal SAH annually in the United States. SAH is a serious event with the potential for high mortality and morbidity. Approximately 10% of patients will die rapidly after a SAH and only one-third of patients are functional survivors. Three major factors determining eventual outcome are the severity of the initial hemorrhage, the potential for rebleeding from the aneurysm, and the onset of cerebral vasospasm. Early diagnosis is imperative, yet one out of four patients is initially misdiagnosed and presents late, often following a second hemorrhage.

Following aneurysmal rupture, the extravasation of blood into the subarachnoid space evokes the classic presenting symptom of the abrupt onset of severe headache. Commonly associated signs and symptoms are vomiting, a transient loss of consciousness, photophobia, meningismus, and the onset of neurologic dysfunction. The clinician must be aware that more subtle presentations of aneurysmal hemorrhage occur. A relatively minor but persistent headache localized to the neck region in the absence of a chronic headache history should prompt careful consideration.

In the absence of an intracranial hematoma, the patient's level of consciousness is the most important indicator of prognosis. Patients with milder presenting symptoms such as a headache with nuchal rigidity, confusion, drowsiness, and mild focal neurologic signs generally have a favorable prognosis. Few patients who present in a coma or a moribund condition survive.

If the patient's history and clinical examination raise any suspicion of SAH, CT of the head, with or without contrast, should be obtained immediately. In 89% of cases, CT will demonstrate the presence of blood in the subarachnoid space. Analysis of the distribution and density of blood may indicate the source of hemorrhage, and aneurysms greater than 1 cm in diameter may be highlighted by intravascular contrast. Further information regarding ventricular size and the presence of cerebral edema or infarction is acquired with imaging.

When the CT results are equivocal or negative, direct CSF examination is mandatory. For immediate information following the lumbar puncture, prior to formal laboratory analysis, a vial of CSF can be spun down in the centrifuge. If the supernatant is xanthochromic when compared with tap water, a diagnosis of SAH is confirmed. A high opening CSF pressure and frank blood in the CSF are not always demonstrated. Laboratory analysis will reveal increased numbers of both red and white blood cells as well as an elevated CSF protein.

Four-vessel angiography is obtained soon after the patient's admission to the hospital in order to pinpoint the location of an aneurysm, rule out the possibility of other aneurysms or arteriovenous malformations, and define the anatomy in preparation for neurosurgical intervention.

The fundamental objectives of preoperative management are to allow the brain to recover from the insult of the hemorrhage while minimizing the risks of rebleeding or cerebral ischemia. Experienced nursing care and observation are essential. If the patient is awake, he should be kept as calm and comfortable as possible with the use of analgesics (acetaminophen, codeine, demerol), sedation (diazepam, phenobarbital), and antiemetics. Anticonvulsants are often used prophylactically (phenobarbital, phenytoin). An adequate bowel program and the prevention of gastric inflammation with the use of antacids and H_2-blocking agents are imperative.

Patients who present with a significant impairment of their level of consciousness, focal neurologic dysfunction, significant hypertension, increased intracranial pressure, medical complications, or progression of deficits must be cared for in a critical care setting. Monitoring of central venous pressure, systemic arterial pressure, and intracranial pressure monitoring instituted as necessary.

Delayed neurologic deficits caused by cerebral ischemia due to vasospasm are seen in up to 30% of patients, most commonly between the fifth and ninth day after the initial hemorrhage. Serial monitoring with noninvasive transcranial Doppler ultrasonography is in use to detect the onset of cerebral vasospasm and monitor cerebral perfusion. The calcium channel–blocking agent nimodipine has been approved for prevention of cerebral vasospasm associated with aneurysmal SAH. Hypervolemic therapy may be necessary for the treatment of clinically evident vasospastic-induced cerebral ischemia. The fundamental need for cerebral perfusion may be at odds with the risks of aneurysmal rebleeding, exacerbation of cerebral edema, and systemic hypertension. The use of epsilon aminocaproic acid (Amicar) is controversial. Its antifibrinolytic action appears to decrease the risk of rebleeding; however, its use has been associated with an increased incidence of both vasospasm and hydrocephalus.

The timing of neurosurgical intervention is critical. Early surgery may be complicated by the presence of blood, cerebral edema, and a medically unstable patient, while later surgery allows the opportunity for the onset of rebleeding and vasospasm. In general, patients with mild neurologic deficits and no evidence of vasospasm are early surgical candidates, while patients with more significant deficits are operated on later following medical stabilization and treatment for vasospasm when indicated.

The hazards and intricacies of caring for patients with aneurysmal subarachnoid hemorrhage are clear and emphasize the need for a highly experienced nursing, medical, and surgical staff.

GUILLAIN–BARRÉ SYNDROME

Acute inflammatory polyradiculoneuropathy, commonly referred to as the Guillain–Barré syndrome (GBS), is a symmetrical, rapidly progressive, demyelinating polyneuropathy that in its most fulminant form may lead to sudden respiratory failure and autonomic instability. It therefore should be considered a neurologic emergency. The mortality rate remains at 3% to 5% despite modern intensive care management.

The classic presentation is a fairly symmetrical, ascending, flaccid paralysis that usually begins in the lower extremities (10% begin in the upper extremities) and progresses upward, with the maximum deficit attained by 4 weeks. In contrast to other more slowly progressive polyneuropathies in which a distal weakness predominates, the greatest weakness in GBS is typically in the proximal muscles. Areflexia is the rule and may precede weakness. Many patients complain of distal paresthesias initially, but formal testing rarely demonstrates a significant sensory loss. In fact, patients with early GBS have been discharged from emergency rooms undiagnosed because of sensory complaints without findings. Facial weakness is seen in about half the cases. Fever should not be present at the onset. A prior history of a recent (within 4 weeks) respiratory or gastrointestinal illness is obtained in about half of the patients. A previous inoculation, surgery, hematologic malignancies, and hepatitis B or mycoplasma infections have also been associated with the syndrome.

CSF analysis within the first week may be normal—the classic albuminocytologic dissociation (increased protein and up to ten mononuclear cells) usually appears after the second week of illness.

Nerve conduction studies may be entirely normal early in the course if the proximal root segments are not studied. The F and H responses measuring the motor and sensory proximal segments, respectively, may be the only abnormality noted early on. Profound slowing of nerve conduction velocity may appear on routine studies after several weeks of illness. Those cases that show evidence of secondary axonal degeneration with denervation on an electromyogram (EMG) will generally have a more protracted recovery.

GBS is a neurologic emergency because of the life-threatening complications of respiratory failure and cardiovascular collapse that sometimes occur within 24 hours of the onset of symptoms. The patient must, therefore, be closely watched in an intensive care unit or an intermediate care unit until the plateau phase of maximum deficit is reached. The vital capacity should be checked every 4 to 6 hours; if it is less than 800 ml, endotracheal intubation should be performed. Artificial ventilation may be required in up to 23% of patients. Autonomic instability may be severe, with marked fluctuations in blood pressure, tachycardia, and malignant arrhythmias. Cardiac arrhythmias are probably the main cause of death in the acute period, hence the need for continuous cardiac monitoring. Hypotension is usually mild and can be controlled with IV fluids; vasopressor agents are rarely needed. Extreme caution should be taken when treating hypertension. Because of the marked lability in blood pressure, only short-acting, easily titratable drugs such as IV nitroprusside should be used. Sustained tachycardia can be treated with small doses of beta blockers if necessary. Corticosteroids, previously widely used in the acute phase of GBS, are no longer advocated, and a randomized double-blind study actually showed significantly slower improvement and more instances of relapse in the steroid-treated group.

One randomized multicenter study has suggested that plasmapheresis, if performed within the first 2 weeks of the onset of symptoms, can significantly shorten the time it takes to attain a functional recovery; however, it does not decrease the incidence of respiratory failure. It is contraindicated in patients with severe autonomic instability. Thus, plasmapheresis, while probably an important treatment modality to invoke early in the course of GBS for long-term goals, is not a valuable therapy for the prevention of its life-threatening complications. A recent Dutch trial comparing high-dose intravenous immune globulin (IIG) with plasma exchange indicated a beneficial effect from prompt institution of gamma globulin, comparable to that seen with plasmapheresis. Although further investigation is needed, IIG may become the treatment of choice for GBS because of its ease of administration, safety profile, and comparable cost.

Several other entities can cause a rapidly progressive and occasionally fatal flaccid paralysis that can mimic GBS (Table 24-3), and these should be differentiated because of variations in acute management.

Acute intermittent porphyria can cause a rapidly ascending flaccid paralysis with respiratory and autonomic involvement, but severe abdominal pain is usually the initial symptom, and seizures and psychosis often occur. Urine porphobilinogen and delta-aminolevulinic acid are elevated. Unlike GBS, the CSF protein is usually normal. Attacks of acute intermittent porphyria may be precipitated by certain drugs such as barbiturates, phenytoin, some of the benzodiazepines, and sulfonamides. Treatment of acute attacks is aimed at the suppression of por-

TABLE 24-3. Disorders That Can Mimic Guillain–Barré Syndrome

Acute intermittent porphyria
Diphtheritic neuropathy
Botulism
Tick-bite paralysis
Poliomyelitis
Arsenic intoxication

phyrin synthesis with a high carbohydrate intake, as well as supportive management of the accompanying complications.

Diphtheritic neuropathy occurs 1 to 2 months after the characteristic pharyngitis. The onset of weakness usually follows pronounced cranial nerve involvement by several weeks, and it may be associated with myocarditis. Unfortunately, by the time neurologic symptoms appear, specific therapy with antitoxin is ineffective and the mainstays of treatment are respiratory support and good nursing care.

The first neurologic symptoms of botulism are usually ocular, with blurred vision and diplopia. Intoxication usually presents with gastrointestinal symptoms. Unlike GBS, the pupillary reflexes are lost and the CSF is normal. Sensation remains intact. The diagnosis is supported by nerve conduction studies with reduced amplitude of compound muscle action potentials and an incremental response following rapid repetitive nerve stimulation. Specific treatment with trivalent botulinum antitoxin is recommended. Nasogastric suctioning and enemas may help remove toxin from the gastrointestinal tract early in the illness. In wound botulism, surgical debridement and penicillin are the essentials of treatment. In food-borne botulism, the role of antibiotics is controversial because of the concern that rapid bacterial destruction might increase the release of toxin.

Tick-bite paralysis is caused by a natural endotoxin that interferes with the release of acetylcholine at the neuromuscular junction. It can present as a rapidly ascending paralysis with respiratory and bulbar involvement. A dramatic improvement occurs after the removal of the offending tick.

Poliomyelitis can produce a flaccid paralysis with respiratory involvement and can thus mimic GBS. However, the weakness of poliomyelitis is characteristically asymmetrical, and the disease usually presents as a febrile illness with gastrointestinal symptoms, myalgias, meningismus, and a CSF pleocytosis. Arsenical neuropathy can present as rapidly developing weakness and areflexia with CSF and nerve conduction studies indistinguishable from GBS. However, the neuropathy is usually accompanied by gastrointestinal, hepatic, and hematologic manifestations of arsenic poisoning. The patient with arsenical neuropathy often complains of burning dysesthesia, a feature not common in GBS.

ACUTE ALTERATION OF MENTAL STATUS

Acute alterations of mental status are the most common neurobehavioral disorders seen in general hospitals. Studies have demonstrated an incidence of between 5% and 15% in hospitalized patients on medical–surgical floors, 20% and 30% in surgical intensive care units, and even higher on geriatric wards. The use of numerous vague and redundant terms to describe this disorder (e.g., organic brain syndrome, acute cerebral insufficiency, organic psychosis, toxic-metabolic encephalopathy, acute confusional state, and exogenous psychosis) reflects the difficulties we encounter in conceptualizing and categorizing these problems.

The most common causes of acute confusional states, often associated with alterations of consciousness, are acquired metabolic disturbances. The metabolic encephalopathies are a diverse group of neurologic disorders characterized by an alteration of mental status caused by the failure of organs other than the brain. Cerebral dysfunction may result from three basic mechanisms: deficiency of a necessary metabolic substrate (e.g., hypoglycemia); disruption of the internal environment of the brain (e.g., dehydration); or the presence of a toxin or accumulation of a metabolic waste product (e.g., drug intoxication or uremia). Although the brain is, in effect, an "innocent bystander," the alterations of personality, behavior, cognitive function, or level of alertness may be the presenting feature that brings the patient to medical attention.

Metabolic encephalopathies are usually characterized by an evolution from the patient's baseline mental status through stages of inattentiveness, disturbed memory, confusion, lethargy, somnolence, obtundation, and coma. The early stages of these deficits will often go unrecognized due to the patient's concurrent loss of insight and judgment.

The disturbance of higher cortical functions is illustrated by a wide range of signs and symptoms. Disorientation, memory impairment, emotional lability, disturbance of the sleep–wake cycle, and either increased or decreased psychomotor activity may be observed. Reduced ability to maintain and shift attention, as well as disorganized thinking with fluctuations over the course of the day are characteristic. Perceptual disturbances may result in illusions, delusions, or hallucinations, which are usually visual and often unpleasant.

The sum total of these disturbances is often characterized by delirium, a clouding of consciousness with reduced ability to sustain attention to environmental stimuli. As a result, the patient is unable to respond to events with the usual clarity, coherence, or speed.

The differential diagnosis of a patient with an unexplained acute alteration of mental status is extensive. The approach to the patient should take into account the three broad areas of structural lesions, toxic–metabolic causes, and psychiatric etiologies. Structural lesions often distinguish themselves with focal or asymmetrical findings on neurologic exam and a more abrupt onset than that seen in metabolic disorders. In addition, the level of consciousness is more likely to fluctuate with metabolic than structural disorders. Inconsistencies on repeated examinations and atypical, nonanatomic findings may raise the suspicion of an underlying psychiatric problem.

Hepatic encephalopathy and uremic encephalopathy are frequent causes of altered mental status in hospitalized patients. Disorders of glucose regulation, osmolarity/sodium homeostasis, and derangement of calcium, magnesium, and phosphorous levels are also frequent offenders. Hypoxic–ischemic encephalopathy is often identified as the causative factor following cardiorespiratory arrest, ventilatory failure, or hypotensive episodes. Endocrine encephalopathies seen in Cushing's syndrome, Addison's disease, and thyroid disease are less common and may be overlooked.

Drug intoxication and drug withdrawal are very common causative factors. Acute alterations of mental status are especially associated with drugs that have anticholinergic properties, including many antidepressants, neuroleptics, antihistamines, antiparkinsonian agents, and over-the-counter cold preparations. High-dose steroids, narcotics, and sedatives may be the offending agent. Abused street drugs associated with violent behavior include amphetamines, cocaine, hallucinogens, minor tranquilizers/sedatives, and, of course, alcohol.

Management of the patient with an acute alteration of mental status involves two stages: identification and treatment of the underlying cause and symptomatic treatment. Significant hypoxia or hypoglycemia demand especially quick recognition and treatment because of the potential for irreversible brain injury. Historical information must be obtained about systemic illnesses, drug or alcohol use, recent trauma, exposure to toxins, the baseline mental status, and the time frame of the change in mental function.

Predisposing factors to acute confusional states are a history of dementia, mental retardation, or preceding brain injury, psychological stress or anxiety, unfamiliar surroundings with loss of daily routine, disruption of sleep–wake cycles, and sensory understimulation or overstimulation. Both the very old and the very young patient are at special risk. Polypharmacy, the simultaneous use of multiple pharmacologic agents, is an especially important contributory factor.

While the alteration in mental states may be the presenting feature that brings the patient to medical attention, evidence of the underlying disorder is usually present on physical examination. A thoughtful examination includes inspection for the stigmata of hepatic, renal, or endocrine disorders. Scrutiny of the states of hydration and nutrition provides important information. Alterations in the patient's vital signs may provide clues to a wide diversity of problems, ranging from sepsis to elevated intracranial pressure. Evidence of head trauma should be sought in the obtunded or comatose patient.

Examination of the patient's mental status should be performed in a reproducible manner to guide subsequent re-evaluations of disease progression and efficacy of therapy. Description of level of consciousness is best limited to a few commonly recognized descriptive terms, such as alert, lethargic, stuporous, and comatose. The arbitrary imposition of labels to a wide continuum of behavior demands precise documentation of the patient's performance on standardized tests of arousability, orientation, attention, and memory. The Folstein Mini-Mental Exam and Glasgow Coma Scale provide convenient quantitative parameters for more precise follow-up.

The neurologic exam includes tests of pupillary control and ocular motility, including the oculocephalic and oculovestibular reflexes, and evaluation of respiratory pattern and motor responses to stimulation. Demonstration of intact brain-stem function makes a structural lesion of the brain stem, including an elevation of intracranial pressure, less likely. Hyperreflexia may be seen in association with metabolic encephalopathy, but other evidence of upper motor neuron dysfunction is usually not demonstrated until advanced stages of alterations of consciousness. Asterixis, generalized tremor, and spontaneous myoclonus are often observed. Toxic encephalopathies should especially be considered in patients with dysarthria, nystagmus, ataxia, tremor, and dilated pupils.

Laboratory evaluation should include a complete blood count, platelet count, prothrombin time (PT), partial thromboplastin time, chemistry profile (electrolytes, glucose, blood urea nitrogen, creatinine, calcium, magnesium, phosphorous), liver function tests, ammonia level, thyroid function tests, arterial blood gas, urinalysis, and drug and toxicology screen. Information gathered during the history and physical exam will provide guidance in choosing from the following additional studies: serum osmolality, plasma cortisol level, fluorescent treponemal antibody (FTA), glucose tolerance test, erythrocyte sedimentation rate, anti-nuclear antibody (ANA), vitamin B_{12}, folate, human immunodeficiency virus, ceruloplasmin, serum copper, urinary copper, and urinary porphobilinogen.

Neuroimaging is required following an acute change in mental status to exclude a structural lesion with increased intracranial pressure. Specific CSF abnormalities are rare in metabolic encephalopathies; however, lumbar puncture may be necessary to rule out meningitis or encephalitis.

An EEG should be routinely obtained in patients with metabolic encephalopathy or altered mental status of uncertain etiology. The EEG recording provides an objective evaluation of the degree of central nervous system (CNS) dysfunction. Disorganization of the normal electroencephalographic patterns and generalized slowing are the most commonly observed changes. Seizure activity, particularly subclinical SE, as well as focal abnormalities may be identified. Oftentimes, the major value of EEG is in the use of serial studies to quantitatively and objectively gauge the degree of cerebral dysfunction.

While it is clear that the term *altered mental status* represents an extensive ensemble of behavior and a spectrum of levels of consciousness, there is a subset of patients who are especially challenging. Patients with disorientation, emotional lability, delusions, hallucinations, paranoid ideation, or intoxication may be agitated, aggressive, violent, and resistant to medical evaluation and treatment. Although it is best to avoid the use of drugs in confused and agitated patients, the patient's behavior may be potentially dangerous, may cause the patient profound distress, and may interfere with the provision of nursing and medical care.

The alternatives of chemical or physical restraints are both fraught with flaws and hazards. Intervention should be individualized and directed at the specific problem (*e.g.*, anxiety, depression, insomnia, disturbance of sleep–wake cycles, agitation, hallucinations, delusions, and assaultiveness). The most commonly used agents are benzodiazepines and neuroleptics. Neuroleptic medications may be an appropriate choice in the acute situation but should not be used in this setting for the long-term management of behavior.

For the patient with acute agitation with psychiatric features haloperidol may be administered in a dosage of 5 mg IM every 4 to 8 hours to a maximum of 15 mg to 30 mg/day. Delirious patients rarely require more than 10 mg of haloperidol daily, and often 2 mg to 4 mg/day will suffice. The therapeutic end point should be a manageable reduction in misperceptions and agitation, not a completely clear sensorium. When the predominant feature is anxiety, benzodiazepines (*e.g.*, diazepam 5 mg to 10 mg IM) are often sufficient.

There are some cautions to keep in mind when using neuroleptics or sedatives for organic cerebral dysfunction, particularly when the underlying etiology is unclear. One should be certain that the patient's level of consciousness is not worsening prior to administration. Intoxication with alcohol, overdosage with sedative or anticholinergic drugs, structural lesions with elevated intracranial pressure and both CNS and systemic infections should be excluded. In some situations these behaviors are a critical guide to the progression of the underlying process and the use of physical restraints is preferable.

While the diagnosis and treatment of the commonplace disorder of alteration of mental status may be challenging and difficult in patients with multiple system failure or irreversible brain injury, a significant proportion of these patients are found to have reversible processes. These encounters, when approached with conversance and proficiency, can be especially rewarding.

ACUTE INTRACRANIAL HYPERTENSION

Brain, blood, and CSF all occupy space within the rigid confines of the skull. Any increase in the volume of one of these components without a corresponding decrease in the volume of the other two will result in raised intracranial pressure that may rise gradually over an extended period of time or suddenly in a matter of minutes to acutely threaten life. The prompt recognition and treatment of acutely raised intracranial pressure are vital to preserve brain-stem function, and they may be lifesaving.

The cranial vault is divided incompletely into compartments by thick, fibrous bands of dura mater. The *tentorium cerebelli* is clinically the most important of these structures. It separates the lower brain stem and cerebellum from the cerebral hemispheres and diencephalon, delineating the infratentorial and supratentorial spaces, respectively. The midbrain lies within an opening in the tentorium called the *tentorial notch*, and it is bound laterally by fascicles of the oculomotor nerve and the medial portion of the temporal lobes (the uncus). This anatomic location renders the midbrain especially vulnerable to compression under conditions of increased intracranial pressure.

An acute rise in intracompartmental pressure, such as occurs with hypertensive hemorrhage, may result in downward displacement and herniation of neural structures. The midbrain, placed centrally in the tentorial notch, may be compressed by surrounding elements, compromising vital brain-stem functions such as respiration, maintenance of consciousness, and cardioregulation. Coma and death may ensue. There are two main types of herniation syndromes: uncal and central. It is important that these syndromes be recognized early and that treatment be urgently instituted before further progression to irreversible brain-stem damage occurs. Some of the mass lesions that can lead to herniation are listed in Table 24-4.

Central herniation occurs when diffusely raised supratentorial pressure compresses central brain-stem structures and produces a progressive impairment of consciousness, respiratory irregularities, abnormal motor responses (posturing), and symmetrical midposition unreactive pupils. Uncal herniation, on the other hand, occurs as a unilateral supratentorial mass lesion displaces the medial temporal lobe toward the tentorial notch. Early on, the oculomotor nerve becomes compressed between the encroaching uncus and the edge of the tentorial opening, producing a larger and less reactive pupil on that side. Hemiparesis may occur ipsilateral to the herniating uncus due to the compression of the contralateral cerebral peduncle against the far edge of the tentorial notch as the midbrain is displaced

laterally (Kernohan's notch syndrome). More commonly, though, the hemiparesis is contralateral to the herniating uncus. In either case, hemiparesis is not a good clinical sign for localizing the side of the herniation. A dilated pupil (oculomotor nerve palsy) is ipsilateral to the herniation 95% of the time, and it is a reliable clinical indicator.

Unlike the situation that occurs with mass lesions, raised intracranial pressure may be distributed equally among the intracranial compartments with little risk of herniation and brain-stem compression. Some of the more common causes of diffuse intracranial hypertension are listed in Table 24-5.

Symptoms and signs of intracranial hypertension are variable and depend on both the etiology and the rapidity with which the pressure increase develops. Headache, for example, is more likely to be a prominent symptom in more acute problems. Vomiting and alteration of consciousness may be seen; papilledema may be present in subacute or chronic conditions. The abducens nerve, by virtue of its extensive intracranial course, is particularly susceptible to traction injury when the intracranial pressure is raised. Sixth nerve palsies, therefore, are frequently seen, but they have no localizing value.

The evaluation of patients with suspected intracranial hypertension should begin with a brief history from available sources and a brief physical examination. Patients who are unresponsive and in danger of herniation should be intubated immediately, and emergency treatment should be begun before diagnostic procedures are undertaken. In such catastrophic situations, mechanical hyperventilation is the fastest way of reducing intracranial pressure. It is desirable to keep the $PaCO_2$ between 25 and 30 mm Hg. The decreased $PaCO_2$ causes cerebral vasoconstriction, thereby reducing cerebral blood volume and intracranial pressure.

Osmotic agents such as mannitol are given to

TABLE 24-4. Mass Lesions Associated with Brain Herniation

Neoplasm (primary or metastatic)
Subdural hematoma
Epidural hematoma
Intraparenchymal hemorrhage
Abscess
Infarction

TABLE 24-5. Causes of Diffuse Intracranial Hypertension with Less Risk of Herniation

Hypoxia
Meningitis
Encephalitis
Head trauma without subdural or epidural hematoma
Subarachnoid hemorrhage
Malignant hyperthermia
Cerebral vein thrombosis
Pseudotumor cerebri
Lead encephalopathy

decrease the water content of the brain. The starting dose is 500 ml of 20% mannitol given IV over 20 to 30 minutes (approximately 1 mg/kg). An indwelling urinary catheter is always inserted. Serum electrolytes and osmolality are monitored closely, using the latter as a guide to further dosing. A mannitol dose of 100 mg to 250 mg can be given every 4 hours as necessary to keep the serum osmolality at 310 to 320 mOsm/liter.

Corticosteroids are administered if considerable vasogenic edema is present. Vasogenic edema occurs in those conditions that involve a breakdown of the blood–brain barrier and is seen commonly with brain neoplasms. Steroids are generally not effective for the type of edema that accompanies cerebral infarction (cytotoxic edema) and thus are not indicated in large hemispheric strokes. Steroids do not begin to work for several hours, so they are usually given concurrently with hyperventilation and hyperosmolar agents in acute situations. Methylprednisolone (Solu-Medrol) 250 mg or dexamethasone (Decadron) 10 mg IV can be used immediately followed by Decadron 4 mg IV every 6 hours.

In some instances of rapidly progressing intracranial hypertension, none of the aforementioned measures are helpful and emergency neurosurgery is the preferred treatment. This is certainly the case with cerebellar hemorrhages or rapidly expanding epidural or subdural hematomas, where surgical decompression and evacuation may be lifesaving.

Only after the patient's clinical status has been stabilized should a further evaluation with a head CT scan proceed. Because of the risk of precipitating herniation, a lumbar puncture should not be performed in any patient suspected of having increased intracranial pressure until a mass lesion is ruled out by a CT scan. A lumbar puncture may have to be performed prior to obtaining a CT scan if the patient is suspected of having bacterial meningitis and focal findings are not seen on the neurologic examination. In this instance, any delay in the diagnosis and administration of appropriate antibiotics may seriously threaten a favorable outcome.

NEUROLEPTIC MALIGNANT SYNDROME

Neuroleptic malignant syndrome (NMS) is a potentially lethal complication associated with the use of agents that block the action of dopamine in the CNS. Although NMS is not exclusively associated with neuroleptic drugs, this syndrome continues to bear a name that reflects the initial circumstances in which it was recognized. Phenothiazines, butyrophenones, and thioxanthenes continue to be the classes of drugs most commonly implicated (Table 24-6). In general, a drug's potential for inducing NMS parallels its antidopaminergic potency. Accordingly, haloperidol, chlorpromazine, and fluphenazine have been identified as the most frequent offenders. Less commonly, NMS has also occurred with the use of a dopamine depleting agent such as tetrabenazine and following the abrupt discontinuation of antiparkinsonian dopaminergic medication.

Due to a scarcity of reliable epidemiologic data, the incidence of NMS is not clearly established. Retrospective studies have documented the incidence of NMS among all patients exposed to neuroleptic drugs to be between 0.5% and 1%. NMS has been reported in all age-groups and in both sexes. It is related neither to the duration of exposure to neuroleptics nor to toxic overdoses of neuroleptics; however, numerous predisposing factors in affected patients have been identified. NMS is associated with the initiation of neuroleptic medications at high dosages, the rapid upward titration of dose, as well as the use of long-acting depot neuroleptic preparations. Metabolic factors such as dehydration, physical exhaustion, and acute agitation with excessive sympathetic discharge have also been implicated.

The four cardinal features of NMS are hyperthermia, muscle rigidity, altered mental status and instability of the autonomic nervous system. An interruption of dopaminergic pathways is believed to be the primary etiology. A blockade of dopa-

TABLE 24-6. Causes of Neuroleptic Malignant Syndrome

Dopamine-blocking agents
   Haloperidol (Haldol)
   Chlorpromazine (Thorazine)
   Fluphenazine (Prolixin)
   Clozapine (Clozaril)
   Thioridazine (Mellaril)
   Thiothixene (Navane)
   Trifluoperazine (Stelazine)
   Metoclopramide (Reglan)
Dopamine-depleting agents
   Tetrabenazine
Abrupt discontinuation of antiparkinsonian dopaminergic medications

minergic receptors in the striatum is thought to cause tonic contraction of skeletal muscles, which generates heat, and a similar blockade in the hypothalamus may disrupt thermoregulatory function. It is proposed that an analogous disruption of dopaminergic function in the mesocorticolimbic system may underlie the alteration of mental status and a blockade of dopamine receptors in the spinal cord may be responsible for the dysautonomia.

Hyperthermia is present in all cases of NMS; however, the height of the temperature elevation is variable. Body temperature above 38°C (100.4°F) was noted in 92% of NMS patients, and higher temperatures, above 40°C (104°F), were recorded in 40%. Muscular hypertonia, commonly described as "lead pipe" rigidity, is generalized in distribution and may be severe enough to compromise chest wall compliance, causing hypoventilation and the need for ventilatory support. Dysphagia may occur due to rigidity of the pharyngeal musculature, placing the patient at risk for aspiration. Other commonly reported motor abnormalities include akinesia, bradykinesia, and involuntary movements, such as tremor and dystonia.

Mental status changes, often described as fluctuating states of consciousness, occur in 75% of affected patients. Progression through stages of agitation to alert mutism, stupor, and coma may be observed. Autonomic dysfunction is universal. Frequently reported manifestations are tachycardia, diaphoresis, blood pressure instability, urinary incontinence, cardiac dysrhythmias, and pallor or flushing of the skin. Infrequent findings include Babinski sign, hyperreflexia, seizures, opisthotonos, oculogyric crisis, chorea, and trismus. The clinical features of NMS typically develop over a 24- to 72-hour period and continue for approximately 5 to 10 days even when the offending agents are discontinued. Symptoms persist two to three times longer when depot preparations of neuroleptics were the etiologic agents.

Laboratory investigations can be instrumental in making the diagnosis of NMS and in recognizing metabolic alterations that mandate diligent monitoring and treatment. Two laboratory abnormalities that are consistently found are elevation of the blood creatinine phosphokinase (CPK) level and a polymorphonuclear leukocytosis. Myonecrosis due to intense sustained muscle contractions underlies the rise in CPK, which can vary widely from slightly elevated into the hundreds of thousands. White blood cell determinations between 10,000 and 30,000 cells/mm^3 are found in the majority of cases.

Electrolyte levels may reveal dehydration, and elevations of liver function tests are commonly seen. Lumbar puncture, when performed, demonstrates either normal CSF parameters or nonspecific changes. CT of the head is typically negative and electroencephalography traces are either normal or consistent with a nonspecific encephalopathy.

The recognition of NMS can be troublesome. It is a clinical diagnosis. Commonly the differential diagnoses of CNS infection (meningitis, encephalitis, postinfectious encephalomyelitis), malignant hyperthermia, acute lethal catatonia, and anticholinergic toxicity must carefully be ruled out. Other disorders with similar presentations include thyrotoxicosis, heat stroke, tetanus, and drug-induced parkinsonism. Most importantly, when the suspicion of NMS is raised, treatment should be initiated without delay. Management of NMS begins with the immediate withdrawal of neuroleptic medications as well as any other dopamine antagonists in use. In the acute setting, IV fluids may be required for volume repletion, metabolic abnormalities may require correction, and ice packs and cooling blankets may be indicated for hyperthermia. The two most commonly used agents for treatment of NMS are dantrolene sodium and bromocriptine. Dantrolene sodium is a directly acting muscle relaxant, and bromocriptine is a centrally acting dopamine agonist. These two medications used alone or in combination promote a reduction of body temperature and serum CPK by lessening skeletal muscle rigidity. Both dantrolene and bromocriptine have been shown to significantly shorten the time of clinical response to therapy as compared with supportive care.

If the syndrome is caused by orally administered neuroleptics, treatment with dantrolene and/or bromocriptine should be continued for at least 10 days, as reoccurrence may develop with early withdrawal from therapy. When depot neuroleptics were used, treatment may be required for 2 to 3 weeks. During this period, supportive care is maintained, with careful monitoring of nutrition, fluid balance, and metabolic parameters. Approximately 40% of patients with NMS suffer from medical complications. Respiratory complications, including ventilatory failure, aspiration pneumonia, pulmonary edema, and pulmonary embolism, are the sequelae of diminished chest wall compliance and prolonged immobility. Cardiovascular complications such as phlebitis, dysrhythmias, myocardial infarction, and cardiovascular collapse may be seen. There is a significant risk of renal failure as a result of the combined effects of volume depletion and myoglobinuria due to rhabdomyolysis.

Mortality may result from the cumulative effects of medical complications. Morbidity and mortality from NMS have decreased over the years; reports document a mortality rate of 25% before 1984 and 11.6% since 1984. The improvement in prognosis is attributed more to early recognition and treatment of the syndrome than to the use of any specific therapeutic agent.

As many patients who recover from NMS continue to require the use of dopamine-blocking agents, the question of the safety of reintroducing neuroleptics is relevant. Experience has shown that neuroleptic agents can be reintroduced safely in the majority of cases. Studies have demonstrated that a reoccurrence of NMS can best be avoided by waiting a sufficient amount of time so that a given episode of NMS has completely resolved, reintroducing low doses of low-potency neuroleptics, and assuring that the patient is well hydrated and metabolically stable.

The diagnosis of NMS should come to mind when encountering any individual receiving neuroleptics who develops unexplained fever associated with muscle rigidity. Although there are numerous alternate diagnoses, the life-threatening potential of NMS demands that treatment should not be delayed if there is significant clinical suspicion.

ACUTE SPINAL CORD COMPRESSION

Acute compression of the spinal cord often presents insidiously with mild sensory disturbance, weakness, or sphincter or sexual dysfunction but may progress rapidly to irreversible paralysis if not corrected. Spinal cord compression is a common complication of metastatic cancer, but it also occurs with other conditions (Table 24-7). The most frequent metastatic tumors causing spinal cord compression include multiple myeloma, lymphoma,

TABLE 24-7. Common Causes of Acute Spinal Cord Compression

Metastatic cancer
Herniated disk
Abscess
Hematoma

and carcinomas of the prostate, lung, breast, kidney, and colon.

Pain is the earliest symptom in the vast majority of patients and may be localized to the involved spinal area or radiate in a dermatomal pattern if the dorsal spinal roots are also involved. Pain may be intensified by actions that increase intrathoracic pressure such as coughing, sneezing, or straining at stool. Percussion tenderness over the spine is often a valuable clinical sign aiding localization.

The development of weakness, sensory loss, or erectile or sphincter dysfunction may progress quickly, and treatment should be started at the first sign of myelopathy. Very high-dose corticosteroids, such as dexamethasone 100 mg IV, is given immediately to reduce the edema caused by the compressing lesion and often provides dramatic pain relief and return of some neurologic function. Dexamethasone is then continued at a dose of 6 mg to 10 mg IV or p.o. every 6 hours until more definitive treatment is completed, with antiulcer prophylaxis given concurrently. An indwelling bladder catheter should be inserted. Bladder and bowel function should be monitored, with stool softeners and laxatives given as needed.

Diagnostic procedures to delineate the etiology and area of involvement should then be pursued. Discerning the cause is usually not difficult in patients with known cancer or recent trauma, but on occasion spinal cord compression may be the initial manifestation of malignancy. Plain x-rays of the spine may show evidence of bony erosion from metastatic disease but are of little help in imaging the soft tissue structures that are invading the epidural or subdural spaces and compressing the spinal cord. Magnetic resonance imaging (MR) is now readily available to most clinicians and is the procedure of choice for visualizing the extent of anatomic involvement and spinal cord compression. It is superior to myelography in most instances because of its noninvasiveness and better resolution of anatomic structures.

Specific treatment directed at the underlying process can begin once the etiology and location are defined. In metastatic disease, radiation therapy is started immediately and is especially valuable for the more radiosensitive tumors such as multiple myeloma and lymphoma. Surgical decompression is the treatment of choice for disk disease, epidural abscess, and hematoma, and is sometimes indicated for metastatic disease in situations in which a tissue diagnosis is needed, spinal stabilization is necessary, or further radiotherapy is not warranted.

A high index of suspicion is required to make the diagnosis of epidural abscess, and a history of recent bacteremia or IV drug abuse is often obtained. The patient may or may not appear septic at the time of presentation. If epidural abscess is suspected, high-dose IV antibiotics should be given immediately (after sending blood and other appropriate cultures) while awaiting radiologic procedures and surgical decompression.

PITUITARY APOPLEXY

Sudden, massive infarction of the pituitary gland, pituitary apoplexy, presents as an acute, severe headache, often with meningismus, vomiting, impaired vision, and altered mentation. The clinical picture and frequent hemorrhagic nature of the infarction often lead to a mistaken diagnosis of aneurysmal rupture. Prompt recognition and treatment are required to avoid permanent visual impairment or death.

Pituitary apoplexy typically occurs in patients not previously suspected of having pituitary adenomas, but it also may occur in patients with known tumors with or without previous endocrinopathy. It may even occur in a baseline normal pituitary gland (*e.g.*, Sheehan's postpartum necrosis).

Symptoms and signs are caused by the abrupt swelling and hemorrhage of the infarcted tissue compressing the parasellar structures and infiltrating the meninges. Effusion of blood and necrotic matter into the subarachnoid space causes meningeal irritation, fever, and obtundation or coma. Sudden expansion in a suprasellar direction results in visual impairment due to compromise of the optic chiasm or optic tracts. Lateral expansion into the cavernous sinus may involve any of the structures lying within. Most common is involvement of the cranial nerves affecting ocular motility (III, IV, and VI), causing varying degrees of ophthalmoparesis. Compression of the ophthalmic division of cranial nerve V in the cavernous sinus may produce facial pain or numbness in that distribution, with impairment of the corneal reflex. Impingement of sympathetic fibers may cause miosis and ptosis of the ipsilateral eye, together with anhidrosis of the forehead (Horner's syndrome). Cerebral hemispheric dysfunction, including seizures and hemiplegia, may occur because of mechanical compression on the carotid siphon. A stroke-like picture may also be seen in the absence of carotid compression due to vasospasm caused by the irritative effects of blood in the subarachnoid space.

Tumors are more prevalent in the anterior portion of the gland than the posterior portion; consequently, infarction may cause deficiencies of prolactin, growth hormone, gonadotropins, thyrotropin, and corticotropin more often than deficiency of vasopressin. Thus, diabetes insipidus is only rarely associated with acute apoplexy.

Apoplexy of the nontumorous pituitary gland often causes no neurologic sequelae other than headache since there is no pre-existing mass lesion to suddenly expand and infiltrate. Hence, this condition may go unrecognized until the endocrinopathies become obvious or until autopsy.

The syndrome of pituitary apoplexy may mimic aneurysmal rupture but may also be confused with bacterial meningitis, cavernous sinus thrombosis, or parasellar tumors such as meningioma or craniopharyngioma. Suspicion of any of these conditions would most likely prompt neurologic and radiologic investigation, leading to the correct diagnosis. Axial and coronal CT scans may reveal an enlarged pituitary fossa with hemorrhagic infarction of sellar contents and extension into the parasellar regions. CSF analysis yields abnormal but nonspecific findings that may be consistent with any of the preceding conditions.

Routine blood studies as well as baseline endocrine testing should be performed during the acute episode before beginning immediate corticosteroid therapy. Levels of growth hormone, thyrotropin, corticotropin, cortisol, prolactin, luteinizing hormone, and follicle-stimulating hormone should be included. High-dose IV corticosteroids should then be given to counteract edema and potentially lethal acute corticotropin deficiency. Some authors recommend early trans-sphenoidal neurosurgical decompression in all patients because of the possibility of rapid deterioration over the ensuing hours to days. Others favor conservative medical management with corticosteroids and appropriate hormonal replacement in less severely affected patients. Evaluation and replacement of hormone deficiencies is a critical therapeutic point with or without underlying tumor and whether or not surgery is performed. This should be done in conjunction with an endocrinologist, whose input will also be helpful in determining the need for future treatment of any remaining tumor with bromocriptine and/or radiotherapy.

QUESTIONS AND DISCUSSION

1. A 21-year-old woman is seen in the emergency room complaining of a feeling of tingling in her feet and hands for 1 day. She has no other neurologic complaints. She denies shortness of breath, exposure to drugs or toxins, or a recent viral illness. An examination reveals diffuse hyporeflexia with absent ankle jerks. Very careful sensory testing is normal despite the patient's complaints. The best course of action would be:

   A. Discharge the patient with the diagnosis of "functional disorder" because of a paucity of objective findings.
   B. Admit her to the hospital for close observation, watching carefully for signs of developing weakness or respiratory difficulty.
   C. Perform a lumbar puncture in the emergency room, suspecting early Guillain–Barré syndrome (GBS), with plans to discharge the patient if the results are normal.

The answer is (B). Paresthesias without objective sensory findings occur commonly and early in GBS, often before a clinical weakness develops. The key features in this case are the sensory complaints in the presence of diffuse hyporeflexia. The typically high CSF protein concentration without pleocytosis may not occur until after a few weeks of illness.

The next day, she complains of difficulty in walking and on examination shows a pulse of 120, diffuse areflexia, and bilateral proximal lower extremity weakness. The best management at this time would be:

   A. Admit her to an ICU with cardiac monitoring, frequent vital capacities with intubation if less than 800 ml, lumbar puncture.
   B. Observe her in a general medical ward with daily vital capacities and steroids.
   C. Admit her to an ICU for cardiac monitoring with monitoring of the vital capacity only if respiratory problems occur.
   D. Admit her to an ICU with vital capacity and cardiac monitoring, and high-dose steroids.

The answer is (A). With weakness now developing, it is clear that the patient has GBS. She should be monitored in an ICU setting and she should be watched closely for the development of cardiac arrhythmias and respiratory compromise. Vital capacities should be checked every 4 to 6 hours, with intubation done if less than 800 ml. Steroids have not been shown to be effective in GBS.

2. A 30-year-old man is brought to the emergency room after suddenly developing a severe generalized headache ("like being struck by lightning") while he was moving furniture. The headache was not associated with nausea or vomiting, photophobia, neck stiffness, or other neurologic complaints. There is no previous history of headaches and no family history. An examination reveals a young man in moderate distress. Temperature is 99°F, blood pressure 140/90, pulse 96. The general physical examination and neurologic examination are unremarkable. Choose the best plan of management:

   A. Intramuscular meperidine, then discharge the patient with a prescription for ergotamine and a follow-up appointment in the neurology clinic
   B. Narcotic analgesics and observation overnight in the emergency room with plans for discharge if symptoms are improved
   C. Immediate CT brain scan
   D. Immediate lumbar puncture

The answer is (C). The sudden onset of a severe headache, especially if it occurs in a patient of this age during exertion, should bring to mind the possibility of aneurysmal subarachnoid hemorrhage. Meningismus or other physical findings may be absent with early sentinel leaks. The diagnostic procedure of choice is a CT brain scan followed by a lumbar puncture if no evidence of subarachnoid blood is seen on the CT.

A CT scan is done and is read as normal. What should be the next step?

   A. Discharge the patient with a follow-up in neurology clinic.
   B. Perform a lumbar puncture.

The answer is (B).

A lumbar puncture is performed and the results are as follows: opening pressure 260 mm of CSF, xanthochromic supernatant, 10 WBC (100% monos), 200 RBC, glucose 70 mg/dl, protein 50 mg/dl. What is the best course of action?

   A. Admit the patient, send for cultures, and begin broad-spectrum antibiotics for presumed bacterial meningitis.

B. Admit the patient to a quiet, closely monitored bed; give sedatives, analgesics, stool softeners, and prophylactic anticonvulsants.

C. Discharge the patient, since the red cells are most likely due to a traumatic tap and the CSF profile is otherwise normal.

The answer is (B). The increased opening pressure, red cells, and xanthochromic fluid are consistent with a subarachnoid hemorrhage. A traumatic tap may have increased red cells but xanthochromia would not be present unless the specimen was left standing for several hours before centrifugation.

3. Generalized status epilepticus should be:

A. Diagnosed in the following situation: A patient has a series of seizures within a 2-hour period. Between fits he is able to state that he recently quit a 2 quart/day vodka habit.

B. Diagnosed in the following situation: A patient has had continuous jerking movements of one limb for 6 hours but no loss of consciousness.

C. Treated aggressively with immediate intubation and neuromuscular blockade to prevent rhabdomyolsis from intense muscular contractions.

D. Treated with a fast-acting benzodiazepine followed immediately by a loading dose of a long-acting anticonvulsant such as phenytoin.

The answer is (D). Generalized status epilepticus, by definition, involves a loss of consciousness as part of the ictus without regaining consciousness in between episodes. Neuromuscular blockade will abolish the motor activity but will have no effect on the underlying persistent epileptiform activity. Following preservation of an airway, blood sampling, and the establishment of intravenous access, first line therapy is aimed at abolishing the epileptiform discharges with anticonvulsants.

4. Spinal cord compression should be considered in all of the following situations except:

A. Sudden onset of right arm and leg weakness accompanied by sensory loss

B. Gradual onset of paraparesis associated with a loss of bowel and bladder function

C. Subacute proximal leg weakness associated with a belt-like sensation across the chest that increases with lifting heavy objects

D. Back pain associated with paraparesis

The answer is (A). In this case, the hemineurologic deficit is most likely secondary to a contralateral hemispheric infarct.

5. All of the following statements are true regarding the management of acute intracranial hypertension except:

A. Reduction of $PaCO_2$ is the quickest way of reducing intracranial pressure.

B. Corticosteroids are especially helpful in reducing the edema associated with infarction.

C. Emergency surgery is the preferred treatment for cerebellar hemorrhages.

D. Osmotic agents are helpful in reducing intracranial hypertension from any cause.

The answer is (B). Steroids are useful when considerable tumor edema (vasogenic edema) is present, but they are not particularly effective on the type of edema associated with cellular damage (cytoxic edema) such as occurs with infarction.

6. All of the following statements concerning the treatment of myasthenic crisis are false except:

A. Aminoglycoside antibiotics are contraindicated.

B. It is not necessary to differentiate a myasthenic from a cholinergic crisis because the emergency management is the same.

C. Anticholinesterase drugs are withdrawn for 48 hours only if a cholinergic crisis is suspected, then restarted at twice the previous dose.

D. Plasmapheresis is an important treatment modality because its effects are always immediate.

E. Although vital capacity monitoring is important prior to intubation it is not helpful in assessing a patient's progress after being placed on a mechanical ventilator.

The answer is (B). Emergency management of a crisis is the same regardless of etiology—the maintenance of adequate ventilation and the withdrawal of anticholinesterase medications. These drugs are then restarted after 48 to 72 hours at smaller doses. Aminoglycoside antibiotics may be used if necessary. Plasmapheresis may be helpful, but its effects are often delayed for several days. Vital capacity monitoring may be a useful tool in assessing the adequacy of therapy in the crisis situation.

SUGGESTED READING

Asbury AK: Diagnostic considerations in Guillain–Barré syndrome. Ann Neurol 9(Suppl):1, 1981.

Asbury AK, Cornblatt DR: Assessment of current diagnostic criteria for Guillain–Barré syndrome. Ann Neurol 27(Suppl):S21, 1990

Biller J, Godersky JL, Adams HP: Management of aneurysmal subarachnoid hemorrhage. Stroke 19:1300, 1988

DeLorenzo RJ: Status epilepticus: Concepts in diagnosis and treatment. Semin Neurol 10:396, 1990

Dickey W: The neurologic malignant syndrome. Prog Neurobiol 36:425, 1991

Drachman DB: Myasthenia gravis, pt. 1. N Engl J Med 298:136, 1976

Factor SA, Singer C: Neuroleptic malignant syndrome. In Weiner WJ (ed): Emergency and Urgent Neurology. Philadelphia, JB Lippincott, 1992

Ferguson IT, Murphy RP, Lascelles RG: Ventilatory failure in myasthenia gravis. J Neurol Neurosurg Psychiatry 45:217, 1982

Fishman RA: Brain edema. N Engl J Med 293:706, 1975

Leppik IE: Status epilepticus: The next decade. Neurology 40(Suppl 2):4, 1990

Lockwood AH: Metabolic encephalopathies: Opportunities and challenges. J Cereb Blood Flow Metab 7:523, 1987

Ohman J, Servo A, Heiskanen D: Risk factors for cerebral infarction in good-grade patients after aneurysmal subarachnoid hemorrhage and surgery: A prospective study. J Neurosurg 74:14, 1991

Plum F, Posner JB: Diagnosis of Stupor and Coma. Philadelphia, FA Davis, 1980

Reid RL, Quigley ME, Yen SS: Pituitary apoplexy. Arch Neurol 42:712, 1985

Ropper AH: The Guillain–Barré syndrome. N Engl J Med 326:1130, 1992

Rosenberg MR, Green M: Neuroleptic malignant syndrome: Review of response to therapy. Arch Intern Med 149:1927, 1989

Van der Meché FG, Schmitz PI: A randomized trial comparing intravenous immune globulin and plasma exchange in Guillain–Barré syndrome. N Engl J Med 326:1123, 1992

Weissman DE: Glucocorticoid treatment for brain metastases and epidural spinal cord compression: A review. J Clin Oncol 6:543, 1988

Neurologic Complications of Human Immunodeficiency Virus Infection

Joseph R. Berger

Peter Portegies

In the spring of 1981 the Centers for Disease Control (CDC) in Atlanta reported on the occurrences of uncommon opportunistic infections (*Pneumocystis carinii* pneumonia) and malignancies (Kaposi's sarcoma) among previously healthy young homosexual men in New York and California. This newly recognized immunodeficiency state was referred to as the *acquired immunodeficiency syndrome (AIDS)*. Shortly afterward, neurologic consequences of this illness were reported.

Within 3 years of its clinical description a retrovirus, initially called lymphadenopathy-associated virus (LAV), human T-cell lymphotropic virus type III (HTLV-III), or AIDS-associated retrovirus (ARV), was convincingly demonstrated to be the etiologic agent. In 1986 this retrovirus was designated as human immunodeficiency virus (HIV). This virus is now referred to as HIV-1 since a second type was isolated from West African patients with AIDS.

HUMAN IMMUNODEFICIENCY VIRUS TYPE 1

The human immunodeficiency virus type 1 (HIV-1) is a member of a unique family of RNA viruses characterized by the presence of RNA-dependent DNA polymerase (reverse transcriptase), an enzyme enabling these RNA viruses to produce a DNA copy of this genome, which can then be incorporated into the host genome. Other characteristics of this family of viruses are their large size, the ability to produce cytopathic changes in infected cells, and the long incubation times before the development of clinical illness, typically, immunologic or neurologic disease. All known lentiviruses are capable of causing neurologic disease. In addition to the neurologic diseases that occur as a direct consequence of HIV-1 infection, a large number of neurologic disorders occur as a result of the accompanying immunosuppression.

SPECTRUM OF NEUROLOGIC DISEASES

Neurologic involvement occurs in at least 70% of patients who meet the CDC's clinical criteria for AIDS, and it is the presenting manifestation in 10% of HIV-infected patients. At autopsy, 80% to 90% are found to have neuropathologic abnormalities.

Each part of the neuraxis may be involved. Some of these neurologic complications occur in the early and clinically "latent" phases of the infection, while others are associated with advanced HIV-1 infection (Table 25-1). Therefore, from a clinical point of view (*e.g.*, differential diagnosis) it is useful to keep in mind the correlation between the neurologic

William J. Weiner and Christopher G. Goetz, eds. *Neurology for the Non-Neurologist*, Third Edition. Copyright © 1994, 1989 by J. B. Lippincott Company. Copyright © 1981 by Harper and Row Publishers, Inc.

TABLE 25-1. Neurologic Complications of HIV-1 Infection

EARLY

Acute syndromes associated with initial infection
Multiple sclerosis–like illness
Aseptic meningitis
Demyelinating neuropathies

LATE

AIDS dementia complex
Vacuolar myelopathy
Peripheral neuropathy
Myopathies
Cerebrovascular complications
Seizures

Opportunistic infections and neoplasms
    Cerebral toxoplasmosis
    Cryptococcal meningitis
    Progressive multifocal leukoencephalopathy
    Cytomegalovirus infections
    Syphilis
    Primary central nervous system lymphoma
    Meningitis lymphomatosis

TABLE 25-2. Incidence of Neurologic Complications in AIDS

Cerebral toxoplasmosis	10–20%
Cryptococcal meningitis	2–10%
Progressive multifocal leukoencephalopathy	2–5%
Cytomegalovirus polyradiculomyelopathy	2%?
Cytomegalovirus encephalitis	<1%?
Primary central nervous system lymphoma	2–13%
Meningitis lymphomatosis	0.5–3%
Aseptic meningitis	<5%?
AIDS dementia complex*	5–33%
Vacuolar myelopathy	20–30%**
Polyneuropathy	10–35%
Myopathy	<10%?

*Incidence of AIDS dementia complex has declined after introduction of zidovudine.
**Autopsy statistic, less frequently recognized on clinical grounds.

complications and the level of immune compromise (CD4 cell count). Furthermore, it is important to appreciate that very often different neurologic complications may occur in one patient. Patients may develop complications additional to those that were previously diagnosed, or several neurologic problems may even occur simultaneously. The physician should not lose sight of the possibility that a given neurologic disorder in these individuals is the result of a more common disorder, unrelated to the underlying HIV-1 infection. The most important neurologic complications in patients with AIDS reported in the literature are given in Table 25-2.

In this chapter, the description of the neurologic disorders accompanying HIV-1 infection will be classified according to their manifestations. The most common etiologies for each of these manifestations will be discussed. Some overlap between the categories occurs. The classification will include meningitis, global encephalopathy, focal neurologic disturbances of central origin, myelopathy, peripheral neuropathy, and myopathy.

MENINGITIS

Meningitis is a frequent occurrence in the patient with HIV-1 infection. Cerebrospinal fluid (CSF) studies are required for a precise identification of the etiology. In the asymptomatic stage of HIV-1 infection, HIV-1 itself is perhaps the most common cause of meningitis in the infected patient. The most important meningeal infection in AIDS patients is caused by *Cryptococcus neoformans*. Other common etiologies of meningitis include tuberculosis, syphilis, and lymphoma (Table 25-3).

HIV-1 MENINGITIS

An aseptic meningitis may occur at the time of seroconversion and in later stages of HIV-1 infection while the patient is systemically well. This aseptic meningitis has been divided in an acute and a chronic form. Patients present with headache, fever, and meningeal signs. Cranial neuropathies,

TABLE 25-3. Meningitides in HIV-1 Infection

HIV-1 meningitis
Cryptococcal meningitis
Tuberculous meningitis
Syphilitic meningitis
Listeria meningitis
Meningitis lymphomatosis (non-Hodgkin's lymphoma)

especially of cranial nerves V, VII, and VIII, and long-tract signs have been noted. The CSF shows a mild mononuclear pleocytosis (<200 cells/mm^3), with slightly elevated protein levels. The meningitis is presumed to result from direct HIV-1 infection of the meninges because HIV-1 can, with the appropriate virologic procedures, be isolated from the CSF. Most cases have a self-limited monophasic course, but the syndrome tends to recur.

It is important to appreciate that a mild mononuclear pleocytosis (usually less <100 cells/mm^3), with or without an elevated protein, is common and well known in HIV-1–infected individuals, even in the absence of neurologic symptoms. It has become increasingly clear that these "background" CSF abnormalities may be confusing in establishing a diagnosis of neurosyphilis, aseptic meningitis, or the inflammatory neuropathies. CSF abnormalities observed with HIV-1 infection should be interpreted cautiously.

CRYPTOCOCCAL MENINGITIS

Cryptococcal meningitis is the most common mycotic infection involving the nervous system in patients with HIV-infection. The fungus *C. neoformans* has a worldwide distribution, is commonly encountered in the feces of pigeons, and is associated with disease in both immunocompetent and immunosuppressed patients. Meningitis results from hematogenous dissemination after a frequently asymptomatic pulmonary infection. The prevalence of this life-threatening opportunistic infection among AIDS patients is 2% to 10%.

Clinically the disease manifests as subacute or chronic meningitis with headache, altered mentation, and fever. Headache may become severe, with nausea and vomiting. Neck stiffness is frequently absent. Papilledema (occasionally with visual loss) and sixth cranial nerve palsy may be present.

The diagnosis is based on CSF analysis: variable mononuclear pleocytosis, with mildly elevated protein and low glucose level. However, these CSF parameters may all be normal in patients with AIDS. The CSF opening pressure is usually increased. The fungus can often be easily recognized in India-ink preparation. Cryptococcal polysaccharide capsular antigen is nearly always positive in the CSF and serum, as are fungal cultures of CSF. Brain computed tomography (CT) scan is usually normal or shows nonspecific abnormalities; occasionally mass lesions (*e.g.*, cryptococcoma) may be present.

Standard therapy with amphotericin B given intravenously (≥0.3 mg/kg/day) with or without oral flucytosine (150 mg/kg/day) is effective in about 60% of cases. The oral triazole fluconazole (400 mg/day) is equally effective as the more toxic regimen of intravenous (IV) amphotericin. However, amphotericin does appear to be superior in patients who are severely ill. Because relapses are so common in AIDS patients, maintenance treatment (after 6 to 8 weeks of induction) is recommended. Fluconzole (100 mg to 200 mg/day) is highly effective in preventing relapses.

TUBERCULOUS MENINGITIS

Mycobacterium tuberculosis and *Mycobacterium avium–intracellulare* (MAI) occur frequently in AIDS and are often extrapulmonary in nature. Involvement of the central nervous system (CNS) is almost always due to *M. tuberculosis*, though atypical mycobacterial infection of the CNS in AIDS has been reported.

Meningitis and mass lesions (tuberculous brain abscess, tuberculomas) due to *M. tuberculosis* have been described. In case of a mass lesion brain biopsy is necessary to confirm the diagnosis. The response of AIDS patients to the standard therapy for *M. tuberculosis* (including isoniazid, rifampin, pyrazinamide, and streptomycin) is generally gratifying. The use of corticosteroids is controversial.

SYPHILITIC MENINGITIS

A retrospective chart review study estimated that neurosyphilis, strictly defined by the presence of reactive CSF VDRL, was present in approximately 1.5% of HIV-1–infected hospitalized patients. Diagnosing neurosyphilis can be quite problematic. First, in 40% to 60% of HIV-1 infected patients the CSF may show a pleocytosis, elevated protein, elevated immunoglobulin G synthesis rate, and oligoclonal bands, making it impossible to use these CSF findings as an indicator of active neurosyphilis. Second, the signs and symptoms of the clinical syndromes caused by HIV-1 infection (meningitis, strokes, myelopathy, dementia) can also occur in neurosyphilis. Third, the CSF serologic tests for neurosyphilis (VDRL and FTA-ABS) may be negative in HIV-1–infected individuals with *Treponema pallidum* in the CSF.

Several diagnostic schemata have been used to establish the diagnosis; however, all have relied on indirect evidence of the presence of *T. pallidum* because the organism is fastidious and requires the rather cumbersome use of animal inoculation for strict verification of its presence. The frequent presence of CSF abnormalities in the HIV-1 infection results in a loss of the specificity of these criteria. Though it is the most specific test for neurosyphilis, the CSF VDRL, as well as other nontreponemal tests, may be insensitive to the diagnosis of neurosyphilis. One suggested approach to the diagnosis of neurosyphilis is as follows: (1) a reactive CSF VDRL in the absence of gross blood contamination of CSF; or (2) a reactive CSF FTA-ABS in the absence of blood contamination occurring in association with a CSF pleocytosis (>5 cells/mm^3), increased protein (>50 mg%), an increased IgG index (>6), or oligoclonal bands in the absence of HIV infection or identifiable neurologic illness; or (3) a reactive CSF FTA-ABS in association with a neurologic illness compatible with neurosyphilis, unexplained by other disease, and responding to penicillin therapy; or (4) *T. pallidum* isolated from the CSF by animal inoculation.

T. pallidum in the CNS may be more aggressive in HIV-1–infected individuals, and the complications may be atypical. In addition to meningovascular syphilis, a polyradiculopathy has also been described. Patients who present with meningovascular syphilis after adequate treatment for primary syphilis, and with neurologic relapse after adequate treatment for secondary syphilis have been described.

Unsuspected neurosyphilis is relatively common in HIV-1–infected individuals, and neurosyphilis should always be considered in the differential diagnosis of neurologic disease in HIV-infected persons. CSF examination should be performed in all HIV-1–seropositive persons with neurologic complaints and a history of syphilis or serologic evidence of syphilis, regardless of prior treatment. If neurosyphilis is suspected, patients should be treated for at least 10 days with aqueous penicillin G, 2 to 4 million units IV every 4 hours (12 to 24 million units each day).

LISTERIA MENINGITIS

Listeria is a gram-positive, rod-shaped, aerobic bacterium that is widespread in nature. Although infection with *Listeria monocytogenes* (usually meningitis, sometimes brain abscess) has been reported in HIV-1–infected individuals and patients with AIDS, the incidence remains low. Diagnosis of *Listeria* meningitis and treatment with high-dose IV penicillin or ampicillin are the same in AIDS patients and in immunocompetent individuals.

LYMPHOMATOUS MENINGITIS

Twelve percent to 33% of AIDS patients with systemic non-Hodgkin's lymphoma (usually high-grade B-cell neoplasms) have leptomeningeal infiltration with a positive CSF cytologic examination at diagnosis. Because of this high incidence, all AIDS patients with systemic lymphoma should have CSF examination as part of their staging evaluation.

Leptomeningeal lymphoma causes headache, encephalopathy, cranial nerve palsies, radicular pain, cauda equina syndrome, or hydrocephalus. A differential diagnostic list of the potential etiologies of cranial neuropathy in AIDS is presented in Table 25-4. Cytologic examination is the single most useful test for leptomeningeal lymphoma. Sometimes subarachnoid nodules or thickened roots can be seen on myelography or by contrast magnetic resonance.

Intrathecal chemotherapy with methotrexate (or cytosine arabinoside) is the primary treatment. An Ommaya reservoir should be inserted. Radiotherapy can be added to the symptomatic region. Corticosteroids may temporarily relieve symptoms.

ENCEPHALOPATHY

Both an alteration in cognitive abilities and a decline in level of consciousness may occur in HIV-1 infection. The former, a direct consequence of HIV-1 infection (AIDS dementia complex, HIV-1 encephalopathy, or HIV-associated cognitive/motor disorder), is usually insidious in nature. The latter is often associated with focal neuro-

TABLE 25-4. Etiologies of Cranial Nerve Palsies with HIV-1 Infection

Infectious meningitis
  Fungal (*Cryptococcus*)
  Bacterial (*M. tuberculosis, L. monocytogenes, T. pallidum*)
  Viral (HIV-1)
Neoplastic meningitis
  Meningitis lymphomatosa
Compression from mass lesion
  Infectious (toxoplasmosis)
  Neoplastic (central nervous system lymphoma)
Vasculitis
Inflammatory
  Guillain–Barré syndrome
  Chronic inflammatory polyradiculoneuropathy
Miscellaneous
  Malignant otitis externa

logic abnormalities and typically results from mass lesions of the brain, usually opportunistic infections or lymphoma. The evaluation of a global encephalopathy complicating HIV-1 infection requires a thorough physical and neurologic examination; laboratory studies that assess electrolytes, renal, liver, and thyroid function, syphilis serologies, vitamin B_{12} and folate levels; MR of the brain, preferably with gadolinium (alternatively, CT may be employed but should be performed as a double-dose, delayed scan); and CSF analysis for routine studies (opening pressure, cell count and differential, protein, glucose) as well as detailed microbiologic studies, including VDRL, and cytology. A differential diagnosis list is given in Table 25-5.

AIDS DEMENTIA COMPLEX

One of the most important neurologic syndromes in patients with AIDS is the AIDS dementia complex (ADC) or HIV-1 encephalopathy. This dementia is characterized by disturbances in cognition, motor performance, and behavior. Patients complain of decreased concentration, forgetfulness, and slowing of thoughts. Tasks take more time to complete and have to be well planned in advance. Patients become apathetic and lose interest in their environment. As a consequence, patients may become socially withdrawn, which is often mistaken for depression. Motor symptoms include clumsiness, tremor, poor balance, unsteadiness of gait, and slowing of rapid alternating movements. Organic psychosis may develop in some patients. Cortical symptoms like aphasia, alexia, and agraphia are lacking. The mini mental state examination is often normal, though responses are delayed. Saccadic and pursuit eye movements are often slowed and inaccurate. Fine finger movements are slowed, snout response is common, and deep tendon reflexes are brisk. With time, increasing psychomotor slowing may progress to severe dementia with

TABLE 25-5. Encephalopathies (Diffuse Brain Disease) in HIV-1 Infection

AIDS dementia complex (= HIV-1 encephalopathy)
Metabolic encephalopathies
Diffuse encephalitis
    Acute HIV-1 encephalitis
    Cytomegalovirus encephalitis
    Herpes simplex virus encephalitis
    Toxoplasmosis (diffuse form)

akinetic mutism, paraparesis, and incontinence. The clinical and neuropsychological abnormalities in ADC are compatible with what has been called a "subcortical dementia."

The epidemiology and course of ADC have not yet been precisely defined and have been influenced by the introduction of zidovudine. The incidence of ADC has declined since the introduction of zidovudine. However, recent prevalence studies suggest that one-third of patients with AIDS eventually develop a mild or severe form of ADC. In patients who develop ADC, there is no protracted decline in neuropsychological performance, but rather a precipitous change first affecting psychomotor speed. This further strengthens existing data suggesting that asymptomatic patients do not have gradually increasing neuropsychological dysfunction. It suggests an acute or subacute rather than a cumulative process affecting the brain over a long period of time as the cause of ADC.

Diagnostic studies are important to exclude treatable infections and tumors. CT scan and MR show cortical atrophy, enlargement of ventricles, or both in most patients. MR may reveal patchy or diffuse increased signal intensity on T2-weighted images, usually in the periventricular white matter and centrum semiovale, without mass effect. However, these neuroradiologic abnormalities may occur in patients who are not demented. CSF analysis may reveal a mononuclear pleocytosis and increased protein level. HIV-1 antibodies may be found, and HIV-1 itself may be cultured from approximately 30% of patients with ADC. HIV-1 p24 core protein in CSF, which is independent of HIV-1 antigen in serum, is detectable in 50% of patients with ADC. In addition to these CSF markers, several immunologic markers support a diagnosis of ADC when other causes have been excluded. These include beta$_2$-microglobulin, neopterin, and quinolinic acid. Beta$_2$-microglobulin and neopterin are markers of immune activation; quinolinic acid is a metabolic product of macrophage activation.

The gross pathology of HIV-1 encephalopathy is characterized by brain atrophy with sulcal widening, ventricular dilatation, and meningeal fibrosis. Histologically, the most common feature of this illness is white matter pallor, chiefly of the periventricular and central white matter. However, multinucleate giant cells, typically located in perivascular spaces, are the pathologic hallmark of this illness. Astrocytosis and perivascular mononuclear inflammation are commonly observed.

Zidovudine remains the best-substantiated treatment for ADC. Zidovudine crosses the blood–

brain barrier, and treatment has been found to be associated with decreasing HIV-1 antigen levels in serum and CSF. Beneficial effects of zidovudine in patients with ADC have been described, and since the introduction of zidovudine the incidence of ADC has declined. Preliminary data on dideoxyinosine (ddI) also suggest that it is effective in improving the neuropsychological deficits found in HIV-1–infected children, but its efficacy in adults is controversial.

CYTOMEGALOVIRUS ENCEPHALITIS

The clinical features of cytomegalovirus (CMV) encephalitis in AIDS are not uniform. Neurologic symptoms may include meningeal signs, disorientation, short-term memory deficits, apathy, dementia, coma, seizures, or brain-stem involvement. CSF examination is often normal. Rarely, CMV can be isolated from the CSF. CT scan may reveal subependymal enhancement compatible with ventriculitis. Often the identification of CMV is based on typical intranuclear inclusions or identification of CMV antigen by immunocytochemistry or both at postmortem neuropathologic examination. The relative importance of CMV infection in many cases is unclear, and CMV often coexists with other infectious agents. Treatment data for neurological disease are not available.

FOCAL NEUROLOGIC DISTURBANCES OF CENTRAL ORIGIN

Focal neurologic disturbances, such as hemianopsia, hemiparesis, and hemianesthesia, occurring with HIV-1 infection may result from a variety of lesions affecting the cerebrum. These lesions can be broadly classified in their order of frequency as opportunistic infections, tumors, and cerebrovascular disease. The most common opportunistic infections are toxoplasmosis and progressive multifocal leukoencephalopathy (PML) (Table 25-6). With rare exception, brain tumors occurring with AIDS are primary central nervous system lymphomas, although other primary CNS tumors and metastatic tumors have been reported. In the HIV-1–infected patient with focal neurologic signs, either a cranial MR with gadolinium or a double-dose, delayed brain CT is mandated. The former is more sensitive, but brain CT scan is more specific, particularly with respect to toxoplasmosis. Therefore, these studies often prove to be complementary.

TABLE 25-6. Histopathology of Focal Brain Lesions in AIDS

1986[1] BEFORE EMPIRIC TOXO-THERAPY		1991[2] AFTER EMPIRIC TOXO-THERAPY (n = 50)	
Toxoplasmosis	50–70%	Toxoplasmosis	14
Lymphoma	10–25%	Lymphoma	14
Progressive multifocal leukoencephalopathy	10–22%	Progressive multifocal leukoencephalopathy	14
Nondiagnostic	10%	Nondiagnostic	4
Candida abscess	3%	HIV encephalopathy	3
Cryptococcoma	2%	Cryptococcoma	1
Kaposi sarcoma	2%	Atypical mycobacteria	1
Tuberculoma	1%	Stroke	1
Herpes simplex	1%	Metastasis	2

[1] De La Paz R, Enzmann D: Neuroradiology of acquired immunodeficiency syndrome. In Rosenblum ML, Levy RM, Bredesen DE (eds): AIDS and the Nervous System, pp 121–154. New York, Raven Press, 1988.
[2] Levy RM, Russel E, Yungbluth M et al: Abstract WB 27, Seventh International Conference on AIDS, Florence, 1991.

CEREBRAL TOXOPLASMOSIS

Infection with the intracellular protozoan *Toxoplasma gondii* has a worldwide distribution, is most often subclinical, and results in seropositivity and chronic, latent infection in immunocompetent individuals. However, it may present with lymphadenopathy or mononucleosis-like illness in otherwise healthy adults. Intracranial mass lesions or diffuse meningoencephalitis sporadically occurs. *Toxoplasma* cysts remain present in all tissues during latent infection. The seroprevalence in adults varies geographically and depends on certain risk factors (*e.g.*, eating habits).

Cerebral toxoplasmosis is the leading cause of focal brain disease in AIDS patients and has a prevalence of 3% to 40%, depending on the seroprevalence of the population studied. Cerebral toxoplasmosis is the presenting opportunistic infection in at least 5% of the AIDS patient population. Clinically patients present with constitutional symptoms, headache, and fever, followed by focal neurologic abnormalities, including focal seizures, aphasia, hemiparesis, and homonymous hemianopsia, depending on the localization of the lesions. This combination of focal abnormalities and signs of a global encephalopathy is very suggestive of cerebral toxo-plasmosis.

Brain imaging is very important in establishing the diagnosis. CT scan normally reveals multiple hypodense areas, usually with mass effect, and contrast enhancement (ring pattern or irregular nodular). MR is more sensitive in detecting lesions. Serology is rarely diagnostic at the time CNS toxo-plasmosis develops: IgM antibodies are rarely demonstrable and a four-fold rise of pre-existing low IgG antibody titer or a high IgG antibody titer (>1:512 in the Sabin–Feldman dye test), consistent with recrudescent infection, is usually absent. Likewise, antibody tests in CSF are rarely diagnostic and may even be negative in many patients. Even negative serology tests in CNS toxoplasmosis have been described.

In AIDS patients with suspected cerebral toxo-plasmosis, based on clinical findings and CT scan abnormalities, empirical treatment is justifiable, reserving brain biopsy for atypical or refractory cases. The most effective therapy is a combination of pyrimethamine (50 mg/day) and sulfadiazine (6 g to 8 g/day). Oral folinic acid is given to prevent hematologic side effects. Corticosteroids may be used for lesions associated with edema and mass effect. A considerable number of patients develop a rash due to the sulfadiazine. In these cases clinda-mycin may represent an alternative therapy. Secondary prophylaxis is mandated because of the high rate of recurrence. For this maintenance treatment the pyrimethamine–sulfa combination is effective, but the value of pyrimethamine alone is controversial.

PROGRESSIVE MULTIFOCAL LEUKOENCEPHALOPATHY

PML is a demyelinating disease of the CNS that results from infection of oligodendrocytes with JC virus, a papovavirus first described in 1958 by Aström, Mancall, and Richardson in patients with lymphoma and leukemia. With rare exception, PML occurs in the clinical setting of cellular immu-nosuppression. Until the AIDS epidemic, the most common underlying illnesses were lympho-proliferative diseases. Since the recognition of the AIDS epidemic in 1981, increasing numbers of individuals with PML have been recognized. Approximately 4% to 5% of all HIV-1–infected patients will develop PML, and in as many as 25% of HIV-1–infected individuals with PML this neuro-logic disease will be the presenting manifestation of AIDS.

The presentation of the AIDS patient with PML does not appear to be substantially different from that of patients with PML complicating other im-munosuppressive conditions. The onset is insidious, with symptoms and signs suggesting multi-focal disease. Hemiparesis is the most common presenting symptom. Headache and seizures are rare, and signs of elevated intracranial pressure are characteristically absent. The diagnosis is strongly supported but not confirmed on the basis of radio-graphic imaging. CT of the brain reveals hypo-dense lesions of the affected white matter that generally do not enhance with contrast administration and exhibit no mass effect. Cranial MR shows a hyperintense lesion on T2-weighted images in the affected regions. As with CT scan, contrast enhancement is an exception. The lesions are not confined to a vascular territory and are less diffusely distributed than MRI abnormalities in AIDS dementia complex. CSF specimens are nondiagnostic. Polymerase chain reaction for JC virus genome in the CSF of affected patients is positive in only about 30%. For the present, diagnostic certainty depends on the demonstration of typical histopathologic abnormalities at brain biopsy and detecting the virus. The histopathologic changes include demyelination, oligodendrocytes with large intranuclear inclusions, and large bizarre astrocytes with hyper-chromatic nuclei. The JC virus can be demonstrated using electron microscopy or by employing immunofluorescence or immunohistochemistry.

Occasionally, prolonged survival and spontaneous partial recovery in AIDS-associated PML have been described. The prognosis in these patients is generally poor, with a mean survival of 4 months. An effective treatment for PML in patients with AIDS has not been identified, but there have been several anecdotal reports of the efficacy of cytarabine (ARA-C) given intrathecally or intravenously.

PRIMARY CENTRAL NERVOUS SYSTEM LYMPHOMA

Primary central nervous system lymphoma (PCNSL) is a non-Hodgkin lymphoma that arises within and is confined to the nervous system. The incidence of PCNSL has increased rapidly over the past 10 years. Of HIV-1–infected patients 0.6% will present with PCNSL, and 2% to 13% can be expected to develop PCNSL. PCNSL is the second most frequent CNS mass lesion in adults with AIDS and is the most frequent in children with AIDS.

Clinically most of the patients present with lethargy, confusion, memory loss, and personality change. The remaining patients present with hemiparesis, dysphasia, seizures, and cranial nerve deficits. CT appearance of PCNSL in AIDS patients is generally described as a mass or multiple masses exhibiting diffuse or ring enhancement with a predilection for the corpus callosum, basal ganglia, and periventricular areas, but toxoplasmosis may also appear as solitary or multiple, ring- or nodular-enhancing masses. It is therefore generally accepted that PCNSL is indistinguishable from toxoplasmosis. In the majority of PCNSLs multiple lesions can be seen on MR or CT. However, among solitary MR lesions there is a predominance of lymphoma.

CSF examination is often not possible because of the mass effect of the tumor. However, up to 25 percent of patients with PCNSL have a positive cytology, and this can eliminate the need for a diagnostic biopsy. At autopsy 100% of patients have leptomeningeal seeding. Histologic confirmation remains essential, and this should preferably be done by stereotactic biopsy. Corticosteroid administration can produce shrinkage of the tumor seen on CT or MR scan due to lysis of tumor cells, but this necrosis in tumor makes it more difficult to establish the diagnosis. So when PCNSL is a diagnostic consideration, corticosteroids should be withheld. Histologically the majority of PCNSLs are large cell and large cell immunoblastic tumors of B-cell origin.

Radiotherapy is the treatment of choice. Patients with PCNSL may respond both clinically and radiologically to whole brain radiotherapy (4000 cG). If possible a boost of 1500 cG to the tumor bed can be added. With radiotherapy, median survival can be prolonged to 4 to 5 months. Leptomeningeal lymphoma should be treated with intrathecal chemotherapy: methotrexate or cytosine arabinoside, using an Ommaya reservoir. Systemic chemotherapy is usually withheld in AIDS patients.

CEREBROVASCULAR COMPLICATIONS

Some patients with AIDS suffer transient ischemic attacks or strokes. Sometimes these cerebrovascular complications occur as the result of an underlying opportunistic infection or lymphoma, or occasionally are secondary to marantic endocarditis. In other cases the underlying condition is not known. In the pathogenesis anticardiolipin antibodies may play an ancillary role since they are frequently found in HIV-infected patients. Treatment is no different from that which is used in the non–HIV-infected patient.

MYELOPATHY

Spinal cord disease is observed frequently in HIV-1 infection. In most instances the disorder is ascribed solely to HIV-1 infection, a condition referred to as HIV-1–related vacuolar myelopathy. The diagnosis of this disorder, like that of HIV-1 encephalopathy, is one of exclusion. A number of other myelopathies may also occur with HIV-1 infection, including infectious myelopathies (CMV, herpes simplex type 2, herpes zoster, HTLV-I, mycobacteria, T. pallidum, and epidural abscesses), vascular myelopathies, epidural and intramedullary tumors, and a demyelinating myelopathy (Table 25-7). Diagnostically, the single most useful study is an MR of the involved area of the spinal cord to exclude the possibility of a mass lesion. The CSF needs to be examined for treatable pathogens, including syphilis and the herpes viruses.

HIV-1–RELATED VACUOLAR MYELOPATHY

A vacuolar myelopathy has been reported in 20% to 25% of AIDS cases. The syndrome is often associated with AIDS dementia complex, but it may occur in isolation. Clinically the syndrome is characterized by a slowly progressive spastic paraparesis, lower extremity hyperreflexia (except when diminished as a result of concomitant peripheral neuropathy), gait ataxia, and impaired sensation with vibratory and position sense being disproportionately affected. A discrete sensory level is distinctly unusual. Sometimes urinary incontinence develops. No treatment has been unequivocally demonstrated to be of value in HIV-related vacuolar myelopathy. Zidovudine seems to have little efficacy, although controlled clinical trials are lacking.

Pathologic changes are most prominent in the thoracic cord and closely mimic the pathology of subacute combined degeneration of the spinal

TABLE 25-7. Myelopathies in HIV-1 Infection

HIV-1–associated vacuolar myelopathy
Cytomegalovirus polyradiculomyelopathy
Varicella-zoster virus radiculomyelopathy
HTLV-I–associated myelopathy
Lymphoma (epidural or intradural)
Vascular insults
Vitamin B_{12} deficiency

cord. There is degeneration of the posterior and lateral columns of the spinal cord. The vacuolation appears to result from swelling within the layers of the myelin sheaths. Microglial nodules and multinucleate giant cells can be detected in the affected spinal cord.

The role of HIV-1 in the pathogenesis of this myelopathy remains unclear. The virus has been demonstrated by *in situ* hybridization and immunohistochemical staining in mononuclear and multinucleated macrophages in the areas of vacuolar myelopathy. However the myelopathy is probably not the result of productive HIV-1 infection.

PERIPHERAL NEUROPATHIES

Several peripheral neuropathies are associated with HIV-1 infection. These include distal symmetrical polyneuropathy or HIV-1–associated predominantly sensory polyneuropathy, the inflammatory demyelinating polyneuropathies, mononeuropathy multiplex, autonomic neuropathy, CMV polyradiculomyelopathy, and the toxic polyneuropathies (associated with ddI and dideoxycytidine [ddC]) (Table 25-8). Some of them, like the inflammatory demyelinating polyneuropathies, occur early in HIV-1 infection and some of them, like the distal symmetrical polyneuropathy and CMV polyradiculomyeloapthy, occur late. The neuromuscular complications of HIV-1 infection are considered common. Several studies suggest that even subclinical neuromuscular involvement occurs frequently. At least one-third of patients with AIDS will develop symptoms of neuropathy.

TABLE 25-8. Neuromuscular Complications of HIV-1 Infection

Neuropathies
   Distal symmetrical polyneuropathy
   Inflammatory demyelinating polyneuropathy (acute and chronic)
   Mononeuropathy multiplex
   Autonomic polyneuropathy
   Toxic neuropathies
   Cytomegalovirus polyradiculomyelopathy
Myopathies
   HIV-1–associated polymyositis
   Zidovudine-associated myopathy
   HIV-wasting syndrome

INFLAMMATORY DEMYELINATING POLYNEUROPATHIES

A demyelinating polyneuropathy may occur acutely or chronically in HIV-infected individuals. These demyelinating neuropathies tend to occur early in the course of HIV infection. The HIV-1–associated acute inflammatory demyelinating polyradiculoneuropathy (HIV-1–associated Guillain–Barré syndrome) is similar to Guillain–Barré syndrome in patients not infected with HIV-1. Patients present with progressive weakness, areflexia, and minor sensory signs. However, CSF examination may reveal a mild mononuclear pleocytosis (and an elevated protein) in HIV-infected patients. The same CSF abnormalities may be found in the HIV-1–associated chronic inflammatory demyelinating polyneuropathy (HIV-1–associated CIDP). Electrophysiologic studies indicate features of primary demyelination and axonal loss. The pathogenesis of the inflammatory demyelinating polyneuropathies may be autoimmune. The clinical course of the neuropathies in HIV-infected individuals is variable, but most patients improve. Plasmapheresis has been suggested as the treatment of choice, but steroids may be effective as well. Some recover spontaneously.

DISTAL SYMMETRICAL POLYNEUROPATHY

Distal symmetrical polyneuropathy, or HIV-1–associated predominantly sensory polyneuropathy (HPSP), is the most common polyneuropathy in HIV-infection. This polyneuropathy has been diagnosed in up to 35% of patients with AIDS. The most frequent symptoms are paresthesias, numbness, pain, and dysesthesias affecting the feet. Ankle reflexes are decreased or absent, there is a decreased sensation to pain and vibration in the feet and legs, and weakness is usually mild. The hands are less often involved. In a small proportion of patients pain is the most prominent feature. Most investigators believe that this painful distal sensory neuropathy is a subgroup of the HPSP. There is some epidemiologic evidence suggesting a relationship with CMV. Electrophysiologic studies demonstrate a polyneuropathy with features of both axonal degeneration and demyelination, but pathologically the abnormalities found are predominantly axonal and the demyelination is largely secondary. HIV has been isolated from peripheral nerves, but the pathogenesis remains unknown. Possible mechanisms include direct viral infection or a cell-mediated immune attack on components of peripheral nerve. Treatment is limited to providing symptomatic relief with tricyclic antidepressants and anticonvulsants. Zidovudine seems to have little efficacy, although clinical trails are lacking.

MONONEUROPATHY MULTIPLEX

Mononeuropathy multiplex is characterized by sensory and motor deficits in the distributions of multiple spinal, cranial, or peripheral nerves. CSF reveals both pleocytosis and elevated protein level. Electrophysiologic studies suggest axonal neuropathy. Nerve biopsies have revealed necrotizing arteritis in some instances.

AUTONOMIC NEUROPATHY

Late in HIV-1 infection a small number of patients develop an autonomic neuropathy that is clinically significant. Patients present with postural hypotension, bowel and bladder dysfunction, impotence, sweating abnormalities, presyncope, and sudden arrhythmias with the risk of death. Numerous factors may contribute to these symptoms, but often these symptoms are due to small-fiber peripheral neuropathy. Extensive autonomic testing reveals both parasympathetic and sympathetic dysfunction in 50% of patients. Treatment is purely symptomatic, with the use of agents such as fludrocortisone for stabilization of blood pressure.

TOXIC POLYNEUROPATHIES

A painful peripheral neuropathy has been associated with the use of the dideoxynucleoside analogues ddI and ddC. The syndrome is characterized by burning pain and tingling in the feet and legs, starting 8 to 27 weeks after initiating ddI treatment. These neuropathic symptoms have generally not been associated with significant abnormalities in nerve conduction studies. Some patients have reported marked improvement in symptoms within 1 to 2 weeks of discontinuing ddI. The neuropathy appears to be related to the total cumulative dose of ddI. DdC neuropathy is clinically similar to ddI neuropathy. This neuropathy is also dose-related, and significant recovery occurs in most patients. The findings in these ddI and ddC neuropathies are consistent with a distal axonopathy primarily affecting sensory fibers.

CMV POLYRADICULOMYELOPATHY

CMV polyradiculomyelopathy or polyradiculitis has been increasingly recognized in patients with AIDS. Patients present with lower extremity and sacral paresthesias or pain, followed by a rapidly progressive flaccid paraparesis, with areflexia and sphincter disturbances. Sensory disturbances are usually mild. The CSF reveals a pleocytosis with predominance of polymorphonuclear leukocytes. CMV has been detected in the CSF by several techniques, including culture, immunohistochemistry, *in situ* hybridization, and the detection of cytomegalic cells by cytologic examination. Myelographic examination may show thickened adherent lumbar nerve roots.

At autopsy, spinal roots have revealed extensive multifocal necrosis, acute inflammatory infiltrates, and vasculitis. Typical CMV inclusions are seen within endoneurial inflammatory cells, Schwann cells, and endothelial cells. Treatment with ganciclovir (DHPG), started early in the course of the disease, may stop progression or even cause some improvement. The ganciclovir regimen recommended is 5 mg/kg intravenously every 12 hours for 2 to 3 weeks, followed by maintenance therapy, 5 mg/kg per day, 5 days per week.

MYOPATHIES

Several myopathies have been described in HIV-1–infected individuals. The most important are HIV-1–associated polymyositis and zidovudine-associated myopathy. Progressive proximal muscle weakness—often associated with myalgia, elevated serum creatinine kinase (CK), myopathic EMG abnormalities, inflammatory infiltrates, and mitochondrial abnormalities (by electron microscopy) in muscle biopsy—may be present in both types, and no features clearly discriminate between them.

HIV-1–associated polymyositis (or some authors prefer HIV-associated myopathy) has been described in all stages of HIV-1 infection. Patients present subacutely with progressive proximal weakness and myalgia, most prominent in the thighs. The weakness involves the legs and neck flexors more than the arms. CK elevation is mild or moderate. Patients usually have myopathic EMG abnormalities, and 50% may have nerve conduction abnormalities indicating an accompanying peripheral neuropathy. Pathologic findings include noninflammatory myofiber degeneration, myofiber necrosis with inflammatory infiltrates, nemaline rod bodies, cytoplasmic bodies, and mitochondrial abnormalities. The pathogenesis is unknown. A T-cell–mediated and major histocompatibility class (MHC-I)–restricted cytotoxic process may be the underlying mechanism. HIV-1–associated polymyositis may respond to corticosteroids.

A zidovudine-associated myopathy occurs in a minority of patients who have been treated with zidovudine for at least 9 to 12 months. Muscle tenderness and weakness are preceded by CK elevation. In this myopathy mitochondrial dysfunction, resulting from drug-induced inhibition of mitochondrial DNA polymerase, has been suggested as the direct cause of the myopathy. The cumulative dose of zidovudine might be important. Pathologically ragged-red fibers, indicative of abnormal mitochondria, coexist with inflammatory changes. Zidovudine-associated myopathy usually (but not always) responds to zidovudine withdrawal.

SUMMARY

In the diagnostic approach to a neurologic problem in an HIV-1–infected individual it is critical to appreciate the following:

1. The degree of advancement of HIV-1 infection (or the level of immune compromise): some neurologic complications occur early in HIV-1 infection, others occur late.
2. The anatomic site of involvement: focal brain lesion or nonfocal disorder? CNS disease or neuromuscular complication?
3. Is there a single disease, or are multiple levels of the neuraxis involved simultaneously?
4. The prevalences of the neurologic complications: some complications are common, others are rare.

CT or MR scanning and CSF examination are the most important tools in confirming a presumed diagnosis and excluding others. Usually lumbar puncture (if not contraindicated) follows CT or MR scanning. Electrophysiologic studies may be helpful in neuromuscular complications. Brain biopsy, muscle biopsy, neuropsychological examination, and electroencephalography may give additional and sometimes essential information in specific problems.

QUESTIONS AND DISCUSSION

1. A patient with AIDS presents with fever and very severe headache. Neurologic examination reveals no abnormalities (including absence of neck stiffness). Give a differential diagnosis and diagnostic approach.

In a patient with AIDS (usually severely immunosuppressed) who presents with severe headache, without focal neurologic abnormalities, cryptococcal meningitis is the most likely diagnosis. This meningitis often results in very severe headaches, due to raised intracranial pressure, without focal abnormalities and in two-thirds of patients without meningeal signs. When there is any doubt about focal abnormalities, CT or MR should precede lumbar puncture. Other causes for meningitis include HIV-1, M. tuberculosis, L. monocytogenes, T. pallidum, and lymphomatous meningitis. HIV-1 (aseptic) meningitis usually occurs early in HIV-1 infection and the others occur less frequently than cryptococcal meningitis. CSF analysis will give the conclusive answer.

2. A patient with AIDS presents with apathy, slowness, and forgetfulness. He has no headache or fever. Can we conclude that the diagnosis is AIDS dementia complex?

No, we cannot. The diagnosis of AIDS dementia complex is one of exclusion. Clinically this patient presents with frontal lobe dysfunction, and so CT or MR should be performed. Frontal lobe toxoplasmosis, PML, and PCNSL have to be excluded. Chronic meningitis (syphilis, M. tuberculosis, Listeria) must also be excluded by CSF examination. If CT or MR and CSF are negative, further support for the diagnosis of AIDS dementia complex can be obtained by neuropsychological examination, which may show abnormalities compatible with "subcortical dementia" and may help to exclude depression. CT or MR and CSF examination may give additional support for a diagnosis of AIDS dementia complex. CT or MR may show atrophy and diffuse white matter abnormalities; CSF analysis may reveal HIV-1 p24 antigen, and increased levels of beta$_2$-microglobulin, neopterin, and quinolinic acid. The diagnosis of AIDS dementia complex can be extremely difficult to make. Sometimes longer follow-up is necessary to make a definite conclusion. If the final conclusion is AIDS dementia complex, zidovudine should be started immediately.

3. An HIV-infected patient presents with headache, fever, aphasia, and a slight right-sided hemiparesis. The day before he had a seizure. His illness developed in 1 week. What is the most likely diagnosis?

The most likely diagnosis in an HIV-infected individual who presents with focal abnormalities is cerebral toxoplasmosis. This is the leading cause of cerebral mass lesions in patients with HIV-infection. A CT or MR scan was performed, which showed multiple ring-enhancing lesions with surrounding edema, compatible with cerebral toxoplasmosis. Because of its high incidence and the fact that toxoplasmosis is easily treatable, empiric treatment is justifiable. Most patients react favorably, both clinically and radiologically, within 2 weeks. The differential diagnosis of focal abnormalities includes PCNSL and PML. PCNSL is clinically and radiologically indistinguishable from toxoplasmosis and has to be confirmed by brain biopsy. PML presents with a more protracted course and is radiologically different (white matter lesions, without contrast enhancement and mass effect). AIDS patients with focal lesions, without a favorable response to empiric anti-toxoplasmosis treatment, require a brain biopsy to make a definite diagnosis.

4. A patient with AIDS presents with slowly progressive gait disturbances. On neurologic examination he has a spastic paraparesis and a sensory ataxia. Give a differential diagnosis.

A slowly progressive spastic paraparesis with a sensory ataxia is usually caused by a myelopathy. There are several etiologic possibilities in a patient with AIDS. Medullary compression (e.g., an epidural tuberculous abscess or lymphoma) has to be excluded by MR, CSF examination should exclude infectious agents, of which the most important are CMV, varicella-zoster virus, HTLV-I and T. pallidum. Vitamin B_{12} deficiency should be ruled out. If MR and CSF are negative for the previously mentioned causes, the most likely diagnosis is HIV-1–related vacuolar myelopathy. This is a slowly progressive myelopathy, which is related to HIV-infection and is often associated with AIDS dementia complex but may occur without dementia. Its pathogenesis is

poorly understood, and zidovudine has no clear efficacy. The diagnosis is one of exclusion.

5. An AIDS patient with CMV retinitis presents with subacute low back pain and radicular pain in the left leg. Do you think this patient has a herniated lumbar disk?

HIV infection does not protect against herniated disks. But be careful! A very aggressive polyradiculomyelopathy caused by CMV has been described in patients with AIDS, and this syndrome may well present like a herniated disk. In this syndrome, in days to weeks after the initial lumbago and radicular pain, a rapidly progressive flaccid paraparesis with sphincter disturbances may develop. The CSF reveals a pleocytosis with predominance of polymorphonuclear leukocytes. CMV may be cultured from the CSF, or CMV may be detected by stop immunohistochemistry or *in situ* hybridization. Treatment with ganciclovir, started early, may stop progression or even cause some improvement. In every AIDS patient with radicular pain in the legs who develops a paresis, a lumbar puncture should be done; when the previously mentioned CSF abnormalities are found, ganciclovir should be started while awaiting CSF culture.

SUGGESTED READING

Price RW, Brew BJ, Sidtis J et al: The brain in AIDS: Central nervous system HIV-1 infection and AIDS dementia complex. Science 239:586, 1988

Rosenblum ML, Levy RM, Bredesen DE (eds): AIDS and the Nervous System. New York, Raven Press, 1988

Rudge P (ed): Bailliere's Clinical Neurology Series: Neurological Aspects of Human Retroviruses. London, Bailliere Tindall, 1992

Sande MA, Volberding PA (eds): The Medical Management of AIDS, 2nd ed. Philadelphia, WB Saunders, 1990

Simpson DM, Wolfe DE: Neuromuscular complications of HIV infection and its treatment. AIDS 5:917, 1991

Neurologic Complications of Pregnancy

Kathleen Shannon

The majority of women who become pregnant do so at times in their lives of relative health and physical fitness. Fortunately, concomitant diseases are relatively rare in this population. However, the childbearing years overlap periods of increased risk for neurologic disorders such as migraine headache, vascular malformations, multiple sclerosis, and myasthenia gravis. Pregnancy enhances susceptibility to some conditions, such as venous and arterial thrombosis, or may be the setting for conditions such as eclampsia, which do not occur in the nongravid state. An understanding of the physiologic changes of pregnancy and how they are likely to influence neurologic diseases forms the foundation upon which decisions about diagnostic and therapeutic interventions are made.

The focus of this chapter is on the evaluation and treatment of neurologic disorders that are commonly encountered during pregnancy. For those conditions that commonly occur in the nongravid population as well, the reader is referred elsewhere in the text for more comprehensive discussion of the disease entities.

TERATOLOGY

Teratologic concerns weigh heavily on the minds of pregnant patients and their physicians. As a result, there is a reluctance to perform neurodiagnostic tests, particularly where ionizing radiation is employed. There is also a popular perception that the risk of malformation consequent to drug ingestion may be as high as 25%, even with drugs not known to be teratogenic. This perception commonly leads to noncompliance with prescribed medications.

Malformations are detected in 2% to 3% of live births; less than 5% are thought to result from exposure to teratogens. The effects of a teratogen depend on the dose reaching the fetus, the duration of exposure, the gestational age of the fetus at the time of the exposure, and simultaneous exposure to other agents. Two major classes of teratogens are of concern to the treating physician: ionizing radiation and drugs.

The effects of radiation on the developing fetus depend on the dose and duration of radiation absorbed by the conceptus and the stage of development at which exposure occurs. With the exception of myelography and fluoroscopy, fewer than 0.1% of neuroradiographic examinations properly performed with abdominal shielding expose the fetus to levels of radiation greater than 1 rad, a level that is not felt to pose significant risk to the fetus. In general, if a radiographic study is indicated for the diagnosis or management of a pregnant woman, the benefits far outweigh the risks to the fetus.

The risks of magnetic resonance imaging (MR) to the fetus are not known. However, in limited studies, it has not shown teratogenic potential and is believed safe for use during pregnancy.

William J. Weiner and Christopher G. Goetz, eds. *Neurology for the Non-Neurologist*, Third Edition. Copyright
© 1994, 1989 by J. B. Lippincott Company. Copyright © 1981 by Harper and Row Publishers, Inc.

Reports of drug teratogenicity are most often based on animal studies, anecdotal reports, or case control studies. Unfortunately, few drugs are known to be entirely without risk in pregnancy, and few are known to be teratogenic. For the majority of compounds, the actual risks to the fetus are unknown.

Because organogenesis mainly occurs during the first trimester, drugs should be avoided whenever possible during this time. Throughout pregnancy, prudent assessment of risk-to-benefit ratios is encouraged.

PERIPHERAL NERVOUS SYSTEM AND MUSCLE DISORDERS IN PREGNANCY

BACK PAIN AND DISK DISEASE

Back pain is almost universal during pregnancy and relates to changes in posture and relaxation of spinal joints and ligaments. The pain is usually localized to the back and buttock, or radiates into the thighs. The cumulative incidence of back pain rises with the duration of pregnancy. Musculoskeletal back pain is treated with bed rest, analgesia, heat, and massage.

Disk disease in pregnancy is rare. Usually, the complaint is of unilateral low back pain radiating through the buttock into the foot. L5 and S1 radiculopathies are most common. Treatment should be conservative, with bed rest, analgesics, heat, and massage. Steroid injections may benefit some who are refractory to conservative management. Surgery should be used only in refractory cases or when there is objective evidence by electromyography or examination of nerve compromise.

PLEXUS DISORDERS, POLYNEUROPATHIES, AND MONONEUROPATHIES

Pregnancy-associated brachial plexus neuropathy may be familial or sporadic. The clinical syndrome consists of pain followed by weakness of the shoulder and arm. Neurologic exam points to a plexus lesion rather than root or nerve lesion. Recovery usually begins 4 to 8 weeks after onset, irrespective of the time of onset relative to the pregnancy. Recovery is complete in 60% at 1 year and in nearly 100% at 3 years. The syndrome may recur during subsequent pregnancies. Treatment is supportive.

Lesions of the lumbosacral plexus or nerves exiting the plexus most commonly are related to traumatic or forceps-manipulated delivery. Most are self-limited, although complete recovery may take many months.

Pregnancy-associated polyneuropathies can result from nutritional deficiencies and resemble those seen in the nonpregnant malnourished.

Acute idiopathic demyelinating polyneuropathy (AIDP, Guillain–Barré syndrome) occurs in women of childbearing age, but pregnancy does not seem to confer added risk of this disorder. AIDP presents as rapidly ascending motor neuropathy with autonomic dysfunction. The presentation and course do not differ from those in the nonpregnant population. AIDP does not adversely affect pregnancy outcome. Depending on the functional status of the patient at term, it may be necessary to assist delivery with forceps or vacuum extraction. Plasmapheresis has been shown to lessen the duration of severe symptoms in AIDP and is permissible during pregnancy. Special attention should be given to avoiding extreme fluid shifts during pheresis.

Chronic idiopathic demyelinating polyneuropathy (CIDP) shares an inflammatory etiology with AIDP. Patients have a chronic motor and large sensory fiber neuropathy with a remitting and relapsing course. CIDP may begin or relapse during pregnancy. For unknown reasons, the relapse rate is increased during pregnancy. Treatment with plasmapheresis may be helpful. Alternative strategies include chronic corticosteroids and human immune globulin administration.

Mononeuropathies in pregnancy result from hormonal and fluid changes as well as disruptions in body mechanics secondary to the gravid uterus. Bell's palsy is an acute, idiopathic unilateral weakness of muscles innervated by the facial nerve. Retroauricular pain is commonly associated. The etiology is obscure, but viral infection, nerve edema, and hormonal influences have been implicated. Most cases occur in the third trimester. The prognosis for complete recovery is good, but some patients with very severe involvement may have residual paralysis. Treatment remains controversial. Prednisone, 40 mg to 60 mg daily for 10 days, has been said to improve long-term outcome.

Carpal tunnel syndrome, presenting as nocturnal pain and burning in the first three digits of the hand, is the most common peripheral neuropathy of pregnancy. The symptoms relate to compression of the median nerve as it traverses the carpal canal. Symptomatic treatment with splinting of the wrist at night and analgesics as needed is adequate for most patients. Because aspirin has been associated with fetal malformations and with complications during labor and delivery, acetaminophen is the preferred analgesic in pregnancy. Persistent carpal tunnel symptoms may require treatment with steroid injection into the tunnel. An occasional patient may need surgical release of the compressed nerve. Usually, symptoms resolve in the postpartum period. Meralgia paresthetica is seen in conditions which place undue pressure on the lateral femoral cutaneous nerve as it passes the inguinal ligament. As in the nonpregnant population, weight gain is largely responsible. Typically, patients notice symptoms beginning in the third trimester. Pain and burning affect the middle third of the lateral thigh. Treatment consists of weight loss if possible, avoidance of binding garments or belts, acetaminophen, and in some instances local injections of analgesics or transcutaneous nerve stimulation. Most patients recover post partum.

DISORDERS OF THE NEUROMUSCULAR JUNCTION OR MUSCLE

Myasthenia gravis (MG) is a disease of women of childbearing age and older men. MG is a disorder of neuromuscular junction transmission that manifests as fatigable weakness in skeletal muscle. MG rarely presents during pregnancy, but in patients with known MG, worsening can be expected in one-third. One-third of patients with MG improve, and one-third remain stable during pregnancy. Although malignant thymoma is no more common during pregnancy than in the general MG population, pregnancy has been associated with an increased risk of widespread metastases. MG is not associated with a poorer outcome of pregnancy. Management of the MG patient who desires to become pregnant should include stabilization of the medication regimen. Corticosteroids may be continued during pregnancy, but immunosuppressants should be discontinued in favor of non-teratogenic therapies. Should thymectomy be indicated, it is best to perform this prior to pregnancy. When pregnancy occurs in the course of therapy, the risks and benefits of continuing the pre-existent management plan should be weighed. There is little to be gained by discontinuing immunosuppressants once the patient has passed the phase of organogenesis, but such patients may be offered ultrasound imaging studies to assess malformations. It is permissible to initiate corticosteroids during pregnancy. Thymectomy may be undertaken if indicated, but the patient should be prepared for this with a course of plasmapheresis. Plasmapheresis may also be needed for disease ex-

acerbations occurring during pregnancy. Anti-cholinesterase agents such as pyridostigmine may be used during pregnancy. They may be particularly helpful, and may be given parenterally, during labor and parturition. It may be necessary to assist delivery with low forceps and vacuum extraction. It is wise to remember that patients on long-term corticosteroids may have adrenal suppression with a blunted response to stress and may require supplemental corticosteroids for delivery. Special attention must be focused on the infant of the myasthenic mother following delivery. Up to 20% of these infants have transient neonatal myasthenia due to transfer of maternal anti-acetylcholine receptor antibody. Such infants are floppy, with poor suck and cry and ventilatory insufficiency. These infants should receive ventilatory assistance as indicated and may require tube feeding. Anticholinesterases may be required in some instances. The disease is self-limited and resolves as antibody titers fall, usually within 30 days of birth.

The course of muscular dystrophies is not altered by pregnancy. Muscular dystrophies do not adversely affect pregnancy outcome, but labor and delivery may be hindered by weakness and fatigability. It may be necessary to assist in the second stage of labor with forceps or vacuum extraction.

Polymyositis is an inflammatory disease involving proximal muscles. Tenderness and proximal muscle weakness, sometimes with rash (dermatomyositis), are accompanied by striking increases in creatinine phosphokinase and erythrocyte sedimentation rate. Other autoimmune diseases may be associated. Treatment is usually with corticosteroids or immunosuppressants. Adverse fetal outcome has been reported in half of pregnancies in polymyositis/dermatomyositis patients. Treatment of the pregnant woman with polymyositis/dermatomyositis stresses avoidance of teratogenic immunosuppressants, attention to steroid replacement peripartum, and support of the second stage of labor as indicated.

CENTRAL NERVOUS SYSTEM DISORDERS IN PREGNANCY

HEADACHE

Headache is the most common neurologic symptom in pregnancy, and rarely does its presence reflect serious underlying pathology. Headaches that present during pregnancy and are severe or atypical, persistently unilateral, or associated with focal findings or papilledema are indications for diagnostic evaluation. The most common headache encountered in the gravid patient is the tension, or muscle contraction, headache. Such headaches are dull and persistent with band- or vise-like pain lasting days. They are commonly associated with tension or spasm in the muscles of the scalp and neck, and may respond in part to nonpharmacologic measures such as relaxation training, massage, and heat. When headaches are disabling, they may be treated with acetaminophen or codeine, which have been found to be safe analgesics in pregnancy. Migraine headaches are severe, throbbing, often unilateral headaches that may be preceded by a visual or sensory aura. They are often associated with nausea and vomiting. Migraine headaches affects 5% to 10% of the general population and a higher percentage of women in the childbearing years. Fifty percent to 74% of women with migraine experience some decrease in the frequency of severity of migraine during pregnancy. However, some are worsened, and migraine may first present during pregnancy, usually during the first trimester. Infrequent migraine headaches are treated with analgesics, as for tension headaches. Ergot preparations, which are the mainstay of abortive migraine therapy outside pregnancy, are not recommended during pregnancy due to their propensity to cause uterine contraction. When disabling headaches occur more frequently than once weekly and adequate control is not achieved with analgesics alone, prophylactic therapy may be indicated. Propranolol 80 mg to 320 mg/day is the treatment of choice for migraine prophylaxis but may be associated with fetal growth retardation, prematurity, respiratory depression, hypoglycemia, and hyperbilirubinemia. Relatively low doses of antidepressants, such as amitriptyline 25 mg may also be helpful.

EPILEPSY

One in every 200 pregnancies occurs in an epileptic woman. At issue in management of these women are the following: the effects of pregnancy on seizure frequency and anticonvulsant pharmacokinetics, the effects of epilepsy on pregnancy and fetal development, and the effects of anticonvulsants on fetal development.

Seizure frequency is increased in 5% to 46%, decreased in 19% to 44%, and unchanged in 35% to 55% of patients. Patients whose epilepsy has been poorly controlled prior to pregnancy are more likely to be poorly controlled during pregnancy. Increased seizure frequency is most likely to occur during the first two trimesters and is often related to changes in serum drug levels (due to altered pharmacokinetics or noncompliance) or to sleep deprivation.

Total concentrations of all anticonvulsants decrease during pregnancy. This reflects changes in dose, body weight, and plasma protein binding (see Table 26-1). Decreased levels are apparent during the first trimester but become more pronounced throughout pregnancy and may be associated with exacerbation of seizures. Changes in protein binding make total drug levels unreliable in monitoring of epileptic patients, as free levels may remain unchanged or may increase. The clinician should use the patient's clinical condition, frequency of seizures, and drug levels to monitor epileptic drug therapy. Whenever possible, free anticonvulsant levels should be used to monitor drug levels.

In prospective studies of epileptic women, stillbirth, prematurity, intrauterine growth retardation, and cesarean section occurred with increased frequency in the pregnancies of patients with sei-

TABLE 26-1. Factors Affecting Drug Pharmacokinetics During Pregnancy

ABSORPTION
Slowed gastric emptying
Increased mucous production
Decreased acid secretion

DISTRIBUTION
Increased intravascular volume
Increased extravascular volume
Increased tissue volume
Changes in plasma protein binding
    Decreased plasma protein concentration
    Decreased binding capacity of albumin
    Increased concentration of endogenous inhibitors of protein binding

LIVER METABOLISM
Induction of microsomal enzymes by circulating steroid hormones
Centrilobular bile stasis

RENAL EXCRETION
Increased renal plasma flow
Increased glomerular filtration rate

zure disorders. There is increased mortality in the neonatal period. There has been no association found between antiepileptic drug therapy and these complications. Although severe and prolonged convulsions may cause fetal heart decelerations, obvious neonatal sequelae of convulsions are rare, even in the case of status epilepticus.

The risk of major congenital malformations in children of epileptic mothers is twice that in the general population. These defects consist mainly of congenital heart malformations, facial clefts, and neural tube defects. Although the risk of major malformation is increased in nontreated epileptics, it is higher still in epileptics receiving anticonvulsant drugs. With the exception of the association between valproic acid and neural tube defects, there is no specific association with a particular drug and resulting malformation. Neural tube defects, ranging from spina bifida to complete failure of fusion of the neuraxis, may be seen in 1% to 2% of children of epileptic mothers treated with valproic acid during the first trimester.

Controlled studies have shown an excess of minor malformations in offspring of epileptic women. The anomalies, which are seen in up to 11% of infants exposed *in utero* to anticonvulsants, include epicanthal folds, hypertelorism, small nose with anteverted nares and low nasal bridge, long philtrum, abnormal ears, low hairline, nail hypoplasia, distal phalangeal hypoplasia, and increased dermal arches. Similar anomalies have been shown to occur in children of epileptic women who have not been exposed to anticonvulsant drugs, which suggests that some of them may be genetically linked to epilepsy. Proposed mechanisms of anticonvulsant teratogenicity include folate deficiency induced by the agents themselves and the effects of toxic intermediate metabolites.

Up to 10% of infants exposed to anticonvulsants *in utero* will develop hemorrhagic complications related to deficiency of vitamin K–dependent coagulation factors. Bleeding usually occurs within the first 24 hours of life and can be prevented in most instances by treating the mother for the last 4 weeks of pregnancy with vitamin K (20 mg orally daily) and by administering parenteral vitamin K to the infant immediately after delivery. Fresh frozen plasma can be used for acute hemorrhage if needed.

Patients in the childbearing years should be encouraged to inform the physician when they begin trying to have children. They should be counseled about the risks of anomalies in their offspring as well as the importance to fetal outcome of careful seizure control during pregnancy. It should be stressed that the likelihood they will have a normal infant is 90%. Vitamin replacement should begin before pregnancy. When possible, seizures should be managed with monotherapy and should be monitored closely to establish the level at which optimal control is achieved. Valproic acid and trimethadione should be avoided in patients likely to have children. With the exception of these two agents, the evidence that one anticonvulsant is less teratogenic than the others is not strong enough to justify removing a patient from a drug regimen under which her seizures are well controlled.

When epileptic patients present after they have become pregnant, there is little to be gained from changing the anticonvulsant regimen, as malformations may have already occurred. Patients who have been exposed to valproic acid during the first trimester should be offered ultrasound and amniocentesis with quantitation of alpha-fetoprotein levels at the 20th week of gestation to detect neural tube defects.

The previously well patient who has a non-eclamptic seizure during pregnancy should have its cause investigated. Most represent coincidental onset of idiopathic epilepsy, but an underlying structural lesion should be excluded. The choice of anticonvulsant should be dictated by the seizure type. Most physicians elect not to initiate anticonvulsants for a single uncomplicated seizure. When anticonvulsants are indicated, monotherapy is desirable; the dose should be optimized to the lowest dose that maintains seizure control.

Pregnant women taking anticonvulsants should have serum levels (preferably free drug levels) monitored on a monthly basis, and the dose of medications should be adjusted to maintain levels in the range of those prepregnancy that controlled seizures. Free drug levels more accurately reflect concentrations of active drug and are useful when seizures prove difficult to manage despite therapeutic serum drug levels.

ISCHEMIC CEREBROVASCULAR DISEASE

The differential diagnosis of stroke in pregnancy is listed in Table 26-2. Sixty percent to 80% of ischemic cerebrovascular events in pregnancy result

TABLE 26-2. Differential Diagnosis of Stroke During Pregnancy

HEMORRHAGIC
Subarachnoid hemorrhage
  Aneurysm
  Arteriovenous malformation
Intracerebral hematoma
  Hypertension
  Eclampsia
  Clotting disorder

ISCHEMIC—ARTERIAL
Embolism
  Cardiac disease
    Valve disease
    Arrhythmia
    Cardiomyopathy of pregnancy
  Systemic venous thromboembolism
  Patent foramen ovale
Thrombosis
  Cervical arterial disease
    Atherosclerosis
    Takayasu's pulseless disease
    Fibromuscular dysplasia
    Carotid artery dissection
  Cranial arterial disease
    Arteritis
    Hypertension

ISCHEMIC—VENOUS
Infectious
Aseptic
  Idiopathic
  Associated with coagulopathy

from arterial occlusion. Most occur during the second and third trimesters and the first postpartum week, and are related to cervical or cranial arterial disease or to cardiac disease with cardiogenic cerebral embolization. Patients with pre-existing hypertension, diabetes mellitus, cigarette smoking, and familial hyperlipidemia are at particular risk for atherosclerotic disease of the cervical and intracranial arteries. Cranial arterial disease may also result from infectious or noninfectious vasculitis or from long-standing hypertension. Coagulopathy may be related to changes in coagulation factors during pregnancy, to underlying sickle cell anemia, or to thrombotic thrombocytopenic purpura. Cardiogenic cerebral emboli originate on infected or damaged cardiac valves or from the cardiac chambers in the presence of hypokinetic wall segments or arrhythmias. Rarely, a patent foramen ovale will be the route for cerebral emboli originating in the systemic venous circulation, or for fat or amniotic fluid emboli.

The evaluation and treatment of arterial occlusion in the pregnant patient differ little from that in the general population. Computed tomography (CT), MR, and arteriography, if indicated, can be performed without significant risk to the fetus. When diagnostic evaluation indicates infarction due to carotid artery disease, a symptomatic, surgically accessible, highly stenosed artery can be approached surgically at a center with acceptably low morbidity and mortality. Conservative treatment with daily low-dose aspirin therapy may be advised as initial therapy for patients with surgically accessible lesions as well as for those with nonsurgical lesions. The only clear indication for systemic anticoagulation is the prevention of recurrent emboli of cardiac origin.

Venous infarction in pregnancy and the puerperium may arise from infectious or noninfectious causes, although the incidence of the former is quite small in the antibiotic age. Most venous infarctions occur in the second to fifth weeks after delivery. Typically, infarction is heralded by severe headache, nausea, and vomiting. Weakness of one or both legs may be accompanied by proximal arm weakness. Focal deficits are commonly progressive and may be accompanied by focal or generalized seizures and increased intracranial pressure. Consciousness is often impaired. Mortality during the acute phase approaches 25%, but the prognosis is good for patients who survive, and recovery is often complete. Diagnosis is based on clinical features, characteristic CT or MR findings, or angiographic studies. Treatment is conservative and includes hospitalization, hydration, and antibiotic and anticonvulsant therapy when indicated. The role of anticoagulation is controversial, but a trial may be indicated for patients who are showing progressive deterioration, early in the course, without evidence of hemorrhage on imaging studies or lumbar puncture.

It should be noted that heparin does not cross the placenta and so is not teratogenic. However, heparin exposure has been associated with an increased risk of prematurity or stillbirth, and also with osteopenia and pathologic fracture in the mother. However, it is the anticoagulant of choice prior to the 13th week of pregnancy. Although it is not without risk in the second and third trimesters, warfarin is a superior anticoagulant and is the drug of choice during the time between the 13th and 36th weeks of gestation. After the 36th week, heparin should again be used to minimize the risk of peripartum hemorrhage.

HEMORRHAGIC CEREBROVASCULAR DISEASE

An underlying arteriovenous malformation or aneurysm can be found in 93% of pregnant patients presenting with subarachnoid hemorrhage, and aggressive and immediate diagnostic evaluation of the pregnant woman presenting with subarachnoid hemorrhage is indicated. Arteriovenous malformations tend to occur in younger primiparous women, bleed during the second trimester, and rebleed during labor, delivery, and subsequent pregnancies (Table 26-3). It is recommended that the patient with arteriovenous malformations be delivered by elective cesarean section, and that the risks of future pregnancy be explained to the patient. Surgical intervention during pregnancy is avoided when possible.

Aneurysms tend to present in older multiparous women. Presentation is usually during the last trimester, and the risk of rebleeding is greatest in the first 2 weeks after initial bleed. Early surgical intervention is recommended. The risk of rebleeding is low during labor and delivery, and vaginal delivery may be allowed. It is recommended that forceps assistance be used in the second stage of labor.

ECLAMPSIA

Although maternal mortality from all causes has declined, preeclampsia and eclampsia continue to account for about 5% of maternal deaths. Eclampsia may have up to 20% maternal mortality and 53% infant mortality. It is largely a disease of nulliparous gravid women. When it occurs in multiparous women, it is usually associated with multiple gestation, chronic hypertension, diabetes, or renal failure. Hypertension (systolic ≥140 mm Hg or increase of ≥30 mm Hg; diastolic ≥90 mm Hg or increase of ≥15 mm Hg), usually occurring after the 20th week of pregnancy, is accompanied by proteinuria and edema. Other symptoms include headache, visual disturbance, epigastric pain, hyperreflexia, and consumptive coagulopathy. Eclampsia is differentiated from preeclampsia by the occurrence of central nervous system signs, usually seizure or coma. Other neurologic manifestations include lethargy, obtundation, flashing lights, cortical blindness, visual hallucinations, and other focal signs.

Gross neuropathologic features of eclampsia are patchy areas of infarction and petechial hemorrhage. Some patients have large hemorrhages in the cortical white matter, deep gray matter structures, or brain stem. Endothelial cell damage, vasospasm, and medial necrosis are seen at the microscopic level. The pathogenesis of preeclampsia and eclampsia remains unknown. Putative causal factors include immunologic, placental or maternal endocrine, genetic, and alterations in prostaglandin metabolism.

The treatment of eclampsia remains controversial and targets multiple signs. First used in 1900 and widely accepted after 1925, magnesium sulfate has been considered the treatment of choice for preeclampsia and eclampsia by the obstetric community, despite the lack of well-controlled scientific data. Although magnesium has been shown to have antiepileptic properties in experimental models of epilepsy, penetration into the central nervous system is poor and there is no evidence of anticonvulsant activity in humans. In light of these findings, it is imprudent to continue to administer magnesium

TABLE 26-3. Subarachnoid Hemorrhage in Pregnancy

	ARTERIOVENOUS MALFORMATION	ANEURYSM
Decade of presentation	3rd	4th
Presentation trimester	1–2	2–3
Rebleeding common	intrapartum	postpartum
Surgery when gravid?	not recommended	recommended
Allow labor?	not recommended	postoperative

sulfate outside the context of a controlled clinical trial.

Clearly, the mainstay of treatment in preeclampsia and eclampsia is control of hypertension. Adequate prenatal care must stress blood pressure surveillance, and immediate action must be taken if the diastolic blood pressure exceeds 75 mm Hg in the second trimester and 85 mm Hg in the third trimester. Conservative measures, such as bed rest, should be supplemented with antihypertensive medications when the former fail. Methyldopa has an established safety record in pregnancy, as has hydralazine. Although less well studied, beta-adrenergic blocking agents and calcium channel blockers are also believed to be safe enough in pregnancy to justify their use as antihypertensives. Acute hypertensive crisis accompanied by other clinical features of preeclampsia or eclampsia should be treated by hospitalization, bed rest, and oral or parenteral antihypertensives. Hydralazine and diazoxide have established roles in the treatment of severe preeclampsia and eclampsia requiring parenteral therapy, but the risk of cyanide toxicity in the neonate dictates against the use of sodium nitroprusside.

Seizures and status epilepticus should be treated aggressively, using standard anticonvulsants as in the nonpregnant patient with acute convulsions. The deleterious effects of convulsions on the fetus far outweigh the central nervous system depression attributed to anticonvulsant drugs. Patients who have had magnesium sulfate therapy are at greater risk of respiratory depression, and should be monitored more closely during treatment with benzodiazepines or barbiturates. Following the acute eclamptic period, it is recommended that anticonvulsants be continued through the 30th postpartum day to prevent seizure recurrence.

SUMMARY

Although as many as 45% of pregnant women are exposed to one or more medications during pregnancy, the majority enjoy uncomplicated pregnancies and are delivered of normal, healthy infants. The physician must function as diagnostician, medication prescriber, and counselor to pregnant women. A coherent approach to care during pregnancy is founded on comprehension of the effects of pregnancy on acute and chronic disease states, working knowledge of pharmacologic and ter-atologic principles, and sensitivity to the concerns of the mother about the outcome of pregnancy.

QUESTIONS AND DISCUSSION

1. A 40-year-old multiparous woman presents during the 32nd week of pregnancy with acute onset of severe headache, neck stiffness, and obtundation. What is the most likely diagnosis?

    A. Ischemic brain-stem stroke
    B. Eclampsia
    C. Subarachnoid hemorrhage due to cerebral aneurysm
    D. Subarachnoid hemorrhage due to arteriovenous malformation

The answer is (C). The symptoms typify subarachnoid hemorrhage, and the usual etiology in a patient of this age and duration of gestation is aneurysm. An emergency CT scan should be performed to confirm this diagnosis.

2. The management of the well-controlled epileptic in her third trimester of pregnancy includes all but which one of the following:

    A. If she is taking phenytoin, this should be changed to phenobarbital to minimize the risk of fetal malformation.
    B. The dose of anticonvulsant should be determined by assessing clinical control of seizures and the presence of side effects, and by following drug levels.
    C. Anticonvulsant levels should be checked approximately once monthly.
    D. She should be given vitamin K supplementation to avoid hemorrhagic complications in the newborn.

The answer is (A). Although it has been believed for some time that phenobarbital is less teratogenic than other anticonvulsants, this is not supported by clinical studies. Patients who are well controlled on phenytoin should be maintained on this agent.

3. A 22-year-old primiparous woman in the 38th week of gestation complains of flashing lights in the visual field and epigastric discomfort. Her blood pressure is 140/85. She has peripheral edema and proteinuria. What is the most responsible course of management?

A. She should be sent home with magnesium supplements.
B. She should be admitted to the hospital and started immediately on parenteral magnesium sulfate.
C. She should be admitted to the hospital and started on bed rest; antihypertensives should be added for continued hypertension.
D. She should be admitted to the hospital and started on phenobarbital, 30 mg t.i.d.

The answer is (C). She is currently preeclamptic, but the visual symptoms indicate impending eclampsia. Despite wide clinical use, there is no convincing evidence that parenteral magnesium is beneficial in preeclampsia or eclampsia. There is also no evidence that prophylactic phenobarbital prevents eclamptic convulsions. Should conservative blood pressure management fail, antihypertensives should be started immediately.

4. A 27-year-old woman in the 30th week of pregnancy complains of 4 days of back pain that radiates into the thighs. Her neurologic examination is normal. What should be your approach?

A. An electromyogram should be ordered to evaluate for acute radiculopathy.
B. CT scan should be ordered to evaluate for acute radiculopathy.
C. Bed rest and analgesics should be prescribed.
D. A neurosurgical evaluation for chymopapain injection should be scheduled.

The answer is (C). Back pain is frequent in pregnancy and usually responds to conservative management. An electromyogram is unlikely to be diagnostic of radiculopathy with this duration of symptoms. CT scan may be abnormal, but interpretation is difficult in the context of this nonspecific syndrome of back pain.

SUGGESTED READING

Dalessio DJ: Seizure disorders and pregnancy. N Engl J Med 312:559, 1985

Donaldson JO: Neurology of Pregnancy. London, WB Saunders, 1989

Gleicher N (ed): Principles of Medical Therapy in Pregnancy. New York, Plenum Publishing, 1985

Hiilesmaa VK: Pregnancy and birth in women with epilepsy. Neurology 42 (Suppl 5):8, 1992

Kaplan PW, Lesser RP, Fisher RS et al: No, magnesium sulfate should not be used in treating eclamptic seizures. Arch Neurol 45:1361, 1983

Stanley FJ, Bower C: Teratogenic drugs in pregnancy. Med J Aust 145:596, 1986

Tanganelli P, Regesta G: Epilepsy, pregnancy, and major birth anomalies: An Italian prospective, controlled study. Neurology 42 (Suppl 5):89, 1992

Wiebers DO: Ischemic cerebrovascular complications of pregnancy. Arch Neurol 42:110, 1985

Yerby MS: Pregnancy and teratogenesis. In Trimble MR (ed): Women and Epilepsy, pp 163–187. New York, John Wiley, 1991

Medical–Legal Issues in the Care of the Patient with Neurologic Illness

Lois Margaret Nora

In recent years, legal aspects of medical practice have assumed greater visibility and importance. This has been particularly apparent in the care of patients with neurologic disease. Although increased attention to medical–legal aspects of patient care are not welcomed by all, it is unlikely that the emphasis will diminish. Knowledge of, and comfort with, legal aspects of medical practice can contribute to optimal medical care.

Medical practice is affected by laws from three major sources, case, statutory, and administrative law. *Case law* (also called common law) is developed in the judicial system through the resolution of various criminal and civil matters. An important role of the courts is to interpret the various statutes passed by different legislative bodies. State and federal courts exist in parallel, and appellate review is available in both systems.

Many physicians are most concerned with this aspect of the legal system because of the recent increase in malpractice lawsuits. Malpractice cases are civil actions. Most malpractice cases allege that the physician was negligent in the care of the plaintiff. In order to win a lawsuit alleging negligence, the plaintiff must demonstrate by a preponderance of the evidence (1) that the physician had a duty of care to the patient; (2) that the physician breached that duty; and (3) that the breach proximately caused injury to the plaintiff. Expert testimony must be used in most medical malpractice cases to establish what the physician's duty was and whether or not it was breached. In addition to proving his case, the plaintiff must also successfully counter any defenses brought by the physician.

It is important to be aware of the other sources of law that affect medical practice. *Statutory law* is developed by local, state, or federal legislative bodies and applies to persons within the jurisdictions of those legislatures. Federal and state laws on medical malpractice, abortion, living wills, and termination of treatment are examples of statutory laws. Variation in laws among different jurisdictions is common. The court system frequently is involved in interpreting statutes and in resolving conflicts that arise between different jurisdictions.

A third source of rules that may affect health care is *administrative law*. Some government agencies are empowered to make and enforce rules related to their specific activities; these rules constitute administrative law. The Internal Revenue Service, for example, has broad authority to make and enforce rules about the collection of taxes. Government agencies whose rulings impact medical practice include the Food and Drug Administration (FDA), state and federal drug enforcement agencies, and the Occupational Health and Safety Administration (OSHA), among others.

This chapter addresses three specific areas where medical and legal matters interface in the care of patients with neurologic illness. First, informed consent, a legal doctrine that affirms patient self-

William J. Weiner and Christopher G. Goetz, eds. *Neurology for the Non Neurologist*, Third Edition. Copyright © 1994, 1989 by J. B. Lippincott Company. Copyright © 1981 by Harper and Row Publishers, Inc.

determination, is presented. The discussion then turns toward the aspects of brain death in clinical practice. The chapter concludes with a discussion of the common problem of licensing drivers with a seizure disorder.

INFORMED CONSENT

Informed consent was first recognized as a legal requirement in 1907.[1] Informed consent doctrine supports individual autonomy and states that patients have the right to understand proposed interventions (diagnostic and therapeutic) and to voluntarily consent to or reject those interventions. Unfortunate instances demonstrate that, even in recent years, medical and scientific practitioners have not always conformed to these expectations.[2,3]

Several assurances are necessary for informed consent. First, the patient must be competent. Second, the patient must be provided with understandable and adequate information about a proposed intervention. Third, the patient's consent must be given voluntarily.

A patient must be competent in order to give informed consent. In order to be competent to give informed consent, the patient must be *both* legally and clinically competent. Adults are presumed to be legally competent unless they have been legally declared incompetent. Some minors are legally competent to provide consent for certain interventions but not for others. For example, in some states, adolescents are legally competent to make reproductive health decisions, despite lacking legal competence to make other medical care decisions. When a person is legally incompetent, the appointed guardian should be approached to obtain consent.

Legal competence, by itself, is not enough. A person must also be clinically competent. Clinical competence is a medical decision. In some situations, not uncommonly in the setting of neurologic illness, a person may be legally competent but not clinically competent. Dementia, encephalopathy, and other conditions may render the patient incapable of providing informed consent for a variable period of time.

In the event of clinical incompetence, medical treatment can proceed in an emergency situation. Attempts should be made to contact members of the patient's family to obtain approval for the intervention, although their consent is not legally necessary if the treatment is a medical necessity.

In situations when consent from an incompetent is not possible, two legal tests have been used to determine whether or not an intervention should proceed. These tests are *substituted judgment* and *best interest*. The substituted judgment test reviews the patient's prior actions, comments, and beliefs in an effort to determine what decision the patient would have made. The best interest approach looks at all the facts of the case and attempts to identify the action that would be in the best interest of the incompetent patient.

A judgment of legal and/or clinical incompetence for certain medical decision making should not preclude the patient's ability to participate in other decisions. Every attempt to allow continued decision making by the patient (*e.g.*, even as basic as what to eat for dinner) should be made.

The second requirement for informed consent is that adequate information be provided to the patient in an understandable fashion. Although other health care personnel may be involved in obtaining consent, the physician remains responsible for ensuring adequate information provision as well as the other aspects of informed consent. Information provided to the patient should include the nature and purpose of the proposed intervention, its risks and anticipated benefits, alternatives to the proposed interventions, prognosis without the intervention, and prognosis with alternative interventions. The patient should be told of his rights to refuse and to withdraw a consent at any time.

The adequacy of information provided to a patient can be an issue in malpractice suits. Two different legal standards of information disclosure are recognized: the *professional standard* and the *material risk standard*. The professional standard requires the physician to give the patient information that other physicians of the same specialty, in the same community, would give to patients considering the same intervention. Expert testimony is necessary to delineate what this information consists of. This is the older of the two standards and is currently the choice of most courts.

The material risk standard requires the physician to provide any information that a reasonable person in the patient's position would want disclosed or would use in making a consent decision. Advocates of this standard identify its emphasis on the patient's need for information. Opponents point to its retrospective application as a major disadvantage.

The most appropriate approach is probably a hybrid. Physicians should communicate those risks that occur with great enough frequency or that are so severe, even if infrequent, that a usual patient would wish to know of them. For example, patients should be advised of the possibility of hirsutism and gingival hyperplasia with phenytoin use and given information about spinal headaches prior to lumbar puncture. In addition, if a physician is aware of a particular characteristic of a patient that would make a potential side effect more important to that patient, this side effect should be communicated, even if not generally discussed. For example, potential teratogenic efects of medications should be discussed with female patients who may become pregnant.

A third requirement of informed consent is that the patient must give consent voluntarily. Coercion invalidates consent. A physician should provide patients with advice and guidance regarding proposed therapies, but this must be done in a noncoercive way. No explicit or implicit threat of loss of medical or nursing care should be linked to a decision.

Consent discussion should be documented in the patient record. A patient-signed consent is not required for valid consent, but it can provide evidence of decision making by the patient. Prepared consent forms can be helpful, but the value of these documents should not be overestimated. Courts are suspicious of complicated documents that appear to be written to protect the physician rather than inform the patient.

Care must be taken that interventions remain within the scope of the consent given by the patient. Consent is given for a particular procedure and other procedures that are within the scope of that procedure or that can be reasonably expected. Consent is usually given to a particular individual and those working with that individual. Care must be taken not to overextend the consent to procedures that are not logically associated with the consent or to personnel not reasonably anticipated by the patient.

In certain circumstances, an intervention can proceed without informed consent. Some exceptions to informed consent exist. In emergency situations when there is significant, immediate risk to the patient, necessary therapy can proceed. A competent patient may waive his right to informed consent; the patient decides to "let the doctor decide." Although courts recognize patient waiver of informed consent, physicians should take care that wavier decisions are documented carefully, and they may wish to have the patient put the waiver in writing.

Therapeutic privilege is another exception to informed consent. This exception is used when the physician determines that an informed consent discussion will prove so detrimental to the patient's health that it should not be done. For example, some physicians have used this exception to justify not disclosing the risk of tardive dyskinesia when neuroleptic medications are prescribed to certain patients whom they fear will refuse a potentially beneficial medication because of a severe, but unlikely, side effect.

Physicians must be extremely cautious in their use of therapeutic privilege. Courts may not be sympathetic to physicians' defending their use of therapeutic privilege when confronted by an uninformed patient who has suffered severe side effects. If a physician feels the use of therapeutic privilege is absolutely necessary, involving the patient's family in the decision may be beneficial. In addition, complete disclosure to the patient at the earliest opportunity is also advisable. The physician should keep contemporaneous clear documentation of reasons for the decision.

The right of a patient to give informed consent carries with it an obvious recognition of the patient's right of informed refusal. Patients have a legal right to refuse interventions, even if the refusal will result in the patient's death. Education and persuasion of the patient are the tools usually available to the physician confronted by a refusal. Physicians must inform patients of potential problems related to refusing a potential intervention, and this should also be documented.

Informed refusal is not an absolute right. Certain exceptions to the patient's right to refuse an intervention have been recognized, and judicial intervention is possible in certain situations. Courts will not permit informed refusal to be used as a means to commit suicide and may override a patient's refusal if deemed necessary for the protection of innocent third parties. The court may modify a patient's refusal in order to protect the standards of the medical profession or of an institution.

Legal proceedings against physicians for failure to obtain informed consent may take two forms. A physician may be sued for battery, an intentional unconsented-to touching of an individual (the patient) by another (the physician). As an intentional tort, punitive damages (monetary damages meant to punish the physician, not just recompense the patient) may be available if a physician is found liable. Except in extreme cases when no consent was obtained or when misrepresentation or fraud was used to obtain the consent, it is unlikely that battery will be alleged. The fact that malpractice insurance coverage is usually not available for intentional torts may also limit the use of a battery action by plaintiffs.

More commonly, failure to obtain informed consent will lead to a negligence suit. In order to win, the plaintiff must demonstrate by a preponderance of the evidence that (1) the injury sustained was a known risk of the therapy, (2) the physician failed to meet the applicable standard of care regarding information about the risk that caused the injury, and (3) the patient would not have consented to the therapy if the information was provided. If these things are proved, the plaintiff can succeed, even if the sustained injury was a known complication of the intervention and did not result through any fault of the physician.

In summary, physicians remain responsible for informed consent even when others are involved in obtaining it. Information given to patients should be adequate and understandable. Patients must be legally and clinically competent, and assent to interventions must be given voluntarily. Written documentation may help provide evidence of patient decision making, although written documentation is neither required nor guaranteed to relieve the physician of liability.

In the case of legal incompetence, guardians should be approached for consent. When a patient is legally competent but clinically incompetent, medical care can proceed in an emergency situation. Intervention by the courts may be necessary in determining nonemergency care for incompetent patients.

In the case of informed refusal, care must be taken to inform the patient of risks of refusal. Although informed refusal is allowed, even when misguided or life threatening, courts do recognize exceptions to the doctrine. Excellent medical and nursing care should continue regardless of a patient's individual treatment decisions.

BRAIN DEATH

Death was traditionally defined clinically by the lack of cardiac and pulmonary functioning. In recent years, medical and technological advances make artificial ventilation and continued cardiac rhythm possible even when death of the brain has occurred. As a result, it is necessary to recognize that irreversible and total brain death is an additional means of demonstrating death of the patient.

The concept that irreversible coma was equivalent to death was first articulated by the Harvard criteria in 1968.[4] A National Institutes of Health Collaborative Study in 1977 studied brain death further, and in 1981 the President's Commission for the Study of Ethical Problems in Medicine and Biomedical and Behavioral Research published a treatise on the issue.[5,6] In 1980, the United States Uniform Determination of Death Act codified brain death as a legally acceptable definition of death, and states were encouraged to adopt this law.[7] These studies and opinions have contributed to a gradual acceptance in the United States of brain death as a medical and legal criterion for death.

The laws of most states currently define death as either the irreversible cessation of circulation and pulmonary functioning *or* the irreversible cessation of complete brain functioning. This does not imply that there are two types of death. Instead, two mechanisms for determining death in a given patient are delineated.

There are two critical aspects in the determination of brain death: (1) the total cessation of total brain functioning, and (2) the irreversibility of the condition. Potential legal difficulties related to brain death can be avoided by a rigorous medical approach to establishing the condition. In addition, careful and considerate communication with the patient's family members contributes to optimal medical care and the avoidance of legal problems.

The diagnosis of brain death should be made by one familiar with doing so. This will usually be a neurologist, neurosurgeon, or critical care specialist. Any physician with a real or perceived conflict of interest in the diagnosis (*e.g.*, member of a transplant team) should not be involved in making the diagnosis.

A diagnosis of brain death is established in three interrelated steps. First, an etiology should be established, and certain conditions that can mimic brain death, but are reversible, must be excluded. The second step is the clinical evaluation of the patient. Third, laboratory tests provide confirmation of the diagnosis and prognosis. Careful attention to these three steps will ensure that complete cessation of brain functioning and its irreversibility are established. Physicians should also be aware of any specific institutional requirements for establishing brain death. For example, some institutions require certain tests or a formal checklist approach.[8]

Certain prerequisites are necessary for a diagnosis of brain death. The brain death criteria to be discussed have been established for adults; these criteria should not be used in children under 5 years of age. Specific consultation with experts in pediatric neurology and critical care should be obtained when diagnosing brain death in a young child.

The reason for the patient's condition must be known. Brain death should not be diagnosed without a clear etiology. The most common causes of brain death are head trauma, intracerebral hemorrhage, and anoxia following a cardiopulmonary arrest. A careful history, examination, and various laboratory tests (*e.g.*, CT scanning) may be helpful in determining the etiology.

Medical conditions that can mimic brain death must be ruled out prior to making a diagnosis of brain death. These include hypothermia, metabolic dysfunction, and drug intoxication. In the setting of hypothermia, the temperature must be corrected prior to a diagnosis. Barbiturate and anesthetic agents are the most frequently implicated drugs in this setting, but tricyclic antidepressants and other medications have also been reported. In the setting of drug intoxication or metabolic dysfunction, brain death can only be established after correction of the problem or with demonstration of lack of cerebral circulation.

The second component of the brain death evaluation is the clinical examination. The clinical examination establishes the total absence of brain (cerebral and brain-stem) functioning and helps rule out those conditions that may mimic brain death. The patient must be in deep coma unresponsive to any external stimuli, including pain. Any form of purposeful response, seizure activity, or decerebrate or decorticate posturing is inconsistent with the diagnosis of brain death.

All activities, including reflexes, mediated by the cortex and the brain stem must be absent. Pupils are dilated but may be midpoint. The light reflex must be absent. Other brain-stem reflexes, including doll's eye, calorics, corneal, gag, swallow, and cough, must be absent.

The brain stem controls respiration, and the evaluation of brain death should include formal apnea testing to rule out the ability of the brain stem to maintain respiration. Following extended ventilation with 90% to 100% oxygen, the patient is discontinued from the respirator. Arterial blood gases are drawn, and an endotracheal catheter with 100% oxygen running at 4 to 6 liters is placed. If the patient has had no spontaneous respiratory efforts after 5 minutes, blood gases are redrawn and the patient placed once again on the ventilator. If a $PaCO_2$ of 55 to 60 is not obtained, testing should

continue with gradual prolongation of the off-ventilator period until this level is reached. If no spontaneous respiratory attempts are made with a $PaCO_2$ of 55 to 60, it can be said with confidence that the patient has no spontaneous respirations.

Although brain-stem reflexes are completely absent with brain death, certain spinal-mediated reflexes can be preserved. The presence of these reflexes does preclude the diagnosis. It is important that members of the health care team and the patient's family are aware that such movements do not constitute purposeful activity.

The third aspect of a brain death evaluation is laboratory testing. These tests can help rule out conditions that can mimic brain death, confirm the neurologic examination, and establish the irreversibility of the condition.

The electroencephalogram (EEG) has been an important part of brain death evaluation for many years. Care must be taken to obtain a technically acceptable EEG when evaluating a patient for brain death; this can be difficult in the intensive care setting. The presence of cortical activity on an EEG is inconsistent with a diagnosis of brain death. Extended electrocerebral silence (ECS), although consistent with brain death, is not pathognomonic for the process. ECS can be seen in certain reversible conditions, including drug overdose.

Evoked potentials can also be helpful in making the diagnosis of brain death. Evoked potentials may be less likely than other EEG activity to be affected in certain metabolic conditions. The presence of cortical and brain stem evoked responses rules out brain death. The absence of evoked potentials is confirmatory, but not absolute, evidence.

The complete cessation of blood flow to the normothermic adult brain for 10 minutes or more is incompatible with life. Blood flow studies that demonstrate no intracranial circulation for 10 minutes or more provide compelling and conclusive evidence of irreversible brain death. Cerebral blood flow studies, by way of angiography or radionuclide imaging, can be very helpful in the diagnosis of brain death.

It is critically important that adequate time be allowed for complete evaluation and serial observations of the patient during the determination of brain death. The time necessary to reach the diagnosis will vary depending upon the etiology of the patient's condition, the clinical expertise of the examiner, and the use of various diagnostic tests. Generally, the patient should be observed for at least 12 hours. In some instances this time period may be shortened, but confirmatory diagnostic testing is critically important in these shorter time periods. Pressure for organ harvesting and other concerns should not prevent the careful and complete process necessary to reach the diagnosis.

Some legal difficulties related to brain death have resulted from poor communication with the patient's family members. Probably the most frequent error in the clinical setting, as well as in literature about brain death, is the suggestion that the brain-dead patient is somehow still alive. This is usually done by referring to the brain as dead but the body as alive. For example, a family member is told the "patient is dead [because of brain death], but we are keeping the body alive [because of desire for organ donor possibilities]." This is confusing information for the family, made more so by the chest movements created by the ventilator and the cardiac rhythm bleeping on a monitor. The situation is further complicated if activities around the patient elicit some form of spinal reflex response.

It is extremely important to communicate that brain death is one way that death is diagnosed and that brain death *is death*. Families must be helped to understand that their loved one is dead. Continued pharmacologic and technological supports should be described in terms of perfusing organs (particularly the specific organs being considered for donation) rather than keeping the body alive. Pharmacologic and technological support should be discontinued as soon as feasible following the diagnosis of brain death; allowing families their goodbyes prior to discontinuation of machinery may be appropriate, but extended technological support of dead bodies is not.

Although organ harvesting is possible in the absence of family consent (*e.g.*, when there is a valid donor card), physicians will usually not do so without family consent. From a risk-management perspective, this is appropriate. When there is a possibility of organ donation, it should be discussed with the family early in the care of the patient by persons uninvolved in diagnostic and treatment decisions about the patient. Many organ procurement programs have personnel specially trained to perform these tasks. In no event should undue pressure be exerted on family members to consent to organ harvesting. One institution was successfully sued for refusing to discontinue organ support systems and release the body of a brain-dead teenager to his family while physicians persisted in encouraging the family to consent to organ harvesting.[9]

Somatic death inevitably follows brain death within several days. When there are no organ harvesting considerations, there may be fewer pressures to declare the patient brain dead and discontinue treatment. This may be a particularly tempting course of action when there is family dissension about terminating organ support systems. Nonetheless, this course of action must be balanced against the ethics of using limited resources (including nursing and medical support staff) to support a corpse.

EPILEPSY AND LICENSING OF DRIVERS

The issue of motor vehicle driving and seizures is complex. Driving a car is an important life activity for most adults, and limitations may have important occupational and social impacts. Most persons with controlled seizure disorders can drive safely and without incident. However, some seizures pose a risk of injury and death to the patient and others if they occur when driving. Persons who have uncontrolled seizures of this type should not drive.

Several areas of legal interest occur in the management of the patient with seizures who wishes to drive. First, what should the physician tell the seizure patient about driving? How should this be documented? Second, what are the state Department of Motor Vehicle (DOMV) requirements and procedures for licensing people with seizures? How does the physician participate in the patient's obtaining a license? Finally, when a person with an active seizure disorder drives against medical advice, how does the physician balance his duty to maintain patient confidences with his duty to warn the state about behavior that places the patient and others in danger?

Physicians should inform patients with seizures of any recommended life-style, recreational, and/or occupational limitations related to the seizure disorder. Abstaining from driving is a common recommendation following a seizure, particularly those that involve an alteration in consciousness or loss of motor control. Most states have a mandatory seizure-free interval, and physicians must be aware of their own state's regulations regarding licensing. In states with a mandatory seizure-free period, requirements vary from 3 months to 2 years. Restricted licenses are available in many states and may represent a way that persons can drive despite not meeting the statutory seizure-free interval. Examples are licenses that allow emergency driving only or limit driving to and from work or limit driving to daylight hours.

Some states do not have a mandatory seizure-free interval prior to licensure; instead, decisions are based on individualized determinations. In such states, important data considered in each decision include the length of time since the last seizure, seizure type, precipitants, and other factors reasonably expected to affect the applicant's ability to control a motor vehicle. The DOMV in these states frequently solicits the recommendation of the treating physician.

The physician should make a medical judgment about necessary driving limitations, incorporating state requirements into his recommendations. If a restricted license or some other exception to the state rules appears appropriate, the physician can work with the patient and the state agency. Recommendations about driving restrictions, as well as other occupational and recreational limits, should be carefully documented in the patient's chart. One effective method of documentation is to have the patient record his understanding of what he has been advised in the chart. This process encourages discussion between the physician and patient and provides clear evidence of patient involvement.

The physician may find that direct interaction with the state's DOMV or similar agency is necessary. In several states, physicians are required to report patients with seizure disorders to the DOMV or another state agency. Mandatory reporting is, however, not common and is considered by many authorities unwise for many reasons. It infantilizes the patient, diminishes patient responsibility, and interposes a third party in the physician–patient relationship. Nonetheless, in these states physicians can be penalized by the state, and can potentially be held liable to third parties who are injured as a result of a seizure, if this reporting activity is not accomplished. Although the physician is immunized from suit for providing such information to the state, the patient should still be told that the information will be transmitted.

In general, no information about a patient's medical condition should be released without the express consent of the patient. Many states require that the physician fill out periodic reports on persons with seizures who drive. Physicians must fill out these forms honestly and are usually immunized from suit for doing so. Nonetheless, it is wise to inform patients that the information is being sent. Office staff should be aware that complying with a state DOMV request does not mean that other requests (*e.g.*, from the patient's employer) should be complied with.

Physicians should be aware of the driver's licensing procedures in their state. Typically, applicants for initial or renewal licensure complete forms developed by the DOMV. These forms may ask generally or specifically about seizure disorders. When a seizure disorder is identified, DOMV personnel may act on available information or may ask for more.

Once adequate information is available, DOMV personnel may grant the license, refuse it, or refer the question to a medical advisory panel, a group of experts who advise the state on the correct procedures as well as individual cases. If DOMV personnel refuse a license, a patient may be able to appeal to the medical advisory panel, which reviews cases and may contact the physician for additional information. Based on its recommendation, the applicant may subsequently be granted or denied licensure. In some settings, negative decisions by the panel may be appealed through the court system.

Perhaps the most difficult problem that a physician can face occurs when a patient with poorly controlled seizures persists in driving despite medical advice. What is a physician to do in such instances? In states with mandatory reporting, the physician is not only able to report such behavior but may be required to do so. In some states, statutory immunities have been granted to physicians who warn of the risky behavior of a patient to third parties. In other states, there is no clear law on the subject. Nonetheless, ethical guidelines of a variety of professional medical groups suggest that in cases in which a patient's behavior creates a clear harm to others, the physician has a strong ethical duty to warn the third party.[10, 11] Some courts have found physicians liable for not warning the potential victim of a patient.[12] The Epilepsy Foundation of America supports the right of physicians to report patients in such a setting.[13] Although the law is not settled, it is unlikely that a court would find a physician liable for breaching confidentiality for notifying the state when a patient refused to comply with medical advice and continued driving despite ongoing seizures that made such behavior unsafe.

Additional information on the status of state and federal laws in this changing area can be obtained from the Epilepsy Foundation of America, 4351 Garden City Drive, Landover, Maryland, 20785-2267, 1-800-EFA-1000.

QUESTIONS AND DISCUSSION

1. In order for informed consent to be valid:

   A. It must be given voluntarily.
   B. It must be given after information is supplied to the patient in an understandable fashion.
   C. The patient must be competent.
   D. It must be accompanied by a witnessed form.

Answers (A) and (C) are correct. (B) is correct unless the patient has waived the information provision or unless the physician has used the therapeutic privilege exception (which should be used only cautiously). (D) is incorrect; although informed consent should be documented, a specific form and witnessing is not absolutely necessary. Informed consent forms may be useful in demonstrating consent, but they are not foolproof and if not "user-friendly" can actually do more harm than good.

2. An adult patient is competent to provide consent unless he has been judged incompetent in legal proceedings.

The answer is false. A patient must be both clinically and legally competent in order to provide informed consent. An adult patient is presumed to be legally competent unless he has been found incompetent in judicial proceedings. Clinical competence is a medical decision. A patient may be clinically incompetent even though legally competent.

3. A 50-year-old man is found collapsed on a city street by paramedics who initiate cardiopulmonary resuscitation and take him to the hospital. One hour later, he is in the emergency room on a ventilator, totally unresponsive to all stimuli, and without brain-stem reflexes. He has a completed donor card. The most appropriate action at this time is:

   A. To pronounce brain death and call the transplant team to come in and recover the organs.
   B. To call the family to see if they agree with the organ donation.
   C. To observe the patient in the emergency department for 2 more hours to ensure that there is no change in the exam.
   D. To transfer the patient to an intensive care setting for further evaluation and work-up.

The answer is (D). The diagnosis of irreversible and total brain death has not been established. There is no clear etiology for this patient's clinical condition, there is no indication that conditions that can produce this clinical picture but be reversible (*e.g.*, drug overdose) have been ruled out. It is unlikely that a complete exam to establish brain death in this setting, including anoxia testing, has been performed. This patient should receive additional evaluation prior to being declared dead.

Although the family's consent for organ retrieval is not absolutely necessary in the presence of a valid organ donor card, most physicians wish to obtain consent of next of kin prior to organ retrieval.

4. In a state with mandatory reporting of persons with seizure disorders, the physician has a duty to inform the patient's family and employer of the diagnosis.

The answer is false. Mandatory reporting requirements apply only to the specific state agency mentioned in the statute. Disclosure to any other person or institution is precluded by the physician's duty to maintain patient confidences.

5. Actions to be taken when a patient with uncontrolled seizures continues to operate a motor vehicle include the following:

   A. Educate the patient about the risks to himself and others.
   B. Carefully document discussions with the patient about driving, and have the patient document his understanding of the discussion in the record as well.
   C. In states with mandatory reporting, conform with the requirements of the applicable statute.
   D. In cases in which patient education has been ineffective and the patient continues to place himself and others at risk by driving despite poor control of seizures, inform the patient of the need to report to the state Department of Motor Vehicles and do so.

The answer is all of the above. Patient education is an important aspect of handling driving restrictions because of uncontrolled seizures. When a patient with uncontrolled seizures persists in driving despite warnings of the risk to self and others, the physician should inform the patient of the need to report to the state. Some states provide immunity for the physician who reports in these instances.

Although not all states provide immunities, it is unlikely that a suit for breach of confidentiality would be successful. In some states, a physician may be found liable for failing to report dangerous behavior on the part of a patient.

SUGGESTED READING

1. *Schloendorff v. Society of New York Hospitals*, 211 N.Y. 125, 105 N.E. 2d 92 (1914)
2. Brandt AM: Racism and research: The case of the Tuskegee Syphilis Study. Hastings Cent Rep 8:21, 1978
3. *Hyman v. Jewish Chronic Disease Hospital*, 251 N.Y.2d 818 (1964), 206 N.E.2d 338 (1965)
4. A definition of irreversible coma: Report of the Ad Hoc Committee of the Harvard Medical School to examine the definition of brain death. JAMA 205:337, 1968
5. National Institutes of Health: A collaborative study: An appraisal of the criteria of cerebral death. A summary statement. JAMA 237:982, 1977
6. President's Commission for the Study of Ethical Problems in Medicine and Biomedical and Behavioral Research: Defining Death: A Report on the Medical, Legal and Ethical Issues in the Determination of Death. 1981.
7. 12 Uniform Laws annotated 237 Cum. Sups. 1983.
8. Young GB: Checklist for brain death. Can Med Assoc J 145(4):294, 1991
9. *Strachan v. John F. Kennedy Memorial Hospital*, 583 A.2d 346 (N.J. 1988)
10. Council on Ethical and Judicial Affairs, American Medical Association: Ethical issues involved in the growing AIDS crisis. JAMA 259:1360, 1988
11. Health and Public Policy Committee, American College of Physicians and Infectious Diseases Society of America: The acquired immunodeficiency syndrome (AIDS) and infection with the human immunodeficiency virus (HIV). Ann Intern Med 108:460, 1988
12. *Tarasoff v. Board of Regents of the University of California*, 17 Cal.3d 425, 551 P.2d 334 (1976)
13. Epilepsy Foundation of America: The Legal Rights of Persons with Epilepsy. 1987

I N D E X

Note: Page numbers followed by the letter *f* refer to figures; numbers followed by *t* refer to tables.

and tardive dyskinesia, 143–144
in tic disorders, 140–141
Dopamine decarboxylase, 113
Drug toxicity, 205–218. *See also* Toxicity
DTRs (deep tendon reflexes), 9
Dysequilibrium, 172, 178–181. *See also* Dizziness;
  Vertigo
Dyskinesia
  dopamine-induced, 115
  tardive, 141–144
Dysthesia, 156
Dystonia
  adult-onset, 123
  childhood-onset, 123
  classification of, 122–123
  craniofacial, 123–124
  idiopathic torsion, 121–127
  pathology and neurochemistry, 126
  primary, 123
  secondary, 125–126, 126t
  spasmodic torticollis, 124–125
  treatment, 126–127
  writer's cramp, 125
Dystrophy
  Duchenne's and Becker's, 246–247
  facioscapulohumeral, 247–248
  limb–girdle, 248
  myotonic, 248–249

E
Ear, vestibular system disorders, 171–181. *See
  also* Dizziness; Vertigo
Eaton–Lambert syndrome, 246
ECG (electrocardiography), in stroke and TIAs,
  56
Eclampsia, 394–395
EEG (electroencephalography)
  in coma, 51
  flat, 19
  interpretation, 17–18
  in sleep disorders, 281f, 282f, 289f, 291f
  in stroke, 58
  technique, 15, 17
Electrocardiography. *See* ECG
  (electrocardiography)
Electromyography. *See* EMG (electromyography)
Electronystagmography. *See* ENG
  (electronystagmography)
Eleptiform activity, 17
Embolism
  cerebral, 60–61
  cerebral paradoxical, 55

Emergencies
  acute alterations of mental status, 365–367
  acute intracranial hypertension, 367–369
  aneurysmal subarachnoid hemorrhage,
    362–363
  Guillain–Barré syndrome, 363–365, 364t
  myasthenia crisis, 361t, 361–362
  neuroleptic malignant syndrome, 369t,
    369–371
  pituitary apoplexy, 372
  status epilepticus, 358–361, 360t
EMG (electromyography), 19–22
  in low back pain, 276
  in neuromuscular disease, 238–239
  in peripheral neuropathy, 160–163
Emotional factors
  in migraine, 72–73, 80
  in multiple sclerosis, 98
Encephalitis, 45t, 353–354
  CMV, 361
  cytomegalovirus, 361
  herpes simplex, 192–193
Encephalomyelitis, vs. multiple sclerosis, 103
Encephalopathy
  in AIDS/HIV infection, 379–381, 380t
  confusional states in, 365–367
  hepatic, 151–152
Endocrine myopathies, 251
ENG (electronystagmography), 173
Ependyomomas, 261
Epidural hematoma, 45t, 223
Epidural spinal cord compression, 263–265, 264f
Epilepsy
  classification, 85–86
  diagnosis, 86–88
  dizziness in, 175
  EEG diagnosis, 17
  licensing of driver's with, 402–403
  post-traumatic, 226
  in pregnancy, 391–392
  status epilepticus, 358–361, 360t
  temporal lobe (psychomotor), 175, 185–188,
    186t, 187t, 188t
  treatment, 88–91, 89t
Epileptic aura, 185–186, 187t
Epsilon aminocaproic acid, 363
Equilibrium disorders, 178–181. *See also* Dizzi-
  ness; Vertigo
Ergot derivatives, in migraine, 73, 76, 79
Erythromycin toxicity, 207
Essential tremor, 125–126
Ethchlovynol toxicity, 214